Pediatric Infection: Prevention and Control

Pediatric Infection: Prevention and Control

Edited by Caroline Francis

AMERICAN
MEDICAL PUBLISHERS
www.americanmedicalpublishers.com

American Medical Publishers,
41 Flatbush Avenue,
1st Floor, New York,
NY 11217, USA

Visit us on the World Wide Web at:
www.americanmedicalpublishers.com

ISBN: 978-1-63927-425-3

Cataloging-in-Publication Data

Pediatric infection : prevention and control / edited by Caroline Francis.
p. cm.
Includes bibliographical references and index.
ISBN 978-1-63927-425-3
1. Infection in children. 2. Infection in children--Prevention. 3. Infection in children--Treatment.
I. Francis, Caroline.

RJ401 .P43 2022

618.92--dc23

Table of Contents

Preface

The main aim of this book is to educate learners and enhance their research focus by presenting diverse topics covering this vast field. This is an advanced book which compiles significant studies by distinguished experts in the area of analysis. This book addresses successive solutions to the challenges arising in the area of application, along with it; the book provides scope for future developments.

Infectious diseases can occur at any stage of life. In children, these may occur in infanthood, childhood and adolescence. The diagnosis, treatment and control of pediatric infectious diseases are under the scope of pediatrics. The timely diagnosis and treatment of acute infections are an important focus of pediatrics. Advancements in medical therapy have resulted in new diagnostics and better therapeutics that have advanced the evaluation, assessment and treatment of infectious diseases. Several diagnostic tests help to ascertain the source of the infection. These may consist of blood cultures, serologic tests, gram staining, genotyping and polymerase chain reaction. In children with chronic infections such as HIV, therapy involves long-term care and assessment. The antimicrobial therapy used to treat an infection depends on the organism that is causing the infections, and accordingly antibiotics, antifungal agents and antiviral agents may be prescribed. This book includes some of the vital pieces of work being conducted across the world, on various topics related to pediatric infections. It provides significant information on pediatric infectious diseases to help develop a good understanding of their prevention and control. The book is appropriate for students seeking detailed information in pediatrics as well as for experts.

It was a great honour to edit this book, though there were challenges, as it involved a lot of communication and networking between me and the editorial team. However, the end result was this all-inclusive book covering diverse themes in the field.

Finally, it is important to acknowledge the efforts of the contributors for their excellent chapters, through which a wide variety of issues have been addressed. I would also like to thank my colleagues for their valuable feedback during the making of this book.

Editor

1

Task Shifting Routine Inpatient Pediatric HIV Testing Improves Program Outcomes in Urban Malawi

Eric D. McCollum[1]*, Geoffrey A. Preidis[2], Mark M. Kabue[3], Emmanuel B. M. Singogo[3], Charles Mwansambo[4], Peter N. Kazembe[3], Mark W. Kline[5]

1 Baylor International Pediatric AIDS Initiative, Baylor College of Medicine, Lilongwe, Malawi, **2** Interdepartmental Program in Translational Biology and Molecular Medicine, Department of Pediatrics, Baylor College of Medicine, Houston, Texas, United States of America, **3** Baylor Children's Foundation-Malawi, Baylor College of Medicine, Lilongwe, Malawi, **4** Department of Pediatrics, Kamuzu Central Hospital, Lilongwe, Malawi, **5** Baylor International Pediatric AIDS Initiative, Baylor College of Medicine, Houston, Texas, United States of America

Abstract

Background: This study evaluated two models of routine HIV testing of hospitalized children in a high HIV-prevalence resource-constrained African setting. Both models incorporated "task shifting," or the allocation of tasks to the least-costly, capable health worker.

Methods and Findings: Two models were piloted for three months each within the pediatric department of a referral hospital in Lilongwe, Malawi between January 1 and June 30, 2008. Model 1 utilized lay counselors for HIV testing instead of nurses and clinicians. Model 2 further shifted program flow and advocacy responsibilities from counselors to volunteer parents of HIV-infected children, called "patient escorts." A retrospective review of data from 6318 hospitalized children offered HIV testing between January-December 2008 was conducted. The pilot quarters of Model 1 and Model 2 were compared, with Model 2 selected to continue after the pilot period. There was a 2-fold increase in patients offered HIV testing with Model 2 compared with Model 1 (43.1% vs 19.9%, $p<0.001$). Furthermore, patients in Model 2 were younger (17.3 vs 26.7 months, $p<0.001$) and tested sooner after admission (1.77 vs 2.44 days, $p<0.001$). There were no differences in test acceptance or enrollment rates into HIV care, and the program trends continued 6 months after the pilot period. Overall, 10244 HIV antibody tests (4779 maternal; 5465 child) and 453 DNA-PCR tests were completed, with 97.8% accepting testing. 19.6% of all mothers (n = 1112) and 8.5% of all children (n = 525) were HIV-infected. Furthermore, 6.5% of children were HIV-exposed (n = 405). Cumulatively, 72.9% (n = 678) of eligible children were evaluated in the hospital by a HIV-trained clinician, and 68.3% (n = 387) successfully enrolled into outpatient HIV care.

Conclusions/Significance: The strategy presented here, task shifting from lay counselors alone to lay counselors and patient escorts, greatly improved program outcomes while only marginally increasing operational costs. The wider implementation of this strategy could accelerate pediatric HIV care access in high-prevalence settings.

Editor: Landon Myer, University of Cape Town, South Africa

Funding: Funding for the PITC program and operational study was provided by Baylor International Pediatric AIDS Initiative (BIPAI) and the Abbott Fund. The funders had no role in study design, data collection and analysis, decision to publish, or preparation of the manuscript.

Competing Interests: The authors have declared that no competing interests exist.

* E-mail: ericdmccollum@gmail.com

Introduction

Globally, an estimated 2.2 million children younger than 15 years of age were HIV-infected (HIV+) in 2007, with 88% living in sub-Saharan Africa [1]. Malawi, a sub-Saharan African country of 13.2 million people, reports an adult HIV prevalence of 11.9% [1]. While 91,000 HIV+ children were estimated to be living in Malawi in 2007 [2], less than 8% of all Malawian children have ever been HIV tested [3]. Additionally, HIV+ children comprised just 8% of all national antiretroviral therapy (ART) recipients, below the 2014 goal of 15% [3]. To address this gap in HIV care, Malawi approved the routine offering of HIV testing, defined here as provider initiated HIV testing and counseling (PITC), in line with global recommendations in 2007 [4]. A high HIV prevalence in hospitalized Malawian children has been reported [5–8]; however, current guidelines do not offer a strategy for pediatric hospital-based PITC in resource-constrained settings [4].

In 2005, the Baylor College of Medicine-Abbott Fund Children's Clinical Centre of Excellence (COE) established a pediatric HIV program in Malawi that included patient care, national capacity building, and technical assistance [9,10]. The COE's outpatient clinic is located adjacent to the Kamuzu Central Hospital (KCH) pediatric inpatient department and has enrolled over 4200 patients to date [Baylor International Pediatric AIDS Initiative, unpublished data]. KCH is a 215 pediatric bed referral hospital located in the capital of Lilongwe with more than 13000 pediatric admissions annually. Severe nurse and clinician shortages strain hospital systems and contribute to pediatric mortality rates that exceed 8% [KCH, unpublished data].

In January 2008, the COE and KCH implemented a PITC program in the pediatric department. In a 24 month period preceding the PITC program, 1613 total children accessed non-routine HIV counseling and testing services offered by lay counselors in the pediatric ward, representing less than 6% of all pediatric inpatients [11]. The PITC program's objectives were the routine offering of confidential and timely HIV testing, enrolling HIV+ and HIV-exposed (HIV-E) hospitalized children into HIV care, and establishing a scalable model.

"Task shifting," or the allocation of tasks to the least costly, capable health worker, is an accepted approach to addressing human resource constraints [12-17]. Our program sequentially piloted two PITC models that utilized different task shifting strategies. Model 1 continued to use lay counselors for HIV testing rather than nurses and clinicians. Model 2 shifted program flow and advocacy tasks from counselors to volunteer parents of HIV+ children, called "patient escorts," while continuing to utilize counselors for testing. One COE clinician provided daily HIV care for all hospitalized HIV+ and HIV-E children. Inpatient care included the prescription of co-trimoxazole preventative therapy, treatment of opportunistic infections, supportive care, and outpatient referral. Outpatient care at the COE consisted of free, comprehensive pediatric HIV services, including ART and co-trimoxazole provision by COE clinicians.

The feasibility, acceptability, and referral of PITC-identified outpatients to HIV care in resource-limited settings have been demonstrated [18–28]. While a referral hospital in Zambia recently described a routine inpatient pediatric HIV testing program using lay counselors [19], no studies to date have investigated whether alternate strategies using volunteers rather than additional professional staff can achieve similar programmatic outcomes while only marginally increasing operational expenses. We hypothesized that a model incorporating lay counselors and additional volunteers would more efficiently achieve this program's objectives in an under-resourced, overburdened hospital.

Methods

Program Implementation and Description

In 2007 a multidisciplinary task force at KCH created a PITC program strategy, program procedural manual [Text S1], and confidential program register [Text S2]. The task force also revised the pediatric department admissions form to include a standing written order for HIV testing as well as a section for documentation of test results. Based on low nurse and clinician staffing levels, high rates of evening admissions when staffing was even lower, and undeveloped triage systems, the task force concluded that HIV testing at admission by nurses and clinicians could not achieve the program objectives and could delay emergent care. Furthermore, the task force decided that a bedside testing model was potentially coercive and inadequate for confidentiality. Instead, the group concluded that a model built around private testing by counselors during inpatient ward rounds, with or without patient escorts, could be immediately piloted.

A program algorithm divided PITC into eight steps [Text S3], and the confidential patient register facilitated referrals and monitoring [Text S2]. All PITC staff worked from 7:30am to 4:00pm Monday through Friday. HIV testing was not available on weekends. Government approval was obtained, and funding was acquired from the Baylor International Pediatric AIDS Initiative. Baylor International Pediatric AIDS Initiative receives primary funding from Bristol Myers Squibb, the Abbott Fund, Texas Children's Hospital, The United Nations Children's Fund, and the Malawi Ministry of Health.

Two rooms within the pediatric department were equipped with partitions and materials to create four private testing spaces. Four nationally certified HIV counselors employed by the COE and Lighthouse Trust were assigned to the program, with one counselor per room. Prior to implementing each model, two half-day departmental orientations took place each preceding month [Text S4, S5, S6]. As a part of the orientation, clinicians and nurses were trained to order HIV testing on all patients during wards rounds, irrespective of clinical symptoms, physical examination, admission diagnosis, or ward location. Counselors also received guidance regarding how to conduct pretest group counseling and opt-out testing.

In both models, counselors followed a PITC opt-out protocol and the Malawi National HIV Counseling and Testing guidelines. National guidelines recommended investigating maternal HIV status before testing the child. Eligible children were tested with a HIV antibody test and/or DNA-PCR test depending upon their age [29]. In some select cases, however, the child was tested first, and the mother was either tested after the child or not at all. If the caregiver produced valid documentation, such as the national health passport, indicating that the child's HIV status was known, then testing information was documented on the patient's admission form and the PITC register was updated. Patients that disclosed their HIV status during ward rounds would not go to the counseling room for testing. Two COE clinicians evaluated all hospitalized HIV+ and HIV-E children using the confidential program register to locate patients, and provided program supervision. Supervision consisted of a weekly review of program registers and monthly PITC meetings within the pediatric department. The meetings provided monitoring feedback to staff and addressed programmatic or staff issues.

The Model 1 pilot period began January 1, 2008 and continued until March 31, 2008. In addition to opt-out HIV testing, Model 1 expected counselors to perform group counseling, team up with providers during ward rounds, interact with patients hospitalized on the ward, and accompany caregivers to the testing rooms.

Four patient escorts were identified for Model 2 and introduced at the Model 2 orientation. The escorts were recruited from a group of pro-active parents of HIV+ children that were attending the COE clinic. Each escort was openly HIV+, compliant with ART, demonstrated proficient oral and written English and Chichewa language skills, and produced documentation confirming completion of primary schooling. All escorts received a half-day orientation [Text S4, S5, S6], as well as pediatric HIV diagnosis [Text S7, S8, S9, S10, S11, S12] and job-related training [Text S13, Text S14], followed by one week of on-the-job supervision by a COE pediatrician. Each volunteer patient escort earned a stipend for work-related transportation and food ($2/day).

The Model 2 pilot period began April 1, 2008 and continued until June 30, 2008. Each escort was assigned to a counselor and KCH clinician for ward rounds, and accompanied patients to the testing room after a provider advised the caregiver about the routine HIV test. If the providers were unavailable or did not advise the caregiver appropriately, escorts would still mentor parents regarding the benefits of pediatric HIV testing and chaperone willing caregivers to the counseling room. Counselors continued to perform group counseling and opt-out HIV testing.

The PITC task force evaluated the pilot models, and selected Model 2 for the programmatic period that started July 1, 2008.

Study Design

The study was approved by the Malawi National Health Sciences Research Committee and Baylor College of Medicine institutional review boards, respectively. Verbal consent for HIV testing was obtained by nationally certified HIV counselors and documented in patient files in accordance with Malawi National HIV Counseling and Testing guidelines [29]. Written consent was not required by study participants since data was collected as a part of routine program monitoring and evaluation. A retrospective review of data from 6318 hospitalized children offered HIV testing from January-December 2008 was conducted. The review was separated into two periods, pilot and programmatic. Disaggregated pre-PITC pediatric ward HIV testing data was unavailable for comparison. A data officer collected maternal and child study data from the PITC register, ward admissions book, and COE electronic medical record. Outcomes data included the proportion of admissions offered HIV testing, the proportion accepting testing, age in months of PITC recipients, days elapsed from admission to testing, maternal HIV antibody test results, child HIV antibody and DNA-PCR test results, mother and child HIV status, and successful enrollment into inpatient and outpatient pediatric HIV care.

Statistical Analysis

Continuous variables were evaluated with the Mann-Whitney U test. Age and time from hospital admission to HIV test were expressed as median months and mean days, respectively, both with interquartile range. For categorical parameters, data were reported as raw value and percentage of the respective group. Pearson's chi-square test was used to determine global significance between Model 1 and Model 2 pilot period data, and post-hoc analyses were performed using pair-wise chi-square tests or Fisher exact tests, with the Bonferroni correction applied to adjust α for multiple variable levels. Only p values smaller than the corrected α were considered statistically significant. All statistical analyses were performed using SPSS software (version 17.0; SPSS Inc., Chicago, IL).

Results

During the one-year study period, 13981 children were admitted to KCH. Overall, 45.2% of children were offered HIV testing, with a 2-fold increase in proportion observed during the Model 2 pilot period (43.1%), compared to Model 1 (19.9%). The HIV testing rate further increased to 64.5% during the programmatic period. "Test offering" was defined as patients offered HIV testing by a clinician or nurse, lay counselor or patient escort within the ward, or by a lay counselor within the testing room. Test acceptance exceeded 96% throughout the pilot and programmatic periods, with no differences observed between the models. Characteristics of children offered testing are described in Table 1. Compared to the Model 1 pilot quarter, children tested during the Model 2 pilot period were 9.4 months younger, with a more than one-half day reduction in the time between hospital admission and an HIV test. These trends continued through the programmatic period. While there was a decrease in the proportion of children previously HIV tested between Model 1 (4.4%) and the pilot quarter of Model 2 (2.2%), a 7-fold increase to 15.5% of children previously HIV tested was observed between the Model 2 programmatic and pilot period. No gender differences were observed between the two models.

HIV antibody and DNA-PCR testing, if applicable, was completed on hospitalized children, and on consenting mothers in accordance with national HIV testing guidelines [29]. Overall, 10244 HIV antibody tests (4779 maternal; 5465 child) and 453 HIV DNA-PCR tests were completed. No test stock-outs were experienced. Maternal test results and HIV status are shown in Table 2 with an overview provided in Figure 1. Cumulatively, 19.6% of mothers were HIV+, with more mothers testing HIV-uninfected during the Model 2 pilot period. Importantly, Model 2 significantly increased the proportion of mothers with an unknown HIV status offered HIV testing. 7.2% of mothers disclosed a valid previous test result during both periods.

Child HIV antibody and DNA-PCR test results are reported in Table 3, and child HIV status is detailed in Table 4. Figure 2 provides an overview of child HIV testing. Overall, 8.5% of children were HIV+ and 6.5% were HIV-E, defined as a child born to an HIV+ mother who was either without a definitive HIV test result or who was DNA-PCR negative but still breastfeeding. While there were no significant differences in HIV-E status between the models, a higher percentage of HIV-E patients were observed during the programmatic period.

Table 5 shows the proportion of children that successfully enrolled into inpatient and outpatient pediatric HIV care. All successfully referred inpatient HIV+ and HIV-E hospitalized children were evaluated by a COE clinician, and were referred to

Table 1. PITC Pediatric Inpatient Characteristics.

Characteristic	Pilot Period Model 1 Jan-Mar 2008	Pilot Period Model 2 Apr-Jun 2008	Programmatic Period Model 2 Jul-Dec 2008	Total Jan-Dec 2008	*p*-Value[1]
Pediatric admissions offered HIV test, *n/N* (%)	830/4172 (19.9)	1689/3919 (43.1)	3799/5890 (64.5)	6318/13981 (45.2)	<0.001
Children offered HIV test with unknown HIV status,[2] *n/N* (%)	793/830 (95.5)	1653/1689 (97.9)	3211/3799 (84.5)	5657/6318 (89.5)	0.001
HIV test acceptance, *n/N* (%)	787/793 (99.2)	1639/1653 (99.2)	3105/3211 (96.7)	5531/5657 (97.8)	0.816
Time from child's admission to HIV test, d, mean (IQR)	2.44 (1–3)	1.77 (1–2)	1.61 (1–2)	1.76 (1–2)	<0.001
Child's age, mos, median (IQR)	26.7 (12.2–50.0)	17.3 (8.7–35.3)	15.8 (7.2–36.0)	17.4 (8.1–37.7)	<0.001
Females, *n/N* (%)	412/830 (49.6)	825/1689 (48.8)	1865/3799 (49.1)	3102/6318 (49.1)	0.708

[1]Pilot Period Model 1 × Pilot Period Model 2; Pearson chi-square test for categorical variables; Mann-Whitney U test for continuous variables.

[2]The patient was not re-tested if they disclosed a documented and valid previous HIV test result. During Pilot Period Model 1, no children offered HIV testing were readmissions with a known HIV status. During Pilot Period Model 2, 5 (0.3%) children offered HIV testing were readmissions with a known HIV status. During Programmatic Period Model 2, 102 (2.7%) children offered HIV testing were readmissions with a known HIV status.

Table 2. Maternal HIV Antibody Test Results and HIV Status.

Characteristic	Category	Pilot Period Model 1 Jan-Mar 2008[2]	Pilot Period Model 2 Apr-Jun 2008[3]	Programmatic Period Model 2 Jul-Dec 2008[4]	Total Jan-Dec 2008	p-Value[1]
Mothers offered HIV test with unknown HIV status, n/N (%)		625/830 (75.3)	1442/1689 (85.4)	2712/3799 (71.4)	4995/6318 (79.1)	<0.001
HIV test acceptance, n/N (%)		610/625 (97.6)	1412/1442 (97.9)	2541/2712 (93.7)	4779/4995 (95.7)	0.647
Maternal HIV antibody test, n/N (%)						0.001
	Positive	120/625 (19.2)	193/1442 (13.4)	348/2712 (12.8)	661/4779 (13.8)	
	Negative	505/625 (80.8)	1249/1442 (86.6)	2364/2712 (87.2)	4118/4779 (86.2)	
Maternal HIV status[5], n/N (%)						0.024
	HIV-infected	141/685 (20.6)	260/1563 (16.6)	711/3430 (20.7)	1112/5678 (19.6)	
	HIV-uninfected	544/685 (79.4)	1303/1563 (83.4)	2719/3430 (79.3)	4566/5678 (80.4)	

[1]Pilot Period Model 1 × Pilot Period Model 2; Pearson chi-square test.
[2]During Pilot Period Model 1, 130 (15.7%) mothers were either unavailable for HIV antibody testing or deceased, 15 (1.8%) declined HIV testing, and 21 (2.5%) and 39 (4.7%) mothers were not retested as they were known HIV-infected and HIV-uninfected, respectively, after disclosing a documented and valid previous HIV test result.
[3]During Pilot Period Model 2, 96 (5.7%) mothers were either unavailable for HIV antibody testing or deceased, 30 (1.8%) declined HIV testing, and 67 (4.0%) and 54 (3.2%) mothers were not retested as they were known HIV-infected and HIV-uninfected, respectively.
[4]During Programmatic Period Model 2, 198 (5.2%) mothers were either unavailable for HIV antibody testing or deceased, 171 (4.5%) declined HIV testing, and 363 (9.6%) and 355 (9.3%) mothers were not retested as they were known HIV-infected and HIV-uninfected, respectively.
[5]Includes newly identified and previously known HIV-infected and HIV-uninfected mothers.

an outpatient HIV clinic at discharge. All patients that received a DNA-PCR, however, were expected to return to the COE for their results whether or not a COE clinician reviewed them during their hospitalization. Overall, inpatient HIV clinicians reviewed 72.9% of HIV+ and HIV-E children during their hospital admission. Of those not previously enrolled into HIV care, 567 accepted outpatient referral to the COE with 68.3% successfully returning and enrolling into care at the clinic. There were no differences in successful inpatient and outpatient pediatric HIV care enrollment rates between the two models.

Discussion

This report reveals that a routine inpatient pediatric HIV testing model incorporating lay counselors and volunteer patient escorts significantly increased the number of children offered testing, maintained high acceptance rates, and shortened the time between hospital admission and HIV testing. These findings suggest that at this crowded, resource-constrained sub-Saharan African hospital, four counselors alone were insufficient to achieve the PITC program objectives. Rather than hire additional counselors and significantly increase operational costs, we improved performance with only a marginal increase in expenses by task-shifting program advocacy and patient flow responsibilities to four capable volunteer patient escorts.

Before the implementation of our model of PITC, clinicians and nurses non-routinely offered HIV testing within the pediatric inpatient wards based upon a patient's clinical findings, otherwise patients independently accessed the service themselves. Less than 6% of pediatric inpatients received HIV tests utilizing this strategy [11].

There are multiple reasons why few inpatients accessed HIV testing before PITC, and also during the Model 1 Pilot Period. The high ratio of patients to providers in the pediatric ward (>25 patients to 1 provider) made it difficult for any clinician or nurse to dedicate the time needed to order HIV testing and continue their other duties. Providers also expressed hesitancy to order testing because they perceived the process as requiring an extensive, specialized counseling session, which they might have felt inadequately trained to convey. Few providers felt comfortable with pediatric HIV care in general, viewing it as a condition for specialists only, and few appreciated the value of knowing a patient's HIV status during the hospitalization. Furthermore, severe human resource constraints and poor retention of pediatric ward staff forced administrators to rely upon temporarily employed clinicians and nurses to provide a majority of patient care. This lack of provider continuity limited the effectiveness of a system that heavily relied upon this cadre of healthcare workers.

While most caregivers readily accepted HIV testing, a minority of parents would require more intensive counseling. These parents expressed a reluctance to go to the testing room for a variety of reasons, including HIV-related stigma, the absence of their spouse's approval, a fear of missing nursing medication rounds, a concern that their child was "too sick" to be tested, a lack of awareness that children could benefit from ART, or a feeling of intimidation by the chaotic, overwhelming hospital environment itself. Thus, for a subset of patients the provider did need to dedicate more time to impart bedside counseling and accompany the patient to the counseling room for testing. Unfortunately, providers rarely made this effort. Furthermore, HIV counselors did little to support providers as they remained inside the HIV testing room and did not actively engage patient caregivers, nurses, or clinicians working on the ward.

While these barriers continued to persist during our intervention, they provide critical insight to explain why patient escorts dramatically improved our program's outcomes, and why Model 1 was only marginally successful. Model 1 expected counselors to proactively collaborate with providers, routinely engage patients at the bedside, and chaperone caregivers to the testing rooms. The contributions of the counselors were inconsistent at best. While the counselors that were willing and motivated routinely succeeded, the patient volume and demand for testing overwhelmed the system.

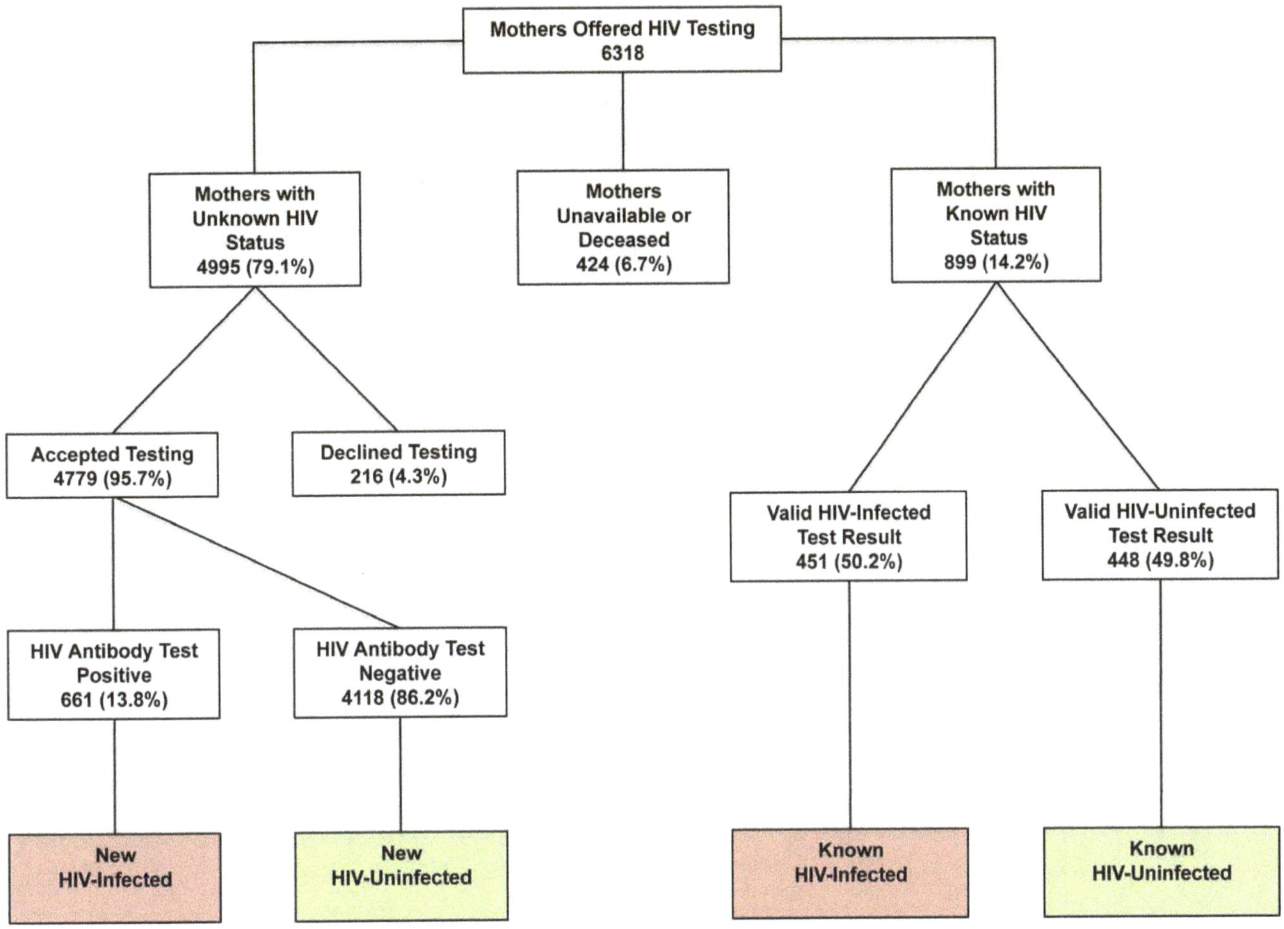

Figure 1. Maternal PITC Overview at Kamuzu Central Hospital; January 1-December 31, 2008. Total HIV-infected mothers (red boxes): 1112/5678 (19.6%); total HIV-uninfected mothers (green boxes): 4566/5678 (80.4%).

Patient escorts effectively bridged the gaps that providers and counselors were unable or unwilling to fill. Compared to providers, the volunteers could spend more time talking with caregivers about the benefits of testing, often motivating them with personal stories. When providers were either unavailable or did not discuss HIV testing with the caregiver, the patient escorts successfully advocated testing to almost all patients, and would subsequently accompany them to the testing room. The escorts also increased the efficiency of the counselors, allowing them to focus upon their more familiar tasks of testing and counseling in their private room rather than managing patient flow on the ward.

Over time, the patient escorts' skills improved and the providers and counselors accepted their contributions warmly. This observation is supported by the continued progress demonstrated during the programmatic period when 64.5% of pediatric admissions were offered HIV testing and the number of patients

Table 3. Child HIV Test Results.

Characteristic	Category	Pilot Period Model 1 Jan-Mar 2008	Pilot Period Model 2 Apr-Jun 2008	Programmatic Period Model 2 Jul-Dec 2008	Total Jan-Dec 2008	*p*-Value[1]
Child HIV antibody test, *n/N* (%)						0.001
	Positive	91/776 (11.7)	126/1633 (7.7)	210/3056 (6.9)	427/5465 (7.8)	
	Negative	685/776 (88.3)	1507/1633 (92.3)	2847/3056 (93.1)	5039/5465 (92.2)	
Child HIV DNA PCR test, *n/N* (%)						0.082
	Positive	42/90 (46.7)	47/134 (35.1)	105/229 (45.9)	194/453 (42.8)	
	Negative	48/90 (53.3)	87/134 (64.9)	124/229 (54.1)	259/453 (57.2)	

[1]Pilot Period Model 1 × Pilot Period Model 2; Pearson chi-square test.

Table 4. Child HIV Status.

Category	Sub-Category	Pilot Period Model 1 Jan-Mar 2008	Pilot Period Model 2 Apr-Jun 2008	Programmatic Period Model 2 Jul-Dec 2008	Total Jan-Dec 2008	*p*-Value[1]
HIV-infected, *n/N* (%)		97/824 (11.8)	108/1675 (6.4)	320/3693 (8.7)	525/6192 (8.5)	0.203
	New	92/97 (94.8)	97/108 (89.8)	201/320 (62.8)	390/525 (74.3)	
	Known[2]	5/97 (5.2)	11/108 (10.2)	119/320 (37.2)	135/525 (25.7)	
HIV-exposed, *n/N* (%)		32/824 (3.9)	98/1675 (5.9)	275/3693 (7.4)	405/6192 (6.5)	1.000
	New	30/32 (93.8)	93/98 (94.9)	129/275(46.9)	252/405 (62.2)	
	Known[2]	2/32(6.3)	5/98 (5.1)	146/275 (53.1)	153/405 (37.8)	
HIV-uninfected, *n/N* (%)		695/824 (84.3)	1469/1675 (87.7)	3098/3693 (83.9)	5262/6192 (85.0)	<0.001
	New	665/695 (95.7)	1449/1469 (98.6)	2775/3098 (89.6)	4889/5262 (92.9)	
	Known[2]	30/695 (4.3)	20/1469 (1.4)	323/3098 (10.4)	373/5262 (7.1)	

[1]Pilot Period Model 1 × Pilot Period Model 2; Pearson chi-square test or Fisher's exact test.
[2]The patient was not re-tested, as they disclosed a documented and valid previous HIV test result.

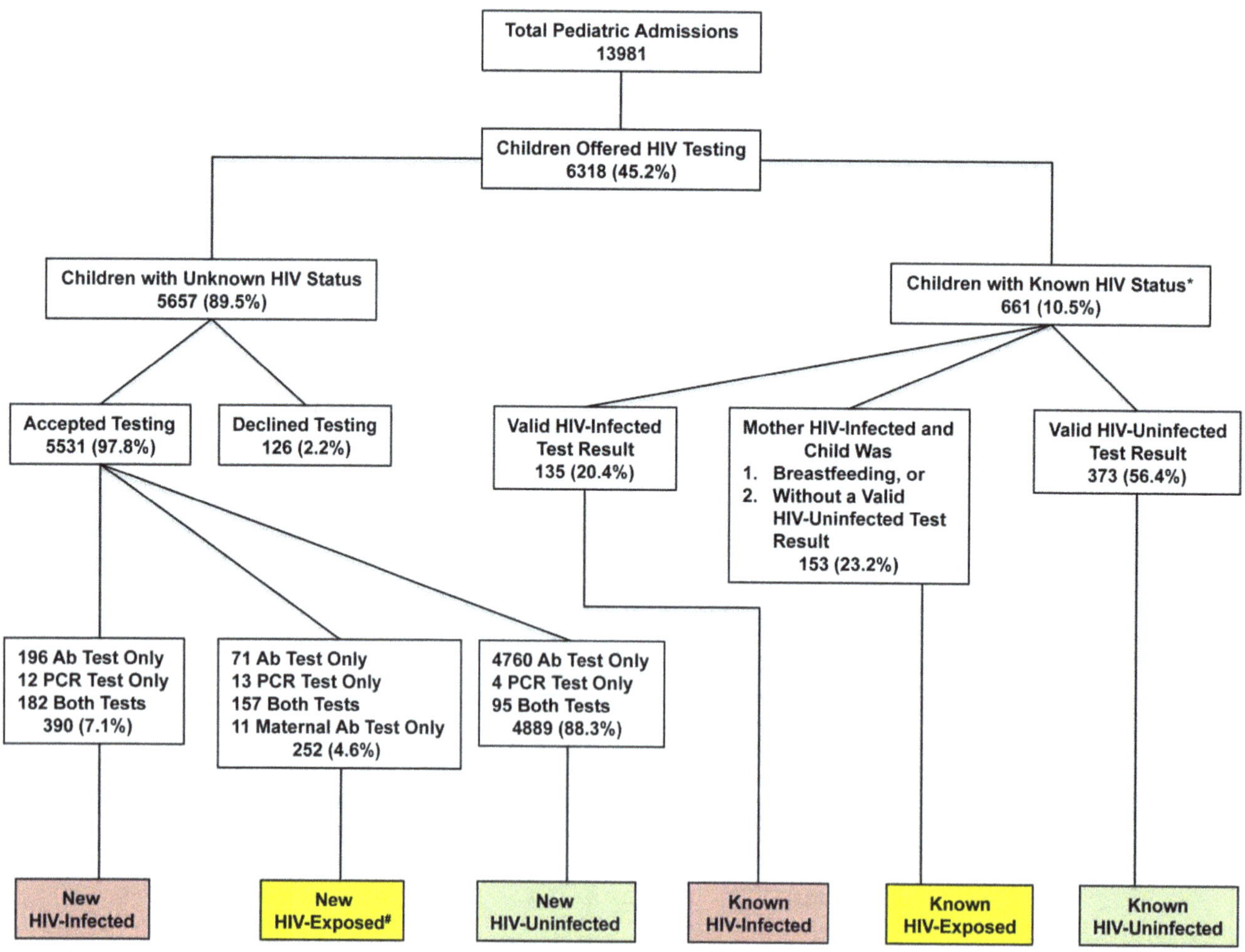

Figure 2. Child PITC Overview at Kamuzu Central Hospital; January 1 - December 31, 2008. Total HIV-infected children (red boxes): 525/6192 (8.5%); total HIV-exposed children (yellow boxes): 405/6192 (6.5%); total HIV-uninfected children (green boxes): 5262/6192 (85.0%). *6 children with known HIV status were incorrectly retested. #158 newly recognized HIV-exposed children had a negative DNA-PCR while breastfeeding, while 12 DNA-PCR results for newly recognized HIV-exposed children were lost. Ab: HIV antibody; PCR: HIV DNA-PCR.

Table 5. Inpatient and Outpatient Pediatric HIV Care Enrollment.

Characteristic	Pilot Period Model 1 Jan-Mar 2008	Pilot Period Model 2 Apr-Jun 2008	Programmatic Period Model 2 Jul-Dec 2008	Total Jan-Dec 2008	*p*-Value[1]
Successful inpatient enrollment, *n/N* (%)	85/128 (66.4)	155/214 (72.4)	438/588 (74.5)	678/930 (72.9)	0.239
Successful outpatient enrollment, *n/N* (%)	75/101 (74.3)	100/147 (68.0)	212/319 (66.5)	387/567 (68.3)	0.290

[1]Pilot Period Model 1 × Pilot Period Model 2; Pearson chi-square test.

disclosing a valid, previously-known HIV status greatly increased. The latter observation, including a 7-fold increase in those known to be HIV+, an 8-fold increase in children known to be HIV-E, and a more than 2-fold increase in those known to be HIV-uninfected, is a notable achievement. Model 2 thus fulfills a vital program objective, as it improves efficiency by reducing unnecessary retesting and ensures that all patients have the opportunity to be reviewed by clinicians after consideration of their HIV status.

There are several limitations to the model presented here. This program relied upon private testing space within the inpatient ward. While this approach maximized discretion and confidentiality, other hospitals may not have space available and would need to create space or modify this strategy. Furthermore, counselors did not staff the department during the weekend, which reduced testing availability. These limitations might be costly to address in many resource-constrained hospitals. While the lack of weekend HIV testing was an identifiable program drawback, these data collection tools were not designed to gather patient-level information about children not offered HIV testing, thus precluding analysis of whether any groups were routinely omitted. This drawback limits the usefulness of our data for detecting program weaknesses. However, when weekend admissions during the programmatic period were excluded, the proportion of pediatric admissions offered testing reached 89.6%.

In addition, the sequential implementation of the models could have biased outcomes in favor of Model 2. However, the immediate two-fold increase and sustained HIV testing levels during the programmatic period more likely reflects the impact of the patient escorts rather than the three additional months of PITC implementation. While the possibility exists that under-reporting of declined HIV testing could have contributed to the high test acceptance rates, it is unlikely that the rates reflect coercion, as this was monitored closely and not detected during unannounced observation visits by a COE pediatrician. Furthermore, a selection bias regarding outpatient care referral is possible, as we were unable to track the proportion of children that enrolled into outpatient HIV care at sites other than the COE. However, all patients, regardless of their follow-up preferences, were provided the same standard of inpatient HIV care and were counseled about outpatient follow-up similarly. Lastly, because no reliable pre-intervention data was available, we were unable to statistically compare either model with the previous HIV testing and counseling approach.

The median length of hospitalization in the KCH general pediatric ward was 3.0 days during both pilot quarters (data not shown), which implies that seasonal changes in the duration of hospitalization did not preferentially bias the increased HIV testing proportion observed in Model 2. Importantly, this program's test acceptance rate compares favorably to other reports [20-25], suggesting that if a similar model were brought to scale in Malawi, the proportion of children ever HIV tested would far surpass current estimates [3]. Importantly, as a substantial proportion of Malawian children die within 2 days of hospital admission, the reduction in time elapsed between hospital admission and HIV testing observed during Model 2 could also allow clinicians to consider a patient's HIV status earlier, provide more directed care for opportunistic infections and other complicating conditions sooner, and improve hospital survival [30].

While the overall proportions of patients enrolled into HIV care were comparable to other published reports [21–23,25,26], this program's 72.9% inpatient and 68.3% outpatient care enrollment rates could be further improved. Of note, these proportions represent actual HIV care received, not simply referral statistics, which are more commonly reported. Programmatic weaknesses that may have reduced these rates include premature hospital discharge by KCH clinicians, inadequate patient defaulter tracking, high transportation costs, weak relationships with community health centers, poor parental understanding of the needs of chronically ill children, and continued HIV-related stigma. Despite the barriers challenging enrollment of any HIV+ child into care, the rates of care demonstrated in this study suggest that pediatric ART recipients, as a percentage of total ART recipients, could more closely approach Malawi's 2014 goal of 15% with broader implementation of this strategy.

Substantial percentages of HIV+ infants suffer from high mortality without early infant diagnosis (EID) and ART initiation irrespective of CD4% [31–36]. Malawi implemented universal ART for all HIV+ children younger than 1 year of age in 2008, highlighting the need to further strengthen EID services with programs that test younger children for HIV. Importantly, Model 2, which incorporated patient escorts, significantly reduced the age of children HIV tested. Cumulatively, hospitalized children at KCH were 2.9 months younger during the Model 2 pilot period compared to Model 1, likely due to documented seasonal increases in lower respiratory tract infection, malaria, and diarrhea at KCH (data not shown). However, this difference does not fully account for the observed 9.4 month median age reduction in children offered HIV testing from Model 1 to Model 2, a reduction that continued during the programmatic period. With wider implementation, the strategy outlined in this report could strengthen EID through the identification and enrollment into care of significantly more HIV+ children younger than 1 year of age, and of more children earlier in their clinical course of disease.

Kankasa et al recently demonstrated that routine HIV testing of children admitted to a referral hospital in Lusaka, Zambia was feasible and acceptable, using a bedside HIV antibody testing strategy that utilized higher numbers of counselors [19]. Our results confirm the acceptability of routine inpatient pediatric HIV testing in a similar setting in Malawi. However, hiring additional nationally certified HIV counselors would have prohibitively increased operational costs for our program, and was determined by the PITC task force to be infeasible at KCH. The task force opted instead to limit the number of paid counselors to four, and to determine whether volunteer patient escorts could improve PITC outcomes compared to lay counselors alone. Furthermore, our overall test acceptance rate of 97.8%, compared to the 87.4% reported by Kankasa et al. [19], suggests that testing performed in a private room could be less stigmatizing than bedside testing in this setting.

This study's overall 8.5% pediatric inpatient HIV prevalence is nearly double the estimated national 4.8% pediatric prevalence reported in 2008 [3], but is less than the 18.9% prevalence reported by Rogerson et al from Blantyre, Malawi in 2000 [5]. The higher prevalence observed by Rogerson et al likely reflects the absence of free public sector ART services at the time of their study as well as differences in HIV prevalence between the southern (i.e. Blantyre) and central regions (i.e. Lilongwe) [37]. Few reports cite the percentage of hospitalized HIV-E children in sub-Saharan Africa. This study's observed 6.5% HIV-E status suggests that many HIV-E children were accessing hospital care without inpatient identification and referral. The hospitalization of this cohort represents a critical opportunity for further prevention of mother-to-child transmission interventions including ongoing breastfeeding counseling [38–43] and initiation of extended maternal and infant post-natal antiretroviral prophylaxis regimens [43–46].

At the time of this study, routine HIV care services in Malawi were primarily restricted to children receiving ART rather than ART-ineligible or HIV-E children. Overall, this study identified a high proportion of hospitalized HIV+ and HIV-E children that were previously identified, suggesting that these children might not be accessing HIV care services after testing or that their quality of outpatient care may be less than adequate. Both scenarios could result in HIV progression requiring hospitalization. Importantly, only 27 HIV+ and 19 HIV-E patients were identified as readmissions during the 12 month study period (data not shown), confirming that most hospital admissions of HIV+ and HIV-E patients were children new to KCH. These findings imply that pediatric HIV and prevention of mother-to-child transmission services must strengthen the linkage between testing and care, and that the hospital is an important care entry point for these patients.

Studies from Uganda and Zambia concluded that inpatient PITC programs provide an ongoing opportunity for HIV testing and care for entire families [19,20]. Our study further supports these conclusions, as 4779 mothers received HIV testing, 13.8% of whom tested positive. While this program did not track outpatient referrals or HIV care enrollment of newly identified HIV+ mothers, we recommended that mothers be evaluated for ART eligibility at their child's outpatient appointment. We also recommended that other undiagnosed siblings attend the outpatient appointment for HIV testing.

In conclusion, the routine inpatient pediatric HIV testing strategy presented here, which incorporates task shifting from lay counselors alone to lay counselors and locally available patient escorts, greatly improved program outcomes while only marginally increasing operational expenses. Based on these results, we recommend that high HIV-prevalence countries suffering from severe human resource limitations implement similar programs as a core component of their national pediatric HIV care strategy. Further studies investigating the characteristics and outcomes of children identified via routine hospital-based HIV testing, counseling quality assessments, patient satisfaction surveys, cost modeling comparisons of alternate routine HIV testing strategies, and further head-to-head studies investigating different inpatient HIV testing approaches in urban and rural hospitals would add additional key information to this critically important area of pediatric HIV care.

Supporting Information

Text S1 Inpatient Pediatric PITC Program - Manual of Procedures. A detailed description of inpatient pediatric PITC program procedures, recommended staffing levels, suggested budget, and program materials.

Text S2 Inpatient Pediatric PITC Program - Register. A confidential inpatient pediatric PITC program register for routine program monitoring and linkage of HIV-infected and HIV-exposed patients to inpatient clinical care.

Text S3 Inpatient Pediatric PITC Program - Overview. A one page overview outlining the eight steps that comprise the Baylor International Pediatric AIDS Initiative inpatient pediatric PITC system.

Text S4 Inpatient Pediatric PITC Program - Orientation. Pediatric department and inpatient pediatric PITC staff orientation presentation. Baylor International Pediatric AIDS Initiative PowerPoint slides 1–7.

Text S5 Inpatient Pediatric PITC Program - Orientation. Pediatric department and inpatient pediatric PITC staff orientation presentation. Baylor International Pediatric AIDS Initiative PowerPoint slides 8–13.

Text S6 Inpatient Pediatric PITC Program - Orientation. Pediatric department and inpatient pediatric PITC staff orientation presentation. Baylor International Pediatric AIDS Initiative PowerPoint slides 14–20.

Text S7 Diagnosis of Pediatric HIV Infection Training. Presentation to train the inpatient pediatric PITC program staff in pediatric HIV diagnosis. Baylor International Pediatric AIDS Initiative PowerPoint slides 1–6.

Text S8 Diagnosis of Pediatric HIV Infection Training. Presentation to train the inpatient pediatric PITC program staff in pediatric HIV diagnosis. Baylor International Pediatric AIDS Initiative PowerPoint slides 7–12.

Text S9 Diagnosis of Pediatric HIV Infection Training. Presentation to train the inpatient pediatric PITC program staff in pediatric HIV diagnosis. Baylor International Pediatric AIDS Initiative PowerPoint slides 13–18.

Text S10 Diagnosis of Pediatric HIV Infection Training. Presentation to train the inpatient pediatric PITC program staff in pediatric HIV diagnosis. Baylor International Pediatric AIDS Initiative PowerPoint slides 19–24.

Text S11 Diagnosis of Pediatric HIV Infection Training. Presentation to train the inpatient pediatric PITC program staff in pediatric HIV diagnosis. Baylor International Pediatric AIDS Initiative PowerPoint slides 25–29.

Text S12 Diagnosis of Pediatric HIV Infection Training - Diagnosis Workshop Session. A small group session to train the inpatient pediatric PITC program staff in pediatric HIV diagnosis. Includes Baylor International Pediatric AIDS Initiative facilitator and participant materials for workshop session.

Text S13 Inpatient Pediatric PITC Program - Patient Escort Training. Presentation to train patient escorts in their roles and responsibilities within the inpatient pediatric PITC program. Baylor International Pediatric AIDS Initiative PowerPoint slides 1–4.

Text S14 Inpatient Pediatric PITC Program - Patient Escort Training. Presentation to train patient escorts in their roles and responsibilities within the inpatient pediatric PITC program. Baylor International Pediatric AIDS Initiative PowerPoint slides 5-8.

Acknowledgments

We would like to offer our gratitude to all of the children and families that we serve in Malawi, as well as to thank our colleagues and partners who contributed to the development and implementation of this program.

Author Contributions

Conceived and designed the experiments: EDM. Performed the experiments: EDM. Analyzed the data: EDM GAP MMK EBS. Wrote the paper: EDM GAP MMK EBS CM PNK MWK.

References

1. Joint United Nations Programme on HIV/AIDS (2008) 2008 Report on the Global AIDS Epidemic. Available: http://data.unaids.org/pub/GlobalReport/2008/JC1511_GR08_ExecutiveSummary_en.pdf. Accessed 7 September 2009.
2. The United Nations Children's Fund (2008) Children and AIDS: Third Stocktaking Report, 2008. Available: http://www.unicef.org/publications/index_46585.html. Accessed 7 September 2009.
3. Ministry of Health Malawi: HIV Unit (2008) Annual Report HIV Unit 2008.
4. World Health Organization (2007) Guidance on provider-initiated HIV testing and counseling in health facilities. Available: http://whqlibdoc.who.int/publications/2007/9789241595568_eng.pdf. Accessed 26 August 2009.
5. Rogerson SR, Gladstone M, Callaghan M, Erhart L, Rogerson SL, et al. (2004) HIV Infection among paediatric in-patients in Blantyre, Malawi. Trans R Soc Trop Med Hyg 98: 544–552.
6. Chinkhumba J, Tomkins A, Banda T, Mkangama C, Fergusson P (2008) The impact of HIV on mortality during inpatient rehabilitation of severely malnourished children in Malawi. Trans R Soc Trop Med Hyg 102: 639–644.
7. Thurstans S, Kerac M, Maleta K, Banda T, Nesbitt A (2008) HIV prevalence in severely malnourished children admitted to nutrition rehabilitation units in Malawi: Geographical & seasonal variations in a cross-sectional study. BMC Pediatr 8(22): doi:10.1186/1471-2431-8-22.
8. Bronzan RN, Taylor TE, Mwenechanya J, Tembo M, Kayira K, et al. (2007) Bacteremia in Malawian children with severe malaria: prevalence, etiology, HIV coinfection, and outcome. J Infect Dis 195: 895–904.
9. Kline MW, Ferris MG, Jones DC, Calles NR, Mizwa MB, et al. (2009) The Pediatric AIDS Corps: responding to the African HIV/AIDS health professional resource crisis. Pediatrics 123: 134–136.
10. Kline MW (2006) Perspectives on the pediatric HIV/AIDS pandemic: catalyzing access of children to care and treatment. Pediatrics 117: 1388–1393.
11. Weigel R, Kamthunzi P, Mwansambo C, Phiri S, Kazembe PN (2009) Effect of provider-initiated testing and counselling and integration of ART services on access to HIV diagnosis and treatment for children in Lilongwe, Malawi: a pre-post comparison. BMC Pediatr 9(80): doi:10.1186/1471-2431-9-80.
12. Sanjana P, Torpey K, Schwarzwalder A, Simumba C, Kasonde P, et al. (2009) Task-shifting HIV counseling and testing services in Zambia: the role of lay counselors. Hum Resour Health 7(44): doi:10.1186/1478-4491-7-44.
13. World Health Organization (2008) Task shifting. Global recommendations and guidelines. Available: http://www.who.int/healthsystems/TTR-TaskShifting.pdf. Accessed 26 August 2009.
14. Zachariah R, Ford N, Philips M, Lynch S, Massaquoi M, et al. (2009) Task shifting in HIV/AIDS: opportunities, challenges and proposed actions for sub-Saharan Africa. Trans R Soc Trop Med Hyg 103: 549–558.
15. McPake B, Mensah K (2008) Task shifting in health care in resource-poor countries. Lancet: 372: 870–871.
16. Mullan F, Frehywot S (2007) Non-physician clinicians in 47 sub-Saharan African countries. Lancet 370: 2158–2163.
17. Huicho L, Scherpbier R, Nkowane A, Victora CG, the Multi-Country Evaluation of IMCI Study Group (2008) How much does quality of child care vary between health workers with differing durations of training? An observational multicountry study. Lancet 372: 910–916.
18. Rollins N, Mzolo S, Moodley T, Esterhuizen T, van Rooyen H (2009) Universal HIV testing of infants at immunization clinics: an acceptable and feasible approach for early infant diagnosis in high HIV prevalence settings. AIDS 23: 1851–1857.
19. Kankasa C, Carter RJ, Briggs N, Bulterys M, Chama E, et al. (2009) Routine offering of HIV testing to hospitalized pediatric patients at university teaching hospital, Lusaka, Zambia: acceptability and feasibility. J Acquir Immune Defic Syndr 51: 202–208.
20. Wanyenze RK, Nawavvu C, Namale AS, Mayanja B, Bunnell R, et al. (2008) Acceptability of routine HIV counseling and testing, and HIV seroprevalence in Ugandan hospitals. Bull World Health Organ 86: 302–309.
21. Nateniyom S, Jittimanee SX, Viriyakitjar D, Jittimanee S, Keophaithool S, et al. (2008) Provider-initiated diagnostic HIV counseling and testing in tuberculosis clinics in Thailand. Int J Tuberc Lung Dis 12: 955–961.
22. Waxman MJ, Kimaiyo S, Ongaro N, et al. (2007) Initial outcomes of an emergency department rapid HIV testing program in western Kenya. AIDS Patient Care STDS 21: 981–986.
23. Pope DS, Deluca AN, Kali P, Hausler H, Sheard C, et al. (2008) A cluster-randomized trial of provider-initiated (opt-out) HIV counseling and testing of tuberculosis patients in South Africa. J Acquir Immune Defic Syndr 48: 190–195.
24. Chandisarewa W, Stranix-Chibanda L, Chirapa E, Miller A, Simoyi M, et al. (2007) Routine offer of antenatal HIV testing ("opt-out" approach) to prevent mother-to-child transmission of HIV in urban Zimbabwe. Bull World Health Organ 85: 843–850.
25. Spensley A, Sripipatana T, Turner AN, Hoblitzelle C, Robinson J, et al. (2009) Preventing mother-to-child transmission of HIV in resource-limited settings: the Elizabeth Glaser Pediatric AIDS Foundation experience. Am J Public Health 99: 631–637.
26. Creek TL, Ntumy R, Seipone K, Smith M, Mogodi M, et al. (2007) Successful introduction of routine opt-out HIV testing in antenatal care in Botswana. J Acquir Immune Defic Syndr 45: 102–107.
27. Cockcroft A, Andersson N, Milne D, Mokoena T, Masisi M, et al. (2007) Community views about routine HIV testing and antiretroviral treatment in Botswana: signs of progress from a cross sectional study. BMC Int Health Hum Rights 7(5): doi:10.1186/1472-698X-7-5.
28. Moses A, Zimba C, Kamanga E, Nkhoma J, Maida A, et al. (2008) Prevention of mother-to-child transmission: program changes and the effect on uptake of the HIVNET 012 regimen in Malawi. AIDS 22: 83–87.
29. Ministry of Health Malawi: HIV Unit (2008) Guidelines for Paediatric HIV Testing and Counseling.
30. Molyneux E, Ahmad S, Robertson A (2006) Improved triage and emergency care for children reduces inpatient mortality in a resource-constrained setting. Bull World Health Organ 84: 314–319.
31. Violari A, Cotton MF, Gibb DM, Babiker AG, Steyn J, et al. (2008) Early antiretroviral therapy and mortality among HIV-infected infants. N Engl J Med 359: 2233–2244.
32. Diaz C, Hanson C, Cooper ER, Read JS, Watson J, et al. (1998) Disease progression in a cohort of infants with vertically acquired HIV infection observed from birth: the Women and Infants Transmission Study (WITS). J Acquir Immune Defic Syndr Hum Retrovirol 18: 221–228.
33. Tovo PA, de Martino M, Gabiano C, Cappello N, E'Elia R, et al. (1992) Prognostic factors and survival in children with perinatal HIV-1 infection: the Italian register for HIV infections in children. Lancet 339: 1249–1253.
34. Newell ML, Coovadia H, Cortina-Borja M, Rollins N, Gaillard P, et al. (2004) Mortality of infected and uninfected infants born to HIV-infected mothers in Africa: a pooled analysis. Lancet 364: 1236–1243.
35. Chilongozi D, Wang L, Brown L, Taha T, Valentine M, et al. (2008) Morbidity and mortality among a cohort of human immunodeficiency virus type 1-infected and uninfected pregnant women and their infants from Malawi, Zambia, and Tanzania. Pediatr Infect Dis J 27: 808–814.
36. Dunn D, HIV Paediatric Prognostic Markers Collaborative Study Group (2003) Short-term risk of disease progression in HIV-1-infected children receiving no antiretroviral therapy or zidovudine monotherapy: a meta-analysis. Lancet 362: 1605–1611.

37. Geubbels E, Bowie C (2006) Epidemiology of HIV/AIDS in adults in Malawi. Malawi Med J 3: 99–121.
38. Kuhn L, Aldrovandi GM, Sinkala M, Kankasa C, Semrau K, et al. (2008) Effects of early, abrupt weaning on HIV-free survival of children in Zambia. N Engl J Med 359: 130–141.
39. Coovadia HM, Rollins NC, Bland RM, Little K, Coutsoudis A, et al. (2007) Mother-to-child transmission of HIV-1 infection during exclusive breastfeeding in the first 6 months of life: an intervention cohort study. Lancet 369: 1107–1116.
40. Kuhn L, Reitz C, Abrams EJ (2009) Breastfeeding and AIDS in the developing world. Curr Opin Pediatr 21: 83–93.
41. Fox MP, Brooks DR, Kuhn L, Aldrovandi G, Sinkala M, et al. (2009) Role of breastfeeding cessation in mediating the relationship between maternal HIV disease stage and increased child mortality among HIV-exposed uninfected children. Int J Epidemiol 38: 569–576.
42. Kuhn L, Aldrovandi GM, Sinkala M, Kankasa C, Semrau K, et al. (2009) Differential effects of early weaning for HIV-free survival of children born to HIV-infected mothers by severity of maternal disease. PLoS One 4(6): e6059. doi:10.1371/journal.pone.0006059.
43. Mofenson LM (2009) Prevention of Breast Milk Transmission of HIV: The Time Is Now. J Acquir Immune Defic Syndr 52: 305–308.
44. Kilewo C, Karlsson K, Massawe A, Lyamuya E, Swai A, et al. (2008) Prevention of mother-to-child transmission of HIV-1 through breast-feeding by treating infants prophylactically with lamivudine in Dar es Salaam, Tanzania: the Mitra Study. J Acquir Immune Defic Syndr 48: 315–323.
45. Kumwenda NI, Hoover DR, Mofenson LM, Thigpen MC, Kafulafula G, et al. (2008) Extended antiretroviral prophylaxis to reduce breast-milk HIV-1 transmission. N Engl J Med 359: 119–129.
46. Six Week Extended-Dose Nevirapine (SWEN) Study Team (2008) Extended-dose nevirapine to 6 weeks of age for infants to prevent HIV transmission via breastfeeding in Ethiopia, India, and Uganda: an analysis of three randomized controlled trials. Lancet 372: 300–313.

2

Prediction of High-Grade Vesicoureteral Reflux after Pediatric Urinary Tract Infection: External Validation Study of Procalcitonin-Based Decision Rule

Sandrine Leroy[1,2,3,4]*, François Bouissou[5], Anna Fernandez-Lopez[6], Metin K. Gurgoze[7], Kyriaki Karavanaki[8], Tim Ulinski[9], Silvia Bressan[10], Geogios Vaos[11], Pierre Leblond[12], Yvon Coulais[5], Carlos Luaces Cubells[13], A. Denizmen Aygun[7], Constantinos J. Stefanidis[8], Albert Bensman[9], Liviana DaDalt[10], Stefanos Gardikis[11], Sandra Bigot[12], Dominique Gendrel[4], Gérard Bréart[3], Martin Chalumeau[3,4]

1 Centre for Statistics in Medicine, Oxford, United Kingdom, **2** Epidemiology of Emerging Diseases Unit, Institut Pasteur, Paris, France, **3** Inserm U953 Unit, Paris, France, **4** Department of Pediatrics, Paris Descartes University, Necker Hospital, AP-HP, Paris, France, **5** Department of Pediatrics, Children's Hospital, Paul Sabathier University, CHU Purpan, Toulouse, France, **6** Department of Pediatrics, Hospital Universitari Arnau de Vilanova, Lleida. Spain, **7** Firat University Faculty of Medicine, Elazig, Turkey, **8** Department of Nephrology "A. and P. Kyriakou" Childen's Hospital, Athens, Greece, **9** Department of Pediatric Nephrology, Trousseau Hospital and University Pierre et Marie Curie, Paris, France, **10** Department of Pediatrics, University of Padova, Padova, Italy, **11** Department of Pediatric Surgery, Alexandroupolis University Hospital, Thrace, Greece, **12** Department of Pediatrics, Jeanne de Flandre Hospital, Lille, France, **13** Department of Pediatrics, Hospital San Joan de Déu., Barcelona, Spain

Abstract

Background: Predicting vesico-ureteral reflux (VUR) ≥3 at the time of the first urinary tract infection (UTI) would make it possible to restrict cystography to high-risk children. We previously derived the following clinical decision rule for that purpose: cystography should be performed in cases with ureteral dilation and a serum procalcitonin level ≥0.17 ng/mL, or without ureteral dilatation when the serum procalcitonin level ≥0.63 ng/mL. The rule yielded a 86% sensitivity with a 46% specificity. We aimed to test its reproducibility.

Study Design: A secondary analysis of prospective series of children with a first UTI. The rule was applied, and predictive ability was calculated.

Results: The study included 413 patients (157 boys, VUR ≥3 in 11%) from eight centers in five countries. The rule offered a 46% specificity (95% CI, 41–52), not different from the one in the derivation study. However, the sensitivity significantly decreased to 64% (95%CI, 50–76), leading to a difference of 20% (95%CI, 17–36). In all, 16 (34%) patients among the 47 with VUR ≥3 were misdiagnosed by the rule. This lack of reproducibility might result primarily from a difference between derivation and validation populations regarding inflammatory parameters (CRP, PCT); the validation set samples may have been collected earlier than for the derivation one.

Conclusions: The rule built to predict VUR ≥3 had a stable specificity (ie. 46%), but a decreased sensitivity (ie. 64%) because of the time variability of PCT measurement. Some refinement may be warranted.

Editor: Guoying Wang, John Hopkins Bloomberg School of Public Health, United States of America

Funding: Sandrine Leroy was funded by a post-doctoral fellowship grant from the French Society of Nephrology, and from la Fondation Bettencourt. The funders had no role in study design, data collection and analysis, decision to publish, or preparation of the manuscript.

Competing Interests: Professors Gendrel and Chalumeau have received unrestricted educational grants for other studies, for a total amount lower than €5000, from Brahms AG, the manufacturer of procalcitonin, in 2007. The funders had no role in study design, data collection and analysis, decision to publish, or preparation of the manuscript. This does not alter the authors' adherence to all the PLoS ONE policies on sharing data and materials.

* E-mail: Sandrine.Leroy @pasteur.fr

Introduction

During the past decade, many European and American pediatric societies have recommended that all young children undergo a cystography after a first febrile UTI [1,2]. This systematic strategy is driven by the belief that VUR, especially moderate and high-grade VUR, is a risk factor for recurrent UTI, then renal scarring and long-term complications, such as recurrent infection, hypertension, poor renal growth, and eclampsia [3]. The systematic strategy is also based on the premise that VUR can be treated and/or children followed to keep them free of complications [1,2]. However, even if systematic cystography offered a nearly 100% sensitivity to identify reflux, it is a truly non-selective strategy, meaning that many children undergo an unnecessary cystography, which is painful, irradiating and expensive, and increases the risk of iatrogenic UTI [4]. Regarding recent publications minimizing the clinical consequences of low-grade VUR [5,6], the low rate of high-grade VUR (only 10% of the children with a first febrile UTI [7]), and the current discussions on the efficacy of high-grade VUR treatment [6,8,9], some new guidelines have proposed to never perform a cystography after a first febrile UTI in children 2 to 24 months old [10,11]. However, these new guidelines have raised some concerns because of the risk of delaying high-grade VUR diagnosis [10]. Moreover, definite evidence about the absence of benefit of antibiotic prophylaxis is still lacking for many clinical situations because of methodological weaknesses of the available trials, and this could make the pendulum swing back towards specific indications of VUR treatment that have to be diagnosed accurately [12]. Furthermore, an American study of clinical practices evaluation measured that only 40% of children who would have benefited from a cystography actually underwent this examination after a first UTI, indicating that a more situational approach would likely be welcomed by parents and clinicians [13].

We believed, then, that there is scope for an evidence-based strategy, one that offered a moderate alternative to two diametrically opposed policies (cystography for all or no children). We derived a predictive tool for moderate and high-grade VUR (grade ≥3), aiming to avoid *a posteriori* unnecessary cystographies and not to miss those patients with high-grade VUR [14]. This predictive decision rule includes procalcitonin (PCT), a validated and sensitive predictor of VUR [15–17], and the ureteral dilation from renal ultrasonography (US) [18]. PCT was initially studied as a predictor of VUR because this sensitive biomarker was demonstrated to correlate with acute pyelonephritis and scars, both related to VUR [19,20]. The rule indicates that in children between one month and four years old with a first febrile UTI, a cystography should be performed in cases with ureteral dilation (i.e. ureter visible on the renal ultrasonography – US) and a serum PCT level (measured at the time of UTI diagnosis) ≥0.17 ng/mL, or without ureteral dilatation (i.e. ureter not visible on the renal US) when the serum PCT level ≥0.63 ng/mL [14]. This rule yielded 86% (95%CI: 74–93) sensitivity with 47% (95%CI: 42–51) specificity; the internal mathematical validation confirmed the derivation predictive ability. However, four steps are involved in the development of a clinical decision rule: the creation of the rule, internal validation, external reproducibility, and assessment of its impact on clinical behavior [21]. Our aim was to evaluate the reproducibility of the prediction rule that we have developed and to perform its external validation.

Results

Patients' characteristics

Eight centres were included [18,22–31]. In all centres, patients underwent a radiological cystography, and had a PCT measurement with the LUMItest PCT immunoluminometric assay or the BRAHMS PCT-Q semiquantitative rapid test (BRAHMS AG, Hennigsdorf, Germany). Half of the centres collected urine with suprapubic aspiration or urethral catheterization for non-toilet trained children, and half used sterile bags (Table 1).

Of the 530 who met the inclusion criteria, 417 were finally included in the analysis (Figure 1). The mean age of the children was 11.9 months (SD: 10.7, median: 8.5, Inter-quartile - IQR: 4.0–16.0); 157 (38%) were boys. VUR was diagnosed in 109 (26%) children and 47 (11%) patients had VUR ≥3. No adverse event was reported in performing PCT measurement, renal US nor cystography. Table 1 provides details on the characteristics of each centre population.

Validity of the rule

When applying the rule to the validation population, 16 (34%) of the 47 patients with VUR ≥3 were misdiagnosed because they presented with either ureteral dilation and PCT <0.17 ng/mL (for one patient – 2%) or without ureteral dilation and PCT <0.63 ng/mL (for the 15–32% - other patients - Figures 2 and 3). We did not find a significant relationship between VUR ≥3 and the clinical decision rule: adjusted OR = 1.5 (95% CI, 0.7–3.4); P = 0.3. On the validation population, the decision rule yielded a 64% (95% CI, 40–76) sensitivity, and a 46% (95% CI, 41–52) specificity (Table 2). Specificity and positive predictive value (46% and 13% respectively) were not significantly different from the derivation set (47%, and 17% respectively), whereas sensitivity and negative predictive value were (64% and 91 respectively for the validation set vs. 86% and 96% respectively for the derivation set-Table 2).

When applying the rounded rule and the rule based on PCT alone to the validation population, we also found a non-significant relationship between VUR ≥3 and the rule, as well as a significant decrease of sensitivity and negative predictive value (Table 2).

In the subgroup of children for whom urine specimens were collected using suprapubic aspiration or urethral catheterization for non-toilet trained children, the relationships between VUR ≥3 and the rules were not significant (Table 3). For the three rules, sensitivities did not differ from those found in the entire population (60 (95% CI, 39–78) in the subgroup *vs.* 64 (95% CI, 50–76) for the entire set for the exact rule), whereas specificities were significantly higher: 58 (95% CI, 51–65) in the subgroup *vs.* 46 (95% CI, 41–52) for the entire set for the exact rule (Table 3).

Comparison of the derivation and validation populations

Because we did not find the similar results between derivation and validation populations, we compared their characteristics. There was no significant difference regarding gender, prevalence of all-grade or high-grade VUR, distribution of age (Table 4). However, CRP was significantly lower in the validation population compared with the derivation population: median = 53.8 mg/L (IQR: 20.0–98.0) *vs.* 77.5 mg/L (IQR: 38.0–140.0), P <0.001. PCT had a trend close to significance to be lower for children with VUR ≥3 in the validation set compared with those in the derivation set: median = 1.5 ng/mL (IQR: 0.3–6.1) *vs.* 2.9 (IQR: 1.2–6.8); P = 0.06. There was also a trend to find more ureteral dilations on renal US in children with VUR <3 in the validation set compared with the derivation one: 23 (6%) *vs.* 16 (4%), P = 0.08.

Discussion

We report the first attempt to evaluate the reproducibility of the decision rule based on PCT and ureteral dilation proposed by our group [14]. In the derivation study, a significant relationship was found between VUR ≥3 and the rule (P <0.0001), even when considering the rounded rule, or the rule based on PCT only. These significant relationships were not found again in the validation set (P >0.1). The 47% specificity (95%CI, 42–51) of the rule for the prediction of VUR ≥3 was confirmed (46%; 95%CI, 41–52), but not the sensitivity: 60% (95% CI, 50–76) in the validation set vs. 86% (95% CI, 74–93) in the derivation population. The results were similarly comparable between validation and derivation populations for the rounded rule and the rule based on PCT only. Applying the rule to the validation set, we would not have prescribed cystography, and then misdiagnosed VUR in 16 patients (15 without ureteral dilation), representing 34% of the patients with VUR ≥3. The rule only had missed 9 (16%) children among those with VUR ≥3 in the derivation study [14].

The first issue to be addressed to investigate the decreases of predictive ability of a rule is the difference in the derivation and

Table 1. Population characteristics according to each center.

Centre*	Urine collection techniques (threshold of the positive bacteriuria)†	n	Male n (%)	Age median (IQR)	All-grade VUR n (%)	Grade ≥3 VUR n (%)	CRP Median (IQR)
Centres using SA or UC (n = 199)							
Alex.	SA (any), UC (10^4), CVM (10^5)	40	9 (23)	10.5 (6.5–12.5)	12 (30)	8 (20)	57.0 (14.5–91.0)
Athens	SA (10^3), UC (10^4), CVM (10^5)	52	26 (50)	6.6 (3.0–9.8)	10 (19)	0 (0)	42.4 (6.1–108)
Barcelona	SA (any), UC (5.10^4), CVM (10^5)	55	22 (41)	6.0 (3.0–9.0)	13 (24)	4 (7)	44.6 (14.1–76.7)
Elazig	UC (10^3), CVM (10^5)	52	25 (48)	6.0 (6.0–36.0)	3 (6)	0 (0)	12.5 (4–40)
Centres using SB (n = 213)							
Lille	SB (10^5)	23	7 (29)	8.5 (4.0–19.0)	14 (58)	3 (13)	52.5 (19–83)
Padova	SB (10^5)	47	17 (38)	6.4 (3.1–11.4)	9 (19)	2 (4)	61.0 (37–120)
Paris	SB (10^5)	52	23 (44)	7.6 (2.8–12.8)	13 (25)	5 (10)	85.0 (53.6–117)
Toulouse	SB (10^5), CVM (10^5)	91	28 (31)	9.2 (5.3–17.7)	35 (38)	17 (19)	75.5 (33.0–117)
Total (n = 413)		413	157 (38)	8.5 (4.0–16.0)	109 (26)	47 (11)	53.8 (20–98)

*Classified according to the urine collection technique in non-toilet-trained children.
†In colony-forming units/mL.
Abbreviations: Alex for Alexandroupolis; CRP, C-reactive protein; CVM, Clean-voided midstream; IQR, Interquartile range; SA, Suprapubic aspiration; SB, Sterile bag; UC, Urethral catheterization; VUR, Vesicoureteral reflux.

validation populations, which would explain why a decision rule could not be transferred across those sets of patients [21]. In the present case, populations were not significantly different ($P > 0.05$) for the classic parameters: gender, prevalence of all-grade and high-grade of VUR. Nevertheless, the validation population had a significantly lower level of inflammatory biomarkers: for CRP for all children, in PCT was also lower in children with VUR ≥3. This result means that the entire distribution of PCT values was moved towards lower values for children with high-grade VUR in the validation population; it could explain why the group of 15 (94%) out of 16 patients with VUR≥3 were missed by the rule, and thus belonged to the rule branch of "patients without ureteral dilation and PCT <0.63 ng/mL". As the weight of the rule is mainly carried by PCT, a lowest distribution of PCT values might have a major influence on the results of the rule validation set; it is demonstrated by that 15 (94%) out of the 16 patients missed by the rule were not rescued by ureteral dilation criterion. Indeed, this hypothesis also may explain why even the rule based on PCT alone failed to reproduce the 85% sensitivity, even though this result had previously been validated in two multicentre cohort studies [16,17]. This significant difference in inflammatory biomarkers distributions between validation and derivation sets could be due to the fact that samples were collected at different time points during UTI course. We were not able to verify this

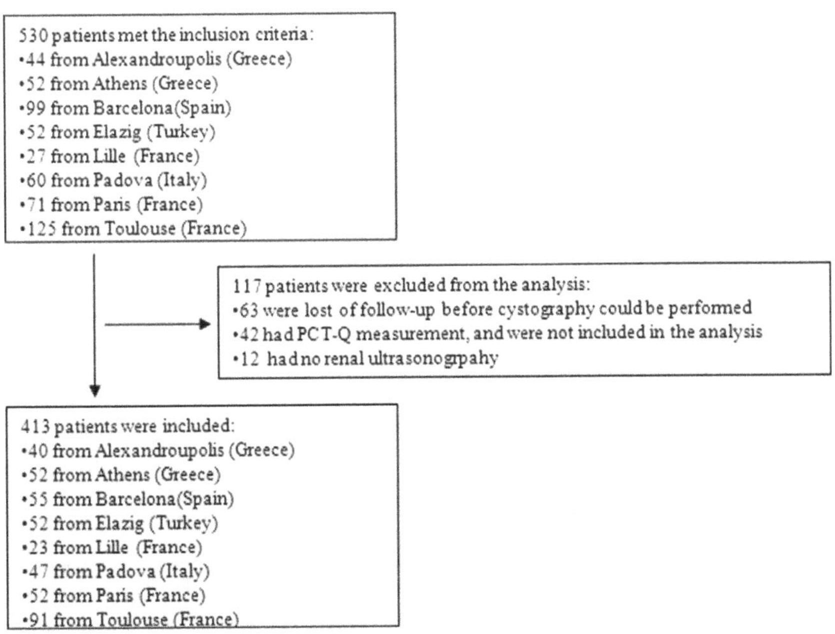

Figure 1. Diagnosis tree and distribution of the study population at each step of the decision rule in the validation population.
Abbreviations: PCT, Procalcitonin; VUR, Vesico-ureteral reflux.

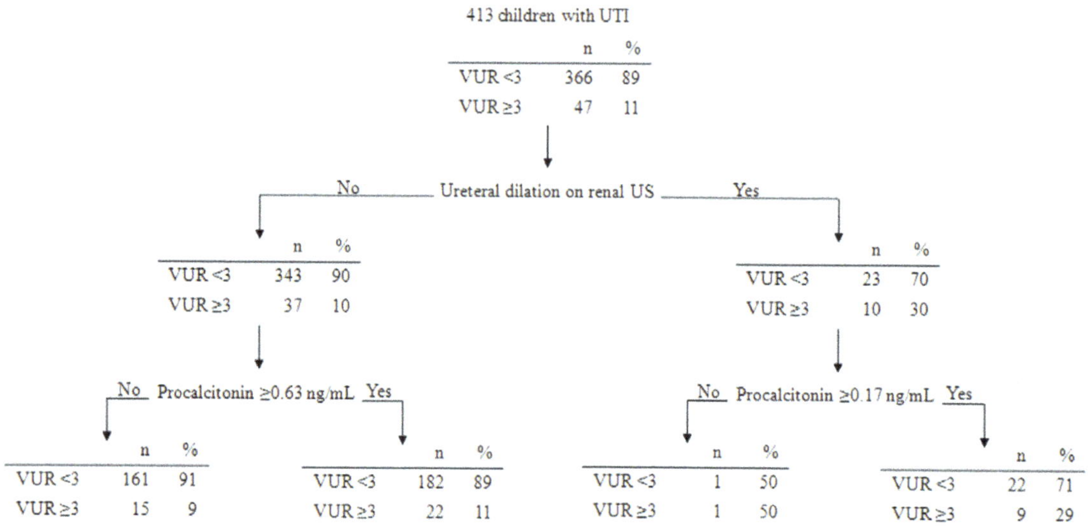

Figure 2. Distribution of Procalcitonin values according to the presence of high-grade VUR and the presence of Ureteral dilation on renal ultrasonography.

suggestion, because the centres identified the exact time of inflammatory markers measurement from the appearance of fever, and this data was not collected. Further study of this time interval would be necessary to improve this rule and to implement it safely. These differences regarding the inflammatory parameters distributions were unpredictable before the study validation, because all centres were European and applied the same standard procedures to diagnose and treat children with UTI. Moreover, there was also a trend ($p = 0.08$) in the difference between derivation and validation sets on the ureteral dilation on renal US

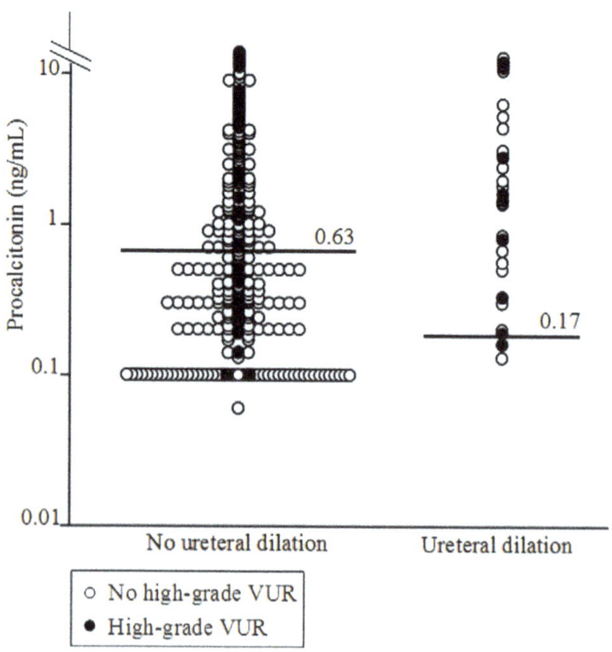

Figure 3. Distribution of Procalcitonin values according to the presence of high-grade VUR and the presence of Ureteral dilation on renal ultrasonography. The horizontal lines are the dichotomization threshold in each group.

Table 2. Sensitivity and specificity of the decision rule in the derivation and validation populations.

	Derivation* (n = 494, prevalence of VUR ≥3: 11%)	Validation (n = 413, prevalence of VUR ≥3: 11%)	Difference†
Clinical decision rule			
aOR**	5.2 (2.4–11.3)	1.5 (0.7–3.4)	
Sensitivity	86 (74–93)	64 (50–76)	22 (5 to 38)
Specificity	47 (42–51)	46 (41–52)	0 (−7 to 7)
PPV	17 (13–22)	13 (10–18)	4 (−3 to 10)
NPV	96 (93–98)	91 (86–94)	5 (1 to 11)
Rounded decision rule			
aOR**	6.8 (0.9–50.0)	1.3 (0.6–3.2)	
Sensitivity	86 (76–94)	62 (47–74)	26 (9 to 41)
Specificity	44 (40–49)	45 (40–50)	1 (−6 to 8)
PPV	17 (13–21)	13 (9–18)	4 (−2 to 10)
NPV	97 (93–98)	90 (85–94)	6 (1 to 12)
Rule based on PCT alone			
aOR**	4.9 (2.3–10.6)	1.3 (0.5–3.4)	
Sensitivity	86 (74–93)	60 (45–72)	28 (11 to 44)
Specificity	45 (40–50)	46 (41–51)	1 (−6 to 8)
PPV	17 (13–21)	12 (9–17)	4 (−2 to 10)
NPV	96 (93–98)	90 (85–93)	7 (2 to 12)

Values are expressed as values or % (95% CI).
Discriminative values were compared using a χ^2 test for unpaired sample.
*Data in the column come from the previously published derivation of the decision rule [34].
**Adjusted OR were calculated with the multi-level logistic regression models.
†Differences are rounded to the closer integer.
Abbreviations: NPV, Negative predictive value; OR, Odd ratio; PCT, Procalcitonin; PPV, Positive predictive value.

Table 3. Sensitivity and specificity of the decision rule in the whole validation population and in the subgroup of children for whom urines were collected using suprapubic aspiration, urethral catheterization or clean-voided midstream sample.

	Whole population	Subgroup*	Difference
Clinical decision rule			
aOR**	1.5 (0.7–3.4)	2.0 (0.4–11.6)	
Sensitivity	64 (50–76)	60 (39–78)	4 (−20 to 28)
Specificity	46 (41–52)	58 (51–65)	11 (2 to 20)
PPV	13 (10–18)	14 (8–22)	1 (−1 to 7)
NPV	91 (86–94)	93 (86–96)	2 (−1 to 8)
Rounded decision rule			
aOR**	1.3 (0.6–3.2)	1.9 (0.3–11.1)	
Sensitivity	62 (47–74)	60 (39–78)	2 (−20 to 26)
Specificity	45 (40–50)	55 (48–62)	10 (1 to 19)
PPV	13 (9–18)	13 (8–21)	0 (−1 to 7)
NPV	90 (85–94)	93 (86–96)	2 (−5 to 9)
Rule based on PCT alone			
aOR**	1.3 (0.5–3.4)	1.9 (0.3–11.1)	
Sensitivity	60 (45–72)	60 (39–78)	0 (−24 to 25)
Specificity	46 (41–51)	56 (49–63)	10 (1 to 18)
PPV	12 (9–17)	13 (8–22)	−1 (−10 to 7)
NPV	90 (85–93)	93 (86–96)	3 (−5 to 9)

Values are expressed as values or % (95% CI).
Discriminative values were compared using a χ^2 test for unpaired sample.
*Subgroup of children for who urines were collected using suprapubic aspiration or urethral catheterization.
**Adjusted OR were calculated with the multi-level logistic regression models.
Abbreviations: NPV, Negative predictive value; OR, Odd ratio; PCT, Procalcitonin; PPV, Positive predictive value.

number in children with VUR <3. This finding may also have added to the differences between the two populations concerning the key variables of the rule. Furthermore, we acknowledge that the rule included ureteral dilation, which is a renal US criterion with no measurement of its inter-operator variability in a multi-case multi-reader study, even if it was found to be the best US renal criterion to predict high-grade VUR [18]. This weakness of the rule needs to be evaluated and corrected.

The second issue concerning the validation's difficulties to reproduce derivation results is the limitations of the external validation study. The validation was a secondary analysis of previously published prospective cohort studies, as was the derivation study. Because our group performed a systematic review and meta-analysis on PCT in UTI in children, we gathered the worldwide published data of children with PCT and VUR [20]. The derivation study was based on the initially published cohort studies, while the validation study was premised on the later ones. We did not, however, believe that the structure of these studies would affect the quality of the data or introduce a bias.

The use of sterile bags for urine collection for the non-toilet trained children in half of the centres might have introduced a selection bias, because this technique is less specific than suprapubic aspiration or urethral catheterization [1]. However, there was no significant difference in the number of children for whom urine were collected by sterile bags, compared with those in the derivation population: 238 (48%) children vs. 214 (52%), P = 0.3 (Table 4). Interestingly, the specificities of the rules were significantly higher in the subgroup of children for whom urine specimens were collected properly than in the whole population. This result can be explained by the lower specificity for UTI diagnosis of sterile bags compared with recommended techniques. Indeed, because VUR is known to be a risk factor for UTI, the use of sterile bags might have increased the number of children with VUR <3 more than those with VUR ≥3. In the same manner, because PCT is positively correlated with the presence and severity of UTI [20], and because the weight of the rule was more carried by PCT than by ureteral dilation [14], the use of sterile bags may have increased the number of children with a negative result than

Table 4. Comparison of the characteristics of the derivation and validation populations.

Variables	Derivation* (n = 494, prevalence of VUR ≥3: 11%)	Validation (n = 413, prevalence of VUR ≥3: 11%)	P-value**
Use of sterile bags	238 (48)	214 (52)	0.3
Male gender	197 (40)	157 (38)	0.6
All grade VUR	126 (26)	109 (29)	0.8
High-grade VUR	56 (11)	47 (11)	1.0
Age (months)	12.1 (±11.2); 8.0 (4.0–17.0)	11.9 (±10.7); 8.5 (4.0–16.0)	0.7
CRP (mg/mL)	94.6 (±74.0); 77.5 (38.0–140.0)	68.4 (±64.1); 53.8 (20.0–98.0)	<0.0001
PCT (ng/mL)	4.2 (±19.3); 0.9 (0.3–2.8)	3.5 (±8.6); 0.8 (0.3–3.1)	0.5
in children with VUR <3	3.6 (±19.3); 0.7 (0.3–2.4)	3.4 (±8.8); 0.8 (0.3–2.5)	1.0
in children with VUR ≥3	8.3 (±18.5); 2.9 (1.2–6.8)	4.4 (±6.5); 1.5 (0.3–6.1)	0.06
Ureteral dilation	25 (5)	33 (8)	0.8
in children with VUR <3	16 (4)	23 (6)	0.08
in children with VUR ≥3	10 (18)	20 (21)	0.7

Values are expressed as n (%) for binary variables (gender, All grade and high-grade VUR, Ureteral dilation), and as: mean (±Standard deviation); median (inter-quartile range) for continuous variables (age, CPR, PCT).
*Data in the column come from the previously published derivation of the decision rule [34].
**Binary variables were compared using a χ^2 test, and continuous variables were compared using the non-parametric Mann-Whitney test.
Abbreviations: CRP, C-reactive protein; PCT, Procalcitonin; U dilation, Ureteral dilation; VUR, Vesico-ureteral reflux.

the one with a positive one. Nevertheless, some centres (e.g. Padova, Italy), in order to decrease the likelihood of false positive results due to bag urine collection, included only children with two consecutive positive urine cultures. The combined increases (in the number of children with VUR <3 and in the number of children with PCT <0.5 ng/mL when sterile bags are used to collected urine) resulted in an underestimate in the specificity in children for whom urine were collected by sterile bags, and thus accounts for the significant difference in specificities. It did not, however, explain the failure to reproduce the sensitivity of the rule, nor the loss of a significant relationship between VUR ≥3 and the rules. To summarize, the validation study may have had some limitations, but none of these limitations appeared to explain fully the failure to validate externally the decision rule.

The validation of the decision rule based on PCT and ureteral dilation on renal US confirmed the rule specificity, but showed a loss of its sensitivity, which led to a misdiagnosis of 34% of children with VUR ≥3. The fact that the rule performed better in the derivation population than in the validation one was predictable, according to the Evidence Based Working Group [21]. However, the decrease in sensitivity might also be primarily due to differences regarding PCT distributions between derivation and validation sets and was thus unpredictable prior to the study. The rule therefore may need greater refinement, particularly regarding the time of PCT measurement and the variability between observers of ureteral dilation. Furthermore, the outcome should also be reconsidered and modified for a composite outcome, including high-grade VUR and renal scars, which are precisely the cause of kidney injuries leading to future complications, and the real goal of any nephroprotection strategy including VUR treatment.

Methods

Study design

We conducted a secondary analysis of already published data on children with UTI, PCT and VUR. Because we had conducted a systematic review and meta-analysis on individual patient data on early and late renal scarring and PCT in children with UTI [16], we knew all the centres possessing data on PCT and VUR in children with UTI. To perform the external validation of the rule, we included all centres [18,22–31] that had not been included in the study to derive the rule [14]. All consecutive children in each center, aged one month to four years and admitted with a first febrile UTI (temperature ≥38°C with a positive bacterial urine culture defined according to each centre criteria – Table 1) were considered for inclusion. Children with an already known uropathy (ie. any urological or urinary tract abnormality, as posterior urethral valves, ectopic ureter, VUR); at the time of the UTI diagnosis, those who had received antibiotics in the 48 hours before diagnosis, and those who had undergone radionuclide cystography (which does not distinguish high-grade from low-grade VUR [32]) were not included. Of note, results of antenatal renal US were not taken into account to include children, insofar as there was no post-natal diagnostic confirmation before UTI diagnosis. Because this study was a secondary analysis of already-published prospective cohort studies, the electronic data files were merged across studies; informed consent had had already been obtained for the initial studies.

Outcome definition

All patients had a voiding cystography, the gold standard examination for the diagnosis and classification of VUR. Cystographies were read according to the "International System of Radiological Grading of Vesicoureteric Reflux" [33] by an experienced senior radiologists in Pediatrics in each centre, and blinded to PCT and renal US results. Moderate and high-grade VUR was a priori defined as a VUR grade ≥3, which means that VUR extends up to the renal pelvis with an increased ureteral dilation with the grade of reflux [7].

Definition of predictors included in the rule

Each child's serum PCT was prospectively measured at admission for febrile UTI (i.e. when children arrived at the Emergency Department), with the LUMItest PCT immunoluminometric assay (BRAHMS, Hennigsdorf, Germany). The other potential predictive variables came from the findings of renal US performed at the time of UTI diagnosis by an experienced senior pediatric radiologist blinded to the PCT measurement, and before cystography was performed: ureteral dilation (defined by ureter visibility during renal US). The imaging studies were reviewed blinded to cystography results, and data were extracted from the radiologist's record.

Statistical analyses

We first described the study population's general characteristics. We then applied the rule to every patient, classifying each one as cystography recommended or not. We also applied the rounded rule (i.e. a cystography should performed in case of ureteral dilation and PCT ≥0.2 ng/mL, or if PCT ≥0.6 ng/mL in absence of ureteral dilation), and the rule based on PCT alone (a cystography should be prescribed if PCT ≥0.6 ng/mL) to each child. We evaluated the relationship between VUR ≥3 and the decision rules with an adjusted OR using a multi-level logistic regression model (where centers were considered as the group level variable). We then calculated for the clinical decision rule, the rounded rule, and the rule based on PCT alone, the sensitivity, specificity, positive and negative predictive values. We ran the same calculation in the subgroup of children for whom urine specimens were collected using "recommended" techniques (i.e. suprapubic aspiration or urethral catheterization for non-toilet trained children and clean-voided midstream for toilet trained children). Discriminative values were compared with those of the derivation population [14]. In case of significant difference, we compared the characteristics of derivation and validation populations using χ^2 tests and non-parametric Mann-Whitney tests. Statistical analyses were performed with Stata 11/SE software (StataCorp, College Station, TX, USA) and Confidence Interval Analysis software (London, UK).

Acknowledgments

The authors thank Dr Deftereos (Department of Radiology, Democritus University of Thrace and University General Hospital of Alexandroupolis Thrace, Greece) Dr Bacchetta (Department of Pediatric Nephrology - Reference Centre for Rare Renal Diseases, Femme Mère Enfant Hospital, University of Lyon, Lyon, France) and Dr Tamara Giles-Vernicke for the Epidemiology Unit of Emerging Diseases in Institut Pasteur, Paris, for helpful discussions.

Author Contributions

Conceived and designed the study: SL MC. Collected the data: FB AF-L MKG KK TU SB GV PL YC CLC ADA CJS AB LD SG SB. Performed the statistical analysis: SL. Interpreted the data: SL. Drafted the manuscript: SL. Critically revised the manuscript for important intellectual content: SL FB AF-L MKG KK TU SB GV PL YC CLC ADA CJS AB LD SG SB DG GB MC. Brought expertise in Epidemiology and Pediatric Infecious Diseses, respectively: GB DG. Obtained funding: SL.

References

1. American Academy of Pediatrics. Committee on Quality Improvement. Subcommittee on Urinary Tract Infection. (1999) Practice parameter: the diagnosis, treatment, and evaluation of the initial urinary tract infection in febrile infants and young children. Pediatrics 103: 843–852.
2. Report of a Working Group of the Research Unit, Royal College of Physicians. (1991) Guidelines for the management of acute urinary tract infection in childhood. J R Coll Physicians Lond 25: 36–42.
3. Williams G, Fletcher JT, Alexander SI, Craig JC (2008) Vesicoureteral reflux. J Am Soc Nephrol 19: 847–862.
4. Guignard JP (1979) Urinary infection after micturating cystography. Lancet 1: 103.
5. Garin EH, Olavarria F, Garcia Nieto V, Valenciano B, Campos A, et al. (2006) Clinical significance of primary vesicoureteral reflux and urinary antibiotic prophylaxis after acute pyelonephritis: a multicenter, randomized, controlled study. Pediatrics 117: 626–632.
6. Roussey-Kesler G, Gadjos V, Idres N, Horen B, Ichay L, et al. (2008) Antibiotic prophylaxis for the prevention of recurrent urinary tract infection in children with low grade vesicoureteral reflux: results from a prospective randomized study. J Urol 179: 674–679.
7. Hoberman A, Charron M, Hickey RW, Baskin M, Kearney DH, et al. (2003) Imaging studies after a first febrile urinary tract infection in young children. N Engl J Med 348: 195–202.
8. Smellie JM, Barratt TM, Chantler C, Gordon I, Prescod NP, et al. (2001) Medical versus surgical treatment in children with severe bilateral vesicoureteric reflux and bilateral nephropathy: a randomised trial. Lancet 357: 1329–1333.
9. Jodal U, Smellie JM, Lax H, Hoyer PF (2006) Ten-year results of randomized treatment of children with severe vesicoureteral reflux. Final report of the International Reflux Study in Children. Pediatr Nephrol 21: 785–792.
10. Mori R, Lakhanpaul M, Verrier-Jones K (2007) Diagnosis and management of urinary tract infection in children: summary of NICE guidance. BMJ 335: 395–397.
11. Subcommittee on Urinary Tract Infection, Steering Committee on Quality Improvement and Management. (2011) Urinary Tract Infection: Clinical Practice Guideline for the Diagnosis and Management of the Initial UTI in Febrile Infants and Children 2 to 24 Months. Pediatrics 128: 595–610.
12. Montini G, Tullus K, Hewitt I (2011) Febrile urinary tract infections in children. N Engl J Med 365: 239–250.
13. Cohen AL, Rivara FP, Davis R, Christakis DA (2005) Compliance with guidelines for the medical care of first urinary tract infection in infants: a population-based study. Pediatrics 115: 1474–1478.
14. Leroy S, Romanello C, Smolkin V, Galetto-Lacour A, Korczowski B, et al. (2010) Prediction of high-grade vesicoureteral reflux after a first febrile urinary tract infection in children: construction and internal validation of a clinical decision rule. Pediatr Nephrol 25: 1852.
15. Leroy S, Gendrel D, Breart G, Chalumeau M (2005) Procalcitonin and vesicoureteral reflux in children with urinary tract infection: In reply. Pediatrics 115: 1262–1263.
16. Leroy S, Romanello C, Galetto-Lacour A, Bouissou F, Fernandez-Lopez A, et al. (2011) Procalcitonin is a Predictor for High-Grade Vesicoureteral Reflux in Children: Meta-Analysis of Individual Patient Data. J Pediatr 159: 644–651.
17. Leroy S, Romanello C, Galetto-Lacour A, Smolkin V, Korczowski B, et al. (2007) Procalcitonin to reduce the number of unnecessary cystographies in children with a urinary tract infection: a European validation study. J Pediatr 150: 89–95.
18. Leroy S, Vantalon S, Larakeb A, Ducou-Le-Pointe H, Bensman A (2010) Vesicoureteral reflux in children with urinary tract infection: comparison of diagnostic accuracy of renal US criteria. Radiology 255: 890–898.
19. Espindola R, Bacchetta J, Cochat P, Leroy S (2011) Vesico-ureteral reflux as a risk factor for acute pyelonephritis and renal damage in children with UTI: systematic review and meta-analysis. Pediatr Nephrol 26: 1589.
20. Leroy S, Fernandez A, Nifkar R, Romanello C, Bouissou F, et al. (2010) Predictive ability of procalcitonin as a predictor for acute pyelonephrtitis and late renal scars in children with UTI: Meta-analysis on individual patient data. Pediatr Nephrol 25: 1844.
21. McGinn TG, Guyatt GH, Wyer PC, Naylor CD, Stiell IG, et al. (2000) Users' guides to the medical literature: XXII: how to use articles about clinical decision rules. Evidence-Based Medicine Working Group. JAMA 284: 79–84.
22. Andreola B, Bressan S, Callegaro S, Liverani A, Plebani M, et al. (2007) Procalcitonin and C-reactive protein as diagnostic markers of severe bacterial infections in febrile infants and children in the emergency department. Pediatr Infect Dis J 26: 672–677.
23. Belhadj-Tahar H, Coulais Y, Tafani M, Bouissou F (2008) Procalcitonin implication in renal cell apoptosis induced by acute pyelonephritis in children. Infect Drug Resist 1: 17–20.
24. Bigot S, Leblond P, Foucher C, Hue V, D'Herbomez M, et al. (2005) Usefulness of procalcitonin for the diagnosis of acute pyelonephritis in children. Arch Pediatr 12: 1075–1080.
25. Bressan S, Andreola B, Zucchetta P, Montini G, Burei M, et al. (2009) Procalcitonin as a predictor of renal scarring in infants and young children. Pediatr Nephrol 24: 1199–1204.
26. Fernandez Lopez A, Luaces Cubells C, Garcia Garcia JJ, Fernandez Pou J (2003) Procalcitonin in pediatric emergency departments for the early diagnosis of invasive bacterial infections in febrile infants: results of a multicenter study and utility of a rapid qualitative test for this marker. Pediatr Infect Dis J 22: 895–903.
27. Fernández López A, Luaces Cubells C, Valls Tolosa C, Ortega Rodríguez J, García García J, et al. (2001) Procalcitonin in the early diagnosis of invasive bacterial infection in febrile infants. An Esp Pediatr 55: 321–328.
28. Gurgoze MK, Akarsu S, Yilmaz E, Gödekmerdan A, Akça Z, et al. (2005) Proinflammatory cytokines and procalcitonin in children with acute pyelonephritis. Pediatr Nephrol 20: 1445–1448.
29. Karavanaki K, Haliotis FA, Sourani M, Kariyiannis C, Hantzi E, et al. (2007) DMSA scintigraphy in febrile urinary tract infections could be omitted in children with low procalcitonin levels. Infect Dis Clin Pract 15: 377–381.
30. Kotoula A, Gardikis S, Tsalkidis A, Mantadakis E, Zissimopoulos A, et al. (2009) Comparative efficacies of procalcitonin and conventional inflammatory markers for prediction of renal parenchymal inflammation in pediatric first urinary tract infection. Urology 73: 782–786.
31. Kotoula A, Gardikis S, Tsalkidis A, Mantadakis E, Zissimopoulos A, et al. (2009) Procalcitonin for the early prediction of renal parenchymal involvement in children with UTI: preliminary results. Int Urol Nephrol 41: 393–399.
32. Fettich J, Colarinha P, Fischer S, Frokier J, Gordon I, et al. (2003) Guidelines for direct radionuclide cystography in children. Eur J Nucl Med Mol Imaging 30: B39–44.
33. Lebowitz RL, Olbing H, Parkkulainen KV, Smellie JM, Tamminen-Mobius TE (1985) International system of radiographic grading of vesicoureteric reflux. International Reflux Study in Children. Pediatr Radiol 15: 105–109.
34. Jodal U (2000) Selective approach to diagnostic imaging of children after urinary tract infection. Acta Paediatr 89: 767–768.

3

WHO 2010 Guidelines for Prevention of Mother-to-Child HIV Transmission in Zimbabwe: Modeling Clinical Outcomes in Infants and Mothers

Andrea L. Ciaranello[1]*, Freddy Perez[2,3], Matthews Maruva[4], Jennifer Chu[5], Barbara Engelsmann[6], Jo Keatinge[4], Rochelle P. Walensky[1,5,7,8], Angela Mushavi[9], Rumbidzai Mugwagwa[9], Francois Dabis[2], Kenneth A. Freedberg[1,5,8], for the CEPAC-International Investigators

1 Division of Infectious Diseases, Massachusetts General Hospital, Boston, Massachusetts, United States of America, **2** INSERM U897 Africa Team, Institut de Santé Publique, d'Epidémiologie et de Développement (ISPED), Université Victor Segalen Bordeaux 2, Bordeaux, France, **3** Pan American Health Organization, HIV/AIDS Unit, Washington, D.C., United States of America, **4** Elizabeth Glaser Pediatric AIDS Foundation: Zimbabwe Country Office, Harare, Zimbabwe, **5** Division of General Medicine, Massachusetts General Hospital, Boston, Massachusetts, United States of America, **6** Organization of Public Health Interventions and Development (OPHID) Trust, Harare, Zimbabwe, **7** Division of Infectious Disease, Brigham and Women's Hospital, Boston, Massachusetts, United States of America, **8** Center for AIDS Research, Harvard Medical School, Boston, Massachusetts, United States of America, **9** Ministry of Health and Child Welfare, Harare, Zimbabwe

Abstract

Background: The Zimbabwean national prevention of mother-to-child HIV transmission (PMTCT) program provided primarily single-dose nevirapine (sdNVP) from 2002–2009 and is currently replacing sdNVP with more effective antiretroviral (ARV) regimens.

Methods: Published HIV and PMTCT models, with local trial and programmatic data, were used to simulate a cohort of HIV-infected, pregnant/breastfeeding women in Zimbabwe (mean age 24.0 years, mean CD4 451 cells/μL). We compared five PMTCT regimens at a fixed level of PMTCT medication uptake: 1) no **antenatal** ARVs (comparator); 2) sdNVP; 3) WHO 2010 guidelines using "Option A" (zidovudine during pregnancy/infant NVP during breastfeeding for women without advanced HIV disease; lifelong 3-drug antiretroviral therapy (ART) for women with advanced disease); 4) WHO "Option B" (ART during pregnancy/breastfeeding without advanced disease; lifelong ART with advanced disease); and 5) "Option B+:" lifelong ART for all pregnant/breastfeeding, HIV-infected women. Pediatric (4–6 week and 18-month infection risk, 2-year survival) and maternal (2- and 5-year survival, life expectancy from delivery) outcomes were projected.

Results: Eighteen-month pediatric infection risks ranged from 25.8% (no **antenatal** ARVs) to 10.9% (Options B/B+). Although maternal short-term outcomes (2- and 5-year survival) varied only slightly by regimen, maternal life expectancy was reduced after receipt of sdNVP (13.8 years) or Option B (13.9 years) compared to **no antenatal ARVs (14.0 years)**, Option A (14.0 years), or Option B+ (14.5 years).

Conclusions: Replacement of sdNVP with currently recommended regimens for PMTCT (WHO Options A, B, or B+) is necessary to reduce infant HIV infection risk in Zimbabwe. The planned transition to Option A may also improve both pediatric and maternal outcomes.

Editor: Landon Myer, University of Cape Town, South Africa

Funding: Funding for this work was provided by the Elizabeth Glaser Pediatric AIDS Foundation (all authors) and the National Institute of Allergy and Infectious Disease (K01 AI078754 (ALC), K24 AI062476 (KAF), and R01 AI058736 (KAF, RPW, RW, JC)). The funders had no role in study design, data collection and analysis, decision to publish, or preparation of the manuscript.

Competing Interests: The authors have declared that no competing interests exist.

* E-mail: aciaranello@partners.org

Introduction

Antiretroviral drugs (ARVs) are highly effective for the prevention of mother-to-child HIV transmission (PMTCT). Without ARV prophylaxis, the risk of transmission by 18 months of age ranges from 25–40% in breastfeeding populations [1–3]. However, recent trials have demonstrated that several ARV regimens, administered to mothers and/or infants during pregnancy and breastfeeding, can reduce transmission to 1–8% at 6–12 months of age [4–10]. The World Health Organization (WHO) now recommends three-drug antiretroviral therapy (ART) for all pregnant women with CD4 cells <350/μL or clinical Stage 3–4 disease. For those with less advanced disease, two options are recommended. "Option A" includes short-course zidovudine during pregnancy and extended infant nevirapine (NVP) prophylaxis throughout breastfeeding. "Option B" includes maternal 3-drug ART during pregnancy and breastfeeding, with cessation after weaning [11]. Select PMTCT programs in sub-Saharan Africa are implementing Option B, and an "Option B+" has also been proposed (lifelong ART for all pregnant, HIV-infected women, regardless of CD4 cell count or disease stage) [12]. However, most programs in sub-Saharan Africa plan to implement the WHO 2010 guidelines by selecting Option A [12].

In 2009, only 53% of pregnant women identified as HIV-infected worldwide received any ARVs for PMTCT, resulting in approximately 370,000 new infant infections [13]. Many of these women received the ARV regimens previously recommended as a "minimum" intervention by WHO: a single dose of nevirapine (sdNVP) to a pregnant woman in labor and her infant after birth [13,14]. Although inexpensive and relatively easy to administer, sdNVP is less effective than currently recommended regimens (18-month transmission risks: 15–25%) [15–17] and can lead to drug-resistant virus that complicates later therapy for both mothers and infected infants [18,19].

Zimbabwe is a low-income country where prolonged breastfeeding is the norm [20,21]. The Zimbabwean Ministry of Health and Child Welfare (MOHCW) has provided sdNVP through the national PMTCT program since 2002, as one of the earliest PMTCT programs in Africa [22]. In 2006–2007, the MOHCW, with the Elizabeth Glaser Pediatric AIDS Foundation and the Organization of Public Health Interventions and Development Trust, demonstrated the feasibility of a pilot program providing the antenatal/intrapartum component of the WHO Option A regimen [23]. Our objective was to use simulation modeling to evaluate the potential benefits to both infants and mothers of replacing sdNVP with WHO 2010-recommended regimens on a national scale in Zimbabwe.

Methods

Analytic overview

We linked two published computer simulation models to project clinical outcomes of five PMTCT strategies in Zimbabwe. First, a model of mother-to-child transmission (MTCT) during pregnancy and delivery [24] was modified to incorporate each step of the "cascade" of PMTCT-related care, from first presentation at antenatal care (ANC) through 18 months postpartum (Figure 1). Second, the Cost-effectiveness of Preventing AIDS Complications (CEPAC)-International model of adult HIV infection [25,26] was used to project clinical outcomes for women following pregnancy, and was expanded to simulate infant outcomes from birth through the first two years of life. The models were linked by using CEPAC results as MTCT model inputs (Text S1). Outcomes of the linked models included risk of infant HIV infection at 4–6 weeks and 18 months of age and 2-year pediatric survival, as well as maternal 2-year survival, maternal 5-year survival, and maternal life expectancy after delivery. Additional details of model structure, data inputs, sensitivity analyses, and results are presented in the Appendix (Text S1).

Population and PMTCT strategies evaluated

We simulated a population of pregnant and breastfeeding women in Zimbabwe who were HIV-infected at the time of conception [27]. For women identified as HIV-infected during ANC, five PMTCT strategies were evaluated (Text S1): 1) A "no antenatal ARVs" strategy, for reference comparison; 2) a single-dose of nevirapine (sdNVP) administered to laboring mothers and infants within 3 days of birth, reflecting the 2002–2009 national Zimbabwe PMTCT program and 2006 WHO "minimum" guidelines for resource-constrained settings [14]; 3) WHO 2010 "Option A:" short-course zidovudine during pregnancy and extended infant nevirapine during breastfeeding for women with CD4 >350/μL and no evidence of WHO stage 3–4 disease, with lifelong ART for women with advanced disease [11]; 4) WHO 2010 "Option B:" ART through pregnancy and breastfeeding regardless of CD4 or disease stage, with continuation after weaning for women with advanced disease [11]; and 5) the "Option B+" under consideration in select locations: lifelong ART for all pregnant, HIV-infected women, for comparison [12,28]. ART-eligible women who linked to HIV-related healthcare after delivery were assumed to receive ART for their own health in all strategies (Text S1). Mothers were assumed to breastfeed their infants for a median duration of 18 months, based on Zimbabwean data [21]. Throughout the manuscript, the term "ARV" refers to any single or dual antiretroviral drug regimen used for PMTCT, while "ART" refers only to three-drug combination therapy (regardless if used for PMTCT or for therapy of maternal disease).

Model structure

MTCT model. The MTCT model is a previously-published decision-analytic simulation of a cohort of pregnant women from conception through delivery [24] (TreeAgePro 2010 software, Williamstown, MA). The model structure was expanded to include key steps in antenatal care, as well as linkage to postnatal maternal and pediatric care (Figure 1 and Text S1). Probabilities of HIV transmission and maternal and infant death before and during delivery were stratified by the severity of maternal HIV infection (ART "eligible," defined as WHO stage 3–4 disease or CD4 350/<μL [11]; "not eligible;" or deceased) and by maternal receipt of postnatal HIV care and ART.

CEPAC adult model. The CEPAC-International model is a first-order Monte Carlo simulation of HIV infection, in which patients are simulated individually from model entry through death. Details of model structure and validation have been published previously [25,26,29] and are further described in the Appendix (Text S1). In brief, disease progression is characterized by a sequence of monthly transitions between health states; these include acute opportunistic and other infections prevalent in

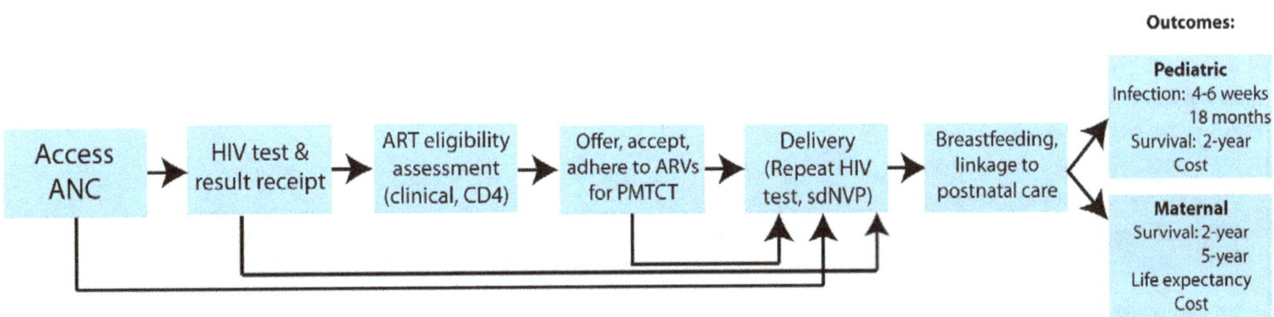

Figure 1. "Cascade" of PMTCT and postnatal HIV care. Opportunities to maximize the effectiveness of PMTCT interventions may be lost at each step in the pathway. ANC: antenatal care, ARVs: antiretroviral drugs, ART: antiretroviral therapy, sdNVP: single-dose nevirapine.

southern Africa, chronic HIV infection, and death. The model records all clinical events during each patient's lifetime. A cohort of ten million women is simulated to produce stable estimates of outcomes (Text S1).

In the CEPAC adult model, current CD4 count, opportunistic infection prophylaxis, and history or absence of previous opportunistic infections determine the monthly risk of opportunistic infections and HIV-related death (Table 1). HIV RNA suppression with effective ART leads CD4 counts to increase, reducing the risks for opportunistic infections and death. Before initiation of ART or after virologic failure on ART, CD4 counts decline at a rate determined by current RNA level; this is accompanied by increased risks of opportunistic infections and death. After planned interruption of suppressive ART at the time of weaning (Option B only), CD4 counts decline more rapidly based on data from ART interruption and PMTCT trials [30–32].

CEPAC infant model. A first-order, Monte Carlo simulation model of infant HIV infection and survival was added to the CEPAC model. Modeled infants enter the postnatal model at birth. Based on events occurring before and during delivery in the MTCT model, infants are assigned one of three HIV categories (HIV-unexposed; HIV-exposed but uninfected; or HIV-infected) and three maternal disease categories (HIV-uninfected; HIV-infected and "ART eligible;" or HIV-infected and "ART non-eligible"). Over a two-year horizon, infants face a monthly probability of four key clinical events: 1) maternal HIV infection, if mother was previously uninfected, causing infants to transition from "unexposed" to "exposed-uninfected;" 2) maternal death, with risks derived from

Table 1. Selected model input parameters for a simulation model of strategies to prevent mother-to-child transmission of HIV in Zimbabwe: Maternal data.

Variable	Base Case Value	Range for sensitivity analyses	Data sources
Baseline maternal cohort characteristics			
Age (mean (SD), in years)	24.0 (5)	20–30	MOHCW [27]
HIV prevalence	16%		MOCHW [27]
HIV incidence	0.96%/year		MOHCW [39]
Mortality during pregnancy	0.7%	0–2%	MOHCW [27]
Live birth	95.7–98%	95–99%	MOHCW [27]
Among HIV-infected women at first ANC visit:			
CD4 count (mean (SD), cells/μL)	451 (50)		ZVITAMBO trial [21] (SD: assumption)
ART eligible	275 (50)		ZVITAMBO trial [21]
Not ART eligible	550 (50)		ZVITAMBO trial [21]
Incident infection in pregnancy	664 (50)		MACS [40]
Initial HIV RNA (mean copies/ml)	72,349		CTAC [41]
Access to PMTCT "cascade"			
Access to ANC	91%	80–100%	MOHCW [27]
HIV testing in ANC	87%	58–95%	MOHCW [23,39]
Receipt of HIV test result in ANC	99%	71–99%	MOHCW [23,39]
Sensitivity of clinical assessment of ART eligibility	36%	20–50%	MTCT-Plus Cohort [43]
Receipt of CD4 test result (Option A)	67%		[79]
Delivery in health care facility	69%	50–100%	MOHCW [23,39]
If HIV status negative/unknown, test in labor	36%		MOHCW [23]
If HIV diagnosed in labor, receive sdNVP	80%		MOHCW [23]
Postnatal HIV Care			
Linkage to postnatal maternal care by 6 weeks postpartum	79%	51–100%	Average and range: [36,44–48]
Loss to follow-up from postnatal maternal care	16% (year 1); 6%/year (years 2+)		[37,80,81]
Maternal antiretroviral therapy			
Efficacy (% HIV RNA suppression at 24 weeks)			
1st-line NVP/ZDV/3TC initiated in pregnancy	90%		[50]
1st-line NVP/d4T/3TC initiated post-partum			
With sdNVP exposure	85%	Difference between sdNVP exposed and unexposed: 0%–16%	OCTANE trial [49] Difference: [18,69,71]
Without sdNVP exposure**	90%		Difference assumed = 5% [50]
2nd-line LPV/r/TDF/FTC	72%		[82]
CD4 decline (6 months after ART interruption)	139 cells	75–139 cells/μL	[30–32]

the adult CEPAC model as described above, after which infants are no longer at risk for HIV infection but are at higher risk of death due to orphanhood [33,34]; **3)** infant HIV infection through breastfeeding, if infant was previously uninfected; and **4)** infant death from any cause. Risks of maternal death and of postnatal HIV transmission are stratified by maternal disease stage and ARV regimen, and risks of infant death are stratified by infant HIV exposure/infection status and receipt of ART if infected.

HIV/AIDS care and ART. For HIV-infected infants, a one-time probability of HIV diagnosis, linkage to HIV care, and ART initiation was modeled [13]. For mothers, care and ART were modeled in greater detail. A one-time probability of linkage to maternal HIV care was incorporated; this parameter reflects the probability that a post-partum mother will present to an HIV clinic for her own healthcare by six weeks postpartum. Women not linking to care within this period were assumed to present to HIV care upon later development of a severe opportunistic infection. Once in postnatal care for her own health, ART eligibility was assumed to be assessed through both CD4 testing and clinical evaluation. For women identified as ART-eligible, both ART and trimethoprim/sulfamethoxazole prophylaxis were initiated [13,35]. For women identified as not yet ART-eligible in postnatal HIV care, medications were administered depending on the modeled breastfeeding prophylaxis regimen: no medications were dispensed for the "no antenatal ARVs" and "sdNVP" regimens; infant nevirapine syrup was dispensed for the "Option A" regimen; and maternal ART was dispensed for the "Option B" and "Option B+" regimens. Specific components of 3-drug ART regimens were simulated to reflect 2009 Zimbabwean guidelines and common current practice in Zimbabwe (Text S1 and Table 1) [35]. ART monitoring and switching strategies are also detailed in the Appendix (Text S1).

Loss to follow-up. During modeled ANC, women could be lost to follow-up (LTFU) at any stage between first presentation (booking) and delivery; if LTFU, no antenatal ARVs were received, but the opportunity to access HIV testing and sdNVP in labor remained. Women could also be LTFU between delivery and six weeks postpartum [36], or after linkage to postnatal HIV care [37,38]. In the absence of specific maternal or pediatric data regarding monthly risks of LTFU and cessation of prophylactic ARVs during breastfeeding, the impact of such events was incorporated in sensitivity analyses via the highest published postnatal transmission estimates for Options A, B and B+. For HIV-infected infants, the impacts of loss to follow-up after established pediatric HIV care were included in cohort-based pediatric survival estimates.

Model input parameters

Maternal cohort characteristics and natural history. Baseline maternal characteristics reflected cohorts of pregnant women in Zimbabwe (Table 1 and Text S1). At first ANC visit, mean age was 24.0 [27] and HIV prevalence was 16% [39]; HIV incidence during pregnancy and breastfeeding was 0.96%/year [39]. Among HIV-infected women, mean CD4 was 275 cells/μL if ART-eligible [21], 550 cells/μL if not ART-eligible [21], and 664 cells/μL if incidently infected during pregnancy [40]. Because detailed clinical data to inform HIV disease progression in the absence of ART were not available from Zimbabwe, these natural history model inputs to the CEPAC model were derived from a clinical cohort in South Africa (Text S1) [41]. For women remaining HIV-negative, life expectancy was projected using UNAIDS cause-deleted mortality rates [42].

Maternal access to care and ART. Modeled rates of access to ANC, HIV and CD4 tests in ANC, ARV drugs for PMTCT, and postnatal care reflected Zimbabwean national estimates whenever available (Table 1). In the sdNVP strategy, women were modeled to undergo clinical ART-eligibility assessment, but not CD4 testing, and to initiate lifelong ART if WHO stage 3–4 disease was identified [11]. The sensitivity of clinical assessment for ART eligibility was 36% [43]. In the base case analysis, to isolate the benefits of each regimen, ARV medications were assumed to be available for, accepted by, and adhered to by all women diagnosed as HIV-infected in ANC, and CD4 testing (but not result return) was assumed for all women under Option A. In addition, sdNVP was modeled to be provided to 80% of women newly HIV-diagnosed in labor [23,39].

The base-case rate of linkage to postnatal maternal HIV care reflected the median of published values; in sensitivity analyses, linkage rates ranged from 51–100%, depending on antenatal care and PMTCT regimen received [36,44–48]. For women in HIV care and receiving ART, the 24-week "efficacy" of first-line, NNRTI-based maternal ART in suppressing HIV RNA to <400 copies/ml was 85% for women with previous sdNVP exposure [49] and 90% (assumed difference of 5%) for women without exposure to sdNVP [50]. In the six months following ART interruption at weaning (Option B), CD4 count was modeled to decline by 139 cells [30,31]. Other modeled ART effects are described in Table 1.

Mother-to-child transmission risks. Mother-to-child HIV transmission risks were derived from randomized clinical trials in several African settings (Table 2) [1,4,5,8–10,15,17,21,51–61]. MTCT risks during the intrauterine and intrapartum period (by 4–6 weeks of age) and postpartum period (6 weeks-18 months) were stratified by maternal HIV stage and by PMTCT regimen received. Postpartum transmission risks were additionally stratified by whether breastfeeding during the first six months of life was exclusive (EBF) or mixed (MBF, including any non-breastmilk liquid or solid) [62].

Pediatric outcomes. Mortality estimates for HIV-unexposed children were derived from UNAIDS HIV-deleted mortality estimates [42] and mortality rates for exposed-uninfected infants were from the ZVITAMBO study in Zimbabwe [63] (Table 2). Mortality rates for untreated HIV-infected children, stratified by timing of HIV infection, were derived from a patient-level analysis of 1,930 children from 12 African PMTCT trials, after removing non-HIV-related causes of death [6]. ART was assumed available for 36% of HIV-infected children [64]. Mortality rates for children treated with ART were from a systematic review of pediatric ART in Africa [65] and a pooled patient-level analysis from 16 African cohorts [66]. For infants of any HIV infection or exposure status, maternal death was assumed to increase mortality 2-fold [33].

Model validation and sensitivity analyses

Model results were validated by comparison to published values (Text S1). Sensitivity analyses, described in detail in the Appendix (Text S1), examined the impact of variations in key maternal clinical and demographic characteristics, highest and lowest published MTCT risks for each regimen, access to ANC and HIV testing in ANC, linkage to postnatal HIV care, ART efficacy and survival following sdNVP exposure, CD4 cell decline following ART interruption, and pediatric and maternal non-HIV-related mortality rates. Parameters leading to substantial changes in model results were identified; a substantial change was defined as 1) a change in the relative order of the outcomes of the PMTCT regimens, or 2) a >10% relative change in the difference between projected outcomes for each ARV regimen (example provided in Text S1). In addition, we projected the impact of each PMTCT regimen on infant infection risk for an annual cohort of women becoming pregnant in Zimbabwe, including both HIV-infected and HIV-uninfected women at conception (Text S1).

Table 2. Selected model input parameters for a simulation model of strategies to prevent mother-to-child transmission of HIV in Zimbabwe: Pediatric data.

II. Mother-to-child transmission risks

Maternal HIV status	Base Case Value (Range for sensitivity analysis) PMTCT regimen received			
Intrauterine/intrapartum period (one-time risks)	**No antenatal ARVs**	**sdNVP***	**scZDV**	**ART**
Mother ART eligible at conception	0.273 [52,83] (0.199–0.322) [54,83,84]	0.176 [21,85] (0.082–0.264) [15,17,86]	0.136 [5] (0.091–0.157) [87,88]	0.033 [89] (0.011–0.041) [10,58]
Mother not ART-eligible at conception	0.175 [52,83] (0.127–0.206) [54,83,84]	0.073 [21,85] (0.033–0.109) [15,17,86]	0.036 [5] (0.024–0.041) [8,88]	0.01 [10] (0.004–0.028) [4,10]
Mother with incident infection during pregnancy	0.30 (assumption)	0.20 (assumption)	0.16 (assumption)	0.033 (assumed = eligible)

Postnatal period (monthly risks, among infants HIV-uninfected at 4–6 weeks of age)	**No postnatal ARVs**	**Maternal ART**	**Extended infant NVP**
Mother ART eligible at conception	0.00758 (EBF) [21,85]; 0.01278 (MBF) [21,85]; (0.00476–0.02336) [53,84]	0.00333[87] (0–0.00534) [4,8,10]	n/a
Mother not ART-eligible at conception	0.00238 (EBF) [85]; 0.00401 (MBF) [21] (0.00149–0.00732) [53,60]	0.00189 (average: [10,46,56,57]) (0–0.00534) [9,10]	0.00221 [9,61] (0.00120–0.00311) [9,61]
Mother with incident infection during pregnancy	0.00758 (EBF) [85]; 0.01278 (MBF) [21,85]; (0.00476–0.02336) [53,84]	n/a	n/a

III. Pediatric inputs

Variable	Base Case Value	Range for sensitivity analyses	Data sources
Postnatal HIV Care			
Probability of linking to pediatric HIV diagnosis, care, and ART	36%	0–100%	WHO [64]

Mortality risks	One-year risk (%)	Two-year cumulative risk (%)	
HIV-unexposed children	5.4	5.9	[42]
HIV-exposed, uninfected children	7.4	9.2	[63]
HIV-infected children, no ART			
Intrauterine/intrapartum infection	51.0	65.0	[6]
Postpartum infection	24.0	38.0	[6]
HIV-infected children, on ART	9.5	12.0	[65,90]
Relative increase in infant mortality if maternal death occurs before 18 m	2-fold increase (range: 1–6-fold increase)		[33,34]

SD: Standard deviation; MOHCW: Zimbabwe Ministry of Health and Child Welfare; MACS: Multicenter AIDS Cohort Study; CTAC: Cape Town AIDS Cohort; ANC: antenatal care; ART: 3-drug, combination antiretroviral therapy; (sd)NVP: (single-dose) nevirapine; scZDV: short-course zidovudine; WHO: World Health Organization; ZDV: zidovudine; 3TC: lamivudine; d4T: stavudine; LPV/r: lopinavir/ritonavir; TDF: tenofovir; FTC: emtricabine; EBF/MBF: exclusive/mixed breastfeeding.

*"Without sdNVP exposure" refers to situations in which sdNVP was not received, or was received in combination with short-course zidovudine or other antenatal/intrapartum medications which may decrease risk of NVP-associated NNRTI-resistant HIV [19].

Role of the funders and ethics approval

The funders had no role in study design, data collection and analysis, decision to publish, or preparation of the manuscript. This analysis was deemed "not human subjects research" by the Partners Healthcare IRB, and was approved as an exempt analysis.

Results

Base-case analyses (fixed levels of ARV uptake for PMTCT)

Pediatric outcomes. Among women HIV-infected at first ANC visit, the risks of infant infection at 4–6 weeks of age were projected to be 20.1% with no **antenatal** ARV prophylaxis, 10.8% with the 2002–2009 sdNVP-based national program, 7.2% with Option A, and 5.4% with Option B and B+ (Table 3, top). At 18 months of age, cumulative risk of infant HIV infection ranged from 25.8% (no antenatal ARVs) to 10.9% (Option B/B+). Two-year pediatric survival similarly ranged from 78.4% (no antenatal ARVs) to 84.9% (Option B/B+).

Maternal outcomes. Postpartum survival among HIV-infected women was projected to range from 92.4% (no antenatal ARVs, sdNVP) to 94.0% (Option B+) at two years, and 79.8% (no antenatal ARVs, sdNVP) to 82.2% (Option B+) at

Table 3. Outcomes of strategies to prevent mother-to-child HIV transmission in Zimbabwe: Base-case model results.

	Model results		
Pediatric outcomes (Infants born to women who are HIV-infected at conception)			
	Risk of HIV infection at 4–6 weeks of age (%)	**Risk of HIV infection at 18 months of age (%)**	**2-year survival (%)**
No **antenatal** ARVs*	20.1	25.8	78.4
Single-dose NVP	10.8	17.2	81.9
Option A	7.2	12.8	83.5
Option B	5.4	10.9	84.9
Option B+	5.4	10.9	84.9
Maternal outcomes after delivery (women who are HIV-infected at conception)			
	2-year survival (%)	**5-year survival (%)**	**Life expectancy (years)**
No **antenatal** ARVs*	92.4	79.8	**14.0**
Single-dose NVP	92.4	79.8	**13.8**
Option A	92.5	79.9	**14.0**
Option B	93.7	80.0	**13.9**
Option B+	94.0	82.2	**14.5**

*"No antenatal ARVs" refers to the receipt of no medications for HIV therapy or for prevention of mother-to-child transmission during the antenatal period. Women who link to postnatal HIV care are assumed to start ART after delivery if CD4 cell count is ≤350/μL or following development of a severe opportunistic infection.

five years after delivery (Table 3, bottom). The impacts of sdNVP-associated resistance and ART interruption manifested primarily after five years postpartum: projected life expectancy was slightly lower following sdNVP (13.9 years) or Option B (13.9 years) than following receipt of no antenatal ARVs or Option A (14.0 years). Projected maternal life expectancy was greatest (14.4 years) with lifelong universal ART (Option B+).

Sensitivity analyses

Sensitivity analyses were performed on all key model input parameters and assumptions (Figures 2 and 3, Text S1). The model input parameters with the greatest influence on pediatric and maternal outcomes are shown in Figure 2 (Figure 2a: 18-month infant infection risk; Figure 2b: maternal life expectancy). Improvements in HIV testing during pregnancy (2a and 2b: scenario 2), linkage to postnatal care (2a and 2b: scenario 3), and reduction in the proportion of women with CD4<350 (2a and 2b: scenario 4) as might result through universal HIV screening acceptance and early ART initiation prior to pregnancy) led to the greatest improvements in both maternal and pediatric outcomes. Lowest published MTCT risks for each regimen (2a: scenario 5) did not change the relative order of the infant outcomes of the PMTCT regimens, but markedly reduced overall transmission risks; lowest projected 18-month infection risks ranged from 8.1% (sdNVP) to 4.5% (Option B/B+).

In the base case (Table 3), maternal life expectancy was slightly shorter following receipt of sdNVP (13.8 years) than if no antenatal ARVs were received for PMTCT (14.0 years). The maternal survival and life expectancy differences between no antenatal ARVs and sdNVP also depended on the degree to which sdNVP exposure was assumed to reduce subsequent 1st-line ART efficacy; at 0% difference, the regimens led to equal maternal outcomes (Appendix); at 16% difference, maternal outcomes associated with each strategy differed substantially (Figure 2b, scenario 5). Base-case maternal life expectancy was also shorter following receipt of Option B than if no antenatal ARVs were received (Table 3). This result did not change when a wide range of reported rates of CD4 decline after ART interruption were incorporated (Appendix) [30–32].

Figure 3 depicts the impact of linkage to postnatal HIV care on maternal life expectancy. In the base case, rates of linkage to postnatal care were assumed to be equal following receipt of any PMTCT regimen. As noted above, resulting maternal life expectancies were slightly lower following the sdNVP and Option B regimens than if no antenatal ARVs were received for PMTCT. However, if the receipt of sdNVP or Option B improved rates of linkage to postnatal care even slightly, compared to ANC without receipt of antenatal ARVs for PMTCT (2.8% increase in linkage for Option B, 3.8% increase for sdNVP), the negative impact of these regimens on life expectancy was overcome.

All other parameters varied in sensitivity analyses are detailed in the Appendix (Text S1). Notably, policy conclusions were insensitive to variations in maternal age, risk of maternal mortality due to pregnancy, probability of live infant birth, delivery location, impact of sdNVP exposure on short-term infant outcomes, and relative risk of infant mortality following maternal death.

Discussion

We linked two validated computer simulation models to project clinical outcomes of improved PMTCT regimens in Zimbabwe. These analyses simultaneously evaluate pediatric and maternal outcomes, a novel approach for model-based investigations of HIV care [67,68], and are likely applicable to other sub-Saharan Africa settings where prolonged breastfeeding is common. Altogether, pediatric outcomes, including HIV infection risk and survival, would be markedly improved by replacing sdNVP-based programs with 2010 WHO guideline-concordant regimens at fixed levels of ARV uptake for PMTCT. However, it is worth noting that the largest improvements in both pediatric and maternal survival may result from a PMTCT program that offers lifelong ART to all pregnant, HIV-infected women regardless of CD4 count or

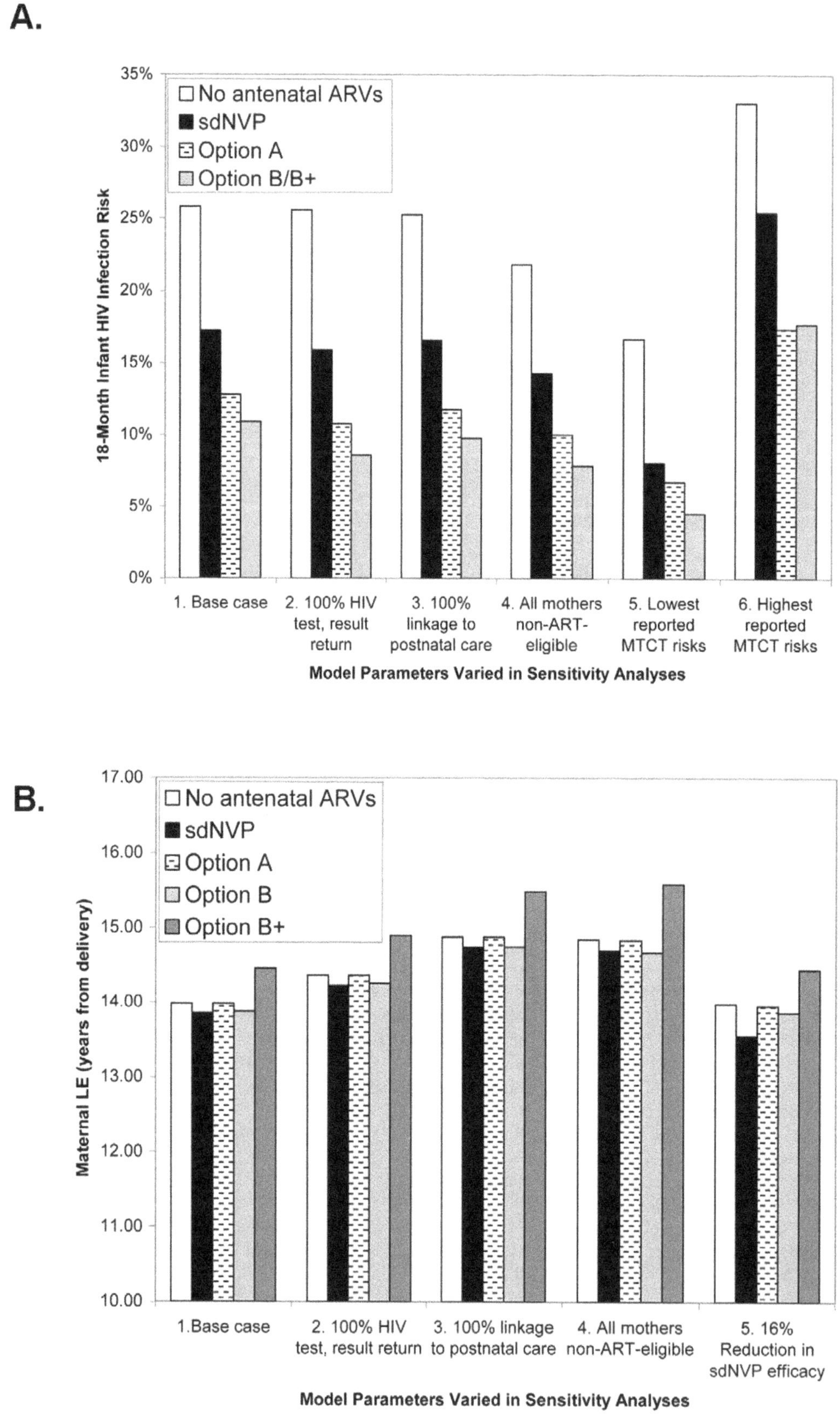

Figure 2. Key sensitivity analyses, identifying selected parameters producing substantial changes in model results. As detailed in the Methods section and Appendix (Text S1), a substantial change in results was defined as: 1) a change in the relative order of the outcomes of the PMTCT regimens, or 2) a >10% relative change in the difference between projected outcomes for each regimen. Panel 2a depicts parameters influencing 18-month mother-to-child HIV transmission risk, and Panel 2b depicts parameters influencing maternal life expectancy from delivery;

these outcomes are shown on the vertical axes. Along the horizontal axes, each group of vertical bars represents a single scenario (numbered 1–6 in 2a and 1–5 in 2b), and each vertical bar represents a PMTCT regimen, as indicated.

disease stage (Option B+), as is currently being investigated [28] and already being considered for implementation in Malawi [12].

The choice of ARV regimen for PMTCT may have important effects on maternal health, important not only in its own right, but also for its impact on pediatric survival [33,34]. First, this analysis underscores the potential long-term impact of sdNVP exposure. The modeled impacts of ARV regimens that are received only briefly during pregnancy or breastfeeding are small in comparison to the impact of lifelong ART for women who link to postnatal HIV care. Nonetheless, the sdNVP-associated life expectancy reduction of **0.1** years is comparable in magnitude to the modeled benefit of trimethoprim/sulfamethoxazole prophylaxis [25]. This life expectancy reduction results from reduced virologic suppression on NNRTI-based ART due to sdNVP-associated NNRTI-resistant virus. The difference in suppression among women with and without sdNVP exposure determines the degree to which sdNVP-based programs create a tradeoff between improved pediatric outcomes and reduced maternal life expectancy. The impact of sdNVP exposure may be negligible if sdNVP is received >12–24 months prior to ART initiation [49,69–71]; in such cases, scale-up of sdNVP-based PMTCT services will improve both maternal and pediatric outcomes. However, absolute reductions in 24-week virologic suppression rates of 16–42% and 12–14% have been reported for women initiating ART <6 months and 6–12 months after sdNVP exposure, respectively [18,49,69] (base-case value for this analysis: 5%). Because protease inhibitor-based first-line ART is not widely available in many settings, the current analysis lends strong support to efforts to expand non-sdNVP-based PMTCT programs to improve both maternal and child health.

In addition to the impact of sdNVP exposure, the ART initiation and discontinuation strategies required by Option B may also impact maternal health. Because ART is recommended for all pregnant, HIV-infected in women in Option B, there may be a health benefit from initiating ART at higher CD4 counts than would prompt therapy in non-pregnant patients. However, it is not yet known whether the adverse effects of ART discontinuation after weaning will outweigh these benefits. When ART is interrupted in men and non-postpartum women, marked increases in viral load, inflammatory markers, and risk for both AIDS- and non-AIDS-related events have been reported [30,72]. The current analysis models rapid CD4 declines, ranging from 75–139 cells/µL, in the 6 months following ART interruption at weaning in Option B [30,32,72]; this results in a decrease in maternal life expectancy of 0.6 years for women who interrupt ART at weaning (then resume when later required for their own health), compared

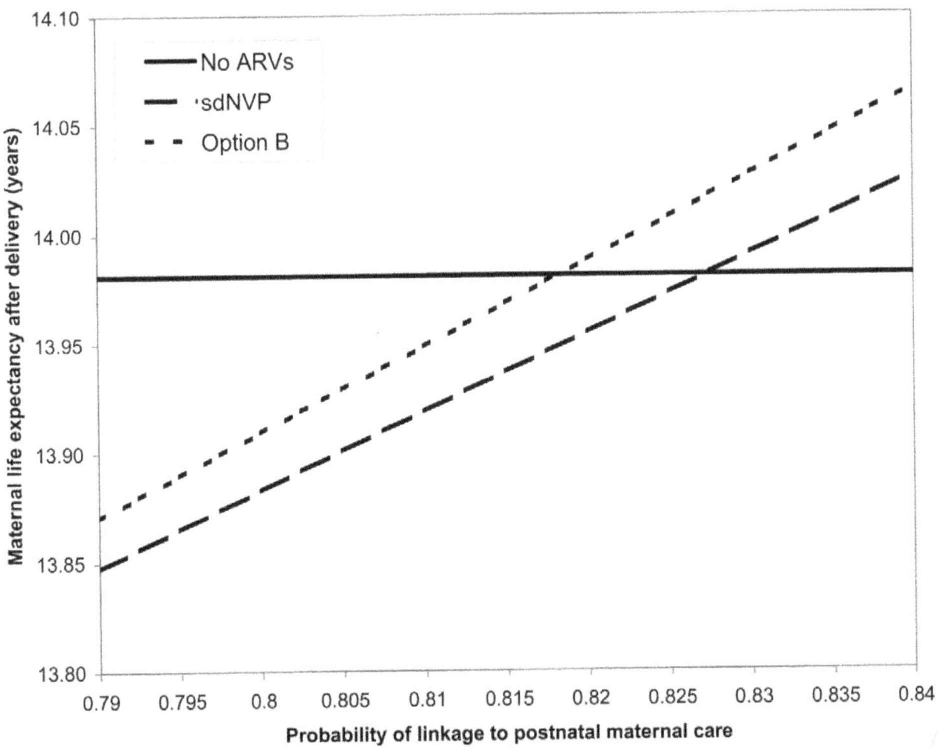

Figure 3. Sensitivity analysis demonstrating the impact on maternal life expectancy of rates of linkage to postnatal HIV care. The vertical axis represents maternal life expectancy, in years from delivery. The horizontal axis depicts the probability of linkage to postnatal HIV care for women who receive the PMTCT regimens shown. This probability of linkage to care is varied from 79% (the base case value) to 85%. In the base case, maternal life expectancy following the sdNVP and Option B regimens is lower than if no antenatal ARVs were received for PMTCT (triangles). This occurs as a result of modeled negative impacts of sdNVP-associated resistance (sdNVP regimen) and ART interruption (Option B regimen). When the probability of linkage to care following Option B is ≥81.8%, as indicated by the open arrow (2.8% more than if no antenatal ARVs are received), the negative impact of ART interruption is overcome. Similarly, when the probability of linkage to care following sdNVP is ≥82.8%, as indicated by the solid arrow (3.8% more than if no ARVs are received), the negative impact of sdNVP-associated resistance is overcome.

to women who continue ART. In the absence of randomized data from postpartum women, we do not specifically simulate additional increased rates of non-AIDS-related events due to interruption; if additional non-AIDS-related risks exist, the negative impact of Option B will be greater than shown here. Data on AIDS- and non-AIDS-related events among postpartum women continuing or interrupting ART are anticipated in the next several years [28], and will more accurately inform the risks and benefits of Option B versus Option B+.

These analyses also highlight that linkage to postnatal maternal HIV care, and thus initiation of ART when needed, is the step in the PMTCT "cascade" that most dramatically influences maternal life expectancy. The impact of improved linkage to care on maternal life expectancy is greater than that of improved access to ANC or HIV testing (holding linkage rates constant for those in care and diagnosed), or any specific PMTCT regimen during pregnancy. Because published rates of linkage to postnatal care range widely and are rarely stratified by PMTCT regimen received [46,47], model-based analyses can highlight areas for future research. For example, if women who receive sdNVP- or Option B-based PMTCT interventions are even slightly more likely to register in postnatal HIV care than are women who receive ANC but no medications for PMTCT (3–4% absolute increases in linkage rates), the life expectancy benefits of this improvement in linkage outweigh the negative effects of sdNVP-associated resistance and ART interruption. However, if receipt of these regimens does not improve linkage to postnatal care compared to ANC services alone, there may be an important tradeoff between long-term maternal and pediatric health with expansion of sdNVP- or Option B- based programs.

Although linkage to postnatal care was the access-to-care parameter with the greatest individual influence on maternal life expectancy, improved uptake at each step in a "cascade" of PMTCT care (including access to ANC, HIV testing and result receipt, and availability and acceptance of ARVs [73]; Figure 1) confers substantial benefits for both infant and maternal health. In fact, improvements in two dimensions are critical: both replacement of sdNVP with more effective regimens and improved uptake of any given PMTCT regimen. While the current analysis addresses the first dimension in greatest detail, further analyses examining the clinical impacts, costs, and cost-effectiveness of interventions to improve uptake are also needed.

This analysis has two main limitations. First, when detailed clinical data to inform modeled maternal and pediatric HIV disease progression were not available from Zimbabwe, data from surrounding southern African countries were used instead. Base-case clinical risks for HIV-infected mothers, such as risks of opportunistic infections and tuberculosis, were derived from South Africa, and might reasonably be expected to be similar in neighboring Zimbabwe. Similarly, risks of MTCT, after stratification by maternal CD4, PMTCT regimen received, and breastfeeding duration, might also be anticipated to be similar across Southern African settings. The impacts of non-Zimbabwean data were tested in extensive sensitivity analyses, as detailed in the Appendix (Text S1), and had little impact on model results. Second, life expectancy projections are subject to uncertainty about events occurring over long time horizons, as healthcare systems and HIV therapy may change substantially in the distant future. Because of the uncertainty inherent in long-term projections, we also report similar findings based on the short-term outcomes of MTCT risks, 2-year pediatric survival, and 2-year and 5-year maternal survival.

Model-projected clinical outcomes are not intended to be interpreted in isolation, but rather as one component of a decision-making framework that incorporates many factors, including feasibility, affordability, and equity. Implementation of more effective PMTCT regimens will be resource-intensive; costs will include not only drug costs, but also infrastructure, personnel, and training costs for clinics and laboratories. However, the 2010-recommended PMTCT regimens may also save money in the future by averting not only costly care for pediatric HIV infection [74], but also the costly morbidity and mortality associated with delayed maternal ART initiation [26,75] or sdNVP-associated resistance [29]. Model-based analyses of pediatric outcomes have suggested that ART for PMTCT is very cost-effective in many settings, compared to sdNVP or to no ARVs [76–78]. Additional budgetary impact and cost-effectiveness analyses, comparing Option A to Option B and incorporating short-term and long-term benefits and costs for both mothers and infants, will comprise an important area of future research. In the interim, model-based analyses can assist policymakers to understand the clinical tradeoffs anticipated to result from the replacement of sdNVP with more effective PMTCT regimens.

Conclusions

Replacing sdNVP with currently WHO-recommended PMTCT regimens at a fixed level of ARV uptake for PMTCT will improve both maternal and pediatric health outcomes in Zimbabwe. The best currently available data suggest that continued dependence on sdNVP-based programs would impact positively on pediatric health, but may worsen long-term maternal outcomes, unless also accompanied by expanded access to postnatal HIV care and ART for eligible women. To avoid an untenable tradeoff between maternal and child health, additional resources are needed to implement WHO guideline-concordant PMTCT programs (Options A, B, or possibly B+) in resource-constrained settings, including Zimbabwe.

Acknowledgments

The authors gratefully acknowledge Ji-Eun Park, BS, and Asinath Rusibamayila, BS, for assistance in model development, analyses, and manuscript preparation; Callie Scott, MPH, Jessica Becker, BS, and Rodrigo Cerda, MD, MPH, for assistance with analyses; Adam Stoler, MS and Erin Rhode, MS for computer programming assistance; and Scott Dryden-Peterson, MD, for comments on the analysis.

We are indebted to the entire CEPAC-International team and investigators for their contributions, including Christine Danel, Thérèse N'Dri-Yoman, Eugène Messou, Raoul Moh, Eric Ouattara, Catherine Seyler, and Siaka Touré (Programme PACCI, Abidjan, Côte d'Ivoire); Yazdan Yazdanpanah (Service Universitaire des Maladies Infectieuses et du Voyageur, Centre Hospitalier de Tourcoing, EA 2694, Faculté de Médecine de Lille, and Laboratoire de Recherches Économiques et Sociales, Centre National de la Recherche Scientifique Unité de Recherche Associée 362, Lille, France); Xavier Anglaret, Delphine Gabillard, Hapsatou Touré (INSERM U897, ISPED, Université Bordeaux 2, Bordeaux, France); Nagalingeswaran Kumarasamy and A. K. Ganesh (Y.R. Gaitonde Centre for AIDS Research & Education, Chennai, India); Catherine Orrell and Robin Wood (University of Cape Town, Cape Town, South Africa); Neil Martinson and Lerato Mohapi (Perinatal HIV Research Unit, WITS Health Consortium, Johannesburg, South Africa); Kara Cotich, Sue J. Goldie, April D. Kimmel, Marc Lipsitch, Alethea McCormick, Chara Rydzak, George R. Seage III, and Milton C. Weinstein (Harvard School of Public Health, Boston, MA, USA); C. Robert Horsburgh (Boston University School of Public Health); Heather E. Hsu (Harvard Medical School, Boston, MA, USA); Timothy Flanigan and

Kenneth Mayer (Miriam Hospital, Providence, RI, USA); A. David Paltiel (Yale University, New Haven, CT, USA); Aima Ahonkhai, Jason Andrews, Ingrid V. Bassett, Melissa A. Bender, Julie Levison, Benjamin P. Linas, Elena Losina, Zhigang Lu, Sarah Lorenzana, Bethany Morris, Mai Pho, Lynn Ramirez, Corina Rusu, Callie A. Scott, Caroline Sloan, Alexis Sypek, Lauren Uhler, Bingxia Wang, and Angela Wong (Massachusetts General Hospital, Boston, MA, USA).

We are also indebted to the CEPAC-International Scientific Advisory Board, including Richard Chaisson, Victor De Gruttola, Joseph Eron, R.R. Gangakhedkar, Jonathan Kaplan, Salim Karim, Thérèse N'Dri Yoman, Douglas Owens, and John Wong.

Author Contributions

Model development: ALC FP JC RPW KAF. Development of research question: ALC FP MM BE JK RPW AM RM FD KAF. Conducted modeling analyses: ALC JC. Critical interpretation of model results: ALC FP MM JC BE JK RPW AM RM FD KAF. Contributed secondary data and selected model input parameters: ALC FP MM JC BE JK AM RM FD. Wrote draft: ALC. Critically reviewed and edited all drafts: ALC FP MM JC BE JK RPW AM RM FD KAF.

References

1. Nduati R, John G, Mbori-Ngacha D, Richardson B, Overbaugh J, et al. (2000) Effect of breastfeeding and formula feeding on transmission of HIV-1: a randomized clinical trial. JAMA 283: 1167–1174.
2. Coutsoudis A, Dabis F, Fawzi W, Gaillard P, Haverkamp G, et al. (2004) Late postnatal transmission of HIV-1 in breast-fed children: an individual patient data meta-analysis. J Infect Dis 189: 2154–2166.
3. Leroy V, Sakarovitch C, Cortina-Borja M, McIntyre J, Coovadia H, et al. (2005) Is there a difference in the efficacy of peripartum antiretroviral regimens in reducing mother-to-child transmission of HIV in Africa? AIDS 19: 1865–1875.
4. Thior I, Lockman S, Smeaton LM, Shapiro RL, Wester C, et al. (2006) Breastfeeding plus infant zidovudine prophylaxis for 6 months vs formula feeding plus infant zidovudine for 1 month to reduce mother-to-child HIV transmission in Botswana: a randomized trial: the Mashi Study. JAMA 296: 794–805.
5. Dabis F, Bequet L, Ekouevi DK, Viho I, Rouet F, et al. (2005) Field efficacy of zidovudine, lamivudine and single-dose nevirapine to prevent peripartum HIV transmission. AIDS 19: 309–318.
6. Marston M, Becquet R, Zaba B, Moulton LH, Gray G, et al. (2011) Net survival of perinatally and postnatally HIV-infected children: a pooled analysis of individual data from sub-Saharan Africa. Int J Epidemiol;Epub ahead of press.
7. Marazzi MC, Liotta G, Haswell J, Zimba I, Nielsen-Saines K, et al. TUAC101: Extended use of highly active antiretroviral therapy (HAART) during pregnancy in Southern Africa is highly protective in HIV-1 prevention of mother-to-child-transmission (PMTCT) also in women with higher CD4 cell counts 5th IAS Conference on HIV Pathogenesis, Treatment and Prevention, Cape Town, South Africa, 2009. Available: http://www.ias2009.org/pag/Abstracts.aspx?AID=2013.
8. Kesho Bora Study Group (2011) Triple antiretroviral compared with zidovudine and single-dose nevirapine prophylaxis during pregnancy and breastfeeding for prevention of mother-to-child transmission of HIV-1 (Kesho Bora study): a randomised controlled trial. Lancet Infect Dis. Epub ahead of press.
9. Chasela CS, Hudgens MG, Jamieson DJ, Kayira D, Hosseinipour MC, et al. (2010) Maternal or infant antiretroviral drugs to reduce HIV-1 transmission. N Engl J Med 362: 2271–2281.
10. Shapiro RL, Hughes MD, Ogwu A, Kitch D, Lockman S, et al. (2010) Antiretroviral regimens in pregnancy and breast-feeding in Botswana. N Engl J Med 362: 2282–2294.
11. World Health Organization (2010) Antiretroviral drugs for treating pregnant women and preventing HIV infection in infants: towards universal access. Available: http://whqlibdoc.who.int/publications/2010/9789241599818_eng.pdf. Accessed February 21, 2011.
12. Schouten E, and Department of HIV and AIDS Ministry of Health M. Making it Happen: Revising national policies to reflect changes in WHO recommendations for preventing vertical transmission of HIV –Malawi. International AIDS Society, Vienna, Austria, 2010. Available: http://www.pedaids.org/Press-Room/Events/2010/IAS-2010-WHO-Satellite-Session/5_Making-it-Happen_-Revising-national-policies-to-r.
13. World Health Organization (2010) Towards universal access: Scaling up priority HIV/AIDS interventions in the health sector. Progress Report. Available: http://www.who.int/hiv/pub/2010progressreport/report/en/index.html. Accessed February 21, 2011.
14. World Health Organization (2006) Antiretroviral drugs for treating pregnant women and preventing HIV infections in infants in resource-limited settings: towards universal access - recommendations for a public health approach. Available: http://www.who.int/hiv/pub/guidelines/pmtct/en/index.html. Accessed March 1, 2009.
15. Mofenson L, Taha T, Li Q, Kumwenda J, Kafulafula G, et al. , for the PEPI Malawi Study Group. TUPEC053: Infant extended antiretroviral (ARV) prophylaxis is effective in preventing postnatal mother-to-child HIV transmission (MTCT) at all maternal CD4 counts International AIDS Society, Cape Town, South Africa, 2009. Available: http://www.ias2009.org/pag/Abstracts.aspx?AID = 1251.
16. Kuhn L, Aldrovandi GM, Sinkala M, Kankasa C, Semrau K, et al. (2008) Effects of early, abrupt weaning on HIV-free survival of children in Zambia. N Engl J Med 359: 130–141.
17. Guay LA, Musoke P, Fleming T, Bagenda D, Allen M, et al. (1999) Intrapartum and neonatal single-dose nevirapine compared with zidovudine for prevention of mother-to-child transmission of HIV-1 in Kampala, Uganda: HIVNET 012 randomised trial. Lancet 354: 795–802.
18. Lockman S, Shapiro RL, Smeaton LM, Wester C, Thior I, et al. (2007) Response to antiretroviral therapy after a single, peripartum dose of nevirapine. N Engl J Med 356: 135–147.
19. Arrive E, Newell ML, Ekouevi DK, Chaix ML, Thiebaut R, et al. (2007) Prevalence of resistance to nevirapine in mothers and children after single-dose exposure to prevent vertical transmission of HIV-1: a meta-analysis. Int J Epidemiol 36: 1009–1021.
20. World Bank (2009) Data and statistics: Country classification. Available: http://web.worldbank.org/WBSITE/EXTERNAL/DATASTATISTICS/0, contentMDK:20420458~menuPK:64133156~pagePK:64133150~piPK:64133175~theSitePK:239419,00.html. Accessed February 1, 2010.
21. Iliff PJ, Piwoz EG, Tavengwa NV, Zunguza CD, Marinda ET, et al. (2005) Early exclusive breastfeeding reduces the risk of postnatal HIV-1 transmission and increases HIV-free survival. AIDS 19: 699–708.
22. Perez F, Orne-Gliemann J, Mukotekwa T, Miller A, Glenshaw M, et al. (2004) Prevention of mother to child transmission of HIV: evaluation of a pilot programme in a district hospital in rural Zimbabwe. BMJ 329: 1147–1150.
23. Engelsmann B, Shumba M, Maruva M, Keatinge J, Miller A, Mahomva A, Mbizvo E, Mashumba S, Perez F, Wilfert C, Dabis F. MOPE0521: Enhancing the uptake of antiretroviral drugs for PMTCT through more complex regimens. International AIDS Society, Mexico City, 2008. Available: http://www.aids2008-abstracts.org/aids2008_book_vol1_web.pdf, page 174.
24. Ciaranello AL, Seage GR, 3rd, Freedberg KA, Weinstein MC, Lockman S, et al. (2008) Antiretroviral drugs for preventing mother-to-child transmission of HIV in sub-Saharan Africa: balancing efficacy and infant toxicity. AIDS 22: 2359–2369.
25. Goldie SJ, Yazdanpanah Y, Losina E, Weinstein MC, Anglaret X, et al. (2006) Cost-effectiveness of HIV treatment in resource-poor settings–the case of Côte d'Ivoire. N Engl J Med 355: 1141–1153.
26. Walensky RP, Wolf LL, Wood R, Fofana MO, Freedberg KA, et al. (2009) When to start antiretroviral therapy in resource-limited settings. Ann Intern Med 151: 157–166.
27. Zimbabwe Ministry of Health and Child Welfare Zimbabwe (2008) Maternal and Perinatal Mortality Study 2007.
28. National Institutes of Health: IMPAACT Trial Network (2010) P1077: The PROMISE Study (Promoting Maternal and Infant Survival Everywhere): Synopsis. Available: http://www.impaactgroup.org/files/IMPAACT_P1077_-Synopsis.doc. Accessed February 21, 2011.
29. Ciaranello A, Lockman S, Freedberg KA, Hughes M, Chu J, et al. (2011) First-line antiretroviral therapy after single-dose nevirapine exposure in South Africa: A cost-effectiveness analysis of the OCTANE trial. AIDS 25: 479–492.
30. El-Sadr WM, Lundgren JD, Neaton JD, Gordin F, Abrams D, et al. (2006) CD4+ count-guided interruption of antiretroviral treatment. N Engl J Med 355: 2283–2296.
31. Danel C, Moh R, Minga A, Anzian A, Ba-Gomis O, et al. (2006) CD4-guided structured antiretroviral treatment interruption strategy in HIV-infected adults in west Africa (Trivacan ANRS 1269 trial): a randomised trial. Lancet 367: 1981–1989.
32. Kesho Bora Study Group. ThLBB105: Impact of Triple-ARV prophylaxis during pregnancy and breastfeeding compared with short-ARV prophylaxis for MTCT prevention on maternal disease progression. International AIDS Society, Vienna, Austria, 2010. Available: http://pag.aids2010.org/Abstracts.aspx?SID=644&AID=17446.
33. Newell ML, Coovadia H, Cortina-Borja M, Rollins N, Gaillard P, et al. (2004) Mortality of infected and uninfected infants born to HIV-infected mothers in Africa: a pooled analysis. Lancet 364: 1236–1243.
34. Zaba B, Whitworth J, Marston M, Nakiyingi J, Ruberantwari A, et al. (2005) HIV and mortality of mothers and children: evidence from cohort studies in Uganda, Tanzania, and Malawi. Epidemiology 16: 275–280.
35. Zimbabwe Ministry of Health and Child Welfare (2009) National Drug and Therapeutics Policy Advisory Committee (NDTPAC) & AIDS and TB Unit. Guidelines for Antiretroviral Therapy in Zimbabwe.
36. Manzi M, Zachariah R, Teck R, Buhendwa L, Kazima J, et al. (2005) High acceptability of voluntary counselling and HIV-testing but unacceptable loss to follow up in a prevention of mother-to-child HIV transmission programme in

rural Malawi: scaling-up requires a different way of acting. Trop Med Int Health 10: 1242–1250.

37. Geng EH, Bangsberg DR, Musinguzi N, Emenyonu N, Bwana MB, et al. (2010) Understanding reasons for and outcomes of patients lost to follow-up in antiretroviral therapy programs in Africa through a sampling-based approach. J Acquir Immune Defic Syndr 53: 405–411.
38. Brinkhof MWG, Dabis F, Myer L, Bangsberg DR, Boulle A, et al. (2008) Early loss of HIV-infected patients on potent antiretroviral therapy programmes in lower-income countries. Bulletin of the World Health Organization 86: 559–567.
39. Zimbabwe Ministry of Health (2009) National HIV Estimates, 2009.
40. Mellors JW, Munoz A, Giorgi JV, Margolick JB, Tassoni CJ, et al. (1997) Plasma viral load and CD4+ lymphocytes as prognostic markers of HIV-1 infection. Ann Intern Med 126: 946–954.
41. Lawn SD, Myer L, Orrell C, Bekker LG, Wood R (2005) Early mortality among adults accessing a community-based antiretroviral service in South Africa: implications for programme design. AIDS 19: 2141–2148.
42. United Nations (2009) World Population Prospects: The 2008 Revision. Available: http://esa.un.org/unpd/wpp2008/index.htm. Accessed February 21, 2011.
43. Carter RJ, Dugan K, El-Sadr WM, Myer L, Otieno J, et al. (2010) CD4+ Cell Count Testing More Effective Than HIV Disease Clinical Staging in Identifying Pregnant and Postpartum Women Eligible for Antiretroviral Therapy in Resource-Limited Settings. J Acquir Immune Defic Syndr 55: 404–410.
44. Ahoua L, Ayikoru H, Gnauck K, Odaru G, Odar E, et al. (2010) Evaluation of a 5-year programme to prevent mother-to-child transmission of HIV infection in Northern Uganda. J Trop Pediatr 56: 43–52.
45. Kaplan R, Orrell C, Zwane E, Bekker LG, Wood R (2008) Loss to follow-up and mortality among pregnant women referred to a community clinic for antiretroviral treatment. AIDS 22: 1679–1681.
46. Peltier CA, Ndayisaba GF, Lepage P, van Griensven J, Leroy V, et al. (2009) Breastfeeding with maternal antiretroviral therapy or formula feeding to prevent HIV postnatal mother-to-child transmission in Rwanda. AIDS 23: 2415–2423.
47. Stinson K, Boulle A, Coetzee D, Abrams EJ, Myer L (2010) Initiation of highly active antiretroviral therapy among pregnant women in Cape Town, South Africa. Trop Med Int Health 15: 825–832.
48. Kumwenda J, Mataya R, Kumwenda N, Kafulafula G, Li Q, Taha T. WEPDD106: Coverage of highly active antiretroviral therapy (HAART) among postpartum women in Malawi International AIDS Society, Cape Town, South Africa, 2009. Available: http://www.ias2009.org/pag/Abstracts. aspx?AID=1938.
49. Lockman S, Hughes MD, McIntyre J, Zheng Y, Chipato T, et al. (2010) Antiretroviral therapies in women after single-dose nevirapine exposure. N Engl J Med 363: 1499–1509.
50. Coetzee D, Hildrebrand K, Boulle A, Maartens G, Louis F, et al. (2004) Outcomes after two years of providing antiretroviral treatment in Khayelitsha, South Africa. AIDS 18: 887–895.
51. Fawzi W, Msamanga G, Spiegelman D, Renjifo B, Bang H, et al. (2002) Transmission of HIV-1 through breastfeeding among women in Dar es Salaam, Tanzania. J Acquir Immune Defic Syndr 31: 331–338.
52. Chigwedere P, Seage GR, Lee TH, Essex M (2008) Efficacy of antiretroviral drugs in reducing mother-to-child transmission of HIV in Africa: a meta-analysis of published clinical trials. AIDS Res Hum Retroviruses 24: 827–837.
53. Coutsoudis A, Pillay K, Kuhn L, Spooner E, Tsai WY, et al. (2001) Method of feeding and transmission of HIV-1 from mothers to children by 15 months of age: prospective cohort study from Durban, South Africa. AIDS 15: 379–387.
54. Petra Study Team (2002) Efficacy of three short-course regimens of zidovudine and lamivudine in preventing early and late transmission of HIV-1 from mother to child in Tanzania, South Africa, and Uganda (Petra study): a randomised, double-blind, placebo-controlled trial. Lancet 359: 1178–1186.
55. Thistle P, Spitzer RF, Glazier RH, Pilon R, Arbess G, et al. (2007) A randomized, double-blind, placebo-controlled trial of combined nevirapine and zidovudine compared with nevirapine alone in the prevention of perinatal transmission of HIV in Zimbabwe. Clin Infect Dis 44: 111–119.
56. Palombi L, Marazzi MC, Voetberg A, Magid NA (2007) Treatment acceleration program and the experience of the DREAM program in prevention of mother-to-child transmission of HIV. AIDS 21 Suppl 4: S65–71.
57. Thomas T, Masaba R, Ndivo R, Zeh C, Borkowf C, et al.,for the Kisumu Breastfeeding Study Team. 45aLB: Prevention of mother-to-child transmission of HIV-1 among breastfeeding mothers using HAART: The Kisumu Breastfeeding Study, Kisumu, Kenya, 2003–2007. Conference on Retroviruses and Opportunistic Infections, Boston, 2008. Available: http://www. retroconference.org/2008/Abstracts/33397.htm.
58. Kilewo C, Karlsson K, Ngarina M, Massawe A, Lyamuya E, et al. (2009) Prevention of mother-to-child transmission of HIV-1 through breastfeeding by treating mothers with triple antiretroviral therapy in Dar es Salaam, Tanzania: the Mitra Plus study. J Acquir Immune Defic Syndr 52: 406–416.
59. Kuhn L, Sinkala M, Kankasa C, Semrau K, Kasonde P, et al. (2007) High uptake of exclusive breastfeeding and reduced early post-natal HIV transmission. PLoS One 2: e1363.
60. Leroy V, Newell ML, Dabis F, Peckham C, Van de Perre P, et al. (1998) International multicentre pooled analysis of late postnatal mother-to-child transmission of HIV-1 infection. Ghent International Working Group on Mother-to-Child Transmission of HIV. Lancet 352: 597–600.
61. Vyankandondera J, Luchters S, Hassink E (2003) N°LB7: Reducing risk of HIV-1 transmission from mother to infant through breastfeeding using antiretroviral prophylaxis in infants (SIMBA-study). International AIDS Society, Paris, France.
62. Coutsoudis A, Pillay K, Spooner E, Kuhn L, Coovadia HM (1999) Influence of infant-feeding patterns on early mother-to-child transmission of HIV-1 in Durban, South Africa: a prospective cohort study. South African Vitamin A Study Group. Lancet 354: 471–476.
63. Marinda E, Humphrey JH, Iliff PJ, Mutasa K, Nathoo KJ, et al. (2007) Child Mortality According to Maternal and Infant HIV Status in Zimbabwe. Pediatr Infect Dis J 26: 519–526.
64. UNAIDS/UNICEF/WHO (2009) Children and AIDS: Fourth stocktaking report, actions and progress. Available: http://www.unicef.org/publications/ index_46585.html. Accessed February 21, 2011.
65. Sutcliffe CG, van Dijk JH, Bolton C, Persaud D, Moss WJ (2008) Effectiveness of antiretroviral therapy among HIV-infected children in sub-Saharan Africa. Lancet Infect Dis 8: 477–489.
66. Kids' ART-LINC Collaboration (2008) Low risk of death, but substantial program attrition, in pediatric HIV treatment cohorts in sub-Saharan Africa. J Acquir Immune Defic Syndr 49: 523–531.
67. Soorapanth S, Sansom S, Bulterys M, Besser M, Theron G, et al. (2006) Cost-effectiveness of HIV rescreening during late pregnancy to prevent mother-to-child HIV transmission in South Africa and other resource-limited settings. J Acquir Immune Defic Syndr 42: 213–221.
68. Beigi RH, Wiringa AE, Bailey RR, Assi TM, Lee BY (2009) Economic value of seasonal and pandemic influenza vaccination during pregnancy. Clin Infect Dis 49: 1784–1792.
69. Stringer JS, McConnell MS, Kiarie J, Bolu O, Anekthananon T, et al. (2010) Effectiveness of non-nucleoside reverse-transcriptase inhibitor-based antiretroviral therapy in women previously exposed to a single intrapartum dose of nevirapine: a multi-country, prospective cohort study. PLoS Med 7: Epub ahead of print.
70. Kuhn L, Semrau K, Ramachandran S, Sinkala M, Scott N, et al. (2009) Mortality and virologic outcomes after access to antiretroviral therapy among a cohort of HIV-infected women who received single-dose nevirapine in Lusaka, Zambia. J Acquir Immune Defic Syndr 52: 132–136.
71. Coovadia A, Hunt G, Abrams EJ, Sherman G, Meyers T, et al. (2009) Persistent Minority K103N Mutations among Women Exposed to Single-Dose Nevirapine and Virologic Response to Nonnucleoside Reverse-Transcriptase Inhibitor-Based Therapy. Clin Infect Dis 48: 462–472.
72. Lundgren JD, Babiker A, El-Sadr W, Emery S, Grund B, et al. (2008) Inferior clinical outcome of the CD4+ cell count-guided antiretroviral treatment interruption strategy in the SMART study: role of CD4+ Cell counts and HIV RNA levels during follow-up. J Infect Dis 197: 1145–1155.
73. Barker PM, Mphatswe W, Rollins N (2010) Antiretroviral drugs in the cupboard are not enough: The impact of health systems' performance on mother-to-child transmission of HIV. J Acquir Immune Defic Syndr 56: e45–48.
74. Meyer-Rath G, Violari A, Cotton M, Ndibongo B, Brenna A, Long L, Panchia R, Coovadia A, Gibb DM, Rosen S THLBB103: The cost of early vs. deferred paediatric antiretroviral treatment in South Africa - a comparative economic analysis of the first year of the CHER trial. International AIDS Society, Vienna, Austria, 2010. Available: http://pag.aids2010.org/Abstracts. aspx?SID=644&AID=17823.
75. Cleary S, Chitha W, Jikwana S, Okorafor OA, Boulle A (2005) Health Systems Trust: South African Health Review. Available: http://www.hst.org.za/ generic/29. Accessed March 15, 2011.
76. Robberstad B, Evjen-Olsen B (2010) Preventing mother to child transmission of HIV with highly active antiretroviral treatment in Tanzania–a prospective cost-effectiveness study. J Acquir Immune Defic Syndr 55: 397–403.
77. Orlando S, Marazzi M, Mancinelli S, Liotta G, Ceffa S, et al. (2010) Cost-effectiveness of using HAART in prevention of mother-to-child transmission in the DREAM-Project Malawi. Journal of Acquired Immune Deficiency Syndromes 55: 631–634.
78. Johri M, Ako-Arrey D (2011) The cost-effectiveness of preventing mother-to-child transmission of HIV in low- and middle-income countries: systematic review. Cost Eff Resour Alloc 9: 3.
79. Mandala J, Torpey K, Kasonde P, Kabaso M, Dirks R, et al. (2009) Prevention of mother-to-child transmission of HIV in Zambia: implementing efficacious ARV regimens in primary health centers. BMC Public Health 9: 314.
80. Brinkhof MW, Dabis F, Myer L, Bangsberg DR, Boulle A, et al. (2008) Early loss of HIV-infected patients on potent antiretroviral therapy programmes in lower-income countries. Bull World Health Organ 86: 559–567.
81. Toro PL, Katyal M, Carter RJ, Myer L, El-Sadr WM, et al. (2010) Initiation of antiretroviral therapy among pregnant women in resource-limited countries: CD4+ cell count response and program retention. AIDS 24: 515–524.
82. Murphy RA, Sunpath H, Lu Z, Chelin N, Losina E, et al. (2010) Outcomes after virologic failure of first-line ART in South Africa. AIDS 24: 1007–1012.
83. Fawzi WW, Msamanga GI, Hunter D, Renjifo B, Antelman G, et al. (2002) Randomized trial of vitamin supplements in relation to transmission of HIV-1 through breastfeeding and early child mortality. AIDS 16: 1935–1944.
84. Leroy V, Karon JM, Alioum A, Ekpini ER, Meda N, et al. (2002) Twenty-four month efficacy of a maternal short-course zidovudine regimen to prevent mother-to-child transmission of HIV-1 in West Africa. AIDS 16: 631–641.
85. Kuhn L, Aldrovandi GM, Sinkala M, Kankasa C, Mwiya M, et al. (2010) Potential impact of new WHO criteria for antiretroviral treatment for prevention

of mother-to- child HIV transmission. AIDS 24: 1374–1377. additional data at http://www.hivpresentation.com/index.cfm?vId=1375BB1328A1344-1423A-F1376F1377-C1370DC1376EC1268CFF1357&cID=1375C1373B1824B-1423A-F1376F1377-C1372E1378CE1379BBF1379B1372D1392&show=slide.

86. Thistle P, Gottesman M, Pilon R, Glazier RH, Arbess G, et al. (2004) A randomized control trial of an Ultra-Short zidovudine regimen in the prevention of perinatal HIV transmission in rural Zimbabwe. Cent Afr J Med 50: 79–84.

87. Kesho Bora Study Group (2010) Eighteen-month follow-up of HIV-1-infected mothers and their children enrolled in the Kesho Bora study observational cohorts. J Acquir Immune Defic Syndr 54: 533–541.

88. Connor EM, Sperling RS, Gelber R, Kiselev P, Scott G, et al. (1994) Reduction of maternal-infant transmission of human immunodeficiency virus type 1 with zidovudine treatment. Pediatric AIDS Clinical Trials Group Protocol 076 Study Group. N Engl J Med 331: 1173–1180.

89. de Vincenzi I, Kesho Bora Study Group (2009) LBPEC01: Triple-antiretroviral (ARV) prophylaxis during pregnancy and breastfeeding compared to short-ARV prophylaxis to prevent mother-to-child transmission of HIV-1 (MTCT): the Kesho Bora randomized controlled clinical trial in five sites in Burkina Faso, Kenya 5th IAS Conference on HIV Pathogenesis, Treatment and Prevention, Cape Town, South Africa. Available: http://www.ias2009.org/pag/Abstracts.aspx?AID=3631.

90. Fassinou P, Elenga N, Rouet F, Laguide R, Kouakoussui KA, et al. (2004) Highly active antiretroviral therapies among HIV-1-infected children in Abidjan, Côte d'Ivoire. AIDS 18: 1905–1913.

4

Can Interferon-Gamma or Interferon-Gamma-Induced-Protein-10 Differentiate Tuberculosis Infection and Disease in Children of High Endemic Areas?

Mohammed Ahmed Yassin[1,2], Roberta Petrucci[1], Kefyalew Taye Garie[2], Gregory Harper[1], Isabel Arbide[3], Melkamsew Aschalew[4], Yared Merid[4], Zelalem Kebede[2], Amin Ahmed Bawazir[1], Nabil Mohamed Abuamer[1], Luis Eduardo Cuevas[1]*

1 Liverpool School of Tropical Medicine, Liverpool, United Kingdom, **2** Faculty of Medicine, University of Hawassa, Awassa, Ethiopia, **3** Bushullo Major Health Centre, Awassa, Ethiopia, **4** Southern Region Health Bureau, Awassa, Ethiopia

Abstract

Background: Diagnosis of childhood tuberculosis (TB) is difficult in high TB burden settings. Interferon-gamma-induced protein 10 (IP10) has been suggested as a marker of TB infection and disease, but its ability to differentiate the two conditions remains uncertain.

Objectives: To describe Interferon-gamma (INFγ) and IP10 expression in children with TB infection and disease and controls to assess their potential to differentiate latent and active TB.

Methods: This was a cross sectional study of 322 1–15 years old children with symptoms of TB (28 *confirmed*, 136 *probable* and 131 *unlikely* TB), 335 children in contact with adults with pulmonary TB and 156 community controls in Southern Ethiopia. The Tuberculin Skin Test (TST) and Quantiferon-In-Tube (QFT-IT) were performed. INFγ and IP10 were measured in plasma supernatants.

Results and Interpretation: Children with *confirmed* and *probable* TB and *contacts* were more likely to have TST+ (78.6%, 59.3% and 54.1%, respectively) than children with *unlikely* TB (28.7%) and *controls* (12.8%) ($p<0.001$). Children with *confirmed* TB (59.3%) and *contacts* (44.7%) were more likely to have INFγ+ than children with *probable* (37.6%) or *unlikely* TB (28.1%) and *controls* (13.1%) ($p<0.001$). IP10 concentrations were higher in INFγ+ children independently of TST ($p<0.001$). There was no difference between IP10 concentrations of children with *confirmed* TB and *contacts* ($p = 0.8$) and children with and without HIV ($p>0.1$). INFγ and IP10 can identify children with TB infection and disease, but cannot differentiate between the two conditions. HIV status did not affect the expression of IP10.

Editor: Laura Ellen Via, National Institute of Allergy and Infectious Disease, United States of America

Funding: This study was funded by a research grant awarded by the Thrasher Foundation, United States of America. The funders had no role in study design, data collection and analysis, decision to publish, or preparation of the manuscript.

Competing Interests: The authors have declared that no competing interests exist.

* E-mail: lcuevas@liv.ac.uk

Introduction

One of the most significant barriers for the appropriate management of Tuberculosis (TB) is the lack of suitable diagnostic tests. This problem is especially critical in settings where facilities are limited and other infections with overlapping clinical presentation are highly prevalent. Childhood TB presentation differs from adult TB as children experience more extra-pulmonary TB (EPTB) and lung involvement is frequently disseminated and without cavitations. Young children are unable to expectorate sputum and the specimens collected, such as gastric aspirates, are often paucibacillary and sometimes contain test inhibitors. Most diagnostics for TB thus perform poorly in children [1,2] and new tests or markers to diagnose TB in children are needed.

Interferon-gamma (INFγ) release assays (IGRAs) were developed in the last decade and are reported to have comparable sensitivity and higher specificity than the Tuberculin Skin Test (TST) to identify latent TB infections (LTBI). Their performance however is less reliable in young children and in patients co-infected with the Human Immunodeficiency Virus (HIV) [3,4,5]. These assays are frequently used by clinicians to support a diagnosis of symptomatic TB [3,6,7], even though they cannot distinguish between LTBI and symptomatic disease. IGRAS are also increasingly used in high TB incidence settings, despite the limited information of their performance in these locations [8,9,10].

INFγ-induced protein 10 (IP10, also known as Chemokine (C-X-C motif) ligand 10 or CXCL10) is another biomarker recently reported to identify LTBI, which, when combined with IGRAS is said to increase the sensitivity of the assays [10]. IP10 expression is putatively less affected by HIV [11] and young age [12,13] and it is said to have potential to differentiate between LTBI and symptomatic infections [12,14].

We have thus conducted a study in Southern Ethiopia to describe INFγ and IP10 concentrations of children presenting with symptoms compatible with TB, asymptomatic children in contact with adults with smear-positive pulmonary TB (PTB) and asymptomatic community controls to explore whether INFγ or IP10 can distinguish between symptomatic and asymptomatic infections in a high TB burden setting and assess whether these markers could be used to support the diagnosis of children with symptoms of TB.

Materials and Methods

This was a cross sectional study of 1 to 15 year old children with symptoms suggestive of TB, children in contact with adults with smear-positive PTB and community controls without known contact with TB. The study was based in Awassa, in the Southern Region of Ethiopia, which has a population of over 15 million.

Children with symptoms of TB (called *symptomatics*) were enrolled consecutively at three health service providers (Awassa Health Centre, Bushullo Major Health Centre and University of Hawassa referral hospital). These included consecutive children with cough or fever for more than 2 weeks, night sweats, anorexia, weight loss, failure to thrive or non-specific symptoms in the presence of a history of contact with an adult with PTB. Children were invited to participate at the time of presentation to the clinic. All children underwent a clinical examination, chest X-rays, TST, three sputum or gastric lavage examinations and fine needle aspiration if enlarged lymph nodes were detected. All specimens were examined using light smear microscopy and culture on Lowenstein Jensen media and children were classified as having *confirmed* (positive smear microscopy or culture), *probable* (negative smear microscopy and culture, clinical and radiological findings consistent with TB, no improvement after a full course of antibiotics and the clinician initiating anti-TB treatment) or *unlikely* TB (children with alternative diagnosis or clinical improvement after a course of broad spectrum antibiotics).

In addition, *contact* children 1–15 year old residing with adults with smear-positive PTB (called *contacts*) were enrolled by identifying adults attending the same study centres with a history of cough for more than 2 weeks duration who had sputum smear-positive PTB. Once a smear-positive adult had been identified, study investigators inquired whether they had children at home and visited the households if the family resided within a 20 km radius from Awassa. All children living under a single roof who shared meal times with the adult were invited to participate after obtaining informed parental consent, unless they had previously received treatment for TB. All children who shared meals at home with the index cases were included, regardless of the duration of contact.

Community *controls* were defined as children residing in the community who did not have a known contact with adults with PTB. *Controls* were selected from Awassa and surrounding *kebeles*, which are the smallest administrative units of Ethiopia and comprise at least five hundred families or 3,500 to 5,000 inhabitants. A list of all villages and *kebeles* located within a 20 Km radius from Awassa was constructed. Controls were enrolled from villages adjacent to the villages where contacts resided. We enrolled more controls from rural villages than from urban areas as the risk of TB transmission from casual contact could be higher among urban residents. Households within a village were selected by spinning a pen in a street somewhere between the centre and the edge of the village and children were enrolled after obtaining informed parental consent. Households were excluded if the parent indicated the family had been in contact with an adult with cough for more than 2 weeks duration in the previous 2 years or if a family member had received treatment for TB. All children were applied a TST using 2 units of Purified Protein Derivate (PPD, RT 23, Statens Serum Institute, Copenhagen, Denmark) using the Mantoux method and indurations were measured using the palpation method 48 to 72 hours later. TST results were graded as negative (<5 mm), intermediate (≥5 and <10 mm) and positive (≥10 mm). Any child with signs and symptoms suggestive of TB was investigated for disease activity and treated. *Contact* children <6 years old were offered INH prophylaxis for 6 months independently of their TST result, following Ethiopian TB Control Programme guidelines.

INFγ and IP10 concentrations were assayed using commercially available Enzyme Linked Immunoassay (ELISA) kits. INFγ was measured using the QuantiFERON-TB Gold In-Tube (QFT-IT) test (Cellestis, Victoria, Australia). Blood samples for QFT-IT were collected in 3 tubes, one containing the *Mycobacterium tuberculosis* ESAT-6, CFP10 and TB7-7 antigens; one with non-specific mytogen (phytohemoagglutinin) to serve as positive control and one blank tube (nil) to serve as negative control. The three tubes were incubated at 37° for 16–24 hours. Supernatant plasma was harvested after centrifugation to separate the blood cells and stored at −70°C. INFγ was measured using the manufacturer's ELISA in a Bio-Rad Plate reader (Model n 550) and read at 450 nm. IGRAs were classified as positive, negative or indeterminate using the manufacturer's software. IP10 concentrations were measured in the same supernatant using a Human IP10 ELISA Construction Kit (Antigenix America Inc, New York, NY). HIV infections were established using two blood-based ELISA methods.

Means and standard deviations (SD) or medians and interquartile ranges (IQR) were used to describe continuous variables. Parametric tests and non parametric tests were used to compare means and medians. The proportion of children in each study category with positive/negative tests compared using Chi-Square and Fisher's exact tests (if expected values were less than<5) and the agreement between TST and INFγ was described using Kappa statistics. IP10 concentrations were described using boxplots stratified by TST and INFγ concordance. The sample size calculations took into account the feasibility to visit about 200 households (of index cases) within the available time and resources and that each household had an average of two children <5 years old and it was expected that 200 children with signs and sypmtoms of TB would attend the health services. It was expected that 50% of the participants would be TST positive and 70% and 30%, of TST-positive children would be INF-γ positive and negative, respectively. It was also assumed that 30% and 70% of TST-negative children would be INF-γ positive and negative, respectively. This sample size would allow estimating the proportion of children with positive and negative INF-γ results by study group with a precision of ±7%. Sample size calculation for the comparison of quantitative data (i.e. differences in IP-10 concentrations by study group) would have required prior information of the dispersion of IP-10 concentrations to estimate standard deviations or medians. As this information was not available, this study should be considered "exploratory", as it might not have enough power for the differences reported. The ability of IP10 to discriminate between children with and without TB infection or disease was evaluated using Receiver Operating Characteristic (ROC) curves using Prism 5 software (GraphPad PRISM, version 5). ROC curves were constructed with children with *confirmed* TB and controls and *contact* children with TST+/INFγ+ and *controls*. Only *controls* with TST-/INFγ- results were included in the ROC analysis to select children unlikely to have TB infection. The area under the curve (AUC) for both *confirmed* and *contact* children were compared to ascertain whether IP10 could discriminate between the two conditions. Statistical tests were considered significant if p values were <0.05.

The study protocol was approved by the Health Bureau of the Southern Region and the Research Ethics Committees of the Liverpool School of Tropical Medicine, Hawassa University and the Sciences and Technology Commission of Ethiopia. The study protocol was registered in the clinicatrials.gov clinical trials register (registration number NCT00456469)

Results

Eight hundred thirteen, 322 *symptomatic*, 335 *contact* and 156 *control* children were enrolled. The flow chart of the three groups is described in Figure 1. Twenty eight (8.7%) of 322 *symptomatic* children had *confirmed*, 136 (42.2%) *probable* and 131 (40.7%) *unlikely* TB and 27 were excluded because a definitive diagnosis was not reached or the child left the hospital before completing the investigations. The 335 *contact* children were recruited from 125 adult index cases who had "scanty" (18, 5.5%), "+" (188, 57%), "++" (109, 33%) or "+++" (15, 4.5%) smear microscopy grades in their sputum smear examination. In five *contacts* the smear result of the adult was not recorded. The median contact duration was 10 hours per week (range of 1 to 41 hours). The characteristics of the participants are shown in Table 1. Children with *probable* TB were more likely to be male (67.6%), while children in the other groups had similar proportions of males and females. Children had similar median age with symptomatic and control children having a median age of 6 years and contacts having a median of 8 years. Although the proportion of children reporting to have received BCG was similar across the groups, BCG scars were found less frequently in children with *confirmed* and *probable* TB (p<0.001). HIV was positive in none of the children with *confirmed* TB, 14 (10.9%) children with *probable* and 8 (6.5%) *unlikely* TB cases, 27 (8.2%) *contacts* and 3 (1.9%) *controls* (p = 0.005). The number of residents per household was higher among children with *symptoms* of TB than among *contacts* and *controls* (means 8, 7.1 and 6.4 persons, respectively, p = 0.003). A significantly high proportion of children had lost one or both parents, with *symptomatic* and *contact* children being more likely to have lost a parent than *controls* (p = 0.01).

TST and INFγ results are shown in table 2. Children with *confirmed* and *probable* TB and *contacts* were more likely to have positive TST (TST+) (78.6%, 59.3% and 54.1%, respectively) than children with *unlikely* TB (28.7%) and *controls* (12.8%) (p<0.001). A high proportion of children had indeterminate INFγ tests, with children with *probable* and *unlikely* TB having a higher proportion of indeterminates than children with *confirmed* TB, *contacts* and *controls*. This problem was mostly due to failure of the positive control tube and was not associated with HIV infection (26/52 (50%) in HIV positive, compared to 256/641 (40%) in HIV-negative children, p = 0.2).

Children with *confirmed* TB (59.3%) and *contacts* (44.7%) were also more likely to have positive INFγ (INFγ+) than children with *probable* (37.6%) or *unlikely* TB (28.1%) and *controls* (13.1%) (p<0.001). Twenty two (78.6%) children with *confirmed*, 73 (53.7%) with *probable* and 68 (52%) with *unlikely* TB, 209 (62.4%) *contacts* and 114 (73.1%) *controls* had paired TST and IFNγ results after exclusion of intermediate TST and indeterminate INFγ tests. Concordance between INFγ and TST varied across the groups. Children with *confirmed* and *probable* TB and *contacts* were more likely to have concordant positive TST and INFγ (15 (68.2%) of 22, 38 (52.1%) of 73 and 87 (41.6%) of 209, respectively), while children with *unlikely* TB and *controls* were more likely to have concordant negative TST and INFγ (29 (42.6%) of 68 and 86 (75.4%) of 114, respectively). Discordant TST+/INFγ− results were more frequent among children with *probable* TB (20.5%) and *contacts* (18.7%) and discordant TST−/INFγ+ results were more frequent among children with *unlikely* TB (22.1%) and *controls* (11.5%). Agreement between TST and IFNγ tests varied from 81% (k = 0.49) in children with *confirmed* TB, 73% (k = 0.40) in *probable* TB and 66% (k = 0.23) in *unlikely* TB, 70% (k = 0.39) in *contacts* and 81% (k = 0.24) in *controls*.

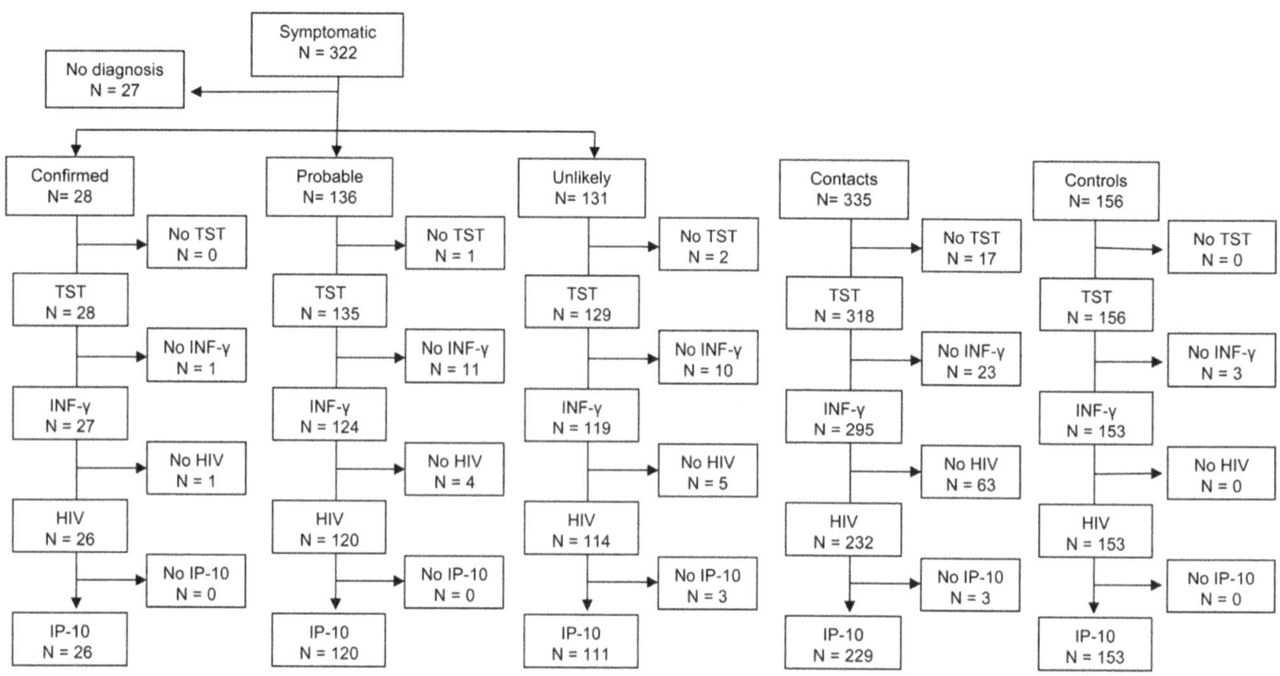

Figure 1. Flow chart of study participants.

Table 1. Characteristics of the study children.

Variables	Symptomatic cases N = 295					
	Confirmed TB N = 28	*Probable TB* N = 136	*Unlikely TB* N = 131	Contacts N = 335	Controls N = 156	p
Male/Female (% Male)	13/15 (46.4)	92/44 (67.6)	67/64 (51.1)	168/166 (50.3)	79/77 (50.6)	
Median age (years)	8	5	7	8	6	<0.001
Range	1–15	1–15	1–15	1–15	1–15	
Received BCG	14 (63.6)	69 (63.3)	82 (70.7)	249 (74.3)	120 (76.9)	0.01
BCG scar present (%)	7 (25)	35 (25.7)	51 (38.9)	174 (51.9)	93 (59.6)	<0.001
Mean (SD) BCG scar (mm)	7.4 (3.2)	5.3 (1.8)	5.5 (2.1)	4.7 (2.4)	5.4 (2.5)	<0.001
Range	4–13	2–9	2–10	1–13	2–13	
HIV status, Pos/tested (%Pos)	0/27 (0)	14/114 (10.9)	8/116 (6.5)	27/231 (8.2)	3/153 (1.9)	0.005
Mean (SD) residents/household	8.3 (7.5)	8.9 (8.3)	7.2 (6.3)	7.1 (2.6)	6.4 (2.4)	0.002
Illiterate Father, N (%)	17 (70.8)	63 (55.8)	55 (48.7)	112 (38.6)	87 (60.4)	<0.001
Mother, N (%)	21 (84)	97 (77.6)	87 (68.5)	170 (52.3)	123 (78.8)	<0.001
Alive Father, N (%)	24 (85.7)	113 (83.1)	113 (86.3)	293 (88.3)	144 (92.3)	0.2
Mother, N (%)	25 (89.3)	124 (92.5)	128 (98.5)	325 (97.6)	156 (100)	<0.001
Both parents, N (%)	23 (82.1)	109 (81.3)	112 (80)	293 (88)	144 (92.3)	0.01

IP10 concentrations are shown in Figure 2. Stimulated concentrations were much higher than non-stimulated concentrations in all groups ($p<0.001$). Non-stimulated concentrations were highest in children with *confirmed* TB and lowest in *controls* (medians 1606 and 386 pg/ml). Stimulated concentrations were higher in children with *confirmed* TB and *contacts* (7812 and 5616 pg/ml, respectively) than in children with *probable* and *unlikely* TB (3680 and 2532 pg/ml, respectively, Kruskal-Wallis, $p=0.02$). The difference of stimulated minus non-stimulated concentrations are shown in Table 3 by TST and INFγ results and study group. Among patients with positive TST, *symptomatic* and *contact* children had higher IP10 concentrations than *controls* ($p=0.03$ and $p<0.001$, respectively). Among children with negative TST, children with *confirmed* TB and *contacts* had higher IP10 concentrations than *controls* ($p=0.02$ and $p=0.001$, respectively. There was no difference in the IP10 concentrations across study groups among children with INFγ− results, while *contact* children with INFγ+ results had the highest IP10 concentrations, followed by *symptomatic* and *control* children. Median (IQR) IP10 concentrations (stimulated minus non-stimulated) are shown in Figure 3 by TST and INFγ concordance. Children with concordant TST+/INFγ+ had higher IP10 concentrations than children with TST−/INFγ− results in all study groups. Children with *confirmed* TB had high IP10 concentrations independently of the TST or INFγ result including two of the three children who had TST−/INFγ− results. In contrast, most *controls* had low IP10 concentrations with the exception of children with TST+/INFγ+ results, who had high IP10 concentrations ($p=0.04$). Children with HIV had similar

Table 2. TST and INFγ results and concordance among the tests by study group.

Variables	Symptomatic cases N = 295				
	Confirmed TB N = 28 (%)	*Probable TB* N = 136 (%)	*Unlikely TB* N = 131 (%)	Contacts N = 335 (%)	Controls N = 156 (%)
TST					
Positive	22 (78.6)	80 (59.3)	37 (28.7)	172 (54.1)	20 (12.8)
Intermediate	0	10 (7.4)	9 (7)	48 (15.1)	15 (9.6)
Negative	6 (21.4)	45 (33.3)	83 (64.3)	98 (30.8)	121 (77.6)
INFγ					
Positive	16 (59.3)	47 (37.6)	34 (28.1)	139 (44.7)	20 (13.1)
Indeterminate	5 (18.5)	47 (37.6)	44 (36.4)	52 (16.7)	25 (16.3)
Negative	6 (22.2)	31 (24.8)	43 (35.5)	120 (38.6)	108 (70.6)
TST/INFγ concordance					
TST+/INFγ+	15 (68.2)	38 (52.1)	14 (20.6)	87 (41.6)	6 (5.3)
TST+/INFγ−	3 (13.6)	15 (20.5)	10 (14.7)	39 (18.7)	10 (8.8)
TST−/INFγ+	1 (4.5)	5 (6.8)	15 (22.1)	24 (11.5)	12 (10.5)
TST−/INFγ−	3 (13.6)	15 (20.5)	29 (42.6)	59 (28.2)	86 (75.4)

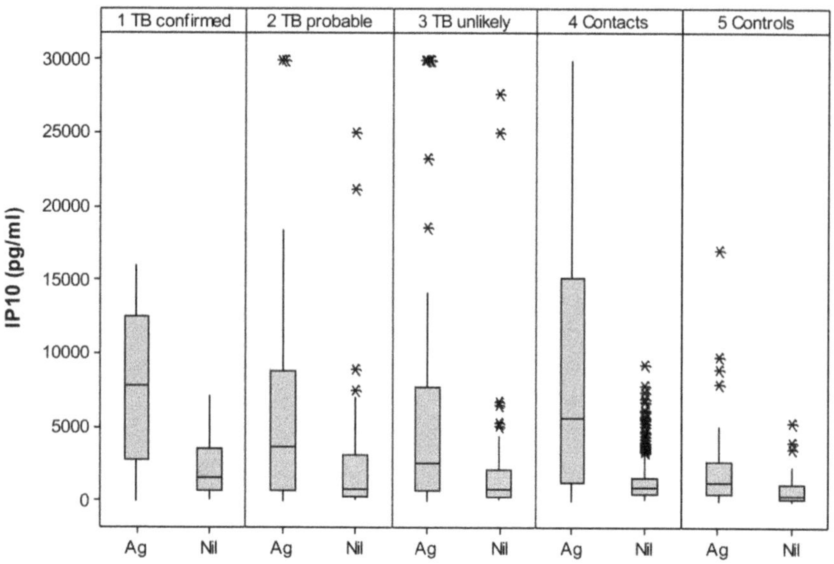

Figure 2. IP10 (pg/ml) concentrations in stimulated (Ag) and non-stimulated (Nil) samples by study group. Box plots describe medians, interquantile values and range. Asterisks depict outliers.

IP10 concentrations than children without HIV across all study groups (p>0.1) as shown in Figure 4.

IP10 concentrations of children with *confirmed* TB (N = 22, median IP10 7774 pg/ml) and *contacts* with TST+ and/or INFγ+ (N = 148, median IP10 12490 pg/ml) where compared against *controls* with TST− and INFγ− (N = 86, median IP10 704 pg/ml) to construct the ROC curves, as shown in Figure 5. The ROC curves for both *confirmed* and *contact* children had the same shape, with cut-off points for best performance being 3128 pg/ml (sensitivity 81.8%, 95%CI = 59.7–94.8, specificity 96.5% 95%CI 90.1–99.3 and area under the curve (AUC) of 0.87%, 95%CI 0.75–0.99) for *confirmed* TB and 3022 pg/ml (sensitivity 77%, 95%CI 69.4–83.5%, specificity 96.5%, 95%CI 90.14–99.3%, and an AUC of 0.87, 95%CI 0.82–0.92) for *contacts*.

Discussion

Despite significant research efforts and technological breakthroughs to develop new diagnostics for TB [15], current diagnostic tests have lower sensitivity in children than in adults [1,2]. New diagnostics are needed to identify children with TB and to differentiate between latent and active TB in high incidence settings with limited resources.

Despite a large body of evidence of the performance characteristics of IGRAs for the diagnosis of LTBI and the identification of individuals infected during TB outbreaks in low TB incidence settings [6,16,17,18,19], there is a small number of studies assessing the IGRAS performance and their utility in high incidence countries [20,21,22]. The data presented here therefore represents a rare opportunity to compare TST, INFγ and IP10 in children with different degrees of exposure to infection and certainty of diagnosis residing in a high TB burden setting.

An important difference to reports from industrialized countries was the high proportion of QFT-IT tests with indeterminate results. Other studies from Africa have reported high rates of indeterminate results [23], and the reason for this high frequency remains unexplained. Our team has conducted similar studies in Nigeria [24], Nepal [8] and Yemen, took care to re-stock tests frequently and used high altitude control tubes provided by the manufacturer. Most indeterminate results however were due to failure of the positive control and further studies are needed to explore whether this was due to a loss of test integrity or an unidentified background morbidity such as parasitic, bacterial or viral infections [25]. The interpretation of the data is also hampered by the lack of reference standards for LTBI. The data however confirms that INFγ, as TST, are more likely to be

Table 3. Medians and interquantile ranges of IP10 concentrations (stimulated minus non-stimulated, in pg/ml) according to the TST and INFγ results by study group.

	TST			INFγ		
	Positive	**Intermediate**	**Negative**	**Positive**	**Indeterminate**	**Negative**
TB confirmed	5116 (2092–9624)	-	6788 (1672–11344)	8848 (4296–11414)	1672 (56–2092)	4560 (8–7496)
TB probable	2592 (64–8272)	768 (0–7424)	512 (84–3348)	7254 (3360–10548)	84 (0–604)	1288 (140–4548)
TB unlikely	2404 (326–8868)	2903 (692–8688)	674 (54–2558)	7594 (3328–12028)	548 (0–2208)	674 (120–1372)
Contacts	9304 (708–14536)	6078 (476–17632)	1486 (308–5544)	13800 (11128–17728)	348 (20–1932)	770 (196–3224)
Controls	528 (72–1392)	1124 (40–2320)	704 (116–1932)	1784 (364–2562)	180 (0–1184)	684 (144–1792)

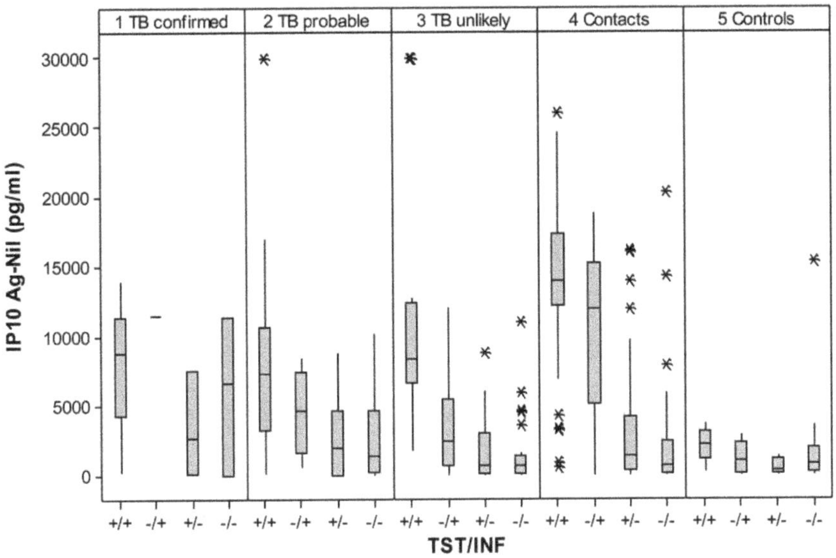

Figure 3. IP10 concentrations (stimulated minus non-stimulated) by TST and INFγ results and study group. Box plots describe medians, interquantile values and range. Asterisks depict outliers.

positive in children with *contact* or *confirmed* TB than in *controls*. Neither INFγ nor TST differentiate between active and latent infections and thus their diagnostic value is restricted to the confirmation of a history of infection [3,19,26]. Given that a number of children had discrepant INFγ/TST results, cost and logistic constrains aside, the use of both TST and INFγ would identify a higher number of children with evidence of infection than a single test alone.

This study also describes IP10 concentrations of children at different risk of infection, and how these concentrations vary with TST, INFγ and HIV. IP10 is a cytokine expressed in response to IFNγ stimulation by cell types involved in delayed-type hypersensitivity [27], including lymphocytes, monocytes, endothelial cells and fibroblasts and is a chemo-attractant to monocytes and activated Th1 lymphocytes [28], promoting selective enhancement of Th1 responses and increasing IFN-γ gene expression [29]. Recent studies have reported that IP10 expression is enhanced in individuals with active TB [30,31] and latent infection [12,13,32] and that combined with INFγ could increase the sensitivity of the IGRAS [9,12]. Although some reports have suggested that this marker could differentiate between active and latent infection [14,33], not all studies have replicated these observations [10,14].

IP-10 concentrations were higher among children with *confirmed* TB and *contacts*, with the highest concentrations observed in *contact* children, which is in agreement with recently recent reports from low incidence settings [12,14]. IP10 concentrations were generally higher among children with INFγ+ results and there was no difference in the median concentrations of children with and without HIV infection. This latter characteristic could have practical applications, increasing the sensitivity of INFγ based tests in areas of high HIV prevalence.

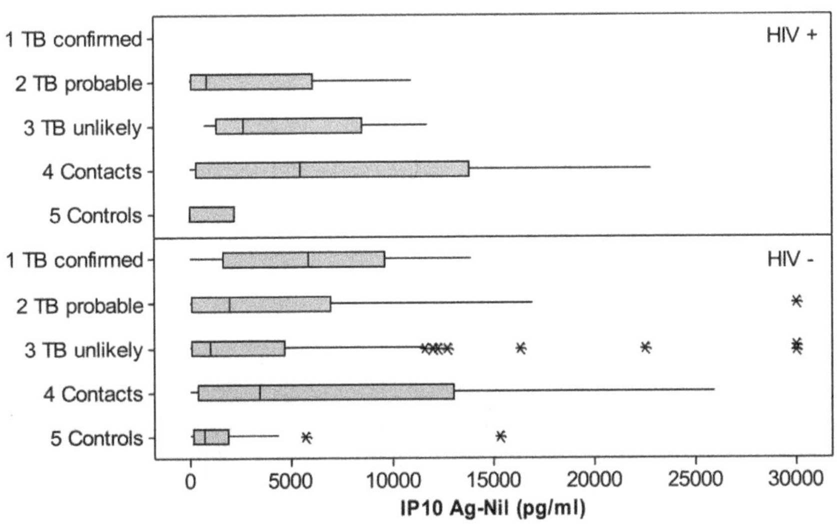

Figure 4. IP10 concentrations (stimulated minus non-stimulated) by HIV status and study group. Box plots describe medians, interquantile values and range. Asterisks depict outliers.

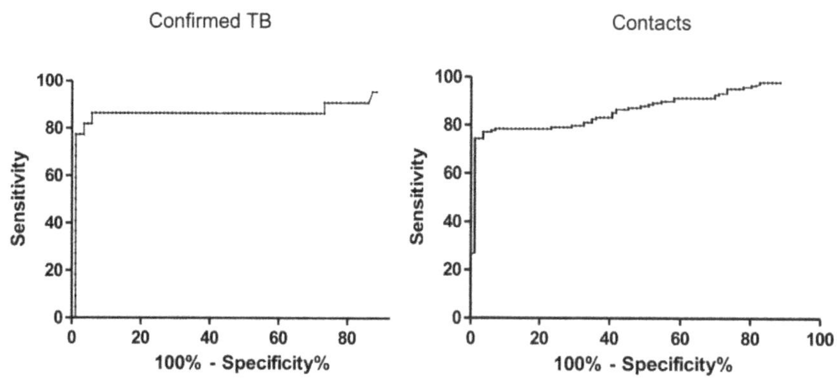

Figure 5. Receiver Operating Characteristic (ROC) curve of IP10 in children with *confirmed* TB and *contacts,* when compared to community *controls* with TST- and INFγ results.

Interestingly, non-stimulated IP10 concentrations were higher in children with *confirmed* TB, resulting in a smaller difference between stimulated and non-stimulated concentrations. Although non-specific IP10 increases have been described in acute and chronic diseases other than TB [34,35,36,37], these findings suggest that IP10 expression may vary during the course of disease progression, maybe with higher expression during the primary stages of granuloma formation, which involves the recruitment of monocytes and Th1 gammadelta T-cells [38] and lower expression in the presence of progressive unchecked infections, in the presence of immunosuppression, as described for INFγ.

The ROC curve analysis however suggested that the cut offs with best test performance to differentiate children with *confirmed* TB and *controls* was similar to the cut offs to differentiate *contacts* and *controls*, with similar AUC. Thus, similar to INFγ and TST, IP10 differentiated between infected and non-infected children but is unable to differentiate between latent and active TB. Data from children residing in a high burden areas is scarce and the sensitivity of 81.8% obtained is lower than reported from Indian adults [10] in Chennai (92.5%, 95%CI: 88.6%–96.4%), which also reported a lower specificity (48%). Ruhwald et. al. [39] selected a cut off of 673 pg/ml for Danish adolescents and adults and Lighter et. al [12] selected a cut off of 732 pg/ml for USA children. Applying Ruhwald et. al., cut off to Ethiopia would increase the sensitivity to 86% and reduce the specificity to 48%, which is similar to those reported by Kabeer et al in India, suggesting that there is more agreement of test performance across settings than suggested by these reports.

This study therefore describes INFγ and IP10 expression in children at different risk of infection and disease in a country with a high incidence of TB. Children with *probable* TB had different tests results patterns than children with *confirmed* TB as the former had more TST but less INFγ positive results, thus reflecting the heterogeneity of this group and underscoring the importance of using clear reporting group categories based on the certainty of diagnosis to facilitate the interpretation of data.

Our findings therefore demonstrate that both INFγ and IP10 identify children with latent and active TB. IP10 is less affected by the presence of HIV co-infection than INFγ and has the potential to increase the sensitivity of the IGRAS when used in combination with INFγ. INFγ, IP10 and TST however are unable to differentiate between latent and active disease.

Longitudinal studies to describe the natural variation of these markers over time and their ability to identify children with latent infections at risk of disease progression or children at risk of poor treatment response after initiation of anti-TB therapy are needed. However, given the high cost of the IGRAS and the high proportion of indeterminate results obtained, control programmes should refrain from incorporating these tests until clear advantages over the TST are demonstrated.

Acknowledgments

We are grateful for the Southern Region Health Bureau's support for this study and the research assistants (Girum Asnake, Habiba Jemal, Tadesse Mamo and Koratu) and laboratory technicians (Tesfaye Tusuna and Kedir Yesuf) who collected the data. Our thanks go to all children and parents participating in the study.

Author Contributions

Conceived and designed the experiments: YM LC. Performed the experiments: YM GH AB NA. Analyzed the data: RP YM LC. Contributed reagents/materials/analysis tools: YM. Wrote the paper: YM LC RP. Coordinated field work and data processing: IA KG MA ZK.

References

1. Zar HJ, Hanslo D, Apolles P, Swingler G, Hussey G (2005) Induced sputum versus gastric lavage for microbiological confirmation of pulmonary tuberculosis in infants and young children: a prospective study. Lancet 365: 130–134.
2. Marais BJ, Pai M (2007) Recent advances in the diagnosis of childhood tuberculosis. Arch Dis Child 92: 446–452.
3. Wallis RS, Pai M, Menzies D, Doherty TM, Walzl G, et al. (2010) Biomarkers and diagnostics for tuberculosis: progress, needs, and translation into practice. Lancet 375: 1920–1937.
4. Bamford AR, Crook AM, Clark JE, Nademi Z, Dixon G, et al. (2010) Comparison of interferon-{gamma} release assays and tuberculin skin test in predicting active tuberculosis (TB) in children in the UK: a paediatric TB network study. Arch Dis Child 95: 180–186.
5. Detjen AK, Keil T, Roll S, Hauer B, Mauch H, et al. (2007) Interferon-gamma release assays improve the diagnosis of tuberculosis and nontuberculous mycobacterial disease in children in a country with a low incidence of tuberculosis. Clin Infect Dis 45: 322–328.
6. Menzies D, Pai M, Comstock G (2007) Meta-analysis: new tests for the diagnosis of latent tuberculosis infection: areas of uncertainty and recommendations for research. Ann Intern Med 146: 340–354.
7. Zar HJ, Connell TG, Nicol M (2010) Diagnosis of pulmonary tuberculosis in children: new advances. Expert Rev Anti Infect Ther 8: 277–288.
8. Petrucci R, Abu Amer N, Gurgel RQ, Sherchand JB, Doria L, et al. (2008) Interferon gamma, interferon-gamma-induced-protein 10, and tuberculin responses of children at high risk of tuberculosis infection. Pediatr Infect Dis J 27: 1073–1077.
9. Ruhwald M, Petersen J, Kofoed K, Nakaoka H, Cuevas LE, et al. (2008) Improving T-cell assays for the diagnosis of latent TB infection: potential of a diagnostic test based on IP-10. PLoS One 3: e2858.

10. Syed Ahamed Kabeer B, Raman B, Thomas A, Perumal V, Raja A (2010) Role of QuantiFERON-TB gold, interferon gamma inducible protein-10 and tuberculin skin test in active tuberculosis diagnosis. PLoS One 5: e9051.
11. Juffermans NP, Verbon A, van Deventer SJ, van Deutekom H, Belisle JT, et al. (1999) Elevated chemokine concentrations in sera of human immunodeficiency virus (HIV)-seropositive and HIV-seronegative patients with tuberculosis: a possible role for mycobacterial lipoarabinomannan. Infect Immun 67: 4295–4297.
12. Lighter J, Rigaud M, Huie M, Peng CH, Pollack H (2009) Chemokine IP-10: an adjunct marker for latent tuberculosis infection in children. Int J Tuberc Lung Dis 13: 731–736.
13. Ruhwald M, Ravn P (2009) Biomarkers of latent TB infection. Expert Rev Respir Med 3: 387–401.
14. Whittaker E, Gordon A, Kampmann B (2008) Is IP-10 a better biomarker for active and latent tuberculosis in children than IFNgamma? PLoS One 3: e3901.
15. Boehme CC, Nabeta P, Hillemann D, Nicol MP, Shenai S, et al. (2010) Rapid molecular detection of tuberculosis and rifampin resistance. N Engl J Med 363: 1005–1015.
16. Ewer K, Deeks J, Alvarez L, Bryant G, Waller S, et al. (2003) Comparison of T-cell-based assay with tuberculin skin test for diagnosis of Mycobacterium tuberculosis infection in a school tuberculosis outbreak. Lancet 361: 1168–1173.
17. Higuchi K, Kondo S, Wada M, Hayashi S, Ootsuka G, et al. (2009) Contact investigation in a primary school using a whole blood interferon-gamma assay. J Infect 58: 352–357.
18. Pai M, Kalantri S, Dheda K (2006) New tools and emerging technologies for the diagnosis of tuberculosis: part I. Latent tuberculosis. Expert Rev Mol Diagn 6: 413–422.
19. Chang KC, Leung CC (2010) Systematic review of interferon-gamma release assays in tuberculosis: focus on likelihood ratios. Thorax 65: 271–276.
20. Dheda K, van Zyl Smit R, Badri M, Pai M (2009) T-cell interferon-gamma release assays for the rapid immunodiagnosis of tuberculosis: clinical utility in high-burden vs. low-burden settings. Curr Opin Pulm Med 15: 188–200.
21. Barth RE, Mudrikova T, Hoepelman AI (2008) Interferon-gamma release assays (IGRAs) in high-endemic settings: could they play a role in optimizing global TB diagnostics? Evaluating the possibilities of using IGRAs to diagnose active TB in a rural African setting. Int J Infect Dis 12: e1–6.
22. Hill PC, Jackson-Sillah DJ, Fox A, Brookes RH, de Jong BC, et al. (2008) Incidence of tuberculosis and the predictive value of ELISPOT and Mantoux tests in Gambian case contacts. PLoS One 3: e1379.
23. Seshadri C, Uiso LO, Ostermann J, Diefenthal H, Shao HJ, et al. (2008) Low sensitivity of T-cell based detection of tuberculosis among HIV co-infected Tanzanian in-patients. East Afr Med J 85: 442–449.
24. Nakaoka H, Lawson L, Squire SB, Coulter B, Ravn P, et al. (2006) Risk for tuberculosis among children. Emerg Infect Dis 12: 1383–1388.
25. Shanaube K, De Haas P, Schaap A, Moyo M, Kosloff B, et al. (2010) Intra-assay reliability and robustness of QuantiFERON(R)-TB Gold In-Tube test in Zambia. Int J Tuberc Lung Dis 14: 828–833.
26. Bianchi L, Galli L, Moriondo M, Veneruso G, Becciolini L, et al. (2009) Interferon-gamma release assay improves the diagnosis of tuberculosis in children. Pediatr Infect Dis J 28: 510–514.
27. Kaplan G, Luster AD, Hancock G, Cohn ZA (1987) The expression of a gamma interferon-induced protein (IP-10) in delayed immune responses in human skin. J Exp Med 166: 1098–1108.
28. Farber JM (1997) Mig and IP-10: CXC chemokines that target lymphocytes. J Leukoc Biol 61: 246–257.
29. Moser B, Loetscher P (2001) Lymphocyte traffic control by chemokines. Nat Immunol 2: 123–128.
30. Ruhwald M, Bjerregaard-Andersen M, Rabna P, Kofoed K, Eugen-Olsen J, et al. (2007) CXCL10/IP-10 release is induced by incubation of whole blood from tuberculosis patients with ESAT-6, CFP10 and TB7.7. Microbes Infect 9: 806–812.
31. Azzurri A, Sow OY, Amedei A, Bah B, Diallo S, et al. (2005) IFN-gamma-inducible protein 10 and pentraxin 3 plasma levels are tools for monitoring inflammation and disease activity in Mycobacterium tuberculosis infection. Microbes Infect 7: 1–8.
32. Ruhwald M, Bjerregaard-Andersen M, Rabna P, Eugen-Olsen J, Ravn P (2009) IP-10, MCP-1, MCP-2, MCP-3, and IL-1RA hold promise as biomarkers for infection with M. tuberculosis in a whole blood based T-cell assay. BMC Res Notes 2: 19.
33. Dheda K, Van-Zyl Smit RN, Sechi LA, Badri M, Meldau R, et al. (2009) Clinical diagnostic utility of IP-10 and LAM antigen levels for the diagnosis of tuberculous pleural effusions in a high burden setting. PLoS One 4: e4689.
34. Korpi-Steiner NL, Bates ME, Lee WM, Hall DJ, Bertics PJ (2006) Human rhinovirus induces robust IP-10 release by monocytic cells, which is independent of viral replication but linked to type I interferon receptor ligation and STAT1 activation. J Leukoc Biol 80: 1364–1374.
35. Dhillon NK, Peng F, Ransohoff RM, Buch S (2007) PDGF synergistically enhances IFN-gamma-induced expression of CXCL10 in blood-derived macrophages: implications for HIV dementia. J Immunol 179: 2722–2730.
36. Jain V, Armah HB, Tongren JE, Ned RM, Wilson NO, et al. (2008) Plasma IP-10, apoptotic and angiogenic factors associated with fatal cerebral malaria in India. Malar J 7: 83.
37. Antonelli A, Ferri C, Fallahi P, Ferrari SM, Sebastiani M, et al. (2008) High values of CXCL10 serum levels in mixed cryoglobulinemia associated with hepatitis C infection. Am J Gastroenterol 103: 2488–2494.
38. Ferrero E, Biswas P, Vettoretto K, Ferrarini M, Uguccioni M, et al. (2003) Macrophages exposed to Mycobacterium tuberculosis release chemokines able to recruit selected leucocyte subpopulations: focus on gammadelta cells. Immunology 108: 365–374.
39. Ruhwald M, Bodmer T, Maier C, Jepsen M, Haaland MB, et al. (2008) Evaluating the potential of IP-10 and MCP-2 as biomarkers for the diagnosis of tuberculosis. Eur Respir J 32: 1607–1615.

5

Serum IgA Responses against Pertussis Proteins in Infected and Dutch wP or aP Vaccinated Children: An Additional Role in Pertussis Diagnostics

Lotte H. Hendrikx[1,2]*, Kemal Öztürk[1], Lia G. H. de Rond[1], Sabine C. de Greeff[1], Elisabeth A. M. Sanders[3], Guy A. M. Berbers[1], Anne-Marie Buisman[1]

1 Centre for Infectious Disease and Control (CIb), National Institute for Public Health and the Environment, Bilthoven, The Netherlands, **2** Research Centre Linnaeus institute, Spaarne Hospital Hoofddorp, Hoofddorp, The Netherlands, **3** Department of Pediatric Immunology and Infectious Diseases, University Medical Centre Utrecht, Utrecht, The Netherlands

Abstract

Background: Whooping cough is a respiratory disease caused by *Bordetella pertussis*, which induces mucosal IgA antibodies that appear to be relevant in protection. Serum IgA responses are measured after pertussis infection and might provide an additional role in pertussis diagnostics. However, the possible interfering role for pertussis vaccinations in the induction of serum IgA antibodies is largely unknown.

Methods/Principal Findings: We compared serum IgA responses in healthy vaccinated children between 1 and 10 years of age with those in children who despite vaccinations recently were infected with *Bordetella pertussis*. All children have been vaccinated at 2, 3, 4 and 11 months of age with either the Dutch whole-cell pertussis (wP) vaccine or an acellular pertussis (aP) vaccine and additionally received an aP booster vaccination at 4 years of age. Serum IgA responses to pertussis toxin (PT), filamentous heamagglutinin (FHA) and pertactin (Prn) were measured with a fluorescent multiplex bead-based immuno-assay. An ELISPOT-assay was used for the detection of IgA-memory B-cells specific to these antigens. Serum IgA levels to all pertussis vaccine antigens were significantly higher in infected children compared with healthy children. High correlations between anti-PT, anti-FHA or anti-Prn IgA and IgG levels were found in infected children and to some degree in wP primed children, but not at all in aP primed children. Highest numbers of IgA-pertussis-specific memory B-cells were observed after infection and generally comparable numbers were found after wP and aP vaccination.

Conclusions: This study provides new insight in the diagnostic role for serum IgA responses against PT in vaccinated children. Since aP vaccines induce high serum IgG levels that interfere with pertussis diagnostics, serum IgA-PT levels will provide an additional diagnostic role. High levels of serum IgA for PT proved specific for recent pertussis infection with reasonable sensitivity, whereas the role for IgA levels against FHA and Prn in diagnosing pertussis remains controversial.

Editor: Geetha P. Bansal, Tulane University, United States of America

Funding: This study is funded by the Dutch government. The funders had no role in study design, data collection and analysis, decision to publish, or preparation of the manuscript.

Competing Interests: The authors have declared that no competing interests exist.

* E-mail: Lotte.Hendrikx@rivm.nl

Introduction

B.pertussis establishes infection by attaching to epithelial cells on the human respiratory tract, where toxins are released that cause local and systemic damage [1]. At the mucosal surface, secretory IgA, a dimeric complex, represents the predominant antibody isotype and functions as a first line of defense. The role of serum IgA is less clear. Circulating serum IgA is mainly monomeric and is considered a second line of defense, mediating elimination of pathogens that have breached the mucosal surface [2]. Serum IgA facilitates antibody-dependent cell-mediated cytotoxity and phagocytosis. However, information about the induction of serum IgA and its role after either pertussis vaccination or infection in children is complicated to interpret. Previous studies showed an increase in serum anti-pertussis IgA responses after infection, but not after whole-cell (wP) vaccination in children and adults [3,4,5,6,7,8,9]. In contrast, others demonstrated increased IgA responses to the pertussis vaccine components after acellular pertussis (aP) vaccination in adolescents and adults [10,11,12]. However, these serum IgA responses might result from earlier priming by (subclinical) infection. Since the last two decades whooping cough is reemerging in countries with widespread pertussis vaccination coverage, especially in the adolescent and adult population. In most of these countries a wP pertussis vaccine was replaced by an aP vaccine in the 1990s. A serum IgG level against PT above 50–100 IU/ml is currently used for pertussis diagnostics [13]. However, aP vaccines also induce high IgG-PT levels that interfere with pertussis diagnostics. Whether the value of anti-pertussis IgA levels could be indicative for recent infection with *B.pertussis* is a long topic of debate and the possible interfering effects of wP and aP vaccinations on the interpretation of IgA results have not been studied before. Therefore, we evaluated the IgA responses to pertussis toxin (PT), filamentous heamagglutinin (FHA) and pertactin (Prn) in children between 1 and 10 years of age who were vaccinated with either the Dutch wP or aP vaccine at 2, 3, 4 and 11 months of age and additionally received an aP preschool booster vaccination. We compared serum IgA levels in healthy vaccinated children with those in vaccinated children of the same ages who despite previous vaccinations recently were infected with *B.pertussis*.

Methods

Ethics Statement

All studies were conducted according to the Declaration of Helsinki, Good Clinical Practice Guidelines with the approval of the relevant ethics review committee (Medisch Ethische Toestingscommissie (METC) in Almere, the Netherlands and the Central Committee on Research Involving Human Subjects (CCMO), the Hague, the Netherlands). Written informed consent was obtained from parents or legal representatives before the start of the study.

Study population

Healthy children of different ages (12 months, 3, 4, 6 and 9 years) included in this study originated from three different cohort studies; (1) 51 children 12 months of age from whom one blood sample was taken at one month after the routine 4th vaccination at 11 months (ISRCTN97785537); (2) 580 children of 3, 4 or 6 years of age with one blood sample at the presented ages or children aged 4 years with one blood sample either before or 10 days or 28 days after the preschool booster vaccination (ISRCTN65428640) [14]; 75 children 9 years of age with sequential blood samples before, one month and one year after a second aP booster vaccination at 9 years of age (ISRCTN64117538) (figure 1). In addition, a fourth cohort consisted of 73 children 1 to 10 years of age who were vaccinated according to the national immunization program (NIP, see below) but in whom a recent pertussis infection was diagnosed [15]. Recent pertussis infection was defined as having a high single serum anti-IgG-PT level (>100 U/ml) or a positive PCR confirmation. One blood sample was taken per child on average 42 days (range 3–119 days) after the first symptoms of whooping cough.

Vaccinations

All healthy and infected children had received either the Dutch whole-cell pertussis vaccine (DTwP-IPV- Hib, NVI, Bilthoven, the Netherlands) or an acellular vaccine (DTaP-IPV- Hib, *Infanrix-IPV-Hib*^{TM}, GlaxoSmithKline Biologicals S.A., Rixensart, Belgium) at 2, 3, 4 and 11 months of age according to the NIP. The Dutch wP vaccine was replaced by an aP vaccine in 2005. Therefore, subgroups of children of 12 months of age had received either 4 injections of wP or 4 of aP vaccines at 2, 3, 4 and 11 months of age and a third subgroup had received 3 wP vaccinations at 2, 3 and 4 months of age and one aP vaccination at 11 months of age. In children 4 years and older, an additional preschool booster vaccination with either ACV-SB or *Infanrix*^{TM} (both from GSK) or with *Triaxis*^{TM} (Sanofi Pasteur, Lille, France) was administered at 4 years of age. ACV-SB and *Infanrix*^{TM} both contained the same amounts of pertussis antigens (high-dose); 25 μg of PT, 25 μg of FHA and 8 μg of Prn, whereas *Triaxis*^{TM} contained 2.5 μg of PT, 5 μg of FHA, 3 μg of Prn and 5 μg of combined fimbriae type 2 and 3 (Fim2/3) (low-dose) [14].

Children 9 years of age had received a second aP booster vaccination, *Boostrix-IPV*^{TM} (GSK), that contained 8 μg of PT, 8 μg of FHA and 2.5 μg of Prn. Of the 73 children who had been infected with *B.pertussis*, 71 children had been vaccinated according to the NIP (63 wP primed children and 8 aP primed children) and 2 children (7 and 8 years of age) had not received any pertussis vaccination before infection.

Serological assays

For measurement of plasma IgA levels directed against the 3 *B. pertussis* vaccine antigens (PT, FHA and Prn) the fluorescent bead-based multiplex immunoassay (MIA) was used as previously described [14,16] with some modifications. To prevent possible inter-immunoglobulin isotype competition, plasma samples were depleted of IgG by adding GullSORB (10:1 vol/vol) (meridian Bioscience Inc., Cincinnati, OH). Moreover, 50 μl of a 1/100 dilution of Goat F(ab′)2-anti-Human IgA was added to each well for 30 minutes before adding 50 μl R-Phycoerythrin conjugated Goat anti-Mouse IgA (Southern Biotechnologies, Alabama). The in-house reference serum was calibrated against the human reference pertussis antiserum lot 3 for PT and FHA and lot 4 for Prn (CBER, FDA). Next to in-house controls in a single dilution, a 3-fold serial dilution of the reference serum was added over 8 wells on each plate. Serum IgA antibodies against a crude cell-membrane preparation of *B.pertussis* were previously measured with an in-house ELISA as described earlier [15].

B-cell isolation, stimulation and ELISPOT-assays

In 149 randomly selected healthy and infected children between 3 and 10 years of age (on average 10 per group, range 5–17), we performed total IgA and at least one pertussis antigen-specific enzyme-linked immunospot (ELISPOT)-assays as previously described [17,18]. Plates were coated with 10 μg/ml anti-human IgA-Fc-specific and incubated the plate with alkaline phosphatase conjugated goat anti-human IgA for the detection of IgA-specific memory B-cells to the pertussis antigens [17,18]. Mean spot values of the non-coated wells were used as negative controls. From all mean spot values of the antigen-coated wells per sample, the negative controls were subtracted. The numbers of antigen-specific IgA-memory B-cells were presented per 10^5 B-cells. Due to low numbers of IgA antigen-specific memory B-cells, we presented the percentage of children with at least 1 antigen-specific memory B-cell and defined this as a positive memory B-cell response.

Statistical methods

Anti-PT, anti-FHA and anti-Prn IgA levels were expressed as geometric mean concentrations (GMCs) with a 95% confidence interval (CI). A positive IgA response was defined as an IgA level above 1 EU/ml for PT, FHA and Prn. The Mann-Whitney-U-test was used for comparison between the different groups. To analyze the correlation between variables Spearman correlations (r_s) and linear regression analysis was used. $P<0.05$ was considered significantly different.

Results

IgA levels after wP or aP vaccinations or pertussis infection

Infected children showed significant higher IgA responses to PT, FHA and Prn than both Dutch wP and aP primed healthy children at 1, 3, 4, 6 and 9 years of age (figure 2). In addition, a positive PT-, FHA- and Prn-specific IgA response was found in 84%, 78% and 80% of the infected children respectively, whereas 6%, 58% and 75% of the wP primed children aged 4 years and

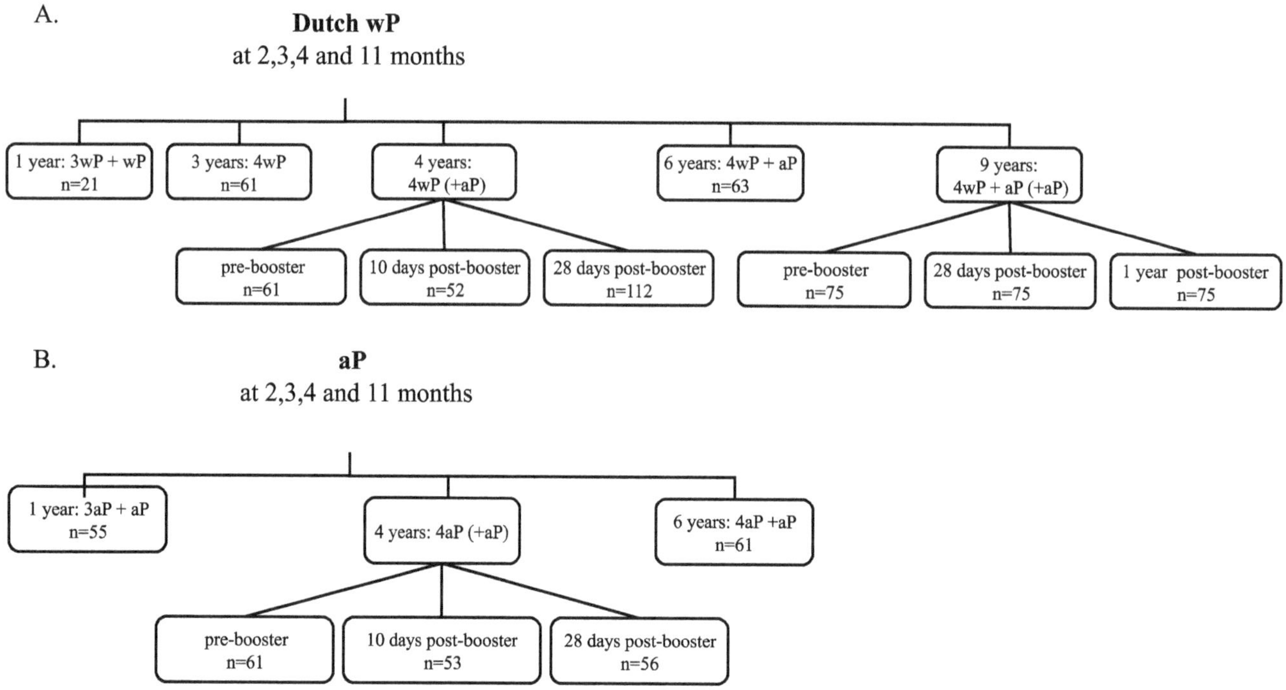

Figure 1. The number of healthy children per age group. (A) children primed with the Dutch wP vaccine and (B) children primed with aP vaccines.

0%, 24% and 44% of the aP primed children aged 4 years showed a positive IgA response at day 10 after the preschool booster vaccination, respectively (data not shown). IgA responses to all 3 antigens were positive in 62% of the infected children, but only 9% of all wP primed children (pre- and post-booster) and in 0% of all aP primed children. In wP primed children at 4 years of age significantly higher post-booster FHA- and Prn-responses were observed and at 6 years of age significantly higher FHA-responses were shown compared with aP primed children of the same ages (figure 2). Five years after the preschool booster at 4 years of age in wP primed children of 9 years of age, anti-pertussis IgA responses had returned to pre-booster levels. However, all pertussis-specific IgA responses significantly increased after a second booster vaccination at 9 years of age and after one-year follow-up anti-FHA and anti-Prn IgA levels still significantly exceeded pre-booster levels.

The effect of the time of blood sampling on IgA responses

In infected children that were older than 4 years significantly higher IgA responses to PT and FHA were observed compared with children younger than 4 years, at least in those children where blood sampling had occured within 30–60 days after the start of clinical symptoms of whooping cough (table 1). After 60 days, GMCs of anti-PT, anti-FHA and anti-Prn IgA levels were comparable in children above 4 years of age compared with those younger than 4 years.

Correlation between IgA and IgG levels

High correlations between anti-PT, anti-FHA and anti-Prn IgA and IgG levels were found in infected children and to some degree in Dutch wP primed children, but not in aP primed children (figure 3). For FHA and Prn, highest correlations were observed in infected and wP primed children, while for PT only a high correlation between IgA and IgG levels was found in infected children. Low correlations for FHA and Prn were found in aP primed children.

As IgA levels against pertussis crude cell-membranes (IgA-Bp) were used for pertussis diagnostics in several countries, we correlated these levels with our pertussis vaccine antigen-specific IgA levels in infected children. No correlation between serum IgA-Bp antibodies and serum IgA levels against PT was found, while IgA-Bp levels correlated with anti-FHA IgA levels and to a lesser extent with serum anti-Prn levels (figure 4).

Pertussis-specific IgA memory B-cells responses

The percentage of total IgA-producing memory B-cells in infected children (on average 6.8%) was significantly higher than in the healthy children (on average 3.0%). Also, the number of PT-, FHA- and Prn-specific memory B-cells was significantly higher in infected children as compared to healthy children. Between the healthy Dutch wP and aP primed children of different ages, no differences in percentages of total IgA-producing B-cells and no differences in the number of PT-, FHA- and Prn-specific memory B-cell responses were found (data not shown). In general, about 50% of the children showed a positive PT-, FHA- or Prn-specific memory B-cell response (table 2). The majority of the Dutch wP primed children at 9 years of age showed PT-, FHA- and Prn-specific memory B-cells 28 days after the second booster vaccination. Remarkably, 4/5 of the aP primed children at 4 years of age showed already FHA-specific memory B-cells even before the preschool booster vaccination.

Discussion

In this study we showed an increased serum IgA level against PT in vaccinated children who had recently been infected with *B.pertussis*, but not in healthy aP vaccinated children and only in a few Dutch wP vaccinated children. Remarkably, the high

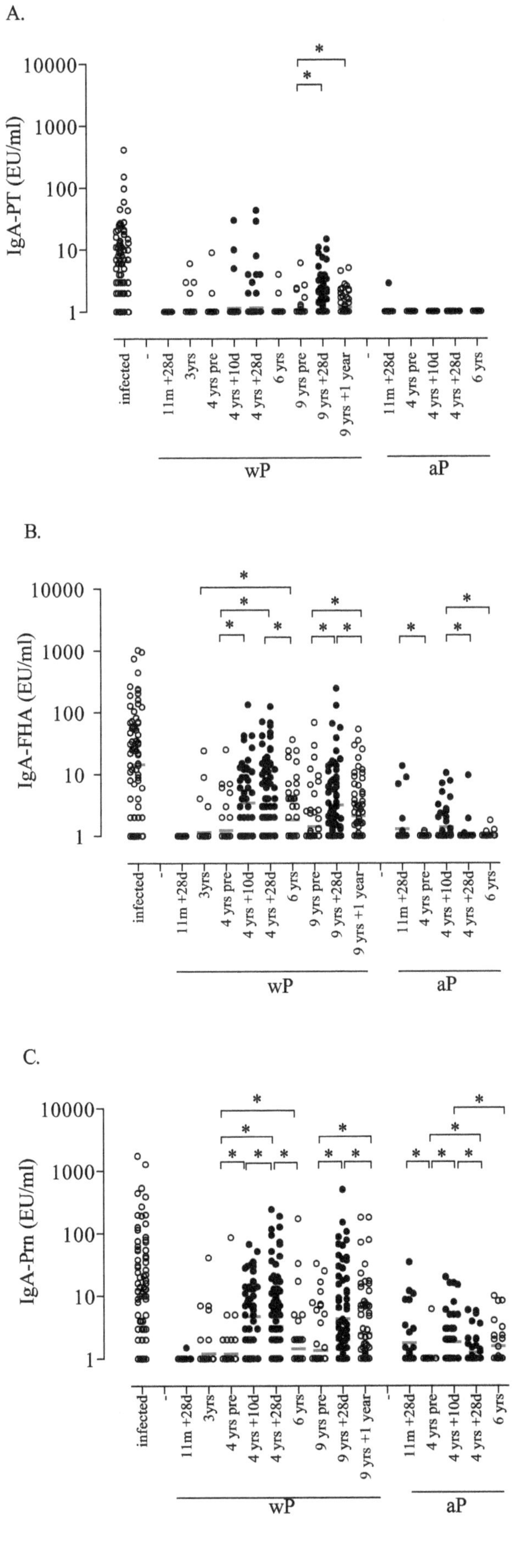

Figure 2. IgA levels. IgA responses specific for PT (A), FHA (B) and Prn (C) for each child in the on the *x*-axis presented group of children. The red horizontal bars indicate the GMC. The 10 and 28 days post-booster responses are indicated by the black circles and all other groups are indicate by open circles. * significant differences ($p<0.05$) are indicated for the healthy children between the presented age groups in similar primed children. Differences between infected children and the various groups of healthy wP and aP primed children are described in paragraph 3.1 of the results section.

correlation between serum IgA and IgG anti-PT antibodies in infected children, but not in the healthy wP and aP vaccinated children, strengthens the role of serum PT-specific IgA as a diagnostic parameter for pertussis also in the vaccinated population. We found that anti-PT IgA levels in serum had a high specificity and a reasonable sensitivity. Since aP vaccinations induce high levels of IgG antibodies against PT, the presence of serum IgA-PT responses will help to differentiate between vaccine induced antibody levels and those induced by natural infection. Only 6% of the Dutch wP primed children showed a positive IgA-response for PT shortly after the preschool booster with an aP vaccine. Interestingly, this percentage is concurrent with the sero-prevalence of pertussis in children in the Netherlands at the time the study was conducted [19]. In these children who might have been primed by previous exposure to *B.pertussis* leading to (subclinical) infection, serum IgA-PT levels could consequently have increased again after re-stimulation by booster vaccination. The overall absence of anti-PT antibodies in aP primed children suggests that infection has not occurred in these children. This implicitly demonstrates that the implementation of the aP vaccine for infant immunization has led to improved protection against whooping cough in young children in the Netherlands as previous data already suggested [19,20]. The absence of a dose-response effect for IgA levels after pertussis booster vaccination with low or high pertussis antigen content in both Dutch wP and aP primed healthy children at 4 years of age actually emphasizes that priming for pertussis-specific IgA responses is induced by infection rather than by vaccination. Moreover, as 6% of the population is suggested to be annually infected with *B.pertussis* [19], about half of our wP primed children 9 years of age should show an elevated serum IgA-PT level at one month after the booster as is confirmed by our data (32/75 children 9 years of age).

The role for IgA levels against the other pertussis antigens FHA and Prn in pertussis diagnostics remains controversial. Serum IgA responses against FHA and Prn were not limited to the infected children only, but were also observed in healthy Dutch wP primed and to a lesser extent in healthy aP primed children. Moreover, serum IgA responses against pertussis crude cell-membranes also lack specificity and correlated with the *B.pertussis* non specific anti-FHA levels, but only marginally with the *B.pertussis* specific anti-PT levels. Since FHA and Prn are adhesion factors of *B.pertussis*, these antibodies might illustrate the ongoing circulation of *B.pertussis*. Moreover, while PT is a toxin unique to *B.pertussis*, Prn antigen also belongs to other *Bordetellae* species [21] and other organisms also induce FHA antibodies [22,23]. As our previous studies already indicated [14,18] the Prn component in the aP vaccine seemed to be highly immunogenic resulting in extremely high IgG-Prn levels after aP vaccination. This high immunogenicity may also explain the small increase in IgA-Prn levels observed in several children in the aP vaccinated groups of 12 months and 6 years of age. The GMCs of the PT, FHA and Prn IgA antibodies in the infected children are in agreement with those previously measured in *B.pertussis* confirmed infected adults with unknown pertussis vaccination-history [7,24]. Moreover, a small increase in

Table 1. The effect of the time of blood sampling since the start of pertussis symptoms on serum IgA responses to PT, FHA and Prn in children younger and older than 4 years of age.

			IgA-PT		IgA-FHA		IgA-Prn	
Children <4 years		**n=**	**GMC**	**95% CI**	**GMC**	**95% CI**	**GMC**	**95% CI**
Timepoint	<30 days	13	4.3	2.3–8.2	7.1	2.9–17.5	13.5	3.2–57.0
	30–60 days	17	7.0	4.2–11.8	14.5	5.5–38.4	15.2	4.6–50.3
	>60 days	9	3.6	1.2–11.1	18.8	1.1–336.2	16.5	0.9–310.5
Children >4 years		**n=**	**GMC**	**95% CI**	**GMC**	**95% CI**	**GMC**	**95% CI**
Timepoint	<30 days	13	11.5	4.4–29.7	16.6	5.0–55.4	11.7	5.5–25.0
	30–60 days	11	14.8*#	8.9–24.4	93.8∫#	41.1–214.1	18.3	8.4–39.7
	>60 days	12	3.4	1.1–10.4	14.6	1.3–163.7	21.5	3.3–139.2

*significantly higher as compared to >60 days GMC.
∫significantly higher as compared to <30 days GMC.
#significantly higher as compared to GMC at same time point in children <4 years of age.

anti-PT IgA levels and a higher increase in anti-FHA and anti-Prn IgA levels after an aP booster vaccination have also been observed in some adolescents and adults [10,11,12] and are in line with our findings in children.

It was previously suggested that serum IgA-PT antibodies represent recent infection, but only 50% of children with pertussis actually showed an IgA-PT response [25]. In an Australian study the sensitivities of whole-cell, PT, FHA or Prn IgA assays varied between 24% and 64% [4]. In our study, however, we found 80% sensitivity of serum anti-PT IgA levels in pertussis infected children that proved independent of the time of blood sampling. As the MIA is a highly accurate and sensitive assay, even in the lower limit of quantification, the minimal defined level of 1 EU/ml for a positive IgA immune response is justified. Future monitoring of serum IgA antibodies in the young aP primed population will be useful to further corroborate the role of serum IgA antibodies in single serum diagnostics for pertussis.

Surprisingly, despite lower serum anti-pertussis IgA levels in healthy aP primed children compared with healthy wP primed children, comparable numbers of children from both groups showed detectable circulating pertussis-specific IgA memory B-cells. Antigen-specific IgA memory B-cells are derived in the mucosa associated lymphoid tissue and migrate via the blood to the secretory effector sites, e.g. the oral mucosa where sIgA is locally produced after antigen challenge [26]. This might explain why both wP and aP vaccinated children have comparable numbers of pertussis-specific IgA memory B-cells, since the contact with *B.pertussis* will be similar for both groups due to the high

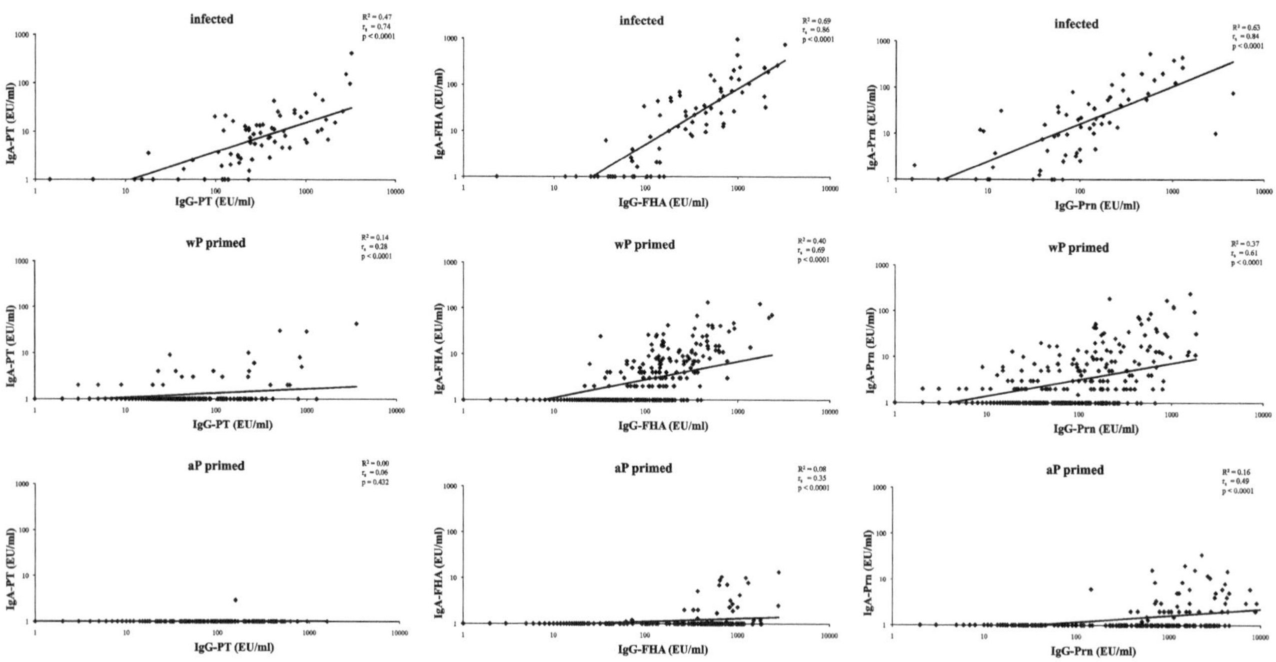

Figure 3. Correlations between serum IgA and IgG responses. Spearman correlations and linear regression analysis between serum IgA and serum IgG responses specific for PT, FHA and Prn presented for infected (A), wP (B) and aP (C) primed children.

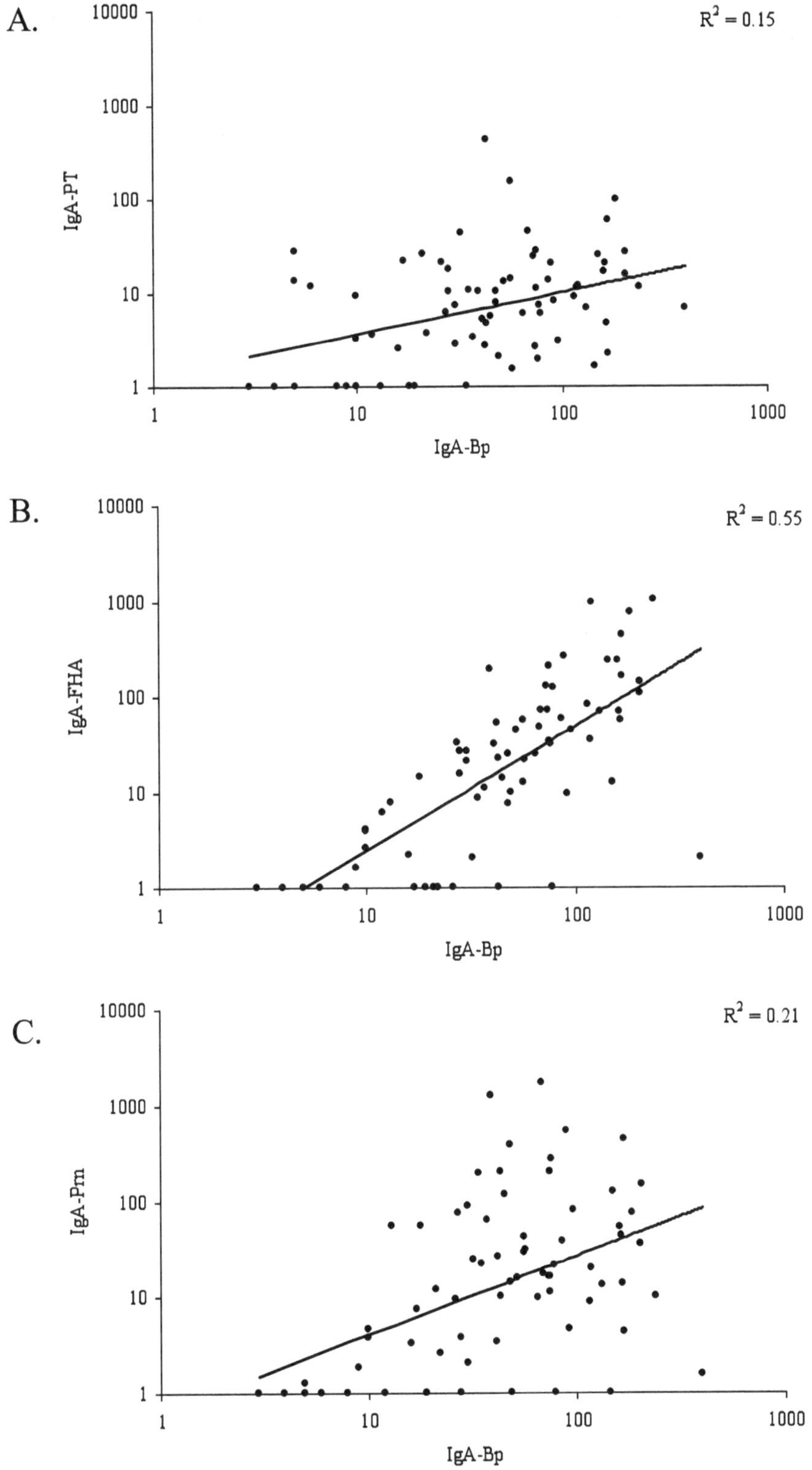

Figure 4. Correlations between serum IgA-Bp and IgA-PT, -FHA and -Prn in infected children. Serum IgA-Bp levels are presented on the *x*-axis and serum IgA-PT (A), -FHA (B) and -Prn (C) on the *y*-axis.

circulation. However, in the wP vaccinated group higher serum IgA responses were observed as compared to aP vaccinated children, probably because infection with *B.pertussis* occurs more frequently in this group. Moreover, we have previously shown that some years after vaccination pertussis specific IgG memory B-cells do not perse correlate with serum IgG levels [18]. In addition, long-lived plasmacells home to the bone marrow and locally produce background serum IgA levels [2]. However, it is unknown

Table 2. Percentages (%) of children with a positive PT-, FHA- and Prn- specific IgA- memory B-cell response in the infected and healthy Dutch wP primed and aP primed children of different ages (number of children per group).

	Infected	Dutch wP at 2, 3, 4 and 11 months								aP at 2, 3, 4 and 11 months			
age	1–10	3	4	4	4	6	9	9	9	4	4	4	6
post-booster	-	-	-	10 days	28 days	-	-	28 days	1 year	-	10 days	28 days	-
PT B-cells	70% (10)	42% (12)	62% (13)	38% (8)	45% (11)	45% (11)	58% (12)	63% (8)	60% (10)	43% (7)	50% (10)	29% (17)	21% (14)
FHA B-cells	70% (10)	22% (9)	54% (13)	17% (6)	29% (7)	50% (12)	33% (6)	60% (5)	40% (5)	80% (5)	13% (8)	33% (12)	50% (14)
Prn B-cells	80% (10)	77% (13)	71% (14)	44% (9)	73% (11)	50% (12)	50% (12)	75% (8)	50% (10)	50% (10)	55% (11)	60% (15)	21% (14)

whether the serum IgA levels are either induced by circulating antigens or polyclonal stimulation or are a result of leakage from the mucosal surfaces into the circulation [26]. Only one study from 20 years ago showed a correlation for FHA and PT between serum IgA and IgA levels in saliva of pertussis-infected individuals. The diagnostic value of salivary IgA seemed rather weak for pertussis [27], whereas circulating pathogen-specific IgA antibodies might reflect those at the mucosal surfaces as demonstrated for rotavirus and poliovirus [28,29,30]. In general, mucosal IgA responses are important in the protection against pathogens as found in newborns and patients with IgA deficiency [31,32]. However, the role for serum IgA in protection against whooping cough remains unresolved. Murine studies showed that IgA exhibits bactericidal effector functions [33], whereas IgA was not required to clear *B.pertussis* [34]. In a recent murine study a superior protection and promising long-term immune response was found after a single intranasal dose of a live-attenuated *B.pertussis* vaccine, named BPZE1, compared to parenterally administred aP vaccines [35]. This suggest an important role for mucosal immune responses in protection against pertussis infection. In our study we found no serum IgA responses after aP vaccinations, whereas protection against pertussis has improved after implementation of these aP vaccines. Therefore, serum IgA antibodies do not seem to be essential for pertussis protection after parentarelly administered vaccines. However, after infection this situation might be different and it is very likely that IgA antibodies play an important role in the clearance of the infection at the mucosa. It will be important to further elucidate anti-PT IgA levels in aP primed individuals who have been infected, to prove the role for serum anti-PT IgA levels in diagnostics. Moreover, the effect of different pertussis vaccinations as well as natural infection on salivary IgA will be important to further elucidate the role of mucosal IgA in protection against whooping cough [31,32,33,34,35].

In conclusion, we demonstrated that a high specificity of serum IgA levels against PT with a reasonable sensitivity recent pertussis infection in Dutch wP and aP vaccinated children. While infection induced anti-PT IgA antibodies, pertussis vaccines clearly did not. Especially in the aP vaccinated population, serum IgA-PT responses will be of great value for the diagnostics of pertussis. A better understanding of serum and mucosal IgA responses and their role in protection against whooping cough should finally result in a further improvement of the pertussis vaccines for infants.

Acknowledgments

We would like to thank all the children who participated in these studies. In addition, we would like to thank all the research staff from the Spaarne Hospital Hoofddorp and from the National Institute for Public Health and the Environment in Bilthoven.

Author Contributions

Conceived and designed the experiments: A-MB GAMB. Performed the experiments: LHH KO LGHdR. Analyzed the data: LHH. Contributed reagents/materials/analysis tools: LHH SCdG. Wrote the paper: LHH A-MB GAMB EAMS.

References

1. Parton R (1999) Review of the biology of Bordetella pertussis. Biologicals 27: 71–76.
2. Woof JM, Kerr MA (2006) The function of immunoglobulin A in immunity. J Pathol 208: 270–282.
3. Nagel J, Poot-Scholtens EJ (1983) Serum IgA antibody to Bordetella pertussis as an indicator of infection. J Med Microbiol 16: 417–426.
4. Poynten M, Hanlon M, Irwig L, Gilbert GL (2002) Serological diagnosis of pertussis: evaluation of IgA against whole cell and specific Bordetella pertussis antigens as markers of recent infection. Epidemiol Infect 128: 161–167.
5. Novotny P, Macaulay ME, Hart TC, Skvaril F (1991) Analysis of antibody profiles in children with whooping cough. Dev Biol Stand 73: 267–273.
6. Heininger U, Cherry JD, Stehr K (2004) Serologic response and antibody-titer decay in adults with pertussis. Clin Infect Dis 38: 591–594.
7. Deen JL, Mink CA, Cherry JD, Christenson PD, Pineda EF, et al. (1995) Household contact study of Bordetella pertussis infections. Clin Infect Dis 21: 1211–1219.
8. Bonhoeffer J, Bar G, Riffelmann M, Soler M, Heininger U (2005) The role of Bordetella infections in patients with acute exacerbation of chronic bronchitis. Infection 33: 13–17.
9. Thomas MG, Ashworth LA, Miller E, Lambert HP (1989) Serum IgG, IgA, and IgM responses to pertussis toxin, filamentous hemagglutinin, and agglutinogens 2 and 3 after infection with Bordetella pertussis and immunization with whole-cell pertussis vaccine. J Infect Dis 160: 838–845.
10. Le T, Cherry JD, Chang SJ, Knoll MD, Lee ML, et al. (2004) Immune responses and antibody decay after immunization of adolescents and adults with an acellular pertussis vaccine: the APERT Study. J Infect Dis 190: 535–544.
11. Littmann M, Hulsse C, Riffelmann M, Wirsing von Konig CH (2008) Long-term immunogenicity of a single dose of acellular pertussis vaccine in paediatric health-care workers. Vaccine 26: 2344–2349.
12. Knuf M, Zepp F, Meyer C, Grzegowski E, Wolter J, et al. (2006) Immunogenicity of a single dose of reduced-antigen acellular pertussis vaccine in a non-vaccinated adolescent population. Vaccine 24: 2043–2048.
13. Guiso N, Berbers G, Fry NK, He Q, Riffelmann M, et al. (2010) What to do and what not to do in serological diagnosis of pertussis: recommendations from EU reference laboratories. Eur J Clin Microbiol Infect Dis.
14. Hendrikx LH, Berbers GA, Veenhoven RH, Sanders EA, Buisman AM (2009) IgG responses after booster vaccination with different pertussis vaccines in Dutch children 4 years of age: effect of vaccine antigen content. Vaccine 27: 6530–6536.
15. de Greeff SC, Mooi FR, Westerhof A, Verbakel JM, Peeters MF, et al. (2010) Pertussis disease burden in the household: how to protect young infants. Clin Infect Dis 50: 1339–1345.

16. van Gageldonk PG, van Schaijk FG, van der Klis FR, Berbers GA (2008) Development and validation of a multiplex immunoassay for the simultaneous determination of serum antibodies to Bordetella pertussis, diphtheria and tetanus. J Immunol Methods 335: 79–89.
17. Buisman AM, de Rond CG, Ozturk K, Ten Hulscher HI, van Binnendijk RS (2009) Long-term presence of memory B-cells specific for different vaccine components. Vaccine 28: 179–186.
18. Hendrikx LH, Ozturk K, de Rond LG, Veenhoven RH, Sanders EA, et al. (2011) Identifying long-term memory B-cells in vaccinated children despite waning antibody levels specific for Bordetella pertussis proteins. Vaccine 29: 1431–1437.
19. de Greeff SC, de Melker HE, van Gageldonk PG, Schellekens JF, van der Klis FR, et al. (2010) Seroprevalence of Pertussis in the Netherlands: Evidence for Increased Circulation of Bordetella pertussis. PLoS One 5: e14183.
20. de Greeff SC, Mooi FR, Schellekens JF, de Melker HE (2008) Impact of acellular pertussis preschool booster vaccination on disease burden of pertussis in The Netherlands. Pediatr Infect Dis J 27: 218–223.
21. Inatsuka CS, Xu Q, Vujkovic-Cvijin I, Wong S, Stibitz S, et al. (2010) Pertactin is required for Bordetella species to resist neutrophil-mediated clearance. Infect Immun 78: 2901–2909.
22. Vincent JM, Cherry JD, Nauschuetz WF, Lipton A, Ono CM, et al. (2000) Prolonged afebrile nonproductive cough illnesses in American soldiers in Korea: a serological search for causation. Clin Infect Dis 30: 534–539.
23. Isacson J, Trollfors B, Taranger J, Lagergard T (1995) Acquisition of IgG serum antibodies against two Bordetella antigens (filamentous hemagglutinin and pertactin) in children with no symptoms of pertussis. Pediatr Infect Dis J 14: 517–521.
24. Cherry JD, Beer T, Chartrand SA, DeVille J, Beer E, et al. (1995) Comparison of values of antibody to Bordetella pertussis antigens in young German and American men. Clin Infect Dis 20: 1271–1274.
25. von Linstow ML, Pontoppidan PL, von Konig CH, Cherry JD, Hogh B (2010) Evidence of Bordetella pertussis infection in vaccinated 1-year-old Danish children. Eur J Pediatr 169: 1119–1122.
26. Brandtzaeg P (2007) Do salivary antibodies reliably reflect both mucosal and systemic immunity? Ann N Y Acad Sci 1098: 288–311.
27. Zackrisson G, Lagergard T, Trollfors B, Krantz I (1990) Immunoglobulin A antibodies to pertussis toxin and filamentous hemagglutinin in saliva from patients with pertussis. J Clin Microbiol 28: 1502–1505.
28. Franco MA, Angel J, Greenberg HB (2006) Immunity and correlates of protection for rotavirus vaccines. Vaccine 24: 2718–2731.
29. Gonzalez R, Franco M, Sarmiento L, Romero M, Schael IP (2005) Serum IgA levels induced by rotavirus natural infection, but not following immunization with the RRV-TV vaccine (Rotashield), correlate with protection. J Med Virol 76: 608–612.
30. Buisman AM, Abbink F, Schepp RM, Sonsma JA, Herremans T, et al. (2008) Preexisting poliovirus-specific IgA in the circulation correlates with protection against virus excretion in the elderly. J Infect Dis 197: 698–706.
31. Hanson LA, Korotkova M (2002) The role of breastfeeding in prevention of neonatal infection. Semin Neonatol 7: 275–281.
32. Brandtzaeg P (1995) The role of humoral mucosal immunity in the induction and maintenance of chronic airway infections. Am J Respir Crit Care Med 151: 2081–2086; discussion 2086–2087.
33. Hellwig SM, van Spriel AB, Schellekens JF, Mooi FR, van de Winkel JG (2001) Immunoglobulin A-mediated protection against Bordetella pertussis infection. Infect Immun 69: 4846–4850.
34. Wolfe DN, Kirimanjeswara GS, Goebel EM, Harvill ET (2007) Comparative role of immunoglobulin A in protective immunity against the Bordetellae. Infect Immun 75: 4416–4422.
35. Feunou PF, Kammoun H, Debrie AS, Mielcarek N, Locht C (2010) Long-term immunity against pertussis induced by a single nasal administration of live attenuated B. pertussis BPZE1. Vaccine 28: 7047–7053.

6

High Prevalence of Extended-Spectrum Beta Lactamases among *Salmonella enterica* Typhimurium Isolates from Pediatric Patients with Diarrhea in China

Fangyou Yu[1], Qiang Chen[2], Xiaojun Yu[2], Qiaoqiao Li[3], Baixing Ding[4], Lehe Yang[3], Cong Chen[4], Zhiqiang Qin[5], Chris Parsons[5], Xueqing Zhang[1], Jinwei Huang[6], Yun Luo[7], Liangxing Wang[3]*, Jingye Pan[4]*

1 Department of Laboratory Medicine, The First Affiliated Hospital of Wenzhou Medical College, Wenzhou, China, **2** Department of Laboratory Medicine, Jiangxi Provincial Children Hospital, Nanchang, China, **3** Department of Respiratory Medicine, The First Affiliated Hospital of Wenzhou Medical College, Wenzhou, China, **4** Department of Intensive Care Unit, The First Affiliated Hospital of Wenzhou Medical College, Wenzhou, China, **5** Division of Infectious Diseases, Department of Medicine, Medical University of South Carolina, Charleston, South Carolina, United States of America, **6** Department of Laboratory Medicine, Lishui Center Hospital, Lishui, China, **7** Department of Microbiology, Zhejiang Provincial Center for Disease Control and Prevention, Hangzhou, China

Abstract

We investigated the extended-spectrum beta lactamases among 62 *Salmonella enterica* Typhimurium isolates recovered from children with diarrhea in a Chinese pediatric hospital. A large proportion of *S. enterica* Typhimurium isolates were resistant to multiple antimicrobial agents, including ampicillin (90.3%), tetracycline (80.6%), trimethoprim/sulfamethoxazole (74.2%), chloramphenicol (66.1%), cefotaxime (27.4%). Forty-nine (79.0%) of *S. enterica* Typhimurium isolates were positive for $bla_{TEM\text{-}1b}$ and resistant to ampicillin. Thirteen *S. enterica* Typhimurium isolates (21.0%) were positive for $bla_{CTX\text{-}M\text{-}1\text{-}group}$ and $bla_{CTX\text{-}M\text{-}9\text{-}group}$, and all isolates harboring $bla_{CTX\text{-}M}$ genes were positive for *IS*Ecp1. Two main clones (PFGE type A and D) accounted for nearly 70% of *S. enterica* Typhimurium isolates, and 7 CTX-M-producing isolates belonged to PFGE type D. Collectively, our data reveal multi-drug resistance and a high prevalence of extended spectrum beta lactamases among *S. enterica* Typhimurium isolates from children in China. In addition, we report the first identification of $bla_{CTX\text{-}M\text{-}55}$ within *Salmonella spp*. Our data also suggest that clonal spread is responsible for the dissemination of *S. enterica* Typhimurium isolates.

Editor: Stefan Bereswill, Charité-University Medicine Berlin, Germany

Funding: This work was supported by Medical Science Fund of Jiangxi Province, China (20094009; 20091256). The funders had no role in study design, data collection and analysis, decision to publish, or preparation of the manuscript.

Competing Interests: The authors have declared that no competing interests exist.

* E-mail: 081101072@fudan.edu.cn (JP); wzyxywlx@163.com (LW)

Introduction

Nontyphoidal *Salmonella* species, particularly *Salmonella enterica* Typhimurium, are the most common bacterial pathogens causing enteric infections among pediatric patients [1]. Antimicrobial agents are required for treating invasive infections caused by *Salmonella spp.*, and third-generation cephalosporins are commonly used to treat invasive infections or severe diarrhea because of their pharmacodynamic properties and the low prevalence of resistance [2]. However, increasing resistance to cephalosporins has been reported worldwide for *Salmonella spp.*, particularly *S. enterica* Typhimurium [3,4,5,6,7]. Resistance to broad-spectrum cephalosporins is often due to production of various plasmid-mediated β-lactamases, especially CTX-M-type extended-spectrum β-lactamases (ESBLs) [4,7,8,9]. Cefotaximases (CTX-M), comprised of five major CTX-M groups (1, 2, 8, 9, and 25), are associated with higher levels of hydrolytic activity against cefotaxime relative to ceftazidime and are distributed among a wide range of bacteria with clinical significance over a wide geographic area [10].

In China, a low prevalence of resistance to third-generation cephalosporins has been reported among *Salmonella spp.*, especially those isolated from pediatric patients [11,12]. The aim of the present study was to investigate the frequency of antimicrobial resistance and cephalosporin resistance genes within *S. enterica* isolates from pediatric inpatients with diarrhea in a Chinese pediatric hospital. However, high prevalence of broad spectrum cephalosporin resistance and ESBLs were found among *S. enterica* Typhimurium isolates from children in China.

Materials and Methods

Bacterial isolates

From May 2007 to March 2009, a total of 62 *S. enterica* Typhimurium isolates were collected from stool samples collected from 62 inpatients aged ranging from 39 days to five years old with diarrhea in Jiangxi provincial pediatric hospital in Nanchang, China. *S. enterica* Typhimurium isolates were identified using standard biochemical tests and commercial typing antiserum according to the manufacturer's instructions. O and H antigens were characterized by slide agglutination with hyperimmune sera (Chengdu Biotech, China) and the serotype was assigned according to the Kauffmann-White scheme. Among 62 inpatients included, 34 and 28 patients were male and female. The ages of the patients were as follows: 39 days −1 year old, 37 patients; 1–2 years old, 10 patients; 2–3 years old, 5 patients; 3–4 years old, 6 patients and 4–5 years old, 4 patients. The antimicrobial agents used for treating the infections by *S. enterica* Typhimurium included penicillin, azithromycin, amoxicillin/sulbactam, latamoxef, cefoperazone/sulbactam, ceftazidime, ampicillin/sulbactam, ceftriaxone, cefazolin, ceftizoxime, and imipenem. Of 62 patients with diarrhea, 7, 4, 4 and 2 patients suffered bronchitis, pharyngitis, acute tonsillitis and meningitis, respectively. After treated by antimicrobial agents, all patients were cured and left hospital. Persistance of diarrhea ranged from 7 to 40 days. Addition to *S. enterica* Typhimurium, *Campylobacter spp*, *enteropathogenic Escherichia coli* and *Shigella spp* were not isolated from the stools of the patients included. This study focused on bacterial, so ethics approval was not needed according to the Ethics Committee of Wenzhou Medical College's regulatioans.

Antimicrobial susceptibility

Antimicrobial susceptibility was determined by the disk diffusion method with 18 antimicrobial agents according to the criteria recommended by the CLSI [13], including including cefotaxime (30 μg), ceftazidime (30 μg), ampicillin (10 μg), aztreonam (30 μg), cefaclor (30 μg), cefoxitin (30 μg), piperacillin plus tazobactam (100/10 μg), imipenem (10 μg), meropenem (10 μg), chloramphenicol (30 μg), trimethoprim/sulfamethoxazole (1.25/23.75 μg), tobramycin (10 μg), gentamicin (10 μg), amikacin (30 μg), tetracycline (30 μg), nalidixic acid (30 μg), ciprofloxacin (5 μg), and levofloxacin (5 μg). MICs for cefotaxime and ceftazidime, were further determined by the agar dilution method in accordance with CLSI guidelines [13]. *Escherichia coli* ATCC 25922 was used as quality control strain for antimicrobial susceptibility testing.

Detection of resistance genes

Total DNA was extracted by boiling. Briefly, a fresh bacterial colony was suspended in 150 μL of sterile distilled water and boiled at 100°C for 10 minutes. After centrifugation at 15000 rpm for 15 minutes at 4°C, the supernatant was removed and stored at −20°C for PCR assays. PCR and DNA sequencing were performed for the detection of ESBL genes in all ampicillin-resistant isolates with oligonucleotide primers previously described, including those for bla_{TEM}, bla_{SHV}, bla_{CTX-M}, bla_{VEB} and bla_{PER} genes [14,15]. All amplicon sequences were compared with those in the GenBank nucleotide database (www.ncbi.nlm.nih.gov/blast/). PCR mapping experiments using combinations of the *ISEcp1* forward primers and the $bla_{CTX-M-1-group}$ or $bla_{CTX-M-9\ group}$ reverse primers were performed to detect the flanking regions of $bla_{CTX-M-1-group}$ and $bla_{CTX-M-9-group}$ genes.

Transfer of resistance genes

In order to determine whether cephalosporin resistance was transferable in *S. enterica* Typhimurium isolates, a conjugation experiment was carried out in Luria-Bertani broth with *E. coli* J53 as the recipient as previously described [16]. Transconjugants were selected on tryptic soy agar plates containing sodium azide (100 μg/mL) for counterselection and cefotaxime (30 μg/mL) for plasmid-mediated cephalosporin resistance selection.

Pulsed-field gel electrophoresis (PFGE)

Chromosomal DNA was prepared from all *S. enterica* Typhimurium isolates and cleaved with 40 U *Xba*I. Electrophoresis was performed on 1% agarose gels in 0.5 M Tris/borate/EDTA buffer on a CHEF-Mapper XA PFGE system (Bio-Rad, Hercules, CA) for 22 h at 14°C, with run conditions of 6 V/cm, a pulse angle of 120° and pulse times from 5 to 20 s. A λDNA ladder (Amersham Biosciences) was used to confirm molecular mass and bands stained with ethidium bromide (0.5 μg/mL) prior to their identification through photography under UV light. Comparison of the PFGE patterns was performed with Bionumerics software (Applied Maths, Sint-Martens-Latem, Belgium) using the Dice Similarity coefficient. Clusters were defined as DNA patterns sharing more than 85% similarity.

Results

Antimicrobial susceptibility

Of the 62 *S. enterica* Typhimurium isolates, 59 (95.2%) were resistant to at least three antimicrobial agents, while only 2 (3.2%) were susceptible to all antimicrobial agents tested. *S. enterica* Typhimurium isolates tested were most commonly resistant to ampicillin (90.3%, 56/62), followed by tetracycline (80.6%, 50/62), trimethoprim/sulfamethoxazole (74.2%, 46/62) and chloramphenicol (66.1%, 41/62). Seventeen (27.4%, 17/62) and 8 (8/62, 12.9%) isolates were resistant to cefotaxime (MIC range from 64 to >256 μg/mL) and ceftazidime (MIC range from 32 to >256 μg/mL), respectively. All ceftazidime-resistant isolates were also resistant to cefotaxime. Twelve isolates (19.4%, 12/62) were highly resistant to ciprofloxacin (MIC≥4 μg/mL). The frequencies of resistance and intermediate to other antimicrobial agents among *S. enterica* Typhimurium isolates were as follows: cefoxitin, 8.1% (5/62) and 1.6% (1/62); aztreonam, 16.1% (10/62) and 12.9% (8/62); cefaclor, 35.5% (22/62) and 0; ampicillin/sulbactam, 51.6% (32/62) and 25.8% (16/62); piperacillin/tazobactam, 19.4% (12/62) and 51.6% (32/62); amikacin, 17.7% (11/62) and 41.9% (26/62); gentamicin, 51.6% (32/62) and 6.5% (4/62); and tobramycin, 56.5% (35/62) and 17.7% (11/62). All isolates were susceptible to imipenem and meropenem.

β-lactam resistance genes

Forty-nine (79.0%) of 62 *S. enterica* Typhimurium isolates were positive for bla_{TEM} and resistant to ampicillin. All bla_{TEM} amplicons were confirmed as bla_{TEM-1b} by DNA sequencing. Thirteen *S. enterica* Typhimurium isolates (21.0%, 13/62) were positive for $bla_{CTX-M-1-group}$ and $bla_{CTX-M-9-group}$ genes (8 for $bla_{CTX-M-14}$, 3 for $bla_{CTX-M-15}$, 1 for $bla_{CTX-M-55}$, and 1 for both $bla_{CTX-M-14}$ and $bla_{CTX-M-55}$). Characteristics of *S. enterica* Typhimurium isolates producing ESBLs were showed in Figure 1.

Among the 8 CTX-M-14- producing isolates with MICs ranging from 128 to 256 μg/mL for cefotaxime, only one was highly resistant to ceftazidime (128 μg/mL) whereas the other 7 exhibited reduced susceptibility to ceftazidime (2–8 μg/mL). Three CTX-M-15- producing isolates with MICs ranging from 32 to 128 μg/mL for ceftazidime were highly resistant to cefotaxime (MIC>256 μg/mL). Two isolates harboring $bla_{CTX-M-55}$ were highly resistant to cefotaxime and ceftazidime (MICs>256 μg/mL). All isolates harboring bla_{CTX-M} genes were positive for *IS*Ecp1. Analysis of the flanking regions of bla_{CTX-M} genes showed that the insertion sequence *IS*Ecp1 was located 48 bp, 45 bp or 42 bp upstream from $bla_{CTX-M-15}$ (accession number GQ330540), $bla_{CTX-M-55}$ (accession number GQ456157) or $bla_{CTX-M-14}$ (accession number GQ385325), respectively.

Transfer of antimicrobial resistance genes

Extended-spectrum cephalosporin resistance could be transferred by conjugation from seven ESBL-producing donors (two isolates harboring $bla_{CTX-M-15}$, six harboring $bla_{CTX-M-14}$, and one harboring both $bla_{CTX-M-14}$ and $bla_{CTX-M-55}$). Seven cephalosporin resistance transconjugants were resistant to chloramphenicol and trimethoprim/sulfamethoxazole and harbored bla_{TEM-1b}.

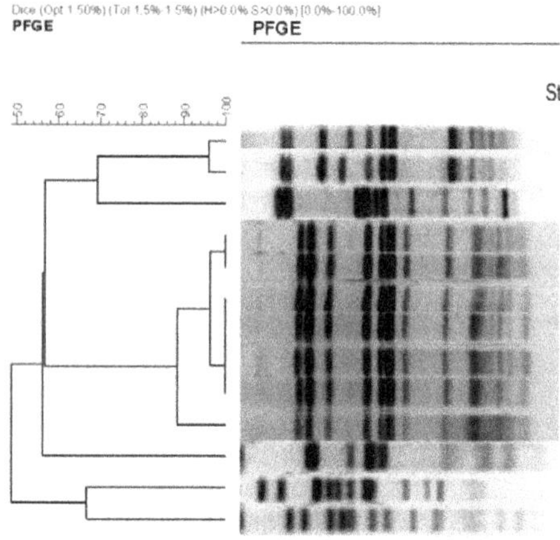

Strains	PFGE	CAZ	CTX	ISEcpl	Resistance phenotype	β-lactamase genes
S6	B	<1	128	+	CTX,CAZ,SAM,ATM,CN,AMP,CEC	blaTEM-1b,blaCTX-M-14
S71	B	8	256	+	CTX,C,SXT,TOB,CIP,TE,SAM,ATM,AMP,TZP,CN,CEC	blaTEM-1b, blaCTX-M-14
S49	H	128	>256	+	CTX,CAZ,C,ATM.AMP,CEC	blaTEM-1b, blaCTX-M-15
S30	D	>256	>256	+	CTX,CAZ,C,SXT,TOB,TE,SAM,ATM,.AMP,TZP,CN,CEC	blaTEM-1b, blaCTX-M-14, blaCTX-M-55
S55	D	4	256	+	CTX,C,SXT,TOB,TE,SAM,AMP,CEC	blaTEM-1b, blaCTX-M-14
S8	D	2	256	+	CTX,SXT,TE,SAM,AMP,CN,CEC	blaTEM-1b, blaCTX-M-14
S33	D	8	256	+	CTX,C,SXT,TOB,TE,SAM,AMP,CN,CEC	blaTEM-1b, blaCTX-M-14
S50	D	4	256	+	CTX,C,SXT,TOB,TE,SAM,ATM,AMP,CEC	blaTEM-1b, blaCTX-M-14
S39	D	>256	>256	+	CTX,CAZ,C,SXT,TE,SAM,AMP,ATM,TZP,CEC	blaTEM-1b, blaCTX-M-55
S16	D	2	128	+	CTX,C,SXT,TOB,TE,SAM,AMPC,CEC	blaTEM-1b, blaCTX-M-14
S65	F	128	256	+	CTX,CAZ,SXT,SAM,FOX,ATM,AMP,TZP,CN,CEC	blaTEM-1b, blaCTX-M-14
S26	I	32	>256	+	CTX,CAZ,ATM,AMP,CEC	blaTEM-1b, blaCTX-M-15
S67	G	128	>256	+	CTX,CAZ,C,SXT,TOB,TE,SAM,ATM,AMK,TZP,CEC	blaTEM-1b, blaCTX-M-15

Figure 1. Characteristics of *S. enterica* Typhimurium isolates producing ESBLs. CTX: cefotaxime; CAZ: ceftazidime; SXT: trimethoprim/sulfamethoxazole; TE: tetracycline; SAM: ampicillin plus sulbactam; AMP: ampicillin; CEC: cefaclor; TOB: tobramycin; CN: gentamicin; AMK: amikacin; TZP: piperacillin plus tazobactam; C: chloramphenicol.

PFGE

Ten different PFGE clusters were identified among the 62 *S. enterica* Typhimurium isolates. PFGE types A, B, and D accounted for 19.4% (12/62), 9.7% (6/62) and 50% (31/62) of these isolates, respectively. Thirteen ESBLs-producing isolates distributed in six FPGE clusters listed in Figure 1. Of the 8 CTX-M-14-producing *S. enterica* Typhimurium isolates, 5, 2 and 1 belonged to PFGE type D, B and I, respectively. Three CTX-M-15-producing isolates belonged to three different PFGE types (F, G and H). One CTX-M-55-producing isolate and both CTX-M-14 and CTX-M-55-producing isolates belonged to PFGE type D.

Discussion

The majority of *S. enterica* Typhimurium isolates in our study were resistant to multiple antimicrobial agents, indicating that fewer antibiotics may be useful for treating *S. enterica* Typhimurium infections. Carbapenems exhibit high antimicrobial activity against *S. enterica* Typhimurium isolates *in vitro* in our studies. The CLSI recommends that for fecal isolates of *Salmonella* and *Shigella spp.*, only ampicillin, fluoroquinolone, and trimethoprim/sulfamethoxazole sensitivities should be reported routinely, whereas for extraintestinal isolates of *Salmonella spp.*, only sensitivities to chloramphenicol and third-generation cephalosporins should be reported [13]. However, *S. enterica* Typhimurium resistance rates for ampicillin, trimethoprim/sulfamethoxazole and chloramphenicol were very high (more than 60%) in our studies. In addition, although no patient had received fluoroquinolones prior to isolation of *Salmonella spp.* from their stool, 48% and 19% of *S. Typhimurium* isolates exhibited low- or high-level resistance to ciprofloxacin, respectively. Therefore, our data suggest that ampicillin, trimethoprim/sulfamethoxazole, chloramphenicol and fluoroquinolones should be used with caution for the treatment of *S. enterica* Typhimurium infections in the pediatric population. ESBL- and AmpC-mediated resistance has been reported for nontyphoidal *Salmonella* isolates in many geographic areas [5,17,18,19]. However, reported resistance of nontyphoidal *Salmonella* isolates to broad-spectrum cephalosporins remains low [12,20,21]. In the study conducted in Wuhan, China using clinical samples from children ages 0–3 years, only 7 of 221 (3.2%) *S. enterica* isolates were resistant to ceftriaxone (10). In another study from the Henan province, only 2.1% of *S. enterica* Typhimurium patient isolates were resistant to ceftiofur over a 2-year timeframe [11,12]. Relative to these studies, the rates of resistance to broad-spectrum cephalosporins for *S. enterica* Typhimurium isolates in our study was very high.

Broad-spectrum cephalosporins are commonly used to treat serious *Salmonella* infections. ESBLs are the predominant cause of resistance to broad- spectrum cephalosporins in Enterobacteriaceae, particularly *E. coli* and *Klebsiella spp.* Therefore, understanding patterns and mechanisms for interspecies and intraspecies transfer of ESBLs is of great interest. The TEM-, SHV- and CTX-M-type ESBLs are the most widely distributed worldwide. Published reports indicate that CTX-M-type ESBLs are the most prevalent in China [22,23]. $bla_{CTX\text{-}M\text{-}14}$ and $bla_{CTX\text{-}M\text{-}15}$ genes have been identified in *S. enterica* Typhimurium isolates from many areas including China [4,7,11,12,24]. In the present study, CTX-M-type ESBLs, mainly CTX-M-14, were detected in *S. enterica* Typhimurium isolates, indicating that CTX-M-type ESBLs were the predominant cause of resistance to broad-spectrum cephalosporins for *S. enterica* Typhimurium isolates in our study. The mobile genetic element *IS*Ecp1, a single copy insertion sequence responsible for mobilization of *bla* genes and identified upstream of several $bla_{CTX\text{-}M}$ genes carried by *E. coli* and *Klebsiella spp* isolates, was found in association with all of our isolates. We speculate that the *S. enterica* Typhimurium isolates in China could have acquired the $bla_{CTX\text{-}M}$ genes from *E. coli* and *Klebsiella spp* in the community, and that subsequent spread of these genes among *S. enterica* Typhimurium isolates may have occurred. Future epidemiologic studies may confirm whether these genes were transmitted in this or perhaps other sequences, and the potential clinical implications of ESBL-mediated resistance for gastrointestinal and/or invasive infections caused by *S. Typhimurium*.

$bla_{CTX\text{-}M\text{-}55}$, which increases the catalytic efficiency against ceftazidime, is a variant of the $bla_{CTX\text{-}M\text{-}15}$ gene and previously found only in *E. coli* and *K. pneumonia spp.* in China and Thailand [25,26,27]. Interestingly, we found that two *S. enterica* Typhimurium isolates with resistance to both cefotaxime and ceftazidine harbored $bla_{CTX\text{-}M\text{-}55}$, and one of these harbored both $bla_{CTX\text{-}M\text{-}14}$ and $bla_{CTX\text{-}M\text{-}55}$. To our knowledge, this is the first report of $bla_{CTX\text{-}M\text{-}55}$ in *Salmonella spp.* Recently, 24 (24.5%) of 98 *E. coli* isolates recovered from pets in South China were found to harbor $bla_{CTX\text{-}M\text{-}55}$, among which 6 isolates harbored both $bla_{CTX\text{-}M\text{-}14}$ and $bla_{CTX\text{-}M\text{-}55}$ [25]. The partial DNA sequence of *IS*Ecp1 found 45 bp upstream of $bla_{CTX\text{-}M\text{-}55}$ in the single isolate in our study harboring both $bla_{CTX\text{-}M\text{-}14}$ and $bla_{CTX\text{-}M\text{-}55}$ was 100% identical to the corresponding sequences of $bla_{CTX-M-55}$ genes harbored by *E. coli* isolates from the pets in this study. We speculate that *E. coli* which either colonize or cause clinically apparent infection in pets may serve as a reservoir for $bla_{CTX-M-14}$ and $bla_{CTX-M-55}$ genes and, ultimately, cause clinically apparent infections in pediatric patients. Confirmation of this hypothesis, and the development of subsequent clinical strategies for limited these infections, would require additional comprehensive surveillance efforts among communities in China and elsewhere.

In our study, two main clusters (PFGE types A and D) were found, indicating that gastrointestinal infections in children were caused mainly by clonally related *S. enterica* Typhimurium isolates and clonal spread was responsible for the dissemination of *S. enterica* Typhimurium. Because 5 isolates harboring $bla_{CTX-M-14}$ genes and two isolates harboring $bla_{CTX-M-55}$ genes belonged to the same PFGE cluster (D), the spread of $bla_{CTX-M-14}$ and $bla_{CTX-M-55}$ genes was also associated with clonal spread.

In conclusion, the present study demonstrates significant multi-drug resistance among *S.enterica* Typhimurium within a pediatric population in China, including a higher prevalence of broad-spectrum cephalosporin resistance and expression of bla_{CTX-M} genes among *S. enterica* Typhimurium isolates than what has previously been reported. Moreover, the present study is the first report of the presence of $bla_{CTX-M-55}$ genes in *Salmonella spp.* Finally, our data suggest that clonal spread is responsible for the dissemination of *S. enterica* Typhimurium isolates and $bla_{CTX-M-14}$ genes in this population.

Acknowledgments

We are grateful to Dr. Xiaogan Xu and Professor Minggui Wang, Huashan Hospital, Fudan University, for the determination of PFGE.

Author Contributions

Conceived and designed the experiments: FY QC LW JP. Performed the experiments: XY QL LY BD CC. Analyzed the data: ZQ CP. Contributed reagents/materials/analysis tools: XZ JH. Wrote the manuscript: FY. Assisted with dealing with figures: YL.

References

1. Chyou SC, Leu YJ, Huang FY, Lee HC, Yang DI (1988) An etiological study of infectious diarrhea in infants and children in Taipei area. Zhonghua Min Guo Xiao Er Ke Yi Xue Hui Za Zhi 29: 213–220.
2. Guerrant RL, Van Gilder T, Steiner TS, Thielman NM, Slutsker L, et al. (2001) Practice guidelines for the management of infectious diarrhea. Clin Infect Dis 32: 331–351.
3. Archambault M, Petrov P, Hendriksen RS, Asseva G, Bangtrakulnonth A, et al. (2006) Molecular characterization and occurrence of extended-spectrum beta-lactamase resistance genes among Salmonella enterica serovar Corvallis from Thailand, Bulgaria, and Denmark. Microb Drug Resist 12: 192–198.
4. Batchelor M, Hopkins K, Threlfall EJ, Clifton-Hadley FA, Stallwood AD, et al. (2005) bla(CTX-M) genes in clinical Salmonella isolates recovered from humans in England and Wales from 1992 to 2003. Antimicrob Agents Chemother 49: 1319–1322.
5. Gonzalez-Sanz R, Herrera-Leon S, de la Fuente M, Arroyo M, Echeita MA (2009) Emergence of extended-spectrum beta-lactamases and AmpC-type beta-lactamases in human Salmonella isolated in Spain from 2001 to 2005. J Antimicrob Chemother 64: 1181–1186.
6. Hamidian M, Tajbakhsh M, Walther-Rasmussen J, Zali MR (2009) Emergence of extended-spectrum beta-lactamases in clinical isolates of Salmonella enterica in Tehran, Iran. Jpn J Infect Dis 62: 368–371.
7. Rotimi VO, Jamal W, Pal T, Sovenned A, Albert MJ (2008) Emergence of CTX-M-15 type extended-spectrum beta-lactamase-producing Salmonella spp. in Kuwait and the United Arab Emirates. J Med Microbiol 57: 881–886.
8. Touati A, Benallaoua S, Gharout A, Amar AA, Le Magrex Debar E, et al. (2008) First report of CTX-M-15 in Salmonella enterica serotype Kedougou recovered from an Algerian hospital. Pediatr Infect Dis J 27: 479–480.
9. Usha G, Chunderika M, Prashini M, Willem SA, Yusuf ES (2008) Characterization of extended-spectrum beta-lactamases in Salmonella spp. at a tertiary hospital in Durban, South Africa. Diagn Microbiol Infect Dis 62: 86–91.
10. Bonnet R (2004) Growing group of extended-spectrum beta-lactamases: the CTX-M enzymes. Antimicrob Agents Chemother 48: 1–14.
11. Cui S, Li J, Sun Z, Hu C, Jin S, et al. (2009) Characterization of Salmonella enterica isolates from infants and toddlers in Wuhan, China. J Antimicrob Chemother 63: 87–94.
12. Xia S, Hendriksen RS, Xie Z, Huang L, Zhang J, et al. (2009) Molecular characterization and antimicrobial susceptibility of Salmonella isolates from infections in humans in Henan Province, China. J Clin Microbiol 47: 401–409.
13. CLSI (2008) Performance standards for antimicrobial susceptibility testing, 18th informational supplement (M100-S18). Clinical and Laboratory Standards Institute, Wayne, PA, USA.
14. Yu Y, Ji S, Chen Y, Zhou W, Wei Z, et al. (2007) Resistance of strains producing extended-spectrum beta-lactamases and genotype distribution in China. J Infect 54: 53–57.
15. Jiang X, Ni Y, Jiang Y, Yuan F, Han L, et al. (2005) Outbreak of infection caused by Enterobacter cloacae producing the novel VEB-3 beta-lactamase in China. J Clin Microbiol 43: 826–831.
16. Wang M, Tran JH, Jacoby GA, Zhang Y, Wang F, et al. (2003) Plasmid-mediated quinolone resistance in clinical isolates of Escherichia coli from Shanghai, China. Antimicrob Agents Chemother 47: 2242–2248.
17. Bouallegue-Godet O, Ben Salem Y, Fabre L, Demartin M, Grimont PA, et al. (2005) Nosocomial outbreak caused by Salmonella enterica serotype Livingstone producing CTX-M-27 extended-spectrum beta-lactamase in a neonatal unit in Sousse, Tunisia. J Clin Microbiol 43: 1037–1044.
18. Izumiya H, Mori K, Higashide M, Tamura K, Takai N, et al. (2005) Identification of CTX-M-14 {beta}-lactamase in a Salmonella enterica serovar enteritidis isolate from Japan. Antimicrob Agents Chemother 49: 2568–2570.
19. Verdet C, Arlet G, Barnaud G, Lagrange PH, Philippon A (2000) A novel integron in Salmonella enterica serovar Enteritidis, carrying the bla(DHA-1) gene and its regulator gene ampR, originated from Morganella morganii. Antimicrob Agents Chemother 44: 222–225.
20. Li WC, Huang FY, Liu CP, Weng LC, Wang NY, et al. (2005) Ceftriaxone resistance of nontyphoidal Salmonella enterica isolates in Northern Taiwan attributable to production of CTX-M-14 and CMY-2 beta-lactamases. J Clin Microbiol 43: 3237–3243.
21. Cheung TK, Chu YW, Chu MY, Ma CH, Yung RW, et al. (2005) Plasmid-mediated resistance to ciprofloxacin and cefotaxime in clinical isolates of Salmonella enterica serotype Enteritidis in Hong Kong. J Antimicrob Chemother 56: 586–589.
22. Liu W, Chen L, Li H, Duan H, Zhang Y, et al. (2009) Novel CTX-M {beta}-lactamase genotype distribution and spread into multiple species of Enterobacteriaceae in Changsha, Southern China. J Antimicrob Chemother 63: 895–900.
23. Yin J, Cheng J, Sun Z, Ye Y, Gao YF, et al. (2009) Characterization of two plasmid-encoded cefotaximases found in clinical Escherichia coli isolates: CTX-M-65 and a novel enzyme, CTX-M-87. J Med Microbiol 58: 811–815.
24. Abdelghani SM, Moland ES, Black JA, Hanson ND, Goering RV, et al. (2009) First Report of CTX-M-14 Producing Clinical Isolates of Salmonella serovar Typhimurium from Egypt. J Infect Dev Ctries 4: 58–60.
25. Sun Y, Zeng Z, Chen S, Ma J, He L, et al. (2009) High prevalence of bla extended-spectrum beta(CTX-M)-lactamase genes in Escherichia coli isolates from pets and emergence of CTX-M-64 in China. Clin Microbiol Infect.
26. Shi WF, Zhou J, Qin JP (2009) Transconjugation and genotyping of the plasmid-mediated AmpC beta-lactamase and extended-spectrum beta-lactamase genes in Klebsiella pneumoniae. Chin Med J (Engl) 122: 1092–1096.
27. Kiratisin P, Apisarnthanarak A, Saifon P, Laesripa C, Kitphati R, et al. (2007) The emergence of a novel ceftazidime-resistant CTX-M extended-spectrum beta-lactamase, CTX-M-55, in both community-onset and hospital-acquired infections in Thailand. Diagn Microbiol Infect Dis 58: 349–355.

7

Interventions to Influence Consulting and Antibiotic use for Acute Respiratory Tract Infections in Children

Talley Andrews[1], Matthew Thompson[2]*, David I. Buckley[1], Carl Heneghan[2], Rick Deyo[1], Niamh Redmond[3], Patricia J. Lucas[4], Peter S. Blair[5], Alastair D. Hay[3]

1 Department of Family Medicine, Oregon Health and Science University, Portland, Oregon, United States of America, **2** Department of Primary Care Health Sciences, University of Oxford, Oxford, United Kingdom, **3** Academic Unit of Primary Health Care, School of Social and Community Medicine, University of Bristol, Bristol, United Kingdom, **4** School for Policy Studies, University of Bristol, Bristol, United Kingdom, **5** School of Social and Community Medicine, St Michael's Hospital, University of Bristol, Bristol, United Kingdom

Abstract

Background: Respiratory tract infections (RTIs) are common in children and generally self-limiting, yet often result in consultations to primary care. Frequent consultations divert resources from care for potentially more serious conditions and increase the opportunity for antibiotic overuse. Overuse of antibiotics is associated with adverse effects and antimicrobial resistance, and has been shown to influence how patients seek care in ensuing illness episodes.

Methodology/Principal Findings: We conducted a systematic review and meta-analysis to assess the effectiveness of interventions directed towards parents or caregivers which were designed to influence consulting and antibiotic use for respiratory tract infections (RTIs) in children in primary care. Main outcomes were parental consulting rate, parental knowledge, and proportion of children subsequently consuming antibiotics. Of 5,714 references, 23 studies (representing 20 interventions) met inclusion criteria. Materials designed to engage children in addition to parents were effective in modifying parental knowledge and behaviour, resulting in reductions in consulting rates ranging from 13 to 40%. Providing parents with delayed prescriptions significantly decreased reported antibiotic use (Risk Ratio (RR) 0.46 (0.40, 0.54); moreover, a delayed or no prescribing approach did not diminish parental satisfaction.

Conclusions: In order to be most effective, interventions to influence parental consulting and antibiotic use should: engage children, occur prior to an illness episode, employ delayed prescribing, and provide guidance on specific symptoms. These results support the wider implementation of interventions to reduce inappropriate antibiotic use in children.

Editor: Daniel Morgan, University of Maryland, School of Medicine, United States of America

Funding: This article presents independent research commissioned by the National Institute for Health Research (NIHR) under its Programme Grants for Applied Research funding scheme (RP-PG-0608-10018). The funders had no role in study design, data collection and analysis, decision to publish, or preparation of the manuscript.

Competing Interests: MT and CH receive financial compensation for conducting evidence-based training, workshops, and developing an iPhone application with the CEBMi and the BMJ Publishing Group. MT was reimbursed for travel and accommodation to give a plenary talk at ESPID meetings in 2010 and 2011 by the European Society for Pediatric Infectious Disease and has received financial compensation to teach evidence-based medicine courses by Isis Consulting. Two reviewers (MT and TA) were reimbursed for travel to meetings to discuss work leading to this review (NIHR RP-PG-0608-10018). RD received honoraria for attending board meetings of the Foundation for Informed Medical Decision Making and honoraria for writing on back pain topics for UpToDate. This does not alter the authors' adherence to all the PLoS ONE policies on sharing data and materials.

* E-mail: matthew.thompson@phc.ox.ac.uk

Introduction

Respiratory tract infections (RTIs) are common in children and drive the majority of antibiotic prescribing for this population [1]. On average, a third of all children in the United Kingdom and United States are seen in primary care for RTIs or related symptoms each year [2,3]. When parental time off work is added to the costs of health care, RTIs pose a major financial burden [1,2,3,4]. Clinical uncertainty regarding the diagnosis and management of RTIs is illustrated by wide variations in antibiotic use in primary care between individual clinicians, general practitioner (GP) practices, and countries [5,6,7,8]. Antibiotics can cause side effects in children, such as rash or diarrhoea, and rarely allergic reactions [9]. Overuse of antibiotics in primary care contributes to resistance [10], thus reducing the benefits of antibiotics, and can lead to subsequent "medicalisation of illness" where patients believe they need to consult when similar symptoms recur [11] – thereby creating a 'vicious cycle'. Combined with a slowing in the development of new antibiotics, resistance constitutes a major threat to public health [12]. Although public education campaigns are ongoing in many countries [13], targeted efforts are also needed at the practice and patient level to reduce population-wide risk of antibiotic resistance.

In the UK, the Department of Health Standing Medical Advisory Committee's 'Path of Least Resistance' report (1998) outlined the pivotal role primary care must play to avert the public health disaster of ineffective antibiotics for serious infections [14]. Recent guidelines highlight the need for patients and primary care professionals to stop seeing a role for antibiotics in the symptomatic relief of RTIs, and to adopt "no or delayed antibiotic" prescribing for the majority of patients [15]. To apply these recommendations, knowledge translation strategies are needed at the parental level to influence consulting behaviour and use of antibiotics, and at the primary care interface to influence consultation skills and prescribing behaviour.

Our goal was to systematically review the evidence for the effectiveness of interventions directed towards parents and/or caregivers to promote more appropriate consulting and antibiotic use for children with RTIs. We originally intended to also include interventions targeted to clinicians designed to change antibiotic prescribing, but decided to focus on interventions targeted to parents and caregivers based on feedback during peer review as research in this area had not been synthesised previously. The systematic review was based on a conceptual model (**Figure S1**) developed by the research team (consisting of qualitative and quantitative researchers, primary care clinicians, and parents) that incorporates knowledge, beliefs, and attitudes regarding decisions to consult and to use antibiotics for RTIs. These factors are often informed by past experience; for example, receiving antibiotics for a previous cough or cold may reinforce the belief that antibiotics are indicated and the decision to consult [16]. As such, repeated consultation and antibiotic prescribing experiences can contribute to 'vicious' or 'virtuous' cycles.

Our rationale for adopting a comprehensive approach to interventions rather than focussing more narrowly on individual components (e.g. delayed prescribing) takes account of the relatedness of the interventions and their effects at multiple points within the parent-doctor interaction. We therefore identified interventions that are applicable to multiple components of the parent-doctor interaction surrounding consultations, including parental knowledge of when to consult, and antibiotic use (measured by parental report of filling prescriptions or giving antibiotics to their child), including parental knowledge and attitudes related to use of antibiotics.

Methods

Search

We searched MEDLINE/PubMed [1966–November 2011], EMBASE [1974–March 2011], CINAHL [1981–March 2011], PsycINFO, and the Cochrane Library using a combination of terms on respiratory tract infection, children and parents, education, antibiotic prescription, and consultation (**Table S1**). No limits were applied for language. One author (TA) independently screened titles and abstracts based on the inclusion criteria to identify potentially relevant studies. Following the initial search, TA reviewed reference lists of selected studies and searched related citations to identify additional references. Two authors (TA and MT) reviewed the full-text of all potentially relevant studies to determine final inclusion. Disagreements were settled through discussions with a third author (CH or DB). Review protocol is available by request.

Selection

We included studies that used randomised, cluster randomised, or non-randomised controlled designs, or one group pre/post-test designs, to assess the effect of educational or behavioural interventions directed at caregivers to influence consulting or antibiotic use for acute RTIs in children (birth to 18 years), in developed countries (based on OECD member classification [17]). Comparisons included no-treatment or alternate treatment controls. We excluded studies that did not report outcomes for children with RTIs; study designs without a control group; evaluations of national treatment guidelines, public health interventions targeting multiple stakeholders at the population level, or diagnostic tests; studies of hospitalised children or those with serious comorbidities (e.g. cystic fibrosis, cancer, or other causes of immunocompromise); or studies from less developed countries (as the generalizability of the data from 'less developed' countries where the risk of severe complications from infection is higher will be limited).

Study characteristics

We sought data on three primary outcomes related to RTIs in children: 1) parental knowledge related to consultations or parental consultation rate, 2) parental knowledge or attitudes related to antibiotic use, and 3) antibiotic use. Secondary outcomes included adverse effects, health outcomes, and costs of interventions.

Data abstraction

Two reviewers (TA, MT) independently extracted data from included studies, using a predetermined extraction form, for study design, setting, patient population, definitions of included illnesses, intervention and comparison, theoretical framework, outcome(s) assessed, and method of assessment. Disagreements were resolved by discussion with a third author (DB or CH). When necessary we contacted study authors for additional information. Reviewers were not blinded to any aspect of the studies.

Validity assessment

Two review authors (TA and MT) independently assessed study quality using a framework adapted from the Cochrane Handbook risk of bias tool [18]. Our framework included a set of criteria selected to assess educational and behavioural interventions. For randomized or cluster randomized trials we assessed risk of bias based on the following criteria: randomization (description of method, differences between experimental groups), blinding, description of intervention (content and mode of delivery), exposure to intervention (and consistency in delivery), and generalisability (to primary care practice). Non-randomized controlled trials were assessed on the basis of comparability of groups, intervention description, exposure to intervention, and generalisability. One-group designs were assessed on the basis of intervention description, exposure to intervention, and generalisability. A judgment of "low", "high", or "unclear" was made regarding the risk of bias for each criterion; based on this, each study was then given an overall judgement of "minimum", "likely", or "high" risk of bias (**Table S2**). The overall quality assessments were used to interpret the main findings.

Quantitative data synthesis

For interventions which measured changes in mean or median numbers we calculated mean differences with 95% confidence intervals (CI), and for changes in rates we calculated odds ratios (OR) with 95% CI, using Yates's correction and Fisher's exact test where an expected cell was below five, for each of the study outcomes (EpiInfo version 3.4.3). Where raw data were unavailable, we presented proportional or mean differences. When possible we pooled outcomes and calculated risk ratio using a random effects model; we then calculated heterogeneity using I^2 and where it was greater than 50% looked for clinical and

Table 1. Effectiveness of interventions to influence parent knowledge related to consulting for respiratory tract infections in children.

Study	Age	Outcome	Intervention	Control	OR [95% CI]	NNT	Mean difference	Significance	Risk of bias
Francis*	6 mo-4 yr	% "intends to consult if their child has similar illness in future"	133/246 (54%)	201/263 (76.4%)	0.36 [0.24–0.54]	5		<0.001	Min.
Herman**	<18 yr	% would visit GP or ED for:							Likely
		earache	40/61 (66%)	101/113 (89%)	0.24 [0.09–0.54]	4	-	<0.001	
		cough	20/61 (31%)	73/113 (64%)	0.27 [0.13–0.54]	3	-	<0.001	
Isaacman***	<3 yr	Mean knowledge score of:							Likely
		how to administer medication	Verbal: 97.6	92.7	-	-	4.9	*NS*	
			Written + verbal: 96.9		-	-	4.2	*NS*	
		signs of symptom improvement	Verbal: 60	44	-	-	16	*<0.05 (vs. C)*	
			Written + verbal: 73.2		-	-	29.2	*<0.05 (vs. both)*	
		signs to reconsult	Verbal: 38.7	22.4	-	-	16.3	*<0.05 (vs. C)*	
			Written + verbal: 44.4		-	-	22.4	*<0.05 (vs. C)*	
Morrell, Anderson	0–4 yr	% with correct responses for: symptom management							Likely
		cough	15/51 (29.4%)	11/47 (23.4%)	1.36 [0.50–3.71]	17	-	0.66	
		runny nose	5/51 (9.8%)	2/47 (4.3%)	2.45 [0.39–19.31]	18	-	0.44¶	
		sore throat	13/51 (25.5%)	10/47 (21.3%)	1.27 [0.45–3.59]	24	-	0.8	
Robbins	<6 mo	% know when to consult for snuffles							Likely
		routine basis	48/49 (98%)	35/43 (81.4%)	10.97 [1.28–244.62]	6	-	0.01¶	
		urgent basis	48/49 (98%)	39/43 (90.7%)	4.92 [0.48–120.59]	14	-	0.18¶	

Table 1. Cont.

*cluster randomised controlled trial;
**pre/post design: intervention = post; control = pre;
***non-randomised controlled trial;
¶using Fisher's Exact Test; ED: emergency department; GP: general practitioner; mo: month; Min: minimum; NNT: number needed to treat; OR: odds ratio; yr: years.
Italicized p-values were those reported in original study.

statistical explanations. Considerable statistical and clinical heterogeneity prevented pooling of most outcomes; therefore results of each study are presented individually and interpreted using narrative analysis.

Results

Flow of included studies

From 5,714 initial studies, 137 met the criteria for full-text review, of which 114 were excluded (**Figure S2**). A total of 23 studies (representing 20 interventions) were included in the review; 12 interventions were from the US, six from the UK, and two from Israel. (Characteristics of included studies are reported in **Table S3**).

1. Interventions to influence parental consulting

We identified nine studies of eight interventions which aimed to change the number or rate of parental consultations for paediatric RTIs, involving a total of 1488 parents, 1580 families, and 558 children [19,20,21,22,23,24,25,26,27]. Interventions were delivered at home in four studies [22,24,26,27], and at GP surgeries or emergency departments in the remainder. All interventions involved written material (e.g. book, pamphlet), complemented by brief verbal education in five studies [19,20,21,24,25]. In three of these studies, intervention materials included cartoons and/or illustrations [22,25,27]. The studies measured change in rate or number of consultations or re-consultations for RTIs [19,21,22, 25,26,27], or change in knowledge about reasons to consult [19,20,21,23,24], Follow-up periods ranged from 3 days to 17 months. Results are shown in **Table 1** and **2**.

Knowledge related to consulting. Outcomes were mixed in the five studies that assessed change in parent knowledge in relation to consulting [19,20,21,23,24] (**Table 1**). Interventions significantly improved parents' knowledge about RTIs compared to controls in two studies [21,23], but did not measure effects on actual consultations. Similarly, the three studies which measured future consultation intentions also found significantly increased knowledge about appropriate reasons to consult, but again their impact on actual consultations was not measured [19,20,24].

Consultation rate. Six studies assessed the effects of interventions designed to reduce the number of consultations for RTIs [19,21,22,25,26,27] (**Table 2**). Three studies found that providing parents with informative, illustrated booklets prior to their child becoming ill resulted in lower rates of consulting for sore throat, cough, respiratory tract infection and otitis media [22,25,27]. Usherwood et al found that consultations per household decreased nearly 16% for sore throat ($p = 0.0002$) and 13% for cough ($p = 0.013$) [27]. In the study by Roberts, there was a relative reduction of 40% in the number of consultations per person/year for acute otitis media and other RTIs [25]. In one study, parents received books with information on multiple symptoms of respiratory infection (for example, cough, sore throat, and runny nose), yet consulting decreased significantly among all age groups only for sore throat ($p < 0.05$) [22]. The method of randomization was not reported in two of these studies, and generalisability may be limited given they were published 20–30 years ago [22,27]. Thomson et al provided mothers of infants in the intervention group with a guide for assessing severity of illness, and found similar numbers of infants subsequently had RTIs recorded by a clinician (52% vs. 50%, $p = 0.718$), however infants in the intervention group were more likely to receive prescriptions for oral antibiotics (OR 1.43 [95%CI 1.07–1.91]) [26]. Two studies assessed interventions delivered at point of consulting and designed to reduce re-consultations within a given illness episode; neither found significant differences in proportions re-consulting between intervention and control groups [19,21]. Adverse events (hospital admission ≤2 nights) were reported in one trial and were similar among intervention and control [19]. Adverse effects were generally not assessed, however Roberts et al noted a non-significant reduction in "necessary" consultations (those for more severe symptoms of respiratory infection, defined by the authors as "symptom clusters suggesting that diagnostic testing or drug therapy might be cost-effective") among African American and Medicaid patients receiving the intervention [25].

2. Interventions to influence parents' decision towards use of antibiotics

We identified 10 studies of nine interventions designed to influence antibiotic use for RTIs in children (**Table 3**, **4**, and **5**) [28,29,30,31,32,33,34,35,36,37]. Studies involved 2,916 participants with follow-up periods ranging from 1 day to 36 weeks. The majority of interventions took place during the consultation, with only two [29,30] designed to influence parental attitudes or knowledge before their children became ill.

Knowledge of appropriate antibiotic use. Five of the studies were set in primary care [28,31,33,34,37] and two in emergency departments [32,36]; the remaining interventions took place at home or in day care centres (**Table 3**). Interventions most often used video or written materials (pamphlets or handouts). Four [31,32,33,34] of the five studies which measured the effects of interventions on parental knowledge of appropriate antibiotic use (using a variety of different scores) found significant increases compared to the control groups, though in one study improvement only occurred among parents with college education [30], and two studies [31,33] had higher risk of bias due to weak study design (pre/post test) and low rates of exposure to the intervention. Three of these studies used interventions designed to engage children as well as their parents, such as cartoon-animation videos and colouring books [30,31,32]. Schnellinger et al found that parental knowledge increased immediately and was maintained at one month ($p < 0.001$) following a three minute cartoon-animated video, compared to parents only given pamphlets in whom knowledge improved immediately, but significantly waned at one month ($p = 0.002$) [32]. One study, however, found no improvement when parents were given a video and brochure (prior to an illness episode) and instructed to view it at home as often as they preferred [29]. It is unclear if the lack of effect was

Table 2. Effectiveness of interventions to change parent consulting rate for respiratory tract infections in children.

Study	Age	Outcome	Intervention	Control	OR [95% CI]	NNT	Mean difference	Significance	Risk of bias
Francis*	6 mo-4 yr	% reconsulting by 2 wk follow-up	33/256 (12.9%)	44/272 (16.2%)	0.77 [0.46–1.28]	30	-	0.34	Min.
Isaacman***	<3 yr	% reconsulting to PED by 3 day follow-up	Verbal: 1/41 (2.2%)	8/78 (10.1%)	0.22 [0.01–1.84]	13	-	0.16¶ (vs. C)	Likely
			Written + verbal: 2/49 (3.8%)		0.37 [0.05–2.02]	16	-	0.31¶ (vs. C)	
Morrell, Anderson §		Mean consultations/ patient/yr****							Likely
	0–4 yr	Sore throat	0.16	0.27	-	-	0.11	*NR*	
		Cough	1.08	1.20	-	-	0.12	*NR*	
		Runny/stuffy nose	0.10	0.10	-	-	0	*NR*	
	5–14 yr	Sore throat	0.19	0.23	-	-	0.04	*NR*	
		Cough	0.31	0.40	-	-	0.09	*NR*	
		Runny/stuffy nose	0.06	0.02	-	-	−0.04	*NR*	
Roberts §	≤18 yr	Consultations/ person/yr (pre vs. post)	0.185	0.303	-	-	0.118	*NR*	Likely
		Unnecessary consultations/ person/yr	0.064	0.141	-	-	0.077	*NR*	
Thomson	<6 mo	Infants receiving RTI diagnoses	242/467 (51.8%)	236/468 (50.4%)	1.06 [0.81–1.38]	72	-	0.72	Min.
		Infants receiving oral antibiotics	161/467 (34.5%)	126/468 (26.9%)	1.43 [1.07–1.91]	13	-	0.02	
Usherwood	2–12 yr	Consultations/ household							Likely
		Sore throat	32/210 (15.2%)	65/209 (31.1%)	0.26 [0.16–0.42]	6	-	<0.001	
		Cough	90/210 (43%)	116/209 (56%)	0.60 [0.40–0.90]	8	-	0.01	

*cluster randomised controlled trial;
***non-randomised controlled trial;
****adjusted for children at risk for part of study year;
¶using Fisher's Exact Test;
§no absolute numbers given; mo: month; Min: minimum; NNT: number needed to treat; NR: not reported; OR: odds ratio; PED: paediatric emergency department; RTI: respiratory tract infection; wk: weeks; yr: years. Italicized p-values were those reported in original study.

due to the home setting, or to specific attributes of the video (e.g. length of video was 20 minutes).

Attitudes towards antibiotic use. Two studies measured effects on parental attitudes towards antibiotic use (**Table 4**). Taylor et al found that a 'personalised' video intervention (featuring a paediatrician from the local clinic) was more effective in changing attitudes about when not to use antibiotics for specific illnesses (e.g. nasal discharge) and less effective in

Table 3. Effectiveness of interventions to improve parent knowledge of appropriate antibiotic use for respiratory tract infections in children.

Study	Age	Outcome	Intervention	Control	OR [95%CI] or difference	NNT	Mean difference	Significance	Risk of bias
Alder	1–10 yr	Change in parental communication efficacy							Likely
			Communication	-	-	-	-	0.02	
			AB information	-	-	-	-	0.34	
			Interaction	-	-	-	-	0.62	
Bauchner	6 mo-3 yr	Post-test adjusted knowledge score (range 0–11)	8.04	7.82	-	-	0.22	0.31	Likely
Croft*	<5 yr	Median knowledge score (range 0–9)							High
		College graduates	7	6.5	0.5	-	-	<0.01	
		Non-college graduates	6	6	0		-	0.20	
Maor**	8 d-16 yr	Knowledge of AB treatment (>50% correct answers)	45.1%	36.1%	9%	-	-	0.01	Likely
Schnellinger	<18 yr	Knowledge score (range 1–10) (baseline vs. following intervention vs. 1 mo)	I1. Pamphlet: (8, 10, 9) I2. Video: (9, 10, 10)	(8, 8, 8)	-	-	-	I1: 0.32*** I2: 0.002*** C: 0.26***	Min.

*cluster randomised controlled trial;
**Pre/post design: intervention = post; control = pre;
***within-group significance; AB: antibiotics; d: days; mo: month; Min: minimum; NNT: number needed to treat; OR: odds ratio; yr: years.

changing general perspectives about antibiotics (e.g. threat of antibiotic resistance) [34]. A video intervention studied by Wheeler et al [33] demonstrated moderate success in increasing the proportion of parents with appropriate attitudes towards antibiotic use (i.e. fewer parents wanting antibiotics, OR 0.20 [0.10–0.39]); however less than 60% of surveyed parents reported exposure to the intervention at any time. Despite significant improvements in parental attitudes toward judicious use of antibiotics, neither study found changes in antibiotic prescribing rates over follow-up periods of 6 to 12 months (data not shown).

Satisfaction with a 'no prescribing' approach. Two studies [36,37] assessed parent satisfaction with a 'watchful waiting,' or no prescribing approach, neither of which found significant differences in parent satisfaction between intervention and control groups (**Table 5**). In addition, McCormick et al [37] found no difference in persistence of acute otitis media symptoms at 30 days, and that more children in the control group reported adverse events (side effects of antibiotics). Treatment costs for children in the intervention group (watchful waiting) averaged $11.43 per child compared to $47.41 per child in the immediate antibiotic group. Chao et al reported no adverse events or increase in consultations related to intervention [36].

3. Interventions to influence antibiotic use in children with RTIs

We found six studies of five interventions that reported the effects of interventions to influence antibiotic use in children with RTIs [19,36,38,39,40,41]; all but one assessed the effect of delayed prescribing or watchful waiting therapy for AOM, the other study [19] involved a book for parents of children with RTIs.

Use of antibiotic prescriptions. Each of the five interventions designed to influence antibiotic use was effective

Table 4. Effectiveness of interventions to improve parental attitudes toward appropriate antibiotic use for respiratory tract infections in children.

Study	Age	Outcome	Intervention	Control	OR [95% CI] or difference	NNT	Mean difference	Significance	Risk of bias
Taylor	<24 mo	Parental attitude score (group mean) (range 1–6; 6 = "completely agree")							Min.
		"Too many children are treated with AB when not necessary"	5.18	4.86	-	-	0.32	0.07	
		"Parents should not try to persuade a doctor to prescribe AB"	5.26	4.99	-	-	0.27	0.08	
		"Physicians should never prescribe AB when they are unnecessary"	5.64	5.47	-	-	0.17	0.10	
		"Overuse of AB can make bacteria more resistant to AB"	5.78	5.52	-	-	0.26	0.021	
		(range 1–6, 1 = "completely disagree")			-	-			
		"Giving an AB to a child with cold symptoms can prevent an infection from occurring"	1.86	2.16	-	-	0.3	0.005‡	
		"It is worth trying an AB when my child has cold symptoms for 5 days"	1.93	2.34	-	-	0.41	0.001‡	
		"Treatment with AB is necessary when a child's nasal discharge turns from yellow to green in color"	2.61	3.47	-	-	0.86	0.001‡	
		"AB help a child's cold symptoms clear up more quickly"	1.64	2.01	-	-	0.37	0.001‡	
		"AB are helpful in treating colds"	1.52	1.87	-	-	0.35	<0.001‡	
Wheeler**	<18 yr	% of parents in agreement with:							High
		"Antibiotics should be used always or mostly" (for children with cold and fever)	9/126 (7.1%)	34/114 (29.8%)	0.18 [0.08–0.42]	4	-	<0.001	
		"Yes, I want	18/130	51/115	0.20	3	-	<0.001	

Table 4. Cont.

Study	Age	Outcome	Intervention	Control	OR [95% CI] or difference	NNT	Mean difference	Significance	Risk of bias
		antibiotics"	(13.8%)	(44.3%)	[0.10–0.39]				

**Pre/post design: intervention = post; control = pre;
‡"Statistically significant P values after correcting for multiple tests"; AB: antibiotics; mo: month; Min: minimum; NNT: number needed to treat; OR: odds ratio; yr: years.

compared to control, with a combined RR 0.39 (0.29, 0.53) (not shown in table). Combining a delayed or no prescribing strategy with brief education significantly decreased antibiotic use in four studies [36,38,40,41], and an interactive book [19] resulted in 19% fewer children taking antibiotics during the two weeks following consultation compared to controls ($p<0.001$) (**Table 6**). In pooled analyses we found significant heterogeneity ($p = 0.002$, $I^2 = 77\%$) due to one study [38] in which nearly 100% of parents in the control group reported antibiotic use. After removal of this study, parents in the intervention groups were still significantly less likely to report antibiotic use, combined RR 0.46 (0.40, 0.54) ($p = 0.51$, $I^2 = 0\%$) (**Figure S3**). Although the duration of acute otitis media symptoms was slightly shorter among children prescribed immediate antibiotics [38,41], follow-up did not show significant differences in increased risk of relapse at either three months or one year [39]. More adverse outcomes related to antibiotic use (diarrhoea) were reported in one study among children in the control group than those receiving the intervention [41].

Discussion

We systematically reviewed and synthesised the evidence for the effectiveness of interventions targeted at parents to modify consulting behaviour and antibiotic use for children with RTIs. To the best of our knowledge, this is the first systematic review of interventions to increase appropriate care-seeking behaviour in parents of children with acute respiratory tract infections. Providing educational materials to parents reduced rates of consulting by up to 40% in three studies; however all were published nearly 20 years ago and therefore may not translate to contemporary primary care [22,25,27]. Interventions may be more successful when delivered prior to the child's illness rather than during consultations [19,22,25,27], and when focussed on specific symptoms rather than generic messages about antibiotic overuse and resistance [34]. Effects were more consistent for certain symptoms (e.g. sore throat) than others (e.g. cough), which may reflect features specific to certain RTIs (particularly duration of illness which is short for sore throat and longer for cough), or merely the studies we identified [22,27]. Delayed or no prescribing interventions reduced rates of antibiotic use by up to half. Finally, educational materials that include cartoons and illustrations and which engage the child as well as their parents may be more successful than text-only materials; this approach was successful in several studies from different settings [22,25,27,30,31,32].

Previous reviews [42,43,44,45] have approached the problem of antibiotic overuse by assessing effectiveness of interventions to reduce clinician antibiotic prescribing. Our review, in contrast, has focussed on interventions targeted to parents or caregivers. In practice, change is needed by clinicians and parents and/or patients to reduce antibiotic use and control resistance. Our finding that framing education around specific presenting symptoms may be more meaningful to parents than less focussed approaches echoes a review by Glascoe [46] of general health education interventions directed toward parents. As with reviews by Arroll [47] and Spurling [48] which assessed the effect of delayed prescriptions in patients of all ages, we also found this strategy reduces antibiotic use in children as reported by their parents; importantly, our review demonstrates that parents accept this approach.

Our review adds to the literature by integrating the research on parental consulting and antibiotic use; we feel it is crucial to consider these elements together as they influence one another, often as part of a 'vicious cycle' of consulting and antibiotic-seeking. Decisions to consult or use antibiotics are not isolated events. Rather, they involve interactions between several stakeholders (e.g. parents, clinicians), in multiple situations (e.g. home, GP surgery), and at multiple moments in time (RTIs occur

Table 5. Change in parental satisfaction with a 'no prescribing' intervention.

Study	Age	Outcome	Intervention	Control	OR [95% CI] or difference	NNT	Mean difference	Significance	Risk of bias
Chao	2–12 yr	Proportion of parents reporting "very or extremely satisfied"	91/100 (91%)	101/106 (95%)	0.50 [0.14–1.74]	23	-	0.345	Min.
McCormick	6 mo-2 yr	Parent satisfaction score (range 0–52)	44.6/52	44.6/52	-	-	0	*NS*	Min.

mo: month; Min: minimum; NNT: number needed to treat; NS: not significant; OR: odds ratio; yr: years. Italicized p-values were those reported in original study.

Table 6. Effectiveness of interventions to influence filling antibiotic prescription for children with respiratory tract infections.

Study	Age	Outcome	Intervention	Control	OR [95% CI] or difference	NNT	Significance	Risk of bias
Reduction in number of children taking antibiotics								
Chao	2–12 yr	Number of children taking AB or re-consulting for ABx	13/100 (13%)	40/106 (37.7%)	0.25 [0.11–0.52]	4	<0.0001	Min.
Francis*	6 mo-14 yr	Number of children taking AB	55/246 (22.4%)	111/263 (42.2%)	0.39 [0.26–0.59]	5	<0.0001	Min.
Little ‡	6 mo-10 yr	Number of children taking AB	36/150 (24%)	132/134 (98.5%)	74.5% (66.2%–80.7%)	1	<0.0001	Min.
Pshetizky	3 mo-4 yr	Number of children taking AB	18/44 (40.9%)	32/37 (86.5%)	0.11 [0.03–0.36]	2	<0.0001	Min.
Reduction in number of parents filling antibiotic prescription								
Spiro	6 mo-12 yr	Number of parents filling AB script	50/132 (37.9%)	116/133 (87.2%)	0.09 [0.05–0.17]	2	<0.0001	Min.

*cluster randomised controlled trial;
‡because of the small numbers in one of the cells we calculated proportional difference; AB: antibiotic; ABx: antibiotic prescription; Min: minimum; mo: month; NNT: number needed to treat; OR: odds ratio; yr: year.

repeatedly). Although it increased the complexity of the review, the main strength of our approach is that it allowed us to identify overarching intervention components that appear effective.

Limitations

Our literature search was limited to studies reported in peer-reviewed journals, and therefore we may have missed relevant, unpublished research. To counter publication bias we searched multiple databases and did not limit by language. This review was focussed on studies from OECD countries (and mostly the US), which may limit generalisability to other countries or clinical settings. We included studies which used a range of study designs and follow-up periods, which limited our ability to synthesise results quantitatively. Several of the studies which showed reductions in consultation were published over 20 years ago [22,25,27], when prescribing for RTIs was higher generally, and thus may not apply to contemporary practice where antibiotic use has declined. Of the 20 interventions included in the review, 13 studies reported receipt of funding or support. The majority of funding organizations were governmental (only three studies [32,33,34] reported sole funding from private organizations). Included studies generally lacked explicit diagnostic criteria and excluded children with severe cases of infection or those at higher risk of complication. Thus, our findings may be less generalisable to these populations. Finally, few studies reported harms of interventions (e.g. missed treatment of serious infection).

Conclusions

The key finding of our review for clinicians is that interventions (such as written materials with focussed information for parents) can reduce the number of consultations for RTIs by 10 to 40%, and that use of antibiotics can be reduced by up to half through delayed prescribing. Importantly, reductions in antibiotic use do not seem to occur at the expense of parent satisfaction. Given the high frequency of paediatric consultations in primary care, a change in parental consulting behaviour for RTIs could potentially create a 'virtuous cycle' of reductions in workload and antibiotic use. We found moderate evidence that interventions are more effective when delivered to parents and children. Moreover, our findings have important implications for the content, format, and

Table 7. Implications of findings.

Outcome	Implications for clinical practice and future research	Level of evidence
Parental knowledge related to consulting	▪ Change in knowledge was equivocal; unclear meaning of parental intent to consult due to hypothetical nature of the outcome	Weak
Parental knowledge or attitudes related to antibiotic use	▪ Cartoon-illustrated materials engage children and parents ▪ Information specific to RTI symptoms, rather than general antibiotic use, may be more meaningful to parents	Moderate
Parental consulting	▪ Providing parents with written information (with cartoons and/or illustrations) reduced consulting compared to control ▪ Consulting for certain RTI (e.g. sore throat) may be easier to modify than consulting for other symptoms (e.g. cough)	Moderate
Filling antibiotic prescription	▪ 'Delayed or no prescribing' approach with supporting educational material reduced antibiotic use without diminishing parental satisfaction	Strong

timing of delivery of patient information materials (see **Table 7**). Written information with focussed content (to a specific symptom) appears to be more effective than generic messages about avoiding antibiotics or antibiotic resistance. Furthermore, altering consultations for certain RTIs (e.g. sore throat) seems to be more achievable than for others (e.g. cough). It is unclear whether this simply reflects the studies included in this review, or whether effectiveness differs for different RTIs because of parent (and clinician) perceptions about severity or risk of complications of different RTIs. Clinicians might want to look carefully at the format of the information they hand to parents; those with cartoons or illustrations seemed to be more effective than bland text. The few studies which examined video interventions showed mixed results, and none explored online technologies.

Reducing unnecessary antibiotic use in primary care with the explicit goal of avoiding further spread of antibiotic resistance is a policy priority in many countries. To some extent it has been successful – prescribing of antibiotics fell by 24% in the UK during the 1990 s [1]. Although some clinicians worry that reductions in prescribing have gone "too far" leading to increased incidence of complications of RTIs [49,50], there is broad agreement that prescribing rates remain inappropriately high for many RTIs. Our findings provide policy makers with evidence they need to implement or commission effective interventions in community settings to reduce consultations and antibiotic use. Moreover, interventions to reduce antibiotic use do not seem to occur at the expense of parent satisfaction, although evidence for conditions other than acute otitis media was limited. GPs implementing any of the strategies identified in this review should be mindful of the possibility of unintended adverse effects, such as reducing consultations for illness episodes that ought to be managed by a GP, as seen in the Roberts study [25]. Paradoxically, reducing the overall numbers of consultations for RTIs may filter a higher proportion of children with more severe illness presenting to primary care, highlighting the need for effective strategies to identify children at highest risk of complications and who are most likely to benefit from antibiotics; our group is currently conducting such research (see http://www.targetstudy.org.uk/).

Recommendations for future research

We have several suggestions to improve the primary research in this area. Firstly, reporting should include detailed descriptions of the intervention, the extent of exposure to the intervention, and whether the trial was conducted in communities where public media campaigns related to antibiotics were occurring (see study [29]). Secondly, follow-up periods need to be long enough to measure the longevity of interventions given that RTIs recur frequently. Further, potential outcomes should include number of symptomatic days, hospitalisations, and time off work or school [42,51]; most importantly, adverse outcomes should be assessed and reported. Finally, we urge the use of "head-to-head trials" [42] that compare the effectiveness of several delivery formats [32] (including online resources) for communicating information to parents. Going forward, interventions should be developed to influence consulting and antibiotic use for RTIs in children, rather than address these outcomes in isolation.

RTIs in children are a common cause for consultation and antibiotic use. We found several intervention strategies effective at improving parent knowledge about RTIs and when to consult, decreasing actual number of consultations, and reducing antibiotic use. Implementing one or a combination of the approaches identified in this review may reduce unnecessary consulting and use of antibiotics for children with RTIs in primary care.

Supporting Information

Figure S1 Conceptual framework for consulting and prescribing antibiotics for children with respiratory tract infections: 'virtuous' cycle.

Figure S2 Flow of included studies.

Figure S3 Effects of interventions to influence filling antibiotic prescription for children with respiratory tract infection.

Table S1 Search strategies.

Table S2 Quality assessment of included studies.

Table S3 Characteristics of included studies.

Checklist S1

Acknowledgments

We would like to acknowledge the support of all other members of the TARGET Programme Management Committee, who include: Peter Brindle, Christie Cabral, Hannah Christensen, Brendan Delaney, Margaret Fletcher, Sandra Hollinghurst, Jenny Ingram, Jeremy Horwood, John Leeming, Paul Little, Andrew Lovering, Peter Muir, Sue Mulvenna, Tim Peters, and Hannah Thornton. The views expressed in this publication are those of the author(s) and not necessarily those of the NHS, the NIHR, or the Department of Health.

Author Contributions

Conceived and designed the experiments: ADH MT TA CH DIB RD. Performed the experiments: TA MT CH. Analyzed the data: TA MT CH PSB DIB. Wrote the paper: TA MT CH DIB RD PJL NR PSB ADH.

References

1. Thompson PL, Spyridis N, Sharland M, Gilbert RE, Saxena S, et al. (2009) Changes in clinical indications for community antibiotic prescribing for children in the UK from 1996 to 2006: will the new NICE prescribing guidance on upper respiratory tract infections just be ignored? Arch Dis Child 94: 337–340.
2. Hay AD, Heron J, Ness A (2005) The prevalence of symptoms and consultations in pre-school children in the Avon Longitudinal Study of Parents and Children (ALSPAC): a prospective cohort study. Fam Pract 22: 367–374.
3. Fendrick AM, Monto AS, Nightengale B, Sarnes M (2003) The economic burden of non-influenza-related viral respiratory tract infection in the United States. Arch Intern Med 163: 487–494.
4. Hollinghurst S, Gorst C, Fahey T, Hay AD (2008) Measuring the financial burden of acute cough in pre-school children: a cost of illness study. BMC Fam Pract 9: 10.
5. Stanton N, Francis NA, Butler CC (2010) Reducing uncertainty in managing respiratory tract infections in primary care. Br J Gen Pract 60: e466–475.
6. Ferech M, Coenen S, Malhotra-Kumar S, Dvorakova K, Hendrickx E, et al. (2006) European Surveillance of Antimicrobial Consumption (ESAC): outpatient antibiotic use in Europe. J Antimicrob Chemother 58: 401–407.
7. Ashworth M, Charlton J, Ballard K, Latinovic R, Gulliford M (2005) Variations in antibiotic prescribing and consultation rates for acute respiratory infection in UK general practices 1995–2000. Br J Gen Pract 55: 603–608.
8. Howie JG (1976) Clinical judgement and antibiotic use in general practice. Br Med J 2: 1061–1064.
9. Clavenna A, Bonati M (2009) Adverse drug reactions in childhood: a review of prospective studies and safety alerts. Arch Dis Child 94: 724–728.

10. Costelloe C, Metcalfe C, Lovering A, Mant D, Hay AD (2010) Effect of antibiotic prescribing in primary care on antimicrobial resistance in individual patients: systematic review and meta-analysis. BMJ 340: c2096.
11. Little P, Gould C, Williamson I, Warner G, Gantley M, et al. (1997) Reattendance and complications in a randomised trial of prescribing strategies for sore throat: the medicalising effect of prescribing antibiotics. BMJ 315: 350–352.
12. Hughes JM (2011) Preserving the lifesaving power of antimicrobial agents. JAMA 305: 1027–1028.
13. Huttner B, Goossens H, Verheij T, Harbarth S (2010) Characteristics and outcomes of public campaigns aimed at improving the use of antibiotics in outpatients in high-income countries. Lancet Infect Dis 10: 17–31.
14. Standing Medical Advisory Committee, Sub-Group on Antimicrobial Resistance (1998) The path of least resistance. London: UK Department of Health.
15. NICE Short Clinical Guidelines Technical Team (2008) Respiratory tract infections – antibiotic prescribing. Prescribing of antibiotics for self-limiting respiratory tract infections in adults and children in primary care;London: National Institute for Health and Clinical Excellence.
16. Watson RL, Dowell SF, Jayaraman M, Keyserling H, Kolczak M, et al. (1999) Antimicrobial use for pediatric upper respiratory infections: reported practice, actual practice, and parent beliefs. Pediatrics 104: 1251–1257.
17. The World Bank (2011) Country and Lending Groups: High-income OECD members.
18. Higgins JP, Green S, eds. Cochrane Handbook for Systematic Reviews of Interventions Version 5.0.2: The Cochrane Collaboration.
19. Francis NA, Butler CC, Hood K, Simpson S, Wood F, et al. (2009) Effect of using an interactive booklet about childhood respiratory tract infections in primary care consultations on reconsulting and antibiotic prescribing: a cluster randomised controlled trial. BMJ 339: b2885.
20. Herman A, Young KD, Espitia D, Fu N, Farshidi A (2009) Impact of a health literacy intervention on pediatric emergency department use. Pediatr Emerg Care 25: 434–438.
21. Isaacman DJ, Purvis K, Gyuro J, Anderson Y, Smith D (1992) Standardized instructions: do they improve communication of discharge information from the emergency department? Pediatrics 89: 1204–1208.
22. Morrell DC, Avery AJ, Watkins CJ (1980) Management of minor illness. Br Med J 280: 769–771.
23. Anderson JE, Morrell DC, Avery AJ, Watkins CJ (1980) Evaluation of a patient education manual. Br Med J 281: 924–926.
24. Robbins H, Hundley V, Osman LM (2003) Minor illness education for parents of young children. J Adv Nurs 44: 238–247.
25. Roberts CR, Imrey PB, Turner JD, Hosokawa MC, Alster JM (1983) Reducing physician visits for colds through consumer education. JAMA 250: 1986–1989.
26. Thomson H, Ross S, Wilson P, McConnachie A, Watson R (1999) Randomised controlled trial of effect of Baby Check on use of health services in first 6 months of life. BMJ 318: 1740–1744.
27. Usherwood TP (1991) Development and randomized controlled trial of a booklet of advice for parents. Br J Gen Pract 41: 58–62.
28. Alder SC, Trunnell EP, White GL, Jr., Lyon JL, Reading JP, et al. (2005) Reducing parental demand for antibiotics by promoting communication skills. AM J Health Educ 36: 132–139.
29. Bauchner H, Osganian S, Smith K, Triant R (2001) Improving parent knowledge about antibiotics: a video intervention. Pediatrics 108: 845–850.
30. Croft DR, Knobloch MJ, Chyou P-H, Ellen DV, Janette C, et al. (2007) Impact of a child care educational intervention on parent knowledge about appropriate antibiotic use. WMJ 106: 78–84.
31. Maor Y, Raz M, Rubinstein E, Derazne E, Ringel S, et al. (2011) Changing parents' opinions regarding antibiotic use in primary care. Eur J Pediatr 170: 359–364.
32. Schnellinger M, Finkelstein M, Thygeson MV, Vander Velden H, Karpas A, et al. (2010) Animated video vs pamphlet: comparing the success of educating parents about proper antibiotic use. Pediatrics 125: 990–996.
33. Wheeler JG, Fair M, Simpson PM, Rowlands LA, Aitken ME, et al. (2001) Impact of a waiting room videotape message on parent attitudes toward pediatric antibiotic use. Pedlatrics 108: 591–596.
34. Taylor JA, Kwan-Gett TSC, McMahon EM, Jr. (2003) Effectiveness of an educational intervention in modifying parental attitudes about antibiotic usage in children. Pediatrics 111: e548–554.
35. Taylor JA, Kwan-Gett TSC, McMahon EM, Jr. (2005) Effectiveness of a parental educational intervention in reducing antibiotic use in children: a randomized controlled trial. Pediatric Infectious Disease Journal 24: 489–493.
36. Chao JH, Kunkov S, Reyes LB, Lichten S, Crain EF (2008) Comparison of two approaches to observation therapy for acute otitis media in the emergency department. Pediatrics 121: e1352–1356.
37. McCormick DP, Chonmaitree T, Pittman C, Saeed K, Friedman NR, et al. (2005) Nonsevere acute otitis media: a clinical trial comparing outcomes of watchful waiting versus immediate antibiotic treatment. Pediatrics 115: 1455–1465.
38. Little P, Gould C, Williamson I, Moore M, Warner G, et al. (2001) Pragmatic randomised controlled trial of two prescribing strategies for childhood acute otitis media. BMJ 322: 336–342.
39. Little P, Moore M, Warner G, Dunleavy J, Williamson I (2006) Longer term outcomes from a randomised trial of prescribing strategies in otitis media. Br J Gen Pract 56: 176–182.
40. Pshetizky Y, Naimer S, Shvartzman P, Pshetizky Y, Naimer S, et al. (2003) Acute otitis media–a brief explanation to parents and antibiotic use. Fam Pract 20: 417–419.
41. Spiro DM, Tay KY, Arnold DH, Dziura JD, Baker MD, et al. (2006) Wait-and-see prescription for the treatment of acute otitis media: a randomized controlled trial. JAMA 296: 1235–1241.
42. Ranji SR, Steinman MA, Shojania KG, Gonzales R (2008) Interventions to reduce unnecessary antibiotic prescribing: a systematic review and quantitative analysis. Med Care 46: 847–862.
43. Patel SJ, Larson EL, Kubin CJ, Saiman L (2007) A review of antimicrobial control strategies in hospitalized and ambulatory pediatric populations. Pediatr Infect Dis J 26: 531–537.
44. Arnold SR, Straus SE (2005) Interventions to improve antibiotic prescribing practices in ambulatory care. Cochrane Database Syst Rev. pp CD003539.
45. Boonacker CW, Hoes AW, Dikhoff MJ, Schilder AG, Rovers MM (2010) Interventions in health care professionals to improve treatment in children with upper respiratory tract infections. Int J Pediatr Otorhinolaryngol 74: 1113–1121.
46. Glascoe FP, Oberklaid F, Dworkin PH, Trimm F (1998) Brief approaches to educating patients and parents in primary care. Pediatrics 101: E10.
47. Arroll B, Kenealy T, Kerse N (2003) Do delayed prescriptions reduce antibiotic use in respiratory tract infections? A systematic review. Br J Gen Pract 53: 871–877.
48. Spurling GK, Del Mar CB, Dooley L, Foxlee R (2007) Delayed antibiotics for respiratory infections. Cochrane Database Syst Rev. pp CD004417.
49. Sharland M, Kendall H, Yeates D, Randall A, Hughes G, et al. (2005) Antibiotic prescribing in general practice and hospital admissions for peritonsillar abscess, mastoiditis, and rheumatic fever in children: time trend analysis. BMJ 331: 328–329.
50. Thompson PL, Gilbert RE, Long PF, Saxena S, Sharland M, et al. (2009) Effect of antibiotics for otitis media on mastoiditis in children: a retrospective cohort study using the United kingdom general practice research database. Pediatrics 123: 424–430.
51. Finch RG, Metlay JP, Davey PG, Baker LJ (2004) Educational interventions to improve antibiotic use in the community: report from the International Forum on Antibiotic Resistance (IFAR) colloquium, 2002. Lancet Infect Dis 4: 44–53.

8

Expression of APOBEC3G/3F and G-to-A Hypermutation Levels in HIV-1-Infected Children with Different Profiles of Disease Progression

Nívea D. Amoêdo[1], Adriana O. Afonso[2,3], Sílvia M. Cunha[4], Ricardo H. Oliveira[5], Elizabeth S. Machado[2,5], Marcelo A. Soares[2,6]*

1 Instituto de Bioquímica Médica, Universidade Federal do Rio de Janeiro, Rio de Janeiro, Brazil, **2** Departamento de Genética, Universidade Federal do Rio de Janeiro, Rio de Janeiro, Brazil, **3** Centro de Ciências da Saúde, Universidade Católica de Petrópolis, Petrópolis, Brazil, **4** Hospital Municipal Jesus, Rio de Janeiro, Brazil, **5** Instituto de Puericultura e Pediatria Martagão Gesteira, Universidade Federal do Rio de Janeiro, Rio de Janeiro, Brazil, **6** Programa de Genética, Instituto Nacional de Câncer, Rio de Janeiro, Brazil

Abstract

Objective: Increasing evidence has accumulated showing the role of APOBEC3G (A3G) and 3F (A3F) in the control of HIV-1 replication and disease progression in humans. However, very few studies have been conducted in HIV-infected children. Here, we analyzed the levels of A3G and A3F expression and induced G-to-A hypermutation in a group of children with distinct profiles of disease progression.

Methodology/Principal Findings: Perinatally HIV-infected children were classified as progressors or long-term non-progressors according to criteria based on HIV viral load and CD4 T-cell counts over time. A group of uninfected control children were also enrolled in the study. PBMC proviral DNA was assessed for G-to-A hypermutation, whereas A3G and A3F mRNA were isolated and quantified through TaqMan® real-time PCR. No correlation was observed between disease progression and A3G/A3F expression or hypermutation levels. Although all children analyzed showed higher expression levels of A3G compared to A3F (an average fold of 5 times), a surprisingly high A3F-related hypermutation rate was evidenced in the cohort, irrespective of the child's disease progression profile.

Conclusion: Our results contribute to the current controversy as to whether HIV disease progression is related to A3G/A3F enzymatic activity. To our knowledge, this is the first study analyzing A3G/F expression in HIV-infected children, and it may pave the way to a better understanding of the host factors governing HIV disease in the pediatric setting.

Editor: Roberto F. Speck, University Hospital Zurich, Switzerland

Funding: This work was funded by the Brazilian AIDS Department (Ministry of Health) and by the Brazilian Research Council (CNPq). The funders had no role in study design, data collection and analysis, decision to publish, or preparation of the manuscript.

Competing Interests: The authors have declared that no competing interests exist.

* E-mail: masoares@biologia.ufrj.br

Introduction

Human immunodeficiency virus type 1 (HIV-1) infection in children often progresses rapidly to acquired immunodeficiency syndrome (AIDS). The majority of infected children under 15 years of age develop AIDS, and most die [1]. The risk of pediatric disease progression in mother-to-child transmission (MTCT) has been associated with different factors, such as mother with advanced HIV-1 disease, as well as immunological, virological and host-specific factors [2,3].

A new class of host restriction factors has been described to play an important role in restricting intracellular viral replication. Enzymes of the apolipoprotein B mRNA-editing catalytic polypeptide (APOBEC) family convert cytidine to uridine in the transient (−)ssDNA replication intermediate, which is later reflected as G-to-A changes in the (+)strand [4,5,6,7]. As these mutations usually occur at very high frequency in sequences, this phenomenon is often called hypermutation. Dinucleotide motifs within DNA are preferentially targeted by APOBEC3G (A3G) and APOBEC3F (A3F), resulting in proviral DNA GG to AG and GA to AA substitutions, respectively. A3G and A3F exhibit potent anti-HIV-1 activity [8,9,10,11,12,13] and are expressed in lymphocytes, the major target cells for HIV-1 infection [9,11]. HIV-1 Vif counteracts A3G/F by preventing their encapsidation into virions and by inducing their proteossomal degradation in the producer cell [14,15]. The effects of A3G/F proteins likely modify both the efficiency of HIV-1 transmission and disease progression [16], but their role in these processes is not well understood.

A3G has been referred to as the major contributor to hypermutation *in vivo* and *in vitro* [12,13,17,18,19,20,21,22,23]. However, depending on the HIV genomic region analyzed, varying effects of A3G can be found. For example, hypermutation analyses in the HIV protease (PR) region of the *pol* gene have indicated a proportionally large number of G-to-A changes associated to A3F [24,25].

Evidence suggests that individuals who express high levels of A3G mRNA tend to control the levels of HIV-1 viremia [26,27]. It has also been suggested that levels of A3G expression decrease

Table 1. Demographic and clinical characteristics of HIV-infected children under study.

Patient ID	Age*	Treatment experience*	CDC classification*	Follow-up Data			Sample Data		
				Period	Highest log HIV-1 VL	Lowest CD4 T-cell%	Date	Log HIV-1 VL	CD4⁺ T-cell%
N35/LTNP	10.2	No	A1	1994–2003	4.59	28	04/2003	3.73	27
N52/LTNP	10.6	Yes	A1	1992–2002	4.88	27	11/2002	3.88	33
N64/LTNP	11.3	No	A1	1993–2004	4.40	31	05/2003	4.08	33
N70/LTNP	13.7	No	A1	1996–2004	4.30	30	11/2003	4.34	32
N72/LTNP	7.7#	No	N1	2000–2007	2.58	29	12/2003	2.23	30
N82/LTNP	6.8#	No	N1	1998–2007	4.91	33	07/2004	4.85	34
N48/P	6.3	Yes	A3	2001–2004	4.28	17	02/2004	3.64	19
N58/P	5.8	No	A2	2000–2004	5.49	15	07/2003	5.49	25
N59/P	5.6	Yes	A2	2000–2005	5.04	5	09/2003	4.75	14
N61/P	12.2	Yes	A2	1998–2004	4.77	15	02/2003	2.86	23
N67/P	8.2	Yes	B2	1999–2005	5.28	10	04/2004	2.34	10
N75/P	6.8	Yes	B2	2000–2004	5.15	19	08/2003	1.96	22
N25/P	3.4	Yes	C3	2001–2003	6.45	1	06/2003	5.26	19
N27/P	3.0	Yes	C3	2001–2003	6.41	9	10/2002	5.30	15
N28/P	3.3	Yes	C3	2001–2003	6.97	6	09/2002	5.79	24
N33/P	3.0	Yes	C3	2001–2003	7.53	4	12/2003	4.83	35
N62/P	1.9	Yes	B3	2002–2003	5.49	6	12/2002	5.23	8

*At sample collection.
#Both patients had CD4%>25% at the age of 8 years old.

with disease progression [28]. A recent study showed that the frequency of hypermutated viral genomes in elite suppressors was not significantly different from that observed in patients on highly active antiretroviral therapy (HAART), and no correlation was found between A3G expression and the rate of hypermutation [20]. Differently from the previous report, the level of hypermutation was correlated with A3G expression in other studies [28,29].

In the present study, we analyzed A3G and A3F mRNA expression levels, as well as G-to-A hypermutation contexts in HIV-1 proviral protease sequences from infected children with different profiles of disease progression.

Methods

Ethics Statement

All parents/guardians of the children read and signed an informed consent to participate to this study. This study was approved by the Institutional Review Board of the Federal University of Rio de Janeiro.

Patients and Samples

Seventeen HIV-1-infected children with different profiles of disease progression regularly followed-up at the Pediatric Unit of Federal University of Rio de Janeiro since birth were enrolled in

Table 2. Frequency of G-to-A hypermutation in HIV-1-infected children with distinct profiles of disease progression.

PATIENT GROUP	NO. OF PATIENTS	NO. OF CLONES	HYPERMUTATION (%)		AVERAGE G-to-A CONTEXT (%)	
			Patients	Clones	GG (A3G)	GA (A3F)
LTNP	6	60	3	1 (10)	50	0
				1 (10)	37	83
				1 (10)	39	91
Total	**6**	**60**	**50%**	**10%**	**42%**	**58%**
P	11	121	3	2 (20)	35	5
				6 (60)	26	86
				1 (10)	32	13
Total	**11**	**121**	**27%**	**30%**	**31%**	**35%**

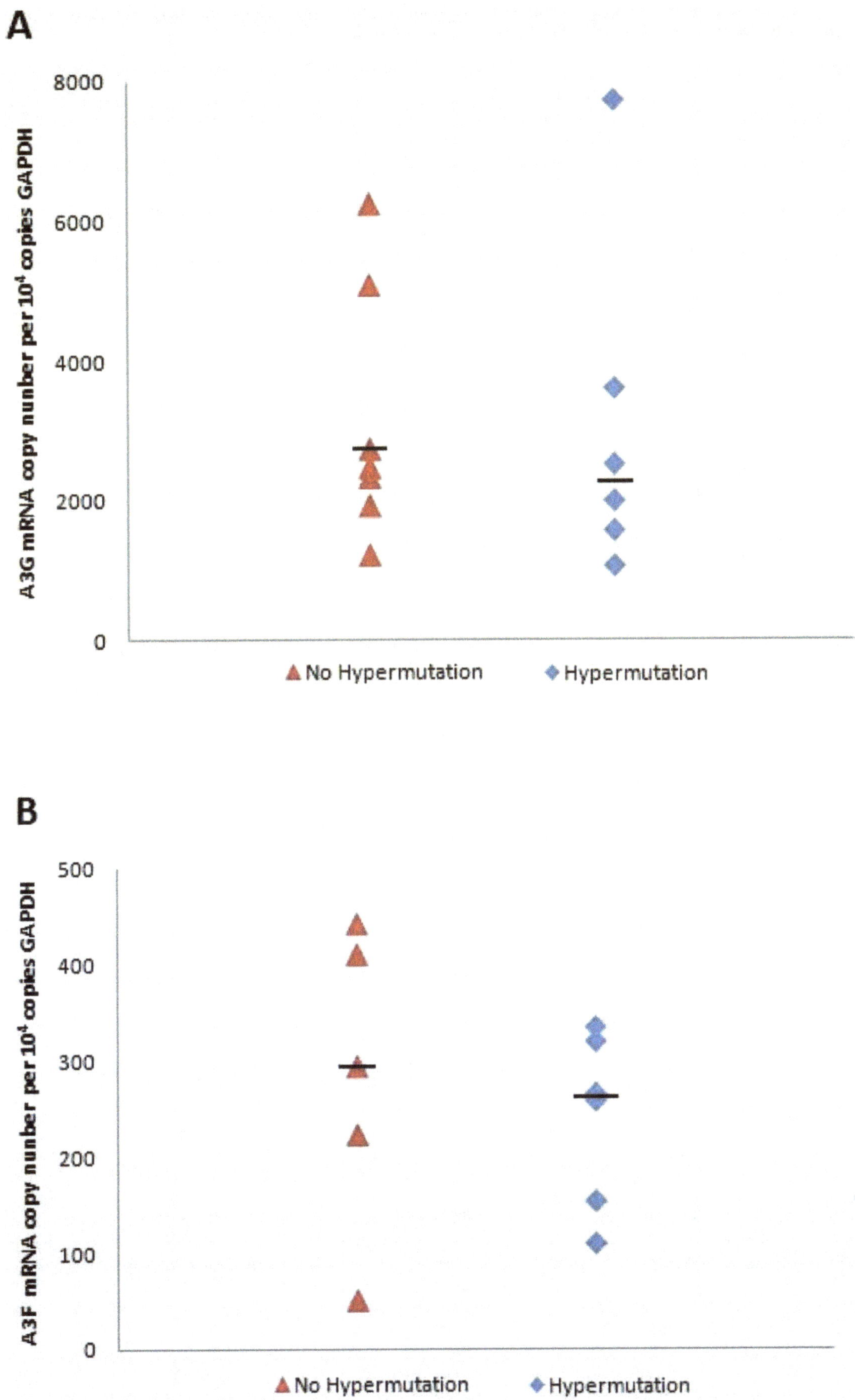
A
8000
6000
4000
2000
0
A3G mRNA copy nunber per 10^4 copies GAPDH
No Hypermutation
Hypermutation
B
500
400
300
200
100
0
A3F mRNA copy nunber per 10^4 copies GAPDH
No Hypermutation
Hypermutation

Figure 1. APOBEC3G (*A*) and APOBEC3F (*B*) mRNA expression levels relative to GAPDH mRNA copy numbers of patients with or without evidenced hypermutation. Horizontal bars depict the median value for each group.

this study. All clinical and laboratory data, including $CD4^+$ T-cell counts and HIV-1 viral load at every 3–4 months, were retrieved from a previous prospective study. All patients have been infected perinatally and therefore had known time of infection. Stored peripheral blood mononuclear cell (PBMC) samples were thawed and used for mRNA and proviral DNA extraction (see below). Six children were classified as long-term nonprogressors (LTNP), defined as over 8 years of age, with CD4≥25%, and under no antiretroviral therapy, a well-accepted definition for pediatric patients [30]; the remaining children (11 patients) were classified as typical progressors. Demographical, clinical, laboratory and follow-up data for all pediatric patients are summarized in Table 1. For A3G and A3F expression level determination, nine samples of HIV-negative children (NC) from the same previous study were used as a negative control group to assess A3G/F expression in the absence of HIV infection.

HIV proviral DNA hypermutation

Genomic DNA from PBMC was isolated using the Illustra Blood GenomicPrep Mini Spin Kit (GE Healthcare). Nested PCR was then performed to amplify the HIV-1 proviral protease (PR) genomic region corresponding to HXB2 coordinates 2268–2564, as previously described [31]. HIV PR region was chosen because the first half of the *pol* gene is a highly frequent target of hypermutation-associated changes [21,23,32]. PCR-amplified products were cloned into pMOSBlue Blunt-ended PCR cloning kit (GE Healthcare) and a minimum of 10 clones from each patient were isolated by colony PCR and sequenced, therefore providing a sensitivity of 10% for detecting hypermutated sequences. Hypermutation was quantified using Hypermut 2.0 [33]. A sequence was considered hypermutated when the *p*-value was ≤0.05 in the Fisher's exact test that compared the number of G-to-A mutations by A3G/F *versus* a control context. In order to avoid overestimation of hypermutation by comparing different viral strains, we have used the plasma-derived genomic viral sequence generated by RT-PCR, representative of each patient's circulating virus, as the control context. We have also used the HIV-1 clone HXB2 as a reference for context in Hypermut for comparison of results. All patients were infected with HIV-1 subtype B viruses, as determined by phylogenetic analysis (not shown). All plasma-derived bulk sequences and proviral clonal sequences analyzed were submitted to the GenBank sequence database and were assigned the accession numbers JF950037 to JF950234.

APOBEC3G and 3F mRNA expression analyses

Patient's PBMC also had their RNA extracted and purified for A3G and A3F mRNA expression analyses through TaqMan®-based real time PCR. Total RNA was extracted with Trizol®, precipitated with lithium chloride and quantified in a Nanodrop® apparatus. Two micrograms of RNA were subject to cDNA synthesis with Superscript RT and oligo-d(T) (Invitrogen, CA). For a subset of the samples, we have also primed the RT reactions with random hexameric primers, using the same amount of RNA. Primers and probes for A3G, A3F and the internal control GAPDH were synthesized through the Assay-on-Demand™ (Applied Biosystems). Real time PCR reactions were conducted in an ABI 7500 apparatus (Applied Biosystems) in triplicate and with three different dilutions for each sample for determination of the reaction efficiency. Only reactions with efficiency superior to 95% were used in the calculations. Results were expressed as the relative number of A3G or A3F mRNA copies per 10^4 copies of GAPDH mRNA.

Statistical analyses

Demographic and laboratory data ($CD4^+$ T-cell counts and HIV viral load) were compared among the two patient groups (typical progressors *versus* non-progressors) using Student's *t* tests, whereas for A3G and A3F expression level comparisons the Mann-Whitney *U* test was used. The definition of HIV-1 hypermutated sequences conducted in Hypermut was implemented within the software package using Fisher's exact tests. We have also compared A3G and A3F mRNA expression levels between patients for which hypermutation was detected and those with no hypermutation. Finally, we have stratified patients according to HIV viral load levels (below and above 10,000 copies/ml) and according to their treatment status (treatment-naïve or experienced), and compared the groups with respect to A3G/F expression. Calculations were performed in StatsDirect v.2.7.2 [34]. In all cases, *p*-values were considered significance at the ≤0.05 level.

Results

Demographic and clinical characteristics of the HIV-infected children analyzed in this study are depicted in Table 1. Among the LTNP children, the lowest $CD4^+$ T-cell percentage values during all time of follow-up ranged from 27 to 33%, whereas for progressors they ranged from 1 to 19%. The average age of the groups at the time of sample collection was 10.0 for LTNP and 5.4 for progressors ($p = 0.005$). As expected, $CD4^+$ counts were higher among LNTP ($p < 0.001$) when compared with the progressor group, but there was no difference in HIV viral load between the 2 groups ($p = 0.50$). Children of the negative control group (NC) averaged 4.7 years of age, ranging from 0.1 to 11.2 years (not shown).

APOBEC3G and 3F G-to-A hypermutation events in HIV proviral sequences were examined in the two disease progression groups of HIV-infected children. An alignment of all proviral clonal sequences referenced by their respective plasma viral bulk sequence can be seen in Figure S1. Hypermutated proviral sequences were detected more frequently among LTNP patients (50%) when compared with the P group (27%) (Table 2 and Figure S1), yet this difference was not statistically significant. Although less frequently, the percentage of clones with hypermuted sequences was higher in the P group patients. Results obtained using HXB2 instead of the patient's consensus plasma HIV sequence as reference for hypermutation determination were not significantly different (not shown). We could not find a clear correlation between hypermutation and the different patterns of disease progression. In both groups, the most frequent changes were <u>G</u>A to <u>A</u>A, surprisingly indicating a predominance of A3F-associated hypermutation (Table 2 and Figure S1). The hypermutated clonal viral sequence with the lowest *p*-value (higher significance) obtained in Hypermut from all patients had evidence of simultaneous A3G and A3F activity with the exception of sample N52-5, for which only A3G activity was detected (Figure S1).

We next investigated whether the G-to-A hypermutation changes were related to the levels of A3G and A3F mRNA expression. All patient samples with detected hypermutation

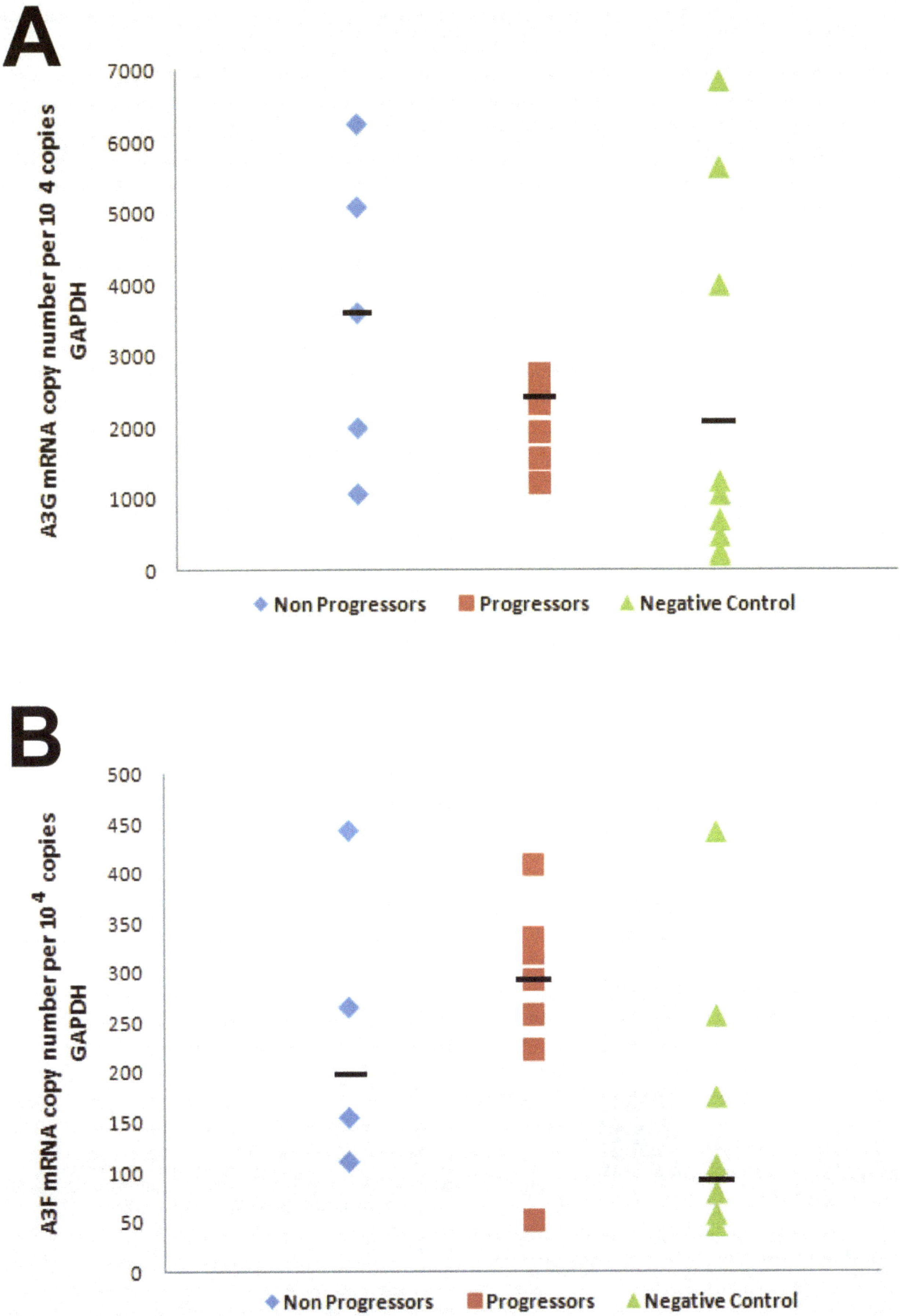
A
7000
6000
5000
4000
3000
2000
1000
0
A3G mRNA copy number per 10 4 copies GAPDH
Non Progressors
Progressors
Negative Control
B
500
450
400
350
300
250
200
150
100
50
0
A3F mRNA copy number per 10 4 copies GAPDH
Non Progressors
Progressors
Negative Control

Figure 2. APOBEC3G (*A*) and APOBEC3G (*B*) mRNA expression levels relative to GAPDH mRNA copy numbers of patients with different profiles of HIV disease progression. Horizontal bars depict the median value for each group.

(n = 6), as well as seven additional, randomly chosen samples of children with no signs of hypermutation, were selected for expression analysis. In all samples, A3G expression was higher than that of A3F ($p<0.0001$; Mann-Whitney *U* test), with fold variations ranging from 5 to 30 X (Figures 1A and B). Levels of both A3G and A3F expression did not differ significantly when comparing subjects with detected hypermutation with those where no hypermutation was detected ($p = 0.84$ and 0.66 for A3G and A3F, respectively; Mann-Whitney *U* test).

We wanted to further assess whether A3G and A3F expression levels were correlated with disease progression in HIV^+ children. Nine samples of uninfected children were used as a negative control (NC) group. Results for A3G and A3F expression in each group are depicted in Figures 2A and B, respectively. There was no clear correlation between both A3G and A3F expression and disease progression in any group comparison done. Of note, when median A3G expression values were compared among groups, we found LTNP to be the highest A3G expressers ($3600 \pm 2131/10^4$ cp GAPDH), followed by progressors (2626 ± 1809) and NC (1049 ± 2302). In our casuistic, the three highest A3G-expressing uninfected children had median expression values significantly higher than the median of the remaining NC ($p = 0.02$; Mann-Whitney *U* test). With respect to A3F expression, the progressors group was the higher expresser ($270 \pm 113/10^4$ cp GAPDH), followed by LTNP (243 ± 148) and NC (157 ± 134). However, none of the median expression values was significantly different when the disease progression groups were compared. Of interest, we also failed to detect a significant correlation between A3G and A3F expression levels in both HIV^+ and NC children groups (data not shown; $R^2 = 0.16$ and 0.03, respectively).

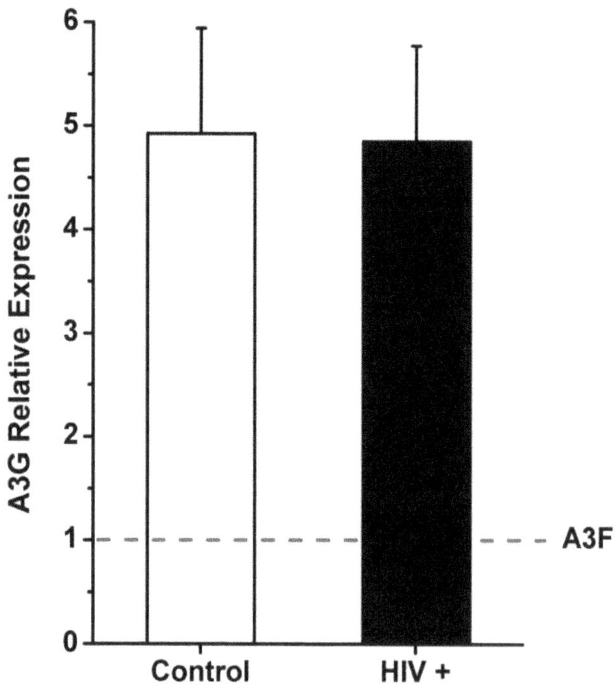

Figure 3. Average APOBEC3G to APOBEC3F mRNA expression levels quantified from eight HIV^+ children (6 progressors and 2 nonprogressors) and five HIV^- controls. A3F expression levels were arbitrarily set at 1.

Recent reports have indicated that A3F mRNA expression levels might be largely underestimated when one uses oligo-d(T)-primed cDNA synthesis, due to the presence of repetitive elements in the long 3′ untranslated region of its mRNA [35]. To test for that possibility, we have subjected a subset of our patient's samples to random hexameric primer-based cDNA synthesis, which is reported to be more efficient under these circumstances [35]. Total RNA from plasma of 6/11 progressors, 2/6 nonprogressors and 5/9 HIV-negative controls were re-synthesized with random primers and subject to the same mRNA A3G and A3F quantification protocol. Indeed, the fold difference between A3G and A3F changed significantly, with an average fold difference of 5x more A3G compared to A3F (range 2–9X) (Figure 3), as opposed to the 15x fold difference seen with oligo-d(T)-primed reactions. These results suggest that A3F mRNA levels were underestimated in the previous experiments. However, the new procedure did not change the relative profiles of A3G and A3F expression among different groups, with HIV^+ subjects displaying higher expression levels than negative controls (data not shown). The differences observed between groups were not statistically significant, as in the previous experiments.

We finally assessed the effect of antiretroviral treatment and of the HIV-1 viral load levels on A3G/F mRNA expression in our casuistic. When children were categorized in treated *versus* untreated, irrespective of their disease progression profile, there were no significant differences in the levels of either A3G or A3F mRNA expression levels (Figure 4A; $p = 0.80$ and 0.16, respectively). Children with low HIV VL (below 10,000 copies/ml) also did not show different levels of A3G/F expression when compared to those with VL above that cut-off (Figure 4B; $p = 0.25$ and 0.71, respectively).

Discussion

Previous studies have addressed G-to-A hypermutation and APOBEC3G sequence variations on disease progression in infected children [36,37]. Our study, however, describes for the first time the analysis of APOBEC3G and 3F mRNA expression levels in an infected pediatric setting. Here, we investigated whether hypermutation and APOBEC expression were associated with different patterns of disease progression in this small cohort of pediatric patients.

We were unable to correlate HIV hypermutation levels to disease progression in children. Although our study has included a small number of individual proviral sequences from each patient, the lack of correlation between delayed disease progression and hypermutation found here is in agreement with recent findings in adults. Gandhi *et al.* found no correlation between hypermutation in elite suppressors when compared to that in HIV^+ patients undergoing HAART, after analyzing a large number of HIV-1 sequences [20]. This observation suggests that hypermutation levels are not directly related to the intrinsic control of viremia seen in LTNP. Indeed, we found one LNTP child with low HIV viral load ($3.73 \log^{10}$/mL of plasma) in which no hypermutation was detected. Conversely, two samples from progressors, with hypermutated sequences, had HIV VL over 5 $\log_{10}$/mL. Our results further suggest a lack of correlation between HIV VL and hypermutation (data not shown). While some other reports have

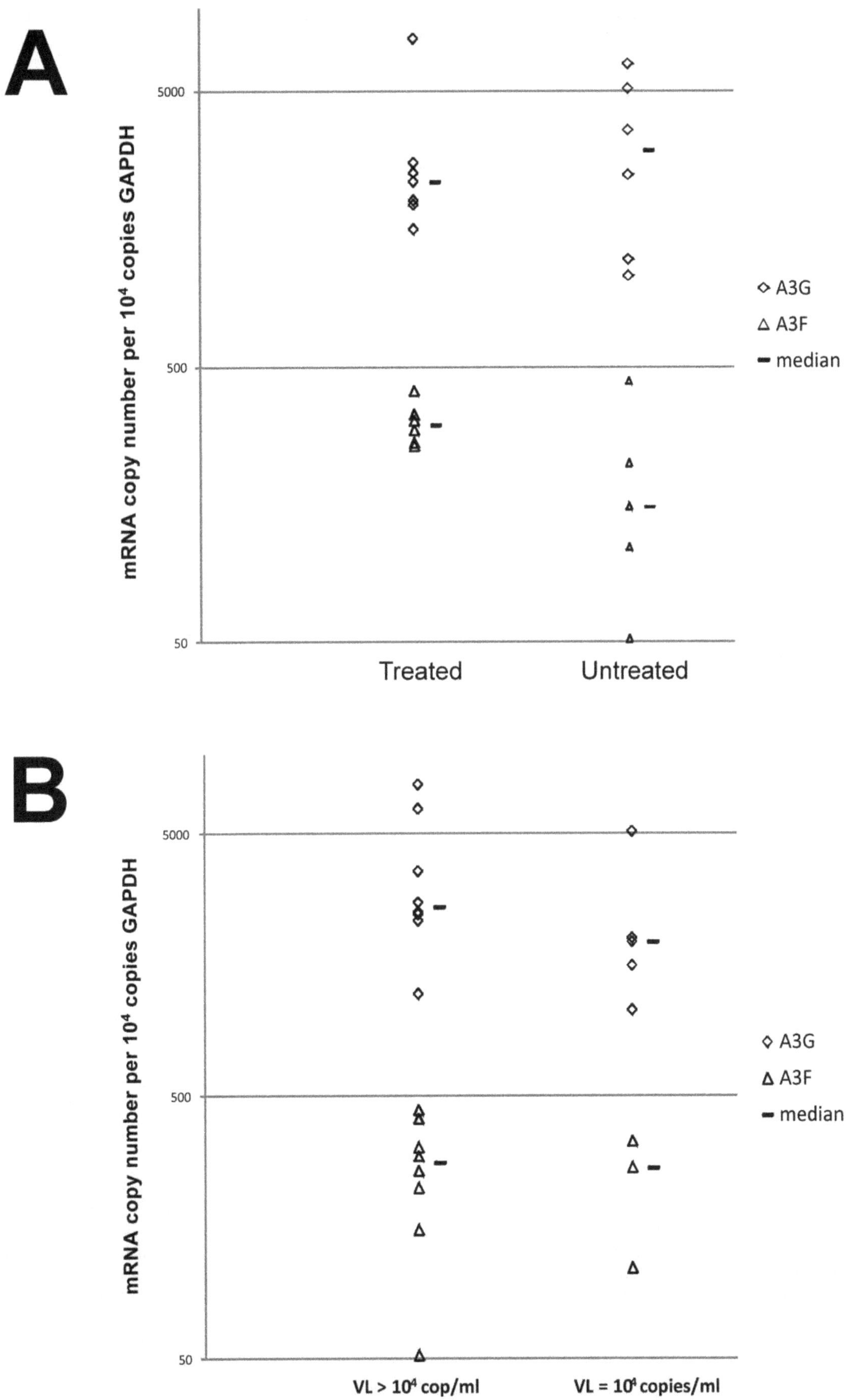
A
mRNA copy number per 10^4 copies GAPDH
5000
500
50
Treated
Untreated
A3G
A3F
median
B
mRNA copy number per 10^4 copies GAPDH
5000
500
50
VL > 10^4 cop/ml
VL = 10^4 copies/ml
A3G
A3F
median

Figure 4. APOBEC3G and APOBEC3F mRNA expression levels relative to GAPDH mRNA copy numbers comparing patients stratified according to antiretroviral treatment exposure (*A*) and HIV viral load (*B*). Horizontal bars depict the median value for each group.

also failed to correlate HIV VL with either A3G-mediated hypermutation [29,38] or to A3G expression levels [20,26,27,39] in adults, different studies showed correlation between A3G mRNA expression or G-to-A hypermutation and disease progression [28,32], and this issue is warranted further investigation.

Of interest, we have found a high contribution of A3F-mediated hypermutation in the HIV-1 PR *pol* genomic region of viruses from our children, a finding previously reported in infected adults. A recent study by Armitage *et al.* has shown that, whereas A3G hypermutates HIV proviruses roughly evenly across the genome, A3F promotes higher numbers of changes at definite regions, the largest being the *pol* PR region [23]. Indeed, A3F-mediated hypermutation in HIV PR has been previously described [9,24]. These observations might explain, at least in part, the relatively high observation of A3F-mediated hypermutation events in our patients.

A re-analysis of A3G and A3F expression levels with random primed-cDNA synthesis in a subset of HIV^+ and negative control children for which cellular RNA was still available showed that the A3F levels were underestimated, with fold differences to A3G levels three times lower than those estimated with oligo-d(T)-primed reactions. This is in agreement with data of Refsland et al. [35], which suggest that the long A3F mRNA 3′UTR presents repetitive elements that can impair oligo-d(T)-primed cDNA synthesis. Moreover, our confirmatory results further corroborate the importance of A3F-mediated hypermutation in the pediatric cohort studied.

Cho *et al.* have previously reported a positive correlation between the expression of A3G and A3F in adults [39]. In our pediatric casuistic, we failed to detect such correlation, both in HIV^+ and in uninfected children. It is plausible that the differences observed between their study and ours are related to the age groups analyzed. Children's immune systems are not completely developed, and HIV infection during development may also impair specific immune components. A3G and A3F expression levels might not correlate well in a partially-developed immune system. In this view, it has been shown that distinct $CD4^+$ T-helper lymphocyte subtypes show differences in the levels of A3G expression [40]. Th1 effector cells express higher levels of A3G and A3F mRNA, and of A3G proteins, than Th2 cells. In addition, HIV-1 virions produced in Th1 cells carry increased amounts of incorporated A3G compared to those produced in Th2 cells [40]. As a result of lower ratios of $CD4^+$ Th1 cells observed in children compared to adults [41], children might have a proportionally higher A3F-mediated hypermutation activity. Finally, differential expression of the A3 proteins has been shown in different human tissues [35]. In particular, tissues such as the thymus and the spleen, which carry a large amount of T cells, and have significantly different activities in children and adults, can explain discrepancies in the levels of A3G and A3F seen in both groups.

We cannot rule out the possibility that differences in A3G and A3F protein activity are due to amino acid polymorphisms, to protein stability or to differential interaction with Vif taking place in the individuals analyzed here. Indeed, a number of Vif mutants have been recently shown to lack A3G-counteracting activity, and even interfere with wild type Vif molecules [42]. Conversely, amino acid changes in several A3 coding regions, including A3G and A3F, also alter susceptibility to HIV-1 Vif [43,44]. Additional studies in the A3G and A3F coding sequences will improve our understanding of the role of each protein in hypermutation. At the protein level, it is recognized that A3G exists in two forms within cells, aggregated into low (LMM) or high molecular mass (HMM) complexes [45]. While the first form is active in virus deamination, the second is inactive. It has been shown that selected cytokines, like IL-2, IL-7 and IL-15, induce a shift of A3G into HMM complexes, rendering $CD4^+$ T-cells more permissive to HIV infection. Other cytokines, such as TNFα, upregulate A3G in cells but leave them in LMM complexes, active against HIV [45]. Again here, differences in the immune system of children compared to that of adults might account for discrepancies in the amount of enzymatically-active forms of A3 proteins.

Another important issue to be considered here is the fact that many different A3 proteins display anti-HIV activity, as reviewed by Albin and Harris [46]. Although A3G and A3F have been recognized as major players in HIV restriction, other members of the APOBEC family such as A3DE and A3H have been shown to harbor anti-HIV activity, as well as sensitivity to lentiviral Vif proteins [43,46,47]. In this scenario, we cannot rule out the possibility that other A3 proteins with similar target contexts to A3F, particularly A3H [48,49], are contributing to the higher non-A3G-mediated hypermutation seen herein.

Previous studies have reported higher levels of A3G expression in subjects infected by HIV or HCV compared to uninfected individuals [27,50]. Our results are in agreement with those studies, and extend this observation to A3F. In our control group, however, the three highest A3G-expressing uninfected children had median expression values significantly higher than the median of the remaining NC, suggesting that A3G expression may vary substantially between individuals depending on various unrelated infections and on other immunological factors. It has been recently shown that infection by influenza A virus upregulates A3G, but not A3F expression in infected cells [51]. Therefore, the possibility that varying, unrecognized clinical conditions might alter A3G expression levels in individuals cannot be ruled out, and may prevent the establishment of clear associations between HIV infection and A3G expression.

We failed to observe any association between HIV VL or treatment experience and A3G/F mRNA expression in our patients. This is agreement with the report by Ulenga *et al.*, which were not able to correlate hypermutation with VL in infected adults [29]. A previous report failed to find differences in A3G-mediated hypermutation between patients with undetectable VL by natural means (among elite supressors) or with the use of antiretroviral therapy [20], indicating that treatment *per se* does not influence A3G expression levels. Further studies are warranted to define specific biological or chemotherapeutical circumstances under which APOBEC expression is modulated.

Overall, we were unable to find any correlations between A3G or A3F expression levels, A3G- or A3F-induced hypermutation and disease progression profiles in HIV-infected children. This is however, to the best of our knowledge, the first study of A3G and A3F mRNA expression conducted in pediatric HIV/AIDS patients. The study of different disease progression profiles in the pediatric setting is also worth mentioning. Interestingly, we found evidence of a more pronounced A3F activity, not previously reported in adults, that merits further investigation. We believe this study helps contributing to a better understanding of the role of restriction factors and host genetics in an infectious disease pediatric setting.

Acknowledgments

We are indebted to Prof. Marcos H. Sorgine (Instituto de Bioquímica Médica, UFRJ) for helpful discussions on the implementation and validation of the real-time PCR experiments. We would also like to thank the HIV/AIDS Staff at the Instituto de Pueircultura e Pediatria Martagão Gesteira, UFRJ, for providing care and clinical information on the HIV-infected children studied here. This study is part of the PhD Thesis by AOA at the Graduate Program in Genetics, UFRJ.

Author Contributions

Conceived and designed the experiments: NDA AOA ESM MAS. Performed the experiments: NDA AOA. Analyzed the data: NDA AOA ESM MAS. Contributed reagents/materials/analysis tools: SMC RHO MAS. Wrote the paper: ESM MAS.

References

1. Foster C, Waelbrouck A, Peltier A (2007) Adolescents and HIV infection. Curr Opin HIV AIDS 2: 431–436.
2. Abrams EJ, Wiener J, Carter R, Kuhn L, Palumbo P, et al. (2003) Maternal health factors and early pediatric antiretroviral therapy influence the rate of perinatal HIV-1 disease progression in children. Aids 17: 867–877.
3. Alexander L, Cuchura L, Simpson BJ, Andiman WA (2006) Virologic and host characteristics of human immunodeficiency virus type 1-infected pediatric long term survivors. Pediatr Infect Dis J 25: 135–141.
4. Harris RS, Bishop KN, Sheehy AM, Craig HM, Petersen-Mahrt SK, et al. (2003) DNA deamination mediates innate immunity to retroviral infection. Cell 113: 803–809.
5. Mariani R, Chen D, Schrofelbauer B, Navarro F, Konig R, et al. (2003) Species-specific exclusion of APOBEC3G from HIV-1 virions by Vif. Cell 114: 21–31.
6. Mangeat B, Turelli P, Caron G, Friedli M, Perrin L, et al. (2003) Broad antiretroviral defence by human APOBEC3G through lethal editing of nascent reverse transcripts. Nature 424: 99–103.
7. Zhang H, Yang B, Pomerantz RJ, Zhang C, Arunachalam SC, et al. (2003) The cytidine deaminase CEM15 induces hypermutation in newly synthesized HIV-1 DNA. Nature 424: 94–98.
8. Bishop KN, Holmes RK, Malim MH (2006) Antiviral potency of APOBEC proteins does not correlate with cytidine deamination. J Virol 80: 8450–8458.
9. Liddament MT, Brown WL, Schumacher AJ, Harris RS (2004) APOBEC3F properties and hypermutation preferences indicate activity against HIV-1 in vivo. Curr Biol 14: 1385–1391.
10. Sheehy AM, Gaddis NC, Choi JD, Malim MH (2002) Isolation of a human gene that inhibits HIV-1 infection and is suppressed by the viral Vif protein. Nature 418: 646–650.
11. Wiegand HL, Doehle BP, Bogerd HP, Cullen BR (2004) A second human antiretroviral factor, APOBEC3F, is suppressed by the HIV-1 and HIV-2 Vif proteins. Embo J 23: 2451–2458.
12. Zennou V, Bieniasz PD (2006) Comparative analysis of the antiretroviral activity of APOBEC3G and APOBEC3F from primates. Virology 349: 31–40.
13. Zheng YH, Irwin D, Kurosu T, Tokunaga K, Sata T, et al. (2004) Human APOBEC3F is another host factor that blocks human immunodeficiency virus type 1 replication. J Virol 78: 6073–6076.
14. Sheehy AM, Gaddis NC, Malim MH (2003) The antiretroviral enzyme APOBEC3G is degraded by the proteasome in response to HIV-1 Vif. Nat Med 9: 1404–1407.
15. Liu B, Sarkis PT, Luo K, Yu Y, Yu XF (2005) Regulation of Apobec3F and human immunodeficiency virus type 1 Vif by Vif-Cul5-ElonB/C E3 ubiquitin ligase. J Virol 79: 9579–9587.
16. Chiu YL, Greene WC (2008) The APOBEC3 cytidine deaminases: an innate defensive network opposing exogenous retroviruses and endogenous retroelements. Annu Rev Immunol 26: 317–353.
17. Bishop KN, Holmes RK, Sheehy AM, Davidson NO, Cho SJ, et al. (2004) Cytidine deamination of retroviral DNA by diverse APOBEC proteins. Curr Biol 14: 1392–1396.
18. Holmes RK, Koning FA, Bishop KN, Malim MH (2007) APOBEC3F can inhibit the accumulation of HIV-1 reverse transcription products in the absence of hypermutation. Comparisons with APOBEC3G. J Biol Chem 282: 2587–2595.
19. Kieffer TL, Kwon P, Nettles RE, Han Y, Ray SC, et al. (2005) G–>A hypermutation in protease and reverse transcriptase regions of human immunodeficiency virus type 1 residing in resting CD4+ T cells in vivo. J Virol 79: 1975–1980.
20. Gandhi SK, Siliciano JD, Bailey JR, Siliciano RF, Blankson JN (2008) Role of APOBEC3G/F-mediated hypermutation in the control of human immunodeficiency virus type 1 in elite suppressors. J Virol 82: 3125–3130.
21. Kijak GH, Janini LM, Tovanabutra S, Sanders-Buell E, Arroyo MA, et al. (2008) Variable contexts and levels of hypermutation in HIV-1 proviral genomes recovered from primary peripheral blood mononuclear cells. Virology 376: 101–111.
22. Land AM, Ball TB, Luo M, Pilon R, Sandstrom P, et al. (2008) Human immunodeficiency virus (HIV) type 1 proviral hypermutation correlates with CD4 count in HIV-infected women from Kenya. J Virol 82: 8172–8182.
23. Armitage AE, Katzourakis A, de Oliveira T, Welch JJ, Belshaw R, et al. (2008) Conserved footprints of APOBEC3G on Hypermutated human immunodeficiency virus type 1 and human endogenous retrovirus HERV-K(HML2) sequences. J Virol 82: 8743–8761.
24. Janini M, Rogers M, Birx DR, McCutchan FE (2001) Human immunodeficiency virus type 1 DNA sequences genetically damaged by hypermutation are often abundant in patient peripheral blood mononuclear cells and may be generated during near-simultaneous infection and activation of CD4(+) T cells. J Virol 75: 7973–7986.
25. Harris RS, Liddament MT (2004) Retroviral restriction by APOBEC proteins. Nat Rev Immunol 4: 868–877.
26. Jin X, Brooks A, Chen H, Bennett R, Reichman R, et al. (2005) APOBEC3G/CEM15 (hA3G) mRNA levels associate inversely with human immunodeficiency virus viremia. J Virol 79: 11513–11516.
27. Ulenga NK, Sarr AD, Thakore-Meloni S, Sankale JL, Eisen G, et al. (2008) Relationship between human immunodeficiency type 1 infection and expression of human APOBEC3G and APOBEC3F. J Infect Dis 198: 486–492.
28. Vazquez-Perez JA, Ormsby CE, Hernandez-Juan R, Torres KJ, Reyes-Teran G (2009) APOBEC3G mRNA expression in exposed seronegative and early stage HIV infected individuals decreases with removal of exposure and with disease progression. Retrovirology 6: 23.
29. Ulenga NK, Sarr AD, Hamel D, Sankale JL, Mboup S, et al. (2008) The level of APOBEC3G (hA3G)-related G-to-A mutations does not correlate with viral load in HIV type 1-infected individuals. AIDS Res Hum Retroviruses 24: 1285–1290.
30. Nielsen K, McSherry G, Petru A, Frederick T, Wara D, et al. (1997) A descriptive survey of pediatric human immunodeficiency virus-infected long-term survivors. Pediatrics 99: E4.
31. Soares EA, Santos AF, Sousa TM, Sprinz E, Martinez AM, et al. (2007) Differential drug resistance acquisition in HIV-1 of subtypes B and C. PLoS ONE 2: e730.
32. Pace C, Keller J, Nolan D, James I, Gaudieri S, et al. (2006) Population level analysis of human immunodeficiency virus type 1 hypermutation and its relationship with APOBEC3G and vif genetic variation. J Virol 80: 9259–9269.
33. Rose PP, Korber BT (2000) Detecting hypermutations in viral sequences with an emphasis on G –> A hypermutation. Bioinformatics 16: 400–401.
34. StatsDirectLtd (2008) StatsDirect statistical software. 2.7.2 ed Liverpool: StatsDirect Ltd.
35. Refsland EW, Stenglein MD, Shindo K, Albin JS, Brown WL, et al. (2010) Quantitative profiling of the full APOBEC3 mRNA repertoire in lymphocytes and tissues: implications for HIV-1 restriction. Nucleic Acids Res 38: 4274–4284.
36. De Maio FA, Rocco CA, Aulicino PC, Bologna R, Mangano A, et al. (2011) Effect of HIV-1 Vif variability on progression to pediatric AIDS and its association with APOBEC3G and CUL5 polymorphisms. Infect Genet Evol 11: 1256–1262.
37. Koulinska IN, Chaplin B, Mwakagile D, Essex M, Renjifo B (2003) Hypermutation of HIV type 1 genomes isolated from infants soon after vertical infection. AIDS Res Hum Retroviruses 19: 1115–1123.
38. Piantadosi A, Humes D, Chohan B, McClelland RS, Overbaugh J (2009) An analysis of the percent of HIV-1 sequences that are hypermutated and markers of disease progression in a longitudinal cohort, including one individual with a partially defective Vif. J Virol.
39. Cho SJ, Drechsler H, Burke RC, Arens MQ, Powderly W, et al. (2006) APOBEC3F and APOBEC3G mRNA levels do not correlate with human immunodeficiency virus type 1 plasma viremia or CD4+ T-cell count. J Virol 80: 2069–2072.
40. Vetter ML, Johnson ME, Antons AK, Unutmaz D, D'Aquila RT (2009) Differences in APOBEC3G expression in CD4+ T helper lymphocyte subtypes modulate HIV-1 infectivity. PLoS Pathog 5: e1000292.
41. Gasparoni A, Ciardelli L, Avanzini A, Castellazzi AM, Carini R, et al. (2003) Age-related changes in intracellular TH1/TH2 cytokine production, immunoproliferative T lymphocyte response and natural killer cell activity in newborns, children and adults. Biol Neonate 84: 297–303.
42. Walker RC, Jr., Khan MA, Kao S, Goila-Gaur R, Miyagi E, et al. (2010) Identification of dominant negative human immunodeficiency virus type 1 Vif

mutants that interfere with the functional inactivation of APOBEC3G by virus-encoded Vif. J Virol 84: 5201–5211.

43. Smith JL, Pathak VK (2010) Identification of specific determinants of human APOBEC3F, APOBEC3C, and APOBEC3DE and African green monkey APOBEC3F that interact with HIV-1 Vif. J Virol 84: 12599–12608.
44. Albin JS, LaRue RS, Weaver JA, Brown WL, Shindo K, et al. (2010) A single amino acid in human APOBEC3F alters susceptibility to HIV-1 Vif. J Biol Chem 285: 40785–40792.
45. Stopak KS, Chiu YL, Kropp J, Grant RM, Greene WC (2007) Distinct patterns of cytokine regulation of APOBEC3G expression and activity in primary lymphocytes, macrophages, and dendritic cells. J Biol Chem 282: 3539–3546.
46. Albin JS, Harris RS (2010) Interactions of host APOBEC3 restriction factors with HIV-1 in vivo: implications for therapeutics. Expert Rev Mol Med 12: e4.
47. Larue RS, Lengyel J, Jonsson SR, Andresdottir V, Harris RS (2010) Lentiviral Vif degrades the APOBEC3Z3/APOBEC3H protein of its mammalian host and is capable of cross-species activity. J Virol 84: 8193–8201.
48. Gourraud PA, Karaouni A, Woo JM, Schmidt T, Oksenberg JR, et al. (2011) APOBEC3H haplotypes and HIV-1 pro-viral vif DNA sequence diversity in early untreated human immunodeficiency virus-1 infection. Hum Immunol 72: 207–212.
49. Li MM, Wu LI, Emerman M (2010) The range of human APOBEC3H sensitivity to lentiviral Vif proteins. J Virol 84: 88–95.
50. Komohara Y, Yano H, Shichijo S, Shimotohno K, Itoh K, et al. (2006) High expression of APOBEC3G in patients infected with hepatitis C virus. J Mol Histol 37: 327–332.
51. Pauli EK, Schmolke M, Hofmann H, Ehrhardt C, Flory E, et al. (2009) High level expression of the anti-retroviral protein APOBEC3G is induced by influenza A virus but does not confer antiviral activity. Retrovirology 6: 38.

9

High Prevalence of Malaria in Zambezia, Mozambique: The Protective Effect of IRS versus Increased Risks due to Pig-Keeping and House Construction

Emmanuel A. Temu[1], Mike Coleman[2]*, Ana Paula Abilio[3], Immo Kleinschmidt[4]

1 London School of Hygiene and Tropical Medicine, London, United Kingdom, **2** Liverpool School of Tropical Medicine, Liverpool, United Kingdom, **3** National Institute of Health, Maputo, Mozambique, **4** Tropical Epidemiology Group, London School of Hygiene and Tropical Medicine, London, United Kingdom

Abstract

Background: African countries are scaling up malaria interventions, especially insecticide treated nets (ITN) and indoor residual spraying (IRS), for which ambitious coverage targets have been set. In spite of these efforts infection prevalence remains high in many parts of the continent. This study investigated risk factors for malaria infection in children using three malaria indicator surveys from Zambezia province, Mozambique. The impact of IRS and ITNs, the effects of keeping farm animals and of the construction material of roofs of houses and other potential risk factors associated with malaria infection in children were assessed.

Methods: Cross-sectional community-based surveys were conducted in October of 2006, 2007 and 2008. A total of 8338 children (ages 1–15 years) from 2748 households were included in the study. All children were screened for malaria by rapid diagnostic tests. Caregiver interviews were used to assess household demographic and wealth characteristics and ITN and IRS coverage. Associations between malaria infection, vector control interventions and potential risk factors were assessed.

Results: Overall, the prevalence of malaria infection was 47.8% (95%CI: 38.7%–57.1%) in children 1–15 years of age, less than a quarter of children (23.1%, 95%CI: 19.1%–27.6%) were sleeping under ITN and almost two thirds were living in IRS treated houses (coverage 65.4%, 95%CI: 51.5%–77.0%). Protective factors that were independently associated with malaria infection were: sleeping in an IRS house without sleeping under ITN (Odds Ratio (OR) = 0.6; 95%CI: 0.4–0.9); additional protection due to sleeping under ITN in an IRS treated house (OR = 0.5; 95%CI: 0.3–0.7) versus sleeping in an unsprayed house without a ITN; and parental education (primary/secondary: OR = 0.6; 95%CI: 0.5–0.7) versus parents with no education. Increased risk of infection was associated with: current fever (OR = 1.2; 95%CI: 1.0–1.5) versus no fever; pig keeping (OR = 3.2; 95%CI: 2.1–4.9) versus not keeping pigs; living in houses with a grass roof (OR = 1.7; 95%CI: 1.3–2.4) versus other roofing materials and bigger household size (8–15 people: OR = 1.6; 95%CI: 1.3–2.1) versus small households (1–4 persons).

Conclusion: Malaria infection among children under 15 years of age in Zambezia remained high but conventional malaria vector control methods, in particular IRS, provided effective means of protection. Household ownership of farm animals, particularly pigs, and living in houses with a grass roof were independently associated with increased risk of infection, even after allowing for household wealth. To reduce the burden of malaria, national control programs need to ensure high coverage of effective IRS and promote the use of ITNs, particularly in households with elevated risks of infection, such as those keeping farm animals, and those with grass roofs.

Editor: Abdisalan Mohamed Noor, Kenya Medical Research Institute - Wellcome Trust Research Programme, Kenya

Funding: This work was funded by the Innovative Vector Control Consortium. The funder had no role in study design, data collection and analysis, decision to publish, or preparation of the manuscript.

Competing Interests: The authors have declared that no competing interests exist.

* E-mail: mcoleman@liverpool.ac.uk

Introduction

Malaria, especially that caused by *Plasmodium falciparum*, remains one of the most important causes of morbidity and early mortality in endemic regions of sub-Saharan Africa [1]. A massive scale-up in malaria control programmes between 2008 and 2010 has resulted in the provision of Insecticide Treated Nets (ITNs) to protect more than 578 million people at risk of malaria in this region [1]. Similarly, Indoor Residual Spraying (IRS) has protected 75 million people in 2009. Due to the scaling up of interventions, the number of deaths caused by malaria is estimated to have decreased from 985,000 in 2000 to 781,000 in 2009 [1]. National strategies to monitor malaria interventions include malaria indicator surveys that measure malaria infection prevalence, coverage and usage of various interventions and changes in knowledge attitude and practices in malaria control [2–4].

Many of the risk factors for malaria are related to access to interventions and inversely related to a household's socio-economic status (SES) with increasing vulnerability of the poorest [5]. In addition, malaria risk varies widely between localities or even households due to their specific characteristics (locations, household possessions, house construction, farm animal ownership and distribution of mosquito breeding sites) that may facilitate human/mosquito contact increasing the likelihood of malaria infection. In regions where the malaria mosquito vectors feed on both animals and humans, the presence of farm animals close to the household may also affect the risk of malaria transmission to humans. The nature of this impact is likely to be vector and site specific [6].

The African Summit on Roll Back Malaria, held in Abuja, Nigeria in 2000, specified that 60% of population at risk of malaria should use ITNs by 2005, a target that was raised to 80% by 2010 [7]. But use of ITNs remains below the target with only 18.5% of African children in stable malaria transmission areas protected by a net in 2007, leaving nearly 90 million unprotected [8].

During the past decade, IRS has been implemented successfully in Mozambique, Eritrea, Ethiopia, Equatorial Guinea, Island of Principe and Madagascar [9–11]. With funding from the President Malaria Initiative (PMI), the Global Fund and the private sector, African countries are expanding ITN and IRS programmes as part of their national malaria control strategies.

In Mozambique malaria is endemic, affecting the entire population of around 23 million people [12] with an estimated 44,000 to 67,000 malaria specific deaths each year across all age groups [13]. Over 90% of reported cases are due to *P falciparum*. Transmission is perennial with peaks during and after rainy seasons. The most important malaria vectors belong to the *Anopheles gambiae* complex and the *An funestus* group [14].

Mozambique is currently promoting ITNs and IRS for malaria prevention. Long lasting insecticidal nets (LLIN), are distributed free to pregnant women and children under five years old. IRS campaign for malaria control has been conducted in Mozambique using various insecticides. Before 2000, pyrethroids were used for IRS but the detection of resistance [14,15] led to the replacement by carbamate. However due to the high cost of using carbamate for IRS, DDT was introduced in 2005 and used until 2008.From 2009, pyrethroids were again used as main insecticide for IRS [16].

In this study, the effects on malarial infection of vector control interventions, house construction, ownership of farm animals, household wealth and other potential risk factors were investigated using malaria indicator survey data from Zambezia province, Mozambique.

Materials and Methods

Study site

Zambezia province is situated in central Mozambique, has an estimated population of 3,794,509 and covers a total area of 103,127 km^2, much of it drained by the Zambezi River [17]. There is considerable forest inland and much of the coast consists of mangrove swamps. Zambezia province is characterized by a seasonal pattern of rainfall from October to June and malaria is perennial with transmission peaking during the rainy season.

In Zambezia province, IRS with DDT was re-introduced in 2006 through the Mozambique National Malaria Control Program (MNMCP), supported by the US Presidents Malaria Initiative [16]. In 2009 there was a change in the insecticide from DDT to pyrethroids. Pyrethroid resistance in *An. funestus* was first reported in southern Mozambique in 2001 [15] and recently (2010) in Zambezia [18].

The ITN used are mostly long lasting types: the Olyset® (active ingredient: 2% permethrin) and PermaNets® (a.i: 50–55 mg/m2 deltamethrin) brands that were distributed in Zambezia since 2004 [16]. From 2004 to 2007, 559,126 LLIN were distributed in Mozambique, the bulk of these were in 2007 with majority of nets distributed in Milange district in Zambezia [16].

Household survey and data preparation

Malaria surveys were conducted annually in October in 2006, 2007 and 2008 in 19 sentinel sites (Figure 1) established for monitoring and surveillance of the malaria control program in 6 districts in Zambezia province. The surveillance was part of the Malaria Decision Support System project (MDSS) [19]. The survey instrument was adapted from the RBM - MERG Malaria Indicator Survey Household Questionnaire [20] to collect information on knowledge of preventive measures; IRS status of houses, net ownership and usage, household assets, house construction and ownership of farm animals. Children between ages of 1 to 15 years gave finger prick blood samples for a rapid diagnostic test (ICT; Global Diagnostics, South Africa), had their temperature taken, and history of fever recorded. Participants who tested positive were treated with Coartem® (Novartis) (Artemether and Lumefantrine) according to Mozambique's national malaria treatment guidelines.

History of fever was defined as parents reporting children who experienced fever in the past 4 weeks. Current fever was defined as body temperature $\geq$37.5°C taken during the survey. Head of household's education was categorised into those without formal education, those with primary/secondary education and those with tertiary education. Knowledge of malaria prevention was classified as adequate if the respondent was aware of malaria preventive measures in addition to IRS and ITN (use of repellents, coils or doom spray; burn leaves or cow dung; close windows and doors; use wire gauze; dispose cans and tyres; and drain water to reduce mosquito breeding). During the interview, respondent provided information on whether the net was treated or not but the ITN status was not verified by the interviewer. Given both IRS and ITN are malaria interventions applied in Zambezia, a composite variable constituting the 4 combinations of vector control interventions was used to develop the risk model as: 1) children in households without IRS and not sleeping under ITN, 2) children in houses with IRS and sleeping under ITN, 3) those protected by IRS but not sleeping under an ITN, and 4) those in unsprayed houses but sleeping under ITN. Socio economic status (SES) for each household was calculated from an index which combined ownership of assets (TV, radio, mobile phones, bicycles, motorcycles, cars and tractors) and house construction materials using principal component analysis [21], divided into quartiles, the 1st quartile being the poorest. Houses were categorized into those covered by a grass roof and those covered with roof materials other than grass. The number of people in the household was grouped into 1–4 people, 5–7 people and 8–15 people.

Statistical analysis

The following risk factors for malaria infection were investigated: whether the house had been sprayed (IRS) in the past 12 months, whether the child slept under a ITN the previous night, the child's sex and age, head of household's level of education, SES quartile, ownership of farm animal, house construction, knowledge of other malaria prevention practices, history of fever and current fever, and number of people in the house. Point estimates, confidence intervals, survey chi-square tests and estimates for odds ratio were derived taking account of the two-stage sample design by using the survey commands in Stata 11 [22] setting sentinel sites as the primary sampling unit (PSU). Data were merged to provide information for each child.

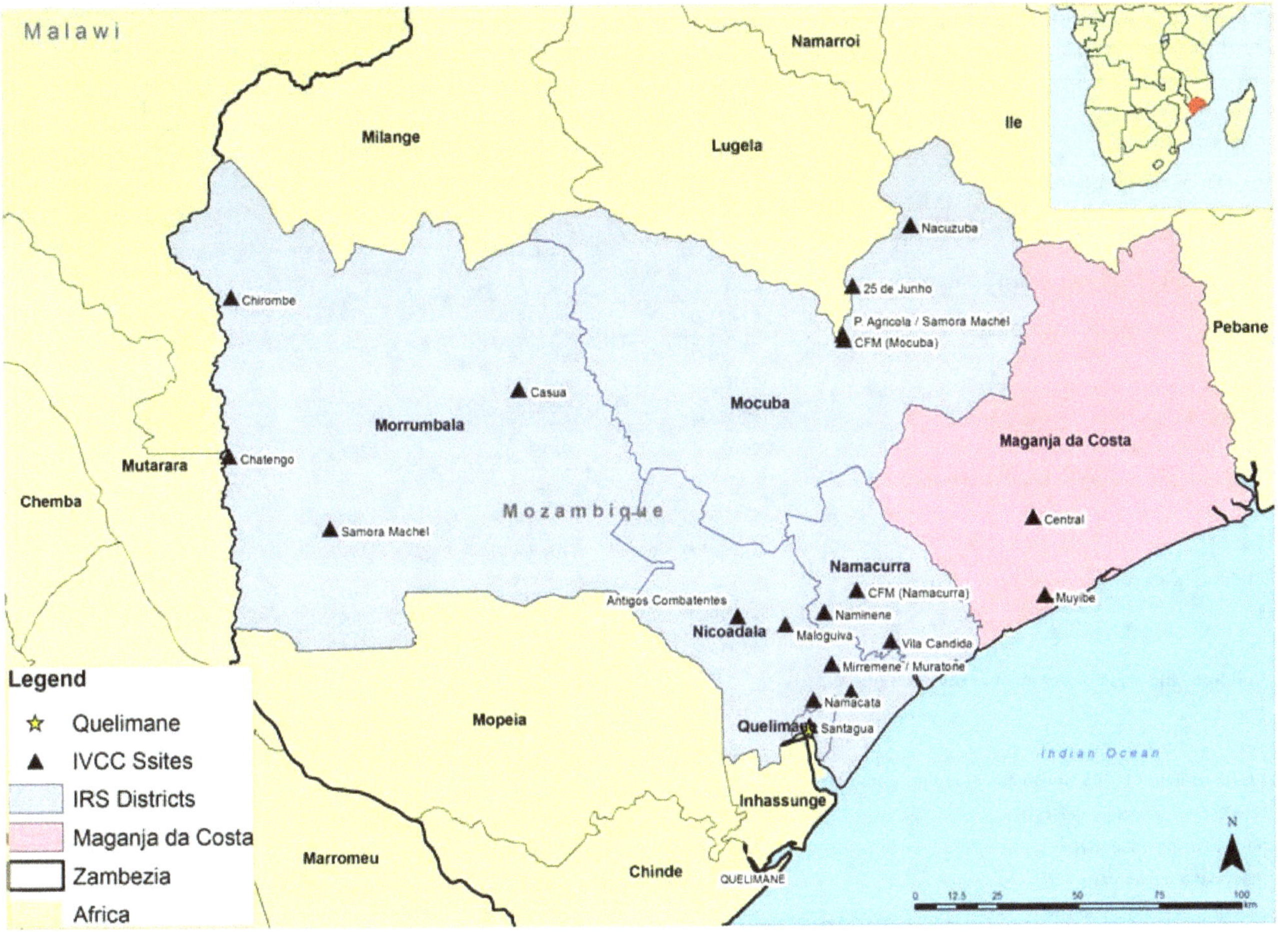

Figure 1. Map of Mozambique showing Zambezia province, the study site.

Crude odds ratio for the association between malaria infection and each explanatory variable were assessed one at a time using logistic regression. Variables with association ($p<0.025$) in the univariate analysis were considered for inclusion in a multivariable logistic regression model. The contribution of each covariate in the risk model was assessed by Wald tests and was included if $p<0.05$ after adjusting for confounders.

Sex and age were used as a priori potential confounders following practice adopted elsewhere [23].

Ethics Approval

Ethics approval for the study was given by the Ministry of Health of Mozambique (Reg: 3622/IMS-2/DNS/06). Written informed consent was obtained from heads of households or responsible adults in each of the participating households.

Results

Characteristics of study population

A total of 2,748 households in 19 villages were surveyed in 2006, 2007 and 2008, with an average of 144 houses per sentinel site [range 99 to 175]. A total of 8,338 children from 1 to below 15 years of age participated, giving an average of 439 children/site.

The majority of children belonged to households whose head was not educated (42.4%) or had primary/secondary education (41.7%). The majority of children lived in houses covered with grass roof (77.6%) (Table 1). The proportion of children living in households with any farm animal was 47.5% (n = 3,957, 95%CI: 36.8–58.3). A high proportion of children were living in households with chickens (44.9%, n = 3,734, 95%CI: 34.7–55.5) compared to those living in houses with pigs (2.7%, n = 225, 95%CI: 1.4–5.1) or sheep (0.2%, n = 19, 95%CI: 0.05–1.1).

Coverage of malaria control measures

The proportion of children who slept under any type of net the previous night increased from 29.8% (95%CI: 26.9%–32.8%) in 2006, to 34.3% (95%CI: 31.4%–37.4%) in 2008. Overall, 32.6% (95%CI: 30.9%–34.4%) of children were reported sleeping under any net the previous night (Table 1). Sixty five percent (95%CI: 63.6%–67.1%) of children were living in IRS treated houses ranging from 59.8% (95%CI: 56.4%–63.1%) in 2006 to 69.6% (95%CI: 66.3%–72.7%) in 2008.

As ITN and IRS campaigns were rolled out in Zambezia province, the proportion of children living in houses with IRS and sleeping under ITNs increased from 12.4% (95%CI: 7.6%–19.7%) in 2006 to 19.0% (95%CI: 13.4%–26.4%) in 2008 (Table 1). Overall, 15.4% (95%CI: 11.0%–21.0%) of children were living in IRS houses and sleeping under ITNs, 49.7% (95%CI: 39.6%–59.9%) were living in sprayed houses without sleeping under ITNs, 7.3% (95%CI: 4.2%–12.4%) were sleeping under ITNs in unsprayed houses and 27.6% (95%CI: 18.9%–38.3%) were neither sleeping under an ITN nor living in a sprayed house.

Table 1. Characteristics of children in Zambezia province.

Characteristics	2006 N(%)*	2007 N(%)*	2008 N(%)*	Total N(%)*
Gender of children tested				
Male	1233(47.8)	1366(48.2)	1297(45.2)	3896(47.0)
Female	1349(52.2)	1466(51.8)	1575(54.8)	4390(53.0)
Age groups of children (years)				
1–3	644(24.7)	690(24.3)	701(24.3)	2035(24.4)
4–6	777(29.7)	884(31.0)	988(34.2)	2649(31.8)
7–9	591(22.6)	651(22.9)	568(19.8)	1810(21.7)
10–15	598(23.0)	620(21.8)	626(21.7)	1844(22.1)
Total Children (below15 years)	2610	2845	2883	8338
Children with history of fever past 4 weeks				
No	1397(55.4)	1649(60.8)	1710(59.8)	4756(58.8)
Yes	1125(44.6)	1062(39.2)	1151(40.2)	3338(41.2)
Children with current fever				
No	2197(84.4)	2436(85.7)	2705(93.9)	7338(88.2)
Yes	405(15.6)	408(14.3)	173(6.1)	986(11.8)
Children who slept under any net previous night				
No	1778(70.2)	1808(66.6)	1867(65.7)	5453(67.4)
Yes	756(29.8)	907(33.4)	975(34.3)	2638(32.6)
Children living in IRS house and sleeping under ITN				
No IRS & not sleeping under ITN	682(31.5)	640(28.0)	559(23.6)	1881(27.6)
IRS & sleeping under ITN	269(12.4)	328(14.4)	450(19.0)	1047(15.4)
IRS & not sleeping under ITN	1027(47.5)	1168(51.1)	1192(50.4)	3387(49.7)
No IRS & sleeping under ITN	185(8.6)	149(6.5)	164(6.9)	498(7.3)
Children living in household practicing other prevention measures than IRS & ITN				
No other prevention practice	1007(38.6)	890(31.3)	850(29.5)	2747(33.0)
Any other prevention practices	1603(61.4)	1955(68.7)	2033(70.5)	5591(67.0)
Size of household in which children live				
1–4 people	510(20.3)	651(22.9)	656(22.7)	1817(22.0)
5–7 people	1367(54.3)	1616(56.9)	1587(55.1)	4570(55.5)
8–15 people	639(25.4)	572(20.2)	640(22.2)	1851(22.5)
Children of parents with different level of education				
None	721(32.3)	895(36.9)	1551(55.0)	3167(42.4)
Primary/Secondary	1141(51.1)	1073(44.2)	902(32.0)	3116(41.7)
Tertiary	371(16.6)	457(18.9)	367(13.0)	1195(15.9)
Children living in household with different wealth index (SES)				
1st quartile (poorest)	792(30.8)	640(22.5)	892(30.9)	2324(28.0)
2nd quartile	544(21.2)	660(23.2)	625(21.7)	1829(22.0)
3rd quartile	667(26.0)	782(27.5)	582(20.2)	2031(24.5)
4th quartile (wealthiest)	565(22.0)	763(26.8)	784(27.2)	2112(25.5)
Roof material of house in which children live				
Without grass roof	406(17.4)	518(20.1)	604(31.4)	1528(22.4)
With grass roof	1927(82.6)	2057(79.9)	1320(68.6)	5304(77.6)
Children living in household with farm animals				
Without farm animal	1425(54.6)	1490(52.4)	1466(50.8)	4381(52.5)
With farm animals	1185(45.4)	1355(47.6)	1417(49.2)	3957(47.5)

*N (%) = number of children and percentage in each category.

The proportion of children whose parents reported knowledge of other malaria preventive measures in addition to IRS or ITN was 67.0% (95%CI: 62.4%–71.4%), increasing from 61.4% (95%CI: 55.5%–67.1%) in 2006, to 70.5% (95%CI: 65.3%–75.2%) in 2008 (Table 1).

Prevalence of malaria infection, ITN use and living in IRS houses

Overall prevalence of *P. falciparum* malaria infection in children (1–15 years) was 47.8% (95%CI: 38.7%–57.1%), of whom 15.8% (95%CI: 12.1%–20.3%) were co-infected with other plasmodial species. Malaria prevalence therefore refers to infections by *P. falciparum* alone or *P. falciparum* with other plasmodia. Malaria infection prevalence among children varied between the 19 villages ranging from 22.1% at Mocuba to 87.2% at 25-de-Junho. The proportion of infected children varied between years of survey from 51.9% in 2006, 60.3% in 2007, to 31.8% in 2008.

There was no evidence of difference in prevalence of malaria infection by sex (p = 0.27) but some evidence that it differed by household size (p = 0.065) and age group (p<0.012) ranging from 43.6% (95%CI: 41.2%–45.9%) in the 1–3 years age group to 51.7% (95%CI: 49.7%–54.1%) in the 7–9 years age group. More children presenting with current fever were infected with malaria (56.7%; 95%CI: 43.7%–68.9%) compared with those without fever (46.7%; 95%CI: 37.6–55.9, p = 0.037).

Malaria infections among children living in IRS houses and not sleeping under ITN were lower (OR = 0.6, 95%CI: 0.4–0.9; p = 0.013) than those in unsprayed (non IRS) houses and without sleeping under ITN. Children living in IRS houses and sleeping under ITN were additionally protected from malaria infection (OR = 0.4, 95%CI: 0.2–0.6, p = 0.001) relative to those not protected by either method. There was no evidence of a lower odds of malaria infection among children sleeping under ITN in unsprayed houses relative to those not protected by either methods (OR = 1.0, 95%CI: 0.7–1.5, p = 0.82) (Table 2).

Risk factors for malaria infection

In univariate analysis, pig-keeping was associated with increased risk of malaria infection for children (OR = 3.1, 95%CI: 2.0–4.7, p<0.001), even after excluding 25 de Junho, the village with highest malaria infection prevalence (87.2%) and highest number of children living in households keeping pigs (29%, 65/225), there was still strong association between pig-keeping and malaria infection (OR = 2.6, 95%CI: 1.8–3.8, p<0.001). In the analysis including all villages, sheep keeping was associated with reduced risk of malaria infection (OR = 0.5, 95%CI: 0.3–1.0, p = 0.042) (Table 2), but the effect was less clear when Mocuba, a village with majority of children living in households keeping sheep (74%, 14/19) and one with the lowest malaria infection prevalence in children (22.1%) was removed from the analysis (OR = 1.3, 95%CI: 0.7–2.3, p = 0.418).

A majority of children (77.6%) were living in houses with a grass roof and these children were at elevated risk of malaria infection compared to those living in houses without a grass roof (OR = 1.8; 95%CI: 1.2–2.7, p = 0.004) (Table 2). Children living in large households with more than 8 people (OR = 1.3; 95%CI: 1.0–1.6, p = 0.027) were at higher risk of malaria infection compared to smaller household.

Children of educated parents (primary/secondary: OR = 0.5, 95%CI: 0.4–0.6, p<0.0001; tertiary: OR = 0.3, 95%CI: 0.2–0.5, p<0.0001) compared to uneducated parents, and those from high SES (wealthiest quartile) (OR = 0.4, 95%CI: 0.3–0.5, p<0.0001) compared to low SES (poorest quartile) were associated with lower odds of malaria infection (Table 2).

The risk model for malaria infection

The multivariable logistic regression model was fitted sequentially starting with variables having an association with malaria infection (p<0.025) (Table 2). Age of child, household SES, year of survey, and the intervention variable (ITN, IRS status of house or both) were included a priori in the model. The model demonstrated that pig-keeping, living in houses with a grass roof, large household size, low parents education level and current fever were associated with an increased risk of malaria infection (Table 3).

In the final model, the risk of malaria infection was much lower among children living in an IRS household and sleeping under an ITN (OR = 0.5, 95%CI: 0.3–0.7) and those living in IRS household and not sleeping under ITN (OR = 0.6, 95%CI: 0.4–0.9) relative to those living in households without either of the two interventions. There was no evidence that sleeping under ITN in an unsprayed house was protective against malaria infection (OR = 1.2, 95%CI: 0.9–1.8, p = 0.238). Children of educated parents were at lower risk of malaria infection (primary/secondary education: OR = 0.6, 95%CI: 0.5–0.7, and tertiary education: OR = 0.4, 95%CI: 0.3–0.6) relative to those with no education.

On the other hand, pig-keeping (OR = 3.2, 95%CI: 2.1–4.9, p<0.0001) was associated with increased risk of malaria infection in children compared to those living in households without pigs. Malaria infection was also associated with children living in houses with a grass roof (OR = 1.7, 95%CI: 1.3–2.4, p = 0.002) relative to children living in houses with a non-grass roof. Overall the risk of malaria infection increased for children living in large households (5–7 people: OR = 1.6, 95%CI: 1.3–2.0, p<0.0001; ≥8 people: OR = 1.6, 95%CI: 1.3–2.1, p = 0.001) relative to those living in small household (1 to 4 people). Children with current fever were more likely to be infected (OR = 1.2, 95%CI: 1.0–1.5, p = 0.076) with malaria than those without fever.

There was no evidence that knowledge of prevention measures other than IRS and ITN was independently associated with risk of infection. The odds of malaria infection for sheep keeping (OR = 1.4, 95%CI: 0.9–2.1, p = 0.158) was in the same direction as pig keeping (OR = 3.2, 95%CI: 2.1–4.9, p<0.001) when sheep keeping was included in the model.

Discussion

In Zambezia province, malaria prevalence is high (47.8%) in children of all age groups below 15 years confirming that malaria remains a major cause of illness during childhood. Likewise, a survey of malaria across Mozambique reported overall malaria prevalence of 49% and relatively high age-specific malaria infection ranging from 39% for 7–10 years to 55% for children 1–2 years [24].

Children living in IRS treated houses and sleeping under an ITN (OR = 0.5, 95%CI: 0.3–0.7, relative to those not protected by either method) were at lower risk of malaria infection than children living in IRS houses and not sleeping under ITN (OR = 0.6, 95%CI: 0.4–0.9, relative to those not protected by either method), p = 0.028. The combined protective effect of IRS and ITN has been reported previously [9,25]. Although the impact of ITN on reducing malaria morbidity and mortality has been confirmed in robust randomised control trials [26], these surveys did not show evidence of protection against malaria infection in children sleeping under ITN in unsprayed houses (OR = 1.2, 95%CI: 0.9–1.8) compared to those not sleeping under ITN in unsprayed houses. This observation could be due to chance, related to irregular compliance or improper use of nets [27], or the result of reverse causation with nets being targeted at

Table 2. Association of malaria infection and other factors in Zambezia province.

Factors		Children N(%)*	Malaria infection %	P value	Trend^	Univariate Analysis OR§, 95%CI, p-value
Gender of children tested						
Male		3896(47.0)	49.0			1
Female		4390(53.0)	46.8	=0.27		0.9(0.8–1.1)p=0.395
Age groups of children (years)						
1–3		2035(24.4)	43.6			1
4–6		2649(31.8)	49.3			1.3(1.1–1.6)p=0.001
7–9		1810(21.7)	51.7			1.5(1.2–1.8)p=0.001
10–15		1844(22.1)	46.6	<0.012	0.013	1.2(0.9–1.5)p=0.14
Children with history of fever past 4 weeks						
No		4756(58.8)	46.4			1
Yes		3338(41.2)	50.5	=0.12		1.2(0.9–1.4) p=0.05
Children with current fever						
No		7338(88.2)	46.7			1
Yes		986(11.8)	56.7	=0.037		1.2(0.8–1.8) p=0.69
Children who slept under any net previous night						
No		5453(67.4)	51.0			1
Yes		2638(32.6)	42.0	=0.005		0.8(0.6–1.0)p=0.048
Children living in IRS house and sleeping under ITN						
No IRS & not sleeping under ITN		1881(27.6)	60.6			1
IRS & sleeping under ITN		1047(15.4)	32.3			0.4(0.2–0.6)p=0.001
IRS & not sleeping under ITN		3387(49.7)	46.2			0.6(0.4–0.9)p=0.013
No IRS & sleeping under ITN		498(7.3)	59.4	=0.0034		1.0(0.7–1.5)p=0.82
Children living in household practicing other prevention measures than IRS & ITN						
No other prevention practice		2747(33.0)	54.4			1
Any other prevention practices		5591(67.0)	44.6	=0.0023		0.8(0.6–0.9)p=0.014
Size of household in which children live						
1–4 people		1817(22.0)	45.3			1
5–7 people		4570(55.5)	49.8			1.3(1.1–1.6)p=0.001
8–15 people		1851(22.5)	45.7	=0.065	0.845	1.3(1.0–1.6)p=0.027
Children if parents with different level of education						
None		3167(42.4)	55.7			1
Primary/Secondary		3116(41.7)	44.6			0.5(0.4–0.6)p<0.0001
Tertiary		1195(15.9)	30.3	<0.0001	<0.0001	0.3(0.2–0.5)p<0.0001
Children living in household with different wealth index (SES)						
1st quartile (poorest)		2324(28.0)	54.4			1
2nd quartile		1829(22.0)	52.2			0.9(0.6–1.1)p=0.286
3rd quartile		2031(24.5)	52.1			0.8(0.6–1.0)p=0.058
4th quartile (wealthiest)		2112(25.5)	33.0	<0.0001	<0.0001	0.4(0.3–0.5) p<0.0001
Roof material of house in which children live						
Without grass roof		1528(22.4)	33.4			1
With grass roof		5304(77.6)	55.2	=0.0004		1.8(1.2–2.7)p=0.004
Children living in households with farm animals						
Chicken(s)	0	4591(55.2)	46.2			1
	≥1	3734(44.8)	49.8	=0.35		1.2(0.9–1.5)p=0.23
Goat(s)	0	7715(92.5)	47.4			1
	≥1	623(7.5)	53.1	=0.25		1.3(0.8–1.9)p=0.253
Sheep	0	8319(99.8)	47.9			1
	≥1	19(0.2)	31.6	=0.12		0.5(0.3–1.0)p=0.042
Cow(s)	0	8319(99.8)	47.8			1

Table 2. Cont.

Factors		Children N(%)*	Malaria infection %	P value	Trend^	Univariate Analysis OR§, 95%CI, p-value
	≥1	19(0.2)	55.6	=0.75		1.0(0.1–7.6)p = 0.98
Pig(s)	0	8113(97.3)	47.2			1
	≥1	225(2.7)	70.1	=0.0014		3.1(2.0–4.7)p<0.001
Year of survey						
2006		2610(31.3)	51.9			1
2007		2845(34.1)	60.3			1.5(1.1–2.0) p = 0.024
2008		2883(34.6)	31.8	<0.0001	<0.0001	0.4(0.3–0.7) p = 0.001

*N(%) = number of children and % in each category.
^P-value based on a non-parametric test for trend.
§Adjusted for age, asset index and year of survey.

communities that have the highest risk of malaria and households burdened by repeated episodes of malaria being more likely to use nets. Recent evidence of pyrethroid insecticide resistance, detected in *An. funestus* [18] in Zambezia could have reduced the protective effect of ITNs, particularly if they were in poor condition [28].

Knowledge of malaria preventive measures other than IRS and ITN (use of repellents, coils or doom spray, burn leaves or cow dung, etc), did not appear to have any protective effect on children, emphasising that conventional methods such as IRS and use of ITNs should be encouraged for public heath use of malaria control.

Keeping farm animals, in particular pigs and to lesser extent sheep was associated with increased risk of malaria infection even after adjusting for confounders such as household wealth, suggesting a possibility that certain farm animals may attract malaria vectors to the houses. Several studies have evaluated the relationship between malaria infection and keeping animals with conflicting results [29,30]. *Anopheles arabiensis*, attracted to animals and displaying opportunistic feeding behaviour [6], was found in Zambezia in low density at the time of the surveys compared to *An. gambiae s.s* and *An. funestus*. Although the latter are inherently endophilic, feeding mainly on human hosts [31,32], there are reports of *An. funestus* being not necessarily entirely anthropophagic [33], which would explain their attraction to houses with animals. . Further investigation into the relationship between farm animals and malaria infections occurring at different seasons may elucidate possible trends.

Malaria risk can vary widely between villages or even households [34] due to their specific characteristics that may facilitate human–mosquito contacts. The majority of children (78%) in Zambezia are living in houses with a grass roof which was associated with a high odds of malaria infection compared to those living in houses with other types of roof. This association confirms previous findings, from Eritrea, of increased risk of malaria infection in houses made with similar material providing micro-environments conducive for mosquitoes, extending their chance of human contact opportunities and survival [35,36]. House modifications and improvements have been associated with a reduction of anopheline mosquitoes entering the house [37] and a decrease of malaria infection prevalence [38] and anaemia [39]. Whilst such interventions are likely to be costly, they should be considered as part of long term preventive measures. In the meantime it is important that IRS spray teams are trained to spray not only the interior walls of houses, but the ceilings and underside of roofs as well, particularly where grass is used for roofing.

Education and smaller household size were associated with lower odds of malaria infection. Educated parents are more likely to encourage their children to sleep under a net because they are better informed and living in smaller household can provide adequate space to hang nets.

The likelihood of a child presenting with fever to be infected with malaria infection was high, with 56.7% of fever cases having malaria infection compared to 46.7% in none fever cases. Other studies have confirmed that malaria infections remain a major cause of febrile illness during childhood [24,40]. Nevertheless, 43% of fever cases were not infected with malaria parasites, highlighting the need to diagnose and treat all fevers among children.

In this study several limitations should be noted. Firstly, the surveys were conducted in October coinciding with the onset of the rainy season with still low mosquito densities and malaria transmission. Also the study does not provide all information on factors determining the risk of malaria infection throughout the year. Secondly, survey sites are mainly located in the southern part of Zambezia province therefore the results are not necessarily representative of the whole province or the country. Thirdly, the malaria rapid tests are subject to limitations in sensitivity and specificity which could have lead to an under-estimation or overestimation of infection prevalence since no blood slides were taken for validation purposes [41,42]. Some answers to question such as enquiring about sleeping under ITNs were reported by the parents and not observed by interviewers. Likewise, it was not possible for the interviewers to verify the ITN status of nets during the survey. Finally, malaria infection is likely to be over-estimated in groups of children remaining at home (possibly sick from malaria) and underestimated in children not found at home (likely to be healthy children, hence attending school).

In conclusion, the malaria burden among children 1 to under 15 years of age is high in Zambezia province. Consequently, health education and treatment should not only target vulnerable groups (children under 5 and pregnant women), but all the age groups. Since almost half (43%) of fever cases were not infected with malarial parasites, this has implications on policy of fever treatment, particularly in rural areas where all febrile cases may be wrongly treated as clinical malaria. Children living in IRS sprayed houses, or living in a sprayed house and sleeping under an ITN were at much lower odds of

Table 3. Multivariable logistical regression model of risk factors for malaria infection in Zambezia province.

Factors	OR*(95%CI)	Wald P-value	Adjusted P-value*
Age groups of children (years)			
1–3	1		
4–6	1.3(1.1–1.5)	=0.01	
7–9	1.4(1.1–1.7)	=0.016	
10–15	1.3(1.0–1.6)	=0.056	
Children with current fever			
No	1		
Yes	1.2(1.0–1.5)	=0.076	
Living in IRS houses and sleeping under ITN			
No IRS & not sleeping under ITN	1		
IRS & sleeping under ITN	0.5(0.3–0.7)	=0.001	
IRS & not sleeping under ITN	0.6(0.4–0.9)	=0.018	
No IRS & sleeping under ITN	1.2(0.9–1.8)	=0.238	0.009
Size of household in which children live			
1–4 people	1		
5–7 people	1.6(1.3–2.0)	<0.0001	
8–15 people	1.6(1.3–2.1)	=0.001	0.0022
Children of parents with different level of education			
None	1		
Primary/secondary	0.6(0.5–0.7)	<0.0001	
Tertiary	0.4(0.3–0.6)	<0.0001	<0.0001
Children living in household with different wealth index (SES)			
1st quartile (poorest)	1		
2nd quartile	0.9(0.7–1.2)	=0.50	
3rd quartile	0.9(0.7–1.3)	=0.723	
4th quartile (wealthiest)	0.5(0.4–0.7)	<0.0001	
Roof material of house in which children live			
Without grass roof	1		
With grass roof	1.7(1.3–2.4)	=0.002	
Children living in household with pig			
No pig	1		
Own pig(s)	3.2(2.1–4.9)	<0.0001	
Year of survey			
2006	1		
2007	1.4(1.0–2.1)	=0.047	
2008	0.4(0.3–0.7)	=0.003	

OR* adjusted for age, year of survey and wealth index. Estimates of OR* for covariates not related with farm animals were done with pig variable in the model.
*P-value derived from Wald test adjusted for the combine effect of categories in the variable.

malaria infection than children living in unsprayed houses and not sleeping under ITN. The risk of malaria infection was associated with keeping farm animals, particularly pigs and living in houses with grass roofs. In addition to ensuring high coverage of IRS, which should include the spraying of grass roofs, and promotion of the use of ITNs, malaria control programs should consider advising owners of farm animals to ensure a reasonable separation between animal sheds and sleeping areas for humans. Households with increased risk of infection, such as those keeping animals, and those with grass roofs should be particularly targeted for ITN use.

Acknowledgments

This project would not have been possible without the participation of people of Zambezia province in Mozambique, and the assistance of the Provincial and National Malaria Control Programmes.

Author Contributions

Conceived and designed the experiments: MC IK. Performed the experiments: MC IK EAT. Analyzed the data: EAT IK. Contributed reagents/materials/analysis tools: MC IK EAT. Wrote the paper: IK EAT. Coordinated the study in Mozambique: APA.

References

1. WHO (2010) World Malaria Report 2010.
2. Korenromp EL, Miller J, Cibulskis RE, Kabir Cham M, Alnwick D, et al. (2003) Monitoring mosquito net coverage for malaria control in Africa: possession vs. use by children under 5 years. Trop Med Int Health 8: 693–703.
3. Muller O, Jahn A (2003) Expanding insecticide-treated mosquito net coverage in Africa: tradeoffs between public and commercial strategies. Trop Med Int Health 8: 853–856.
4. WHO, UNICEF, DHS M, Evaluation M, CDC (2005) Roll Back Malaria: Guidelines for Core Population Coverage Indicators for Roll Back Malaria: To Be Obtained from Household Surveys.
5. Worrall E, Basu S, Hanson K (2005) Is malaria a disease of poverty? A review of the literature. Trop Med Int Health 10: 1047–1059.
6. Mahande A, Mosha F, Mahande J, Kweka E (2007) Feeding and resting behaviour of malaria vector, Anopheles arabiensis with reference to zooprophylaxis. Malar J 6: 100.
7. Simooya O (2005) The WHO 'Roll Back Malaria Project': planning for adverse event monitoring in Africa. Drug Saf 28: 277–286.
8. Noor AM, Mutheu JJ, Tatem AJ, Hay SI, Snow RW (2009) Insecticide-treated net coverage in Africa: mapping progress in 2000-07. Lancet 373: 58–67.
9. Lee PW, Liu CT, Rampao HS, do Rosario VE, Shaio MF (2010) Pre-elimination of malaria on the island of Principe. Malar J 9: 26.
10. Sharp BL, Kleinschmidt I, Streat E, Maharaj R, Barnes KI, et al. (2007) Seven years of regional malaria control collaboration–Mozambique, South Africa, and Swaziland. Am J Trop Med Hyg 76: 42–47.
11. Nyarango PM, Gebremeskel T, Mebrahtu G, Mufunda J, Abdulmumini U, et al. (2006) A steep decline of malaria morbidity and mortality trends in Eritrea between 2000 and 2004: the effect of combination of control methods. Malar J 5: 33.
12. UNPP (2010) World Population Prospects: Population database, The 2010 revision.
13. Bradbury K, Edward A (2005) Community-based solutions for effective malaria control: lessons from Mozambique Baltimore, Maryland: World Relief 289746: 289746.
14. Casimiro SL, Hemingway J, Sharp BL, Coleman M (2007) Monitoring the operational impact of insecticide usage for malaria control on Anopheles funestus from Mozambique. Malar J 6: 142.
15. Brooke BD, Kloke G, Hunt RH, Koekemoer LL, Temu EA, et al. (2001) Bioassay and biochemical analyses of insecticide resistance in southern African Anopheles funestus (Diptera: Culicidae). Bull Entomol Res 91: 265–272.
16. PMI (2010) Presidential Malaria Initiative Operational Plan FY10, Mozambique 2010.
17. Instituto-Nacional-de-Estatística (2008) Total Population By Provinces-2006 Available: Retrieved 2009-08-15. http://www.inegovmz/Ingles/o_pais/populacao_total_prov. (Accessed 2009 Aug 15).
18. Abilio AP, Kleinschmid I, Rehman A, Cuamba N, Ramdeen V, et al. (2011) The emergence of insecticide resistance in central Mozambique and potential threat on the successful Indoor Residual Spraying malaria control programme. Malar J.
19. Hemingway J, Beaty BJ, Rowland M, Scott TW, Sharp BL (2006) The Innovative Vector Control Consortium: improved control of mosquito-borne diseases. Trends Parasitol 22: 308–312.
20. WHO (2005) Malaria Indicator Survey: Basic documentation for survey design and implementation. Roll Back Malaria Monitoring and Evaluation Reference Group.
21. Vyas S, Kumaranayake L (2006) Constructing socio-economic status indices: how to use principal components analysis. Health Policy Plan 21: 459–468.
22. Stata Stata IC 10.1 ed. TX.
23. Bouyou-Akotet MK, Dzeing-Ella A, Kendjo E, Etoughe D, Ngoungou EB, et al. (2009) Impact of Plasmodium falciparum infection on the frequency of moderate to severe anaemia in children below 10 years of age in Gabon. Malar J 8: 166.
24. Mabunda S, Aponte JJ, Tiago A, Alonso P (2009) A country-wide malaria survey in Mozambique. II. Malaria attributable proportion of fever and establishment of malaria case definition in children across different epidemiological settings. Malar J 8: 74.
25. Kleinschmidt I, Schwabe C, Shiva M, Segura JL, Sima V, et al. (2009) Combining indoor residual spraying and insecticide-treated net interventions. Am J Trop Med Hyg 81: 519–524.
26. Lengeler C (2004) Insecticide-treated bed nets and curtains for preventing malaria. Cochrane Database Syst Rev. CD000363.
27. Baragatti M, Fournet F, Henry MC, Assi S, Ouedraogo H, et al. (2009) Social and environmental malaria risk factors in urban areas of Ouagadougou, Burkina Faso. Malar J 8: 13.
28. Rehman AM, Coleman M, Schwabe C, Baltazar G, Matias A, et al. (2011) How much does malaria vector control quality matter: the epidemiological impact of holed nets and inadequate indoor residual spraying. PLoS ONE 6: e19205.
29. Bogh C, Clarke SE, Walraven GE, Lindsay SW (2002) Zooprophylaxis, artefact or reality? A paired-cohort study of the effect of passive zooprophylaxis on malaria in The Gambia. Trans R Soc Trop Med Hyg 96: 593–596.
30. Mahande AM, Mosha FW, Mahande JM, Kweka EJ (2007) Role of cattle treated with deltamethrine in areas with a high population of Anopheles arabiensis in Moshi, Northern Tanzania. Malar J 6: 109.
31. Costantini C, Sagnon N, della Torre A, Coluzzi M (1999) Mosquito behavioural aspects of vector-human interactions in the Anopheles gambiae complex. Parassitologia 41: 209–217.
32. Gillies TM, Coetzee M (1987) Supplement of the Anopheles of Africa South of Sahara (Afrotropical Region). Johannesburg: Publication of The SouthAfrica Institute of Medical Research.
33. Muriu SM, Muturi EJ, Shililu JI, Mbogo CM, Mwangangi JM, et al. (2008) Host choice and multiple blood feeding behaviour of malaria vectors and other anophelines in Mwea rice scheme, Kenya. Malar J 7: 43.
34. Carter R, Mendis KN, Roberts D (2000) Spatial targeting of interventions against malaria. Bull World Health Organ 78: 1401–1411.
35. Ghebreyesus TA, Haile M, Witten KH, Getachew A, Yohannes M, et al. (2000) Household risk factors for malaria among children in the Ethiopian highlands. Trans R Soc Trop Med Hyg 94: 17–21.
36. Sintasath DM, Ghebremeskel T, Lynch M, Kleinau E, Bretas G, et al. (2005) Malaria prevalence and associated risk factors in Eritrea. Am J Trop Med Hyg 2005 72: 682–687.
37. Atieli H, Menya D, Githeko A, Scott T (2009) House design modifications reduce indoor resting malaria vector densities in rice irrigation scheme area in western Kenya. Malar J 8: 108.
38. Lindsay SW, Jawara M, Paine K, Pinder M, Walraven GE, et al. (2003) Changes in house design reduce exposure to malaria mosquitoes. Trop Med Int Health 8: 512–517.
39. Kirby MJ, Ameh D, Bottomley C, Green C, Jawara M, et al. (2009) Effect of two different house screening interventions on exposure to malaria vectors and on anaemia in children in The Gambia: a randomised controlled trial. Lancet 374: 998–1009.
40. Smith T, Charlwood JD, Kitua AY, Masanja H, Mwankusye S, et al. (1998) Relationships of malaria morbidity with exposure to Plasmodium falciparum in young children in a highly endemic area. Am J Trop Med Hyg 59: 252–257.
41. Murray CK, Gasser RA, Jr., Magill AJ, Miller RS (2008) Update on rapid diagnostic testing for malaria. Clin Microbiol Rev 21: 97–110.
42. Nicastri E, Bevilacqua N, Sane Schepisi M, Paglia MG, Meschi S, et al. (2009) Accuracy of malaria diagnosis by microscopy, rapid diagnostic test, and PCR methods and evidence of antimalarial overprescription in non-severe febrile patients in two Tanzanian hospitals. Am J Trop Med Hyg 80: 712–717.

10

Temporal Association of Acute Hepatitis A and *Plasmodium falciparum* Malaria in Children

Peter Klein Klouwenberg[1,2], Philip Sasi[2,3], Mahfudh Bashraheil[2], Ken Awuondo[2], Marc Bonten[1], James Berkley[2], Kevin Marsh[2], Steffen Borrmann[2,4*]

1 University Medical Center Utrecht, Utrecht, The Netherlands, **2** Kenya Medical Research Institute/Wellcome Trust Research Programme, Centre for Geographical Medicine Research – Coast, Kilifi, Kenya, **3** Muhimbili University, Dar es Salaam, Tanzania, **4** Department of Infectious Diseases, Heidelberg University School of Medicine, Heidelberg, Germany

Abstract

Background: In sub-Saharan Africa, *Plasmodium falciparum* and hepatitis A (HAV) infections are common, especially in children. Co-infections with these two pathogens may therefore occur, but it is unknown if temporal clustering exists.

Materials and Methods: We studied the pattern of co-infection of *P. falciparum* malaria and acute HAV in Kenyan children under the age of 5 years in a cohort of children presenting with uncomplicated *P. falciparum* malaria. HAV status was determined during a 3-month follow-up period.

Discussion: Among 222 cases of uncomplicated malaria, 10 patients were anti-HAV IgM positive. The incidence of HAV infections during *P. falciparum* malaria was 1.7 (95% CI 0.81–3.1) infections/person-year while the cumulative incidence of HAV over the 3-month follow-up period was 0.27 (95% CI 0.14–0.50) infections/person-year. Children with or without HAV co-infections had similar mean *P. falciparum* asexual parasite densities at presentation (31,000/μL vs. 34,000/μL, respectively), largely exceeding the pyrogenic threshold of 2,500 parasites/μL in this population and minimizing risk of over-diagnosis of malaria as an explanation.

Conclusion: The observed temporal association between acute HAV and *P. falciparum* malaria suggests that co-infections of these two hepatotrophic human pathogens may result from changes in host susceptibility. Testing this hypothesis will require larger prospective studies.

Editor: Mauricio Martins Rodrigues, Federal University of São Paulo, Brazil

Funding: SB is funded by a Deutsche Forschungsgemeinschaft (DFG) Junior Group grant (SFB 544, A7). This study was supported by the Kenya Medical Research Institute and the Wellcome Trust. The funders had no role in study design, data collection and analysis, decision to publish, or preparation of the manuscript.

Competing Interests: The authors have declared that no competing interests exist.

* E-mail: sborrmann@kilifi.kemri-wellcome.org

Introduction

In Africa, both *Plasmodium falciparum* malaria and hepatitis A virus (HAV) infections are common infections, especially in children [1,2], although concurrent infections of these two highly prevalent human pathogens are likely to occur, knowledge about their prevalence and potential significance is poor. Since both pathogens target the hepatocyte as host cell for intracellular replication (mosquito-transmitted malaria parasites replicate silently in suitable hepatocytes before red blood cell invasion) direct or immunologically mediated interactions in concurrent infections could potentially escalate or inhibit progression of both infections.

Epidemiologically relevant interactions, though with contradictory findings, have previously been shown for *P. falciparum* malaria and hepatitis B (HBV). In a case-control study in The Gambia, the prevalence of HBV was significantly increased amongst children with severe *P. falciparum* malaria compared to matched controls [3]. Barcus et al found a prevalence of HBV infection of 24% in adult Vietnamese patients admitted with severe *P. falciparum* malaria, which was higher than the estimated prevalence of HBV in that area (10%) [4]. In contrast, a study in Papua New Guinea showed that female adults with the highest spleen rates of *Plasmodium* had the lowest prevalence of HBV infection, but there was no correlation with parasitemia [5]. Pasquetto et al showed a reduction of HBV replication rate, and ultimately, clearance of virions, in mice co-infected with *P. yoelii* [6]. It is also known that co-infections of other viruses such as Ebstein-Barr Virus [7,8], and HIV [9] with *P. falciparum* affect the natural course of *P. falciparum* infections.

In this study we aimed to determine the temporal pattern of co-infection of *P. falciparum* malaria and acute HAV in a cohort of Kenyan children under the age of 5 years presenting with uncomplicated *P. falciparum* malaria. We focused on HAV since an initial viral screen (hepatitis A, B, C and D virus) of cases with elevated plasma concentrations of alanine aminotransferase (ALT; an established biomarker for the extent of liver cell damage) patients were positive for HAV, but not for any other hepatitis viruses.

Results

A total of 222 children were included in this study. Forty patients (18.0%) had ALT plasma concentrations above the upper limit of normal for children (36 U/L) at one or more measurements at enrolment or during follow-up, and fifteen patients (6.7%) had ALT levels exceeding 100 U/L. All ten cases of HAV occurred in patient with ALT levels above 36 U/L (range 41–1295 U/L): eight patients had ALT levels ≥100 U/L, and two children had maximal ALT levels between 36–100 U/L (41 and 56 U/L). Demographic and laboratory data of HAV positive and negative children are shown in Table 1.

We also tested the presence of IgM-HAV antibodies in 15 patients with normal ALT levels (≤36 U/L). These children were matched on treatment, study date, gender and age with the 15 patients having ALT levels ≥100 U/L. None of these patients showed a positive reaction for IgM-HAV. In addition, we tested an alternative hypothesis that *falciparum* malaria infections can lead to increased production of unspecific HAV-IgM [10] potentially causing false positive test results. We therefore measured 14 samples with the highest *P. falciparum* parasite density at baseline (of whom six children also belonged to the matched controls). The geometrical mean parasitemia in this subgroup was 196,000 parasites/µL (95% CI = 177,000–217,000; range = 164,000–350,000), and the median ALT level was 28 U/L (range 16–194 U/L). One patient with a parasitemia of 202,000/µL and a maximal ALT level of 41 U/L (case #10 in Table 2) showed a positive reaction. This indicated that elevated ALT plasma concentrations above 100 U/L had acceptable sensitivity (8/15, 53%) and high specificity (61/63, 97%), and levels above 36 U/L had low sensitivity (10/55, 18%) but excellent specificity (23/23, 100%) for detecting HAV infections in our cohort. As all available samples with ALT levels above the cut-off value of 36 U/L were measured, it is unlikely that we missed any additional HAV-positive cases.

Importantly, all but one case coincided with malaria (8 during first week and 1 on malaria reinfection; cases #1–7 and cases #9–10 in Table 2). The other case (case #8) had elevated ALT levels at day 84, indicating that a possible re-infection, if having occurred in this patient, could not have be detected due to end of follow-up. Thus, the number of HAV positive patients in this cohort of children in the 3-month follow-up period was 10 cases per 37.3 person-years (222 children with an average follow-up time of 2.0 months) resulting in a cumulative incidence of 0.27 (95% CI 0.14–0.50) infections per person-year, while during malaria there were 9 HAV-positive cases per 5.4 person-years, resulting in an incidence of 1.7 (95% CI 0.81–3.1) HAV infections per person-year. In the latter case, we calculated the incidence rate based on a 1-week time frame, that is, during and shortly after the malaria episode, and took into account all malaria episodes during baseline and all 73 recurrences that occurred during follow-up of the cohort of 222 children. The choice of a 1-week time frame thus resulted in an artificial saturation of the incidence rate (>1 infection per person-year) in a disease with 100% immunity. However, using this unit we obtained a realistic estimate for the incidence rate of HAV infections in children during the convalescence phase (0.27 per person-year), which is consistent with estimates that nearly all children in this part of Africa will have experienced an infection before the age of 5 years [2]. The proportion of children with elevated ALT levels differed significantly between baseline (60/

Table 1. Comparison of HAV positive and negative patients presenting with uncomplicated *P. falciparum* malaria.

	HAV positive (n = 10)	HAV negative (n = 68)	p-value
Age (months) (mean ± SD)	26.1±11.8	28.9±14.1	0.549#
Weight (kg) (mean ± SD)	10.5±2.13	10.8±2.41	0.734#
Sex (male/female) (number)	6/4	37/31	0.491§
Treatment (DHA-piperaquine/artemether-lumefantrine) (number)	8/2	48/20	0.534§
Baseline laboratory data			
Parasitemia (/µL) (geomean±95%CI)	37,000 (17,000–79,000)∞	48,000 (33,000–64,000)†	0.551*
Hemoglobin (g%) (mean ± SD)	8.1±1.8	9.2±1.4	0.031#
WBC count (/µL) (median, IQR)	8.7 (7.7–14.4)	9.0 (6.7–11.8)	0.774*
Creatinine (µmol/L) (mean ± SD)	38±6.5	43±9.6	0.144#
Total bilirubin (µmol/L) (median, IQR)	14.8 (12.3–23.6)	13.8 (8.8–24.6)	0.679*
ALT (U/L) at			
D0 (median (IQR))	92 (36–173)	29 (22–45)	0.016*
D3 (median (IQR))	64 (40–235)	28 (22–47)	0.028*
D7 (median (IQR))	81 (53–416)	21 (17–52)	0.012*
D28 (median (IQR))	27 (23–64)	23 (18–31)	0.385*
D42 (median (IQR))	21 (19–27)	24 (21–31)	0.270*
D84 (median (IQR))	26 (24–171)	27 (20–36)	0.599*
Recurrent *P .falciparum* infections (number)	5	19	0.374§

Geometric mean parasitemia at baseline were
∞31,000 (15,000–63,000) and
†34,000 (24,000–47,000) when patients with high parasitemia are excluded.
#T-test,
*Mann-Whitney test,
§chi square test.

Table 2. Summary of key laboratory parameters of patients who presented with uncomplicated *P. falciparum* malaria and subsequently found to have anti-HAV IgM indicating acute HAV infection.

Case #	Date of inclusion in study[1]	HAV detected (day)	Age (months)	ALT (U/L)						Baseline asexual parasite density (/μL)	Asexual *P. falciparum* parasite recurrence (day)
				Day 0	Day 3	Day 7	Day 28	Day 42	Day 84		
1	29/05/06	0	11	114	48	-	13	25	26	20,000	-
2	23/01/06	42	17	13	15	82	121	29	-	62,000	49
3	04/05/06	0	18	134	71	39	-	21	25	13,000	-
4	05/05/06	0	22	330	235	123	-	18	-	130,000	42
5	25/05/06	0	22	290	187	58	26	19	24	17,000	28
6	07/04/06	0	26	69	236	1295	45	21	-	126,000	-
7	18/05/06	0	28	118	327	80	27	-	42	19,000	35
8	06/12/05	84	38	25	44	-	-	21	559	20,000	-
9	11/10/05	0	28	40	56	-	-	17	-	14,000	-
10	05/05/06	0	52	41	29	-	27	29	23	202,000	56

[1]One-third of patients were enrolled in May 2006.

222, 27.0%) and follow-up (9/89, 10.1%) (difference, 16.9%; 95%CI 7.6–26.3%; $P=0.001$). A possible explanation could be the aggregation of measurements from baseline to day 7, because when only data from baseline were used, the difference ceased to be significant (39/222; difference, 7.5%, 95%CI −1.4%–16.3%; $P=0.119$), possibly indicating that other factors such as treatment could have caused the additional increase in ALT levels.

Only one child with acute HAV infection showed clinical symptoms of the infection, i.e., jaundice; this patient had the highest ALT plasma concentration (case #6 in Table 2). None of the other children had clinical signs or symptoms suggestive of viral hepatitis infection, apart from fever, which is the main clinical symptom of malaria. Fever clearance times were similar between HAV positive and negative patients (1.0 versus 1.1 days, respectively).

Fifty percent (5/10) of patients with HAV infection had a *P. falciparum* malaria recurrence, compared to 35 percent (19/54) of HAV uninfected patients ($p=0.37$). Of the five patients with a malaria recurrence in the HAV positive group, four were found to be HAV infected at baseline; the other patient had an HAV infection at day 42 and experienced a recurrent *P. falciparum* infection 1 week later. Four patients had a re-infection; the other sample could not be analyzed. Of the 19 HAV negative patients with a malaria recurrence, 17 had a re-infection, 1 had both recrudescent primary and secondary re-infections, and 1 sample could not be analyzed.

Discussion

The present study describes a temporal association between *P. falciparum* malaria and acute HAV in a cohort of pediatric patients. We found that nine out of ten cases of acute HAV infections occurred simultaneously with *P. falciparum* malaria infections.

What are the alternative explanations that could have lead to a potential overestimation of the temporal association of active HAV infections with uncomplicated *P. falciparum* malaria? Firstly, overestimation of the association might have occurred if patients with HAV infections presented primarily for seeking relief for symptoms of HAV infection, and not of malaria. The baseline blood stage density in our study group was high (>37,000 asexual parasites/μL), far exceeding the pyrogenic threshold of 2,500 parasites/μL in this population and thus, minimizing over-diagnosis of malaria as an alternative explanation [11,12]. Moreover, most HAV infections in children below the age of 5 years are known to be asymptomatic [13] and indeed, patients with co-infections did not differ in times to symptom clearance compared to patients with *P. falciparum* mono-infections. Secondly, *P. falciparum* malaria and/or hepatotoxic side effects of antimalarial drugs can also lead to elevated plasma concentrations of liver enzymes, indicating hepatocellular damage [14]. This could have led to an overestimation of the temporal association, as samples were selected based on ALT levels. However, patients with high and low baseline parasite densities had similar ALT levels and HAV infections clustered in patients with elevated ALT concentrations, but not in matched controls (matched on treatment, study date, gender and age). Thirdly, false positive results could have been caused by an induction of unspecific IgM antibody production leading to false positive anti-HAV IgM test results. We addressed this question by measuring IgM antibodies in 14 patients with the highest blood stage parasite density at baseline. This could possibly have led to misclassification bias. However, even if this is true and this patient is regarded to be HAV negative, we still find a significant incidence rate ratio. The risk of more false positive cases is limited, as the three highest parasitemias amongst the HAV positive children are 216,000/μL (the child who tested positive), 130,000/μL, and 125,000/μL. The latter two values are much lower than the parasitemia of the patient who tested positive and also lower than the parasitemia of the patient with the highest parasitemia in the HAV negative group (170,000/μL). In addition, the ALT levels of these patients were among the highest of the group (330 and 1300 UI/L) making an alternative diagnosis than acute HAV very unlikely. Fourthly, an overestimation of the association with malaria may have occurred, if anti-HAV IgM remains positive (long) after viral HAV particles have been cleared from the liver. However, the anti-HAV IgM response becomes undetectable usually within 6 months [15], but HAV RNA can be detected for more than 400–600 days after ALT peak [16,17]. So even if anti-HAV IgM stays positive for a long time after acute infection, viral HAV particles will be residing in hepatocytes during that time period; therefore possibly increasing the likelihood to find concurrence of acute HAV and malaria. We could also rule out the possibility of an outbreak of HAV infection since patients were enrolled continuously from 2005 to 2006 and HAV cases did not cluster during a particular period of the year.

We found that HAV infections were a common cause for elevated plasma concentrations of an established biomarker of liver cell damage (ALT) in these patients. Children from the Kilifi district with *P. falciparum* malaria and elevated ALT concentrations (>100 U/L) had a 53% (8/15) chance of being co-infected with HAV, indicating that almost 50% of elevations could not be explained by HAV infections. This percentage is high and warrants consideration whenever determining the safety profile of antimalarial drugs. This study did not reveal any adverse clinical consequences of concurrent infections, except for a significant lower hemoglobin level. We have no ready explanation for this difference. Unlike *Plasmodium* infections HAV is not known to affect hemoglobin levels. One could speculate that *Plasmodium* infections in co-infected children were protracted and thus caused a slight additional drop in hemoglobin concentrations. Malaria patients co-infected with HAV were as likely as patients without HAV co-infections to clear clinical symptoms and parasites. By extension, this also indicates that most HAV infections were asymptomatic as expected [13]. There was only one HAV case with highly elevated ALT and clinical symptoms suggestive of acute hepatitis, which developed during the treatment of malaria.

The biological mechanism, if any, behind the observed temporal association remains elusive. For instance, *P. falciparum* liver stage and/or blood stage infections could, mediated by unknown immune mechanisms, promote HAV replication and thus, increase the chance to detect active HAV infections. Alternatively, coincidental HAV infection could facilitate parasite survival at the liver stage leading to increased numbers of infective merozoites and higher likelihood of subsequent pathogenic blood stage infection, in a similar way to the suggested mechanism for the observed association between malaria and HBV. In the study by Thursz, the increased incidence of severe malaria that was observed in chronic HBV carriers was explained by reduced expression of HLA class I molecules by hepatocytes during chronic HBV infection [3]. HLA class I molecules are important in the recognition and subsequent lysis of *P. falciparum* infected hepatocytes by cytotoxic T lymphocytes (CTLs). Thus, the lysing of parasite-infected hepatocytes by cytotoxic T lymphocytes (CTLs) may have been impaired in HBV carriers leading to an increased susceptibility to severe malaria. Whether similar mechanisms play a role in the association of acute HAV and falciparum malaria remains unclear.

In conclusion, we provide tentative evidence for a temporal association between *P. falciparum* and HAV infections in children living in an area of high *P. falciparum* and HAV transmission. Unfortunately, there is very limited information available about baseline HAV rates in Kenya, which is needed to draw stronger conclusions. We did not measure this; nevertheless we observed a temporal association between falciparum malaria and HAV. Prospective and larger studies are required to further elucidate the epidemiological interaction between these two important human pathogens. Our data also highlight the need for more comprehensive analyses of the complex interactions of prevalent infectious diseases in endemic countries that contribute to an unacceptably high disease burden.

Materials and Methods

Study site

The study was conducted at the Pingilikani study site of the Kenya Medical Research Institute/Centre for Geographic Medicine Research-Coast (CGMR-C). The Pingilikani study site is located 20 km south of Kilifi town in Kilifi district along the Kenyan coast [18]. *P. falciparum* transmission rates have been estimated to range between 22 and 53 infective bites per person per year [19]. Currently there is no data on the incidence of HAV or any other hepatitis viruses in this age group in Kilifi District.

Study design and patients

This study was nested in an ongoing clinical trial to assess the efficacy and safety of dihydroartemisinin-piperaquine in comparison with artemether-lumefantrine in children with uncomplicated *P. falciparum* malaria [20] and Borrmann *et al* (unpublished data). Ethical approval for this study was granted by the Kenya National Ethics Review Committee, the Oxford Tropical Research Ethics Committee and the Ethics Committee of the Heidelberg University School of Medicine. Children aged 6–59 months presenting to the Pingilikani Health Centre with symptoms suggestive of uncomplicated malaria and a documented *P. falciparum* infection with an asexual parasite density of 2,000–200,000 parasites/μL, were recruited. Written informed consent was obtained from the parents. Patients were monitored daily until parasite and fever clearance was achieved. Active follow-up was on days 3 and 7, then weekly on days 14, 21, 28, 35, 42, 56, and 63 and 84. All subjects were seen on any day between day 0 and 84 upon request. ALT was measured routinely at baseline and at day 3, 7, 28, 42, 84, and at asexual parasite recurrence. Although ALT levels in patients with active HAV infection are typically 4–100 times elevated [21], we determined acute HAV infection status in all available samples with ALT levels of >36 U/L which is the upper limit of normal in children. In order to identify whether false positive tests were occurring at high parasite density, acute HAV infection status was also determined in children who had a baseline parasitemia of >150,000/μL. We used samples from baseline to measure anti-HAV IgM titers in any sample with elevated ALT from baseline up to day 7 as we assumed that the anti-HAV IgM levels would not significantly change during this period. For the other time-points (day 28, 42, and 84) we used blood samples from the respective study days.

Laboratory procedures

Malaria infection was confirmed by Giemsa-stained thick smear [22]. We used a commercial ELISA kit to detect IgM antibodies to HAV (ELISA Kit for IgM Antibody to Hepatitis A Virus, BioChain, USA). The assay was performed according to the manufacturer's instructions.

Statistical analysis

Analysis was carried out using Stata version 9.2 (Statacorp, Texas, USA). Data were entered and checked for inconsistencies by two different persons to reduce faulty entries. The Kolmogorov-Smirnov test was used to verify the normality of distribution of continuous variables. Comparisons between groups were performed using the t-test or two-tailed unpaired Mann-Whitney test for continuous variables evaluated as normally distributed and not-normally distributed, respectively. The chi-square test was used for comparisons between categorical variables. Parasitemia results were summarized using geometrical means and 95% confidence intervals. All the remaining continuous variables were reported with arithmetic means and standard deviation, or by the median and IQR. $P<0.05$ was considered statistically significant. Exact binomial confidence intervals were calculated to compare incidence rates.

Acknowledgments

We are indebted to the children and their parents who participated in the trial. We thank the Pingilikani study team, in particular, Amina Salim, Fauzat Jamal Hamid, Judy Peshu, Ann Kithinji, Crispinah Kaula, Joy Lewa, Fixtan Njuga. Anja Rippert and Elise Schieck shared parasite genotyping results. Stephan Boehm advised on diagnostic tests for hepatitis viruses and tested the initial samples. We would also like to thank Drs. Stephan Urban, Kai Matuschewski, Olivier Sylvie and Johannes Friesen whose comments on earlier versions helped to improve the manuscript. This work is published with the permission of the Director of KEMRI.

Author Contributions

Conceived and designed the experiments: PKK PS M. Bonten JB KM SB. Performed the experiments: PKK PS KA M. Bashraheil SB. Analyzed the data: PKK PS M. Bonten JB KM SB. Contributed reagents/materials/analysis tools: JB KM SB. Wrote the paper: PKK PS M. Bonten JB KM SB.

References

1. Snow RW, Guerra CA, Noor AM, Myint HY, Hay SI (2005) The global distribution of clinical episodes of Plasmodium falciparum malaria. Nature 434: 214–217.
2. Jacobsen KH, Koopman JS (2004) Declining hepatitis A seroprevalence: a global review and analysis. Epidemiol Infect 132: 1005–1022.
3. Thursz MR, Kwiatkowski D, Torok ME, Allsopp CE, Greenwood BM, et al. (1995) Association of hepatitis B surface antigen carriage with severe malaria in Gambian children. Nat Med 1: 374–375.
4. Barcus MJ, Hien TT, White NJ, Laras K, Farrar J, et al. (2002) Short report: hepatitis b infection and severe Plasmodium falciparum malaria in Vietnamese adults. Am J Trop Med Hyg 66: 140–142.
5. Brabin L, Brabin BJ, Dimitrakakis M, Gust I (1989) Factors affecting the prevalence of infection with hepatitis B virus among non-pregnant women in the Alexishafen area of Papua New Guinea. Ann Trop Med Parasitol 83: 365–374.
6. Pasquetto V, Guidotti LG, Kakimi K, Tsuji M, Chisari FV (2000) Host-virus interactions during malaria infection in hepatitis B virus transgenic mice. J Exp Med 192: 529–536.
7. Chene A, Donati D, Guerreiro-Cacais AO, Levitsky V, Chen Q, et al. (2007) A molecular link between malaria and Epstein-Barr virus reactivation. PLoS Pathog 3: e80.
8. Moormann AM, Chelimo K, Sumba OP, Lutzke ML, Ploutz-Snyder R, et al. (2005) Exposure to holoendemic malaria results in elevated Epstein-Barr virus loads in children. J Infect Dis 191: 1233–1238.
9. Abu-Raddad LJ, Patnaik P, Kublin JG (2006) Dual infection with HIV and malaria fuels the spread of both diseases in sub-Saharan Africa. Science 314: 1603–1606.
10. Jimmy EO, Bedu-Addo G, Bates I, Bevan D, Rutherford TR (1996) Immunoglobulin gene polymerase chain reaction to distinguish hyperreactive malarial splenomegaly from 'African' chronic lymphocytic leukaemia and splenic lymphoma. Trans R Soc Trop Med Hyg 90: 37–39.
11. Bejon P, Berkley JA, Mwangi T, Ogada E, Mwangi I, et al. (2007) Defining childhood severe falciparum malaria for intervention studies. PLoS Med 4: e251.
12. Smith T, Schellenberg JA, Hayes R (1994) Attributable fraction estimates and case definitions for malaria in endemic areas. Stat Med 13: 2345–2358.
13. Ciocca M (2000) Clinical course and consequences of hepatitis A infection. Vaccine 18 Suppl 1: S71–74.
14. Anand AC, Puri P (2005) Jaundice in malaria. J Gastroenterol Hepatol 20: 1322–1332.
15. Stapleton JT (1995) Host immune response to hepatitis A virus. J Infect Dis 171 Suppl 1: S9–14.
16. Bower WA, Nainan OV, Han X, Margolis HS (2000) Duration of viremia in hepatitis A virus infection. J Infect Dis 182: 12–17.
17. Normann A, Jung C, Vallbracht A, Flehmig B (2004) Time course of hepatitis A viremia and viral load in the blood of human hepatitis A patients. J Med Virol 72: 10–16.
18. Olotu A, Fegan G, Williams TN, Sasi P, Ogada E, et al. (2010) Defining clinical malaria: the specificity and incidence of endpoints from active and passive surveillance of children in rural Kenya. PLoS One 5: e15569.
19. Mbogo CM, Mwangangi JM, Nzovu J, Gu W, Yan G, et al. (2003) Spatial and temporal heterogeneity of Anopheles mosquitoes and Plasmodium falciparum transmission along the Kenyan coast. Am J Trop Med Hyg 68: 734–742.
20. Bassat Q, Mulenga M, Tinto H, Piola P, Borrmann S, et al. (2009) Dihydroartemisinin-piperaquine and artemether-lumefantrine for treating uncomplicated malaria in African children: a randomised, non-inferiority trial. PLoS One 4: e7871.
21. Jiang XJ, Luo KX, He HT (2000) Intrahepatic transfusion-transmitted virus detected by in situ hybridization in patients with liver diseases. J Viral Hepat 7: 292–296.
22. Mwangi TW, Ross A, Snow RW, Marsh K (2005) Case definitions of clinical malaria under different transmission conditions in Kilifi District, Kenya. J Infect Dis 191: 1932–1939.

11

A Systematic Review on the Diagnosis of Pediatric Bacterial Pneumonia: When Gold is Bronze

Tim Lynch[1], Liza Bialy[2*], James D. Kellner[3], Martin H. Osmond[4], Terry P. Klassen[2], Tamara Durec[2], Robin Leicht[2], David W. Johnson[3]

1 Department of Pediatrics, Children's Hospital, University of Western Ontario, London, Ontario, Canada, **2** Department of Pediatrics, University of Alberta, Edmonton, Alberta, Canada, **3** Department of Pediatrics and Physiology and Pharmacology, University of Calgary and Alberta Children's Hospital, Calgary, Alberta, Canada, **4** Clinical Research Unit, Children's Hospital of Eastern Ontario Research Institute, Ottawa, Ontario, Canada

Abstract

Background: In developing countries, pneumonia is one of the leading causes of death in children under five years of age and hence timely and accurate diagnosis is critical. In North America, pneumonia is also a common source of childhood morbidity and occasionally mortality. Clinicians traditionally have used the chest radiograph as the gold standard in the diagnosis of pneumonia, but they are becoming increasingly aware that it is not ideal. Numerous studies have shown that chest radiography findings lack precision in defining the etiology of childhood pneumonia. There is no single test that reliably distinguishes bacterial from non-bacterial causes. These factors have resulted in clinicians historically using a combination of physical signs and chest radiographs as a 'gold standard', though this combination of tests has been shown to be imperfect for diagnosis and assigning treatment. The objectives of this systematic review are to: 1) identify and categorize studies that have used single or multiple tests as a gold standard for assessing accuracy of other tests, and 2) given the 'gold standard' used, determine the accuracy of these other tests for diagnosing childhood bacterial pneumonia.

Methods and Findings: Search strategies were developed using a combination of subject headings and keywords adapted for 18 electronic bibliographic databases from inception to May 2008. Published studies were included if they: 1) included children one month to 18 years of age, 2) provided sufficient data regarding diagnostic accuracy to construct a 2×2 table, and 3) assessed the accuracy of one or more index tests as compared with other test(s) used as a 'gold standard'. The literature search revealed 5,989 references of which 256 were screened for inclusion, resulting in 25 studies that satisfied all inclusion criteria. The studies examined a range of bacterium types and assessed the accuracy of several combinations of diagnostic tests. Eleven different gold standards were studied in the 25 included studies. Criterion validity was calculated for fourteen different index tests using eleven different gold standards. The most common gold standard utilized was blood culture tests used in six studies. Fourteen different tests were measured as index tests. PCT was the most common measured in five studies each with a different gold standard.

Conclusions: We have found that studies assessing the diagnostic accuracy of clinical, radiological, and laboratory tests for bacterial childhood pneumonia have used a heterogeneous group of gold standards, and found, at least in part because of this, that index tests have widely different accuracies. These findings highlight the need for identifying a widely accepted gold standard for diagnosis of bacterial pneumonia in children.

Editor: Luis Huicho, Universidad Nacional Mayor de San Marcos, Peru

Funding: This study was funded by the Canadian Institutes of Health Research Team Grants Program (CIHR Team in Pediatric Emergency Medicine) (grant #G118160601). The funders had no role in study design, data collection and analysis, decision to publish, or preparation of the manuscript.

Competing Interests: The authors have declared that no competing interests exist.

* E-mail: lbialy@ualberta.ca

Introduction

In developing countries, pneumonia is one of the leading causes of death in children under five years of age and hence timely and accurate diagnosis is critical [1]. In North America, pneumonia is also a common source of childhood morbidity and occasionally mortality [2]. A study from Israel has also shown that there can be significant economic burdens to children and families dealing with community acquired pneumonia, as well as significant reduction in their quality of life [3].

Viruses, atypical, and typical bacteria cause the vast majority of childhood pneumonia [2–4] The distribution of pathogens varies with age and clinical setting. Atypical bacterial microorganisms, such as Mycoplasma and Chlamydia usually occur in children between the ages of five and 15 years [5–7], while the incidence of viral infections typically decreases with age [5]. In hospitalized children, the most frequently diagnosed bacteria are the typical pathogens, such as Streptococcus pneumoniae [5]. It can be difficult to identify whether the cause of pneumonia in a given patient is bacterial or nonbacterial [8,9]. Classic signs unique to bacterial or nonbacterial pneumonia can be helpful in coming to a diagnosis [9]. However, these signs and symptoms are often subjective, and are ultimately imprecise at determining whether antibiotics are truly warranted [4].

A clinically acceptable gold standard for the diagnosis of bacterial pneumonia has not yet been developed [2,5,8]. Often the most readily available means of diagnosing pneumonia are through observations of physical signs and radiological evidence. Diagnostic guidelines have been developed by the World Health Organization for pneumonia and these are generally used in developing countries or in the absence of quick access to laboratory tests [10]. Other diagnostic tests have been used with variable rates of accuracy, such as chest radiographs, laboratory tests (white blood cell count [WBC]) with differential, C-reactive protein (CRP), erythrocyte sedimentation rate (ESR) [8,9], blood cultures and serology [8], and lung puncture [8,9]. The ideal surrogate marker for bacterial pneumonia should be accurate, minimally invasive, and readily available. To date, there is no such gold standard that a physician can rely on to confidently diagnose and subsequently treat bacterial pneumonia [2].

Clinicians traditionally have used the chest radiograph as the gold standard in the diagnosis of pneumonia, but they are becoming increasingly aware that it is not ideal. Numerous studies have shown that chest radiography findings lack accuracy in defining the etiology of childhood pneumonia [2,11,12]. There is no single test that reliably distinguishes bacterial from non-bacterial causes [4]. These factors have resulted in clinicians historically using a combination of physical signs and chest radiographs as a 'gold standard', though this combination of tests has been shown to be imperfect for diagnosis and assigning treatment [5,13].

The objectives of this systematic review are to: 1) identify and categorize studies that have used single or multiple tests as a gold standard for assessing accuracy of other tests, and 2) given the 'gold standard' used, determine the accuracy of these other tests for diagnosing childhood bacterial pneumonia.

Methods

This review has been carried out using methods defined for rigorous systematic reviews [14,15]. The aim was to use these guidelines and other methodological criteria [16–18] to produce a systematic review that is comprehensive and summarizes the data collected (see PRISMA Checklist S1).

Ethics Statement

Data for this study was acquired through previously published work, no patient or hospital data was accessed. Therefore, written consent and institutional ethical review was not required for this research.

Search Strategy and Selection Criteria

Search strategies were developed using a combination of subject headings and keywords, including: "pneumonia", "bacteria", "community acquired pneumonia", "lower respiratory tract infection", "pneumococcal", "diagnosis", "accuracy", "sensitivity", "reliability", "specificity", "false/true positive/negative", "predictive value", "observer variation", "likelihood functions/ratios", "ROC curve", "receiver operating characteristic", "child", "adolescent", "infant", "minors", "pediatrics", "nurseries", "youth", "nursery", "nurseries", "toddler", "clinical trials", "cohort studies", "case-control studies", "comparative", "evaluation studies", "prospective", "retrospective", and "follow up".

These keywords were adapted for each of the 18 electronic bibliographic databases from inception to May 2008 (see Table 1 for full listing). Extended systematic search methods (e.g., hand searches of non-indexed journals, reference list tracking, and contact with experts) were also used (See Table 2 for full listing). No language or date restrictions were applied to the search strategy.

Table 1. Databases and Trials Registers Included in Search.

Source/Database Name	Source/Year
MEDLINE®	(Ovid; 1950–April 2008)
Ovid Medline® In-Process & Other Non-Indexed Citations	(up to April 2008)
Cochrane Central Register of Controlled Trials	(Ovid; 1st Quarter, 2008)
Cochrane Database of Systematic Reviews	(Ovid; 1st Quarter, 2008)
Database of Abstracts of Reviews of Effects (DARE)	(Ovid; 1st Quarter 2008)
EMBASE®	(1988–April 2008)
CINAHL	(EBSCOhost; 1937–April 2008)
HealthSTAR	(Ovid; 1966–April 2008)
Global Health	(Ovid; 1987–April 2008)
Pascal	(Ovid; 1987–April 2008)
BIOSIS Previews®	(via Web of Science® ; 1969–April 2008)
Science Citation Index Expanded™ and Social Science Citation Index®	(via Web of Science®; 1900–April 2008)
PubMed	(1966 to October 2006)
Current Controlled Trials, ClinicalTrials.gov, Clinical Trials in Cardiology	http://www.controlled-trials.com/, http://clinicaltrials.gov/, www2.umdnj.edu/~shindler/trials/trials_a.html
National Research Register	www.update-software.com/National/
Computer Retrieval of Information on Scientific Projects (CRISP)	http://crisp.cit.nih.gov
Australian Clinical Trials Registry	www.actr.org.au
MEDION	www.mediondatabase.nl
NLM (National Library of Medicine) Gateway, BioMed Central, and OCLC PapersFirst were searched for identification of meeting abstracts	

Table 2. Grey Literature Databases/Websites Searched.

Website	URL
Agency for Healthcare Research and Quality (AHRQ)	http://ahcpr.gov
American Academy of Allergy Asthma & Immunology	http://www.aaaai.org/members/annual_meeting
American Academy of Pediatrics	http://www.aap.org/
American College of Chest Physicians	http://www.chestnet.org/
American Thoracic Society	http://www.thoracic.org/sections/meetings-and-courses/index.html
Annual Meeting of the European Society for Paediatric Infectious Diseases (ESPID)	http://www.espid.net/
Annual Meeting of the Infectious Diseases Society of America (IDSA) 2001–2005	http://www.idsociety.org/
Asian Pacific Society of Respirology, 11th APSR Congress	http://www.apsresp.org/
Australian Clinical Trials Registry	http://www.actr.org.au/
Basal Institute of Clinical Epidemiology	http://www.bice.ch/engl/research.htm
Basel Institute for Clinical Epidemiology	http://www.bice.ch/engl/home.htm
Bayes Library of diagnostic Studies and Reviews	http://www.ispm.ch
British Thoracic Society	http://www.brit-thoracic.org.uk/
Conference on Global Lung Health	http://www.worldlunghealth.org/
Database of Promoting Health Effectiveness Reviews (DoPHER)	http://eppi.ioe.ac.uk.cms
Database of Systematic Reviews in Clinical Chemistry and Laboratory Medicine	http://www.ckcjl-mb.nl/ifcc/
European Congress of Clinical Microbiology and Infectious Diseases 2001–2005	http://www.akm.cc/eccmid2001-2005/
European Respiratory Society	http://dev.ersnet.org/
European Society of Clinical Microbiology and Infectious Diseases (ESCMID)	http://www.escmid.org/
GreyLit Report	http://nyam.org/library/grey.shtml
Guidelines International Network	http://www.g-i-n.net
Health Evidence	http://hebs.cf.ac.uk
Health Technology Assessment Database	http://agatha.york.ac.uk/htahp.htm
HTAi vortal Health Technology Assessment International	http://www.htai.org/vortal/
Infectious Diseases Society of America	http://www.idsociety.org/
International Pediatric Association	http://www.ipa-world.org/meetings/meetings.htm
International Society for Infectious Diseases	http://www.isid.org/
Interscience Conference Antimicrobial Agents and Chemotherapy	http://www.icaac.org
LWWOnline: The Pediatric Infectious Disease Journal	http://pidj.com
MEDION	http://www.mediondatabase.nl/
National Institute of Allergy and Infectious Diseases (NIAID)	http://www3.niaid.nih.gov
New York Academy of Medicine Library, Grey Literature Collection	http://www.nyam.org/library/grey.shtml
Oxford Childhood Infection Study	http://www.dphpc.ox.ac.uk/oxcis/
Pediatric Academic Societies Archive 2000–2005	http://www.abstracts2view.com/pasall
Pediatric Critical Care Medicine	http://www.pccmjournal.com
The Society for Clinical Trials	http://www.sctweb.org/
US Department of Health and Human Services, Centers for Disease Control and Prevention	http://www.cdc.gov/ncidod/
World Health Organization (WHO)	http://search.who.int
World Congress on Pediatric Critical Care	http://www.wfpiccs.org/

Inclusion criteria were assessed independently by at least two reviewers (LB and RL). The primary reason for exclusion of articles was documented. Scientific-based publications were included if they: (1) involved children between the ages of 1 month and 18 years of age, (2) provided diagnostic accuracy data to construct a 2×2 table, and (3) compared a gold standard and index test that were both used to make a diagnosis of bacterial pneumonia taken to include both typical and atypical pneumonia. Gold standard and index test categories included radiographic, hematologic, immunologic, microbiologic, virologic, and clinical variables (signs and symptoms). Due to the lack of a defined gold standard that can reliably differentiate bacterial from non-bacterial pneumonia, all combinations of tests assessing the diagnostic accuracy of bacterial pneumonia were included. To assess study quality the Quality Assessment of Studies of Diagnostic Accuracy included in Systematic Reviews (QUADAS) was applied by two independent reviewers (LB and RL) [19,20].

Data Extraction and Analysis

Data was extracted by one reviewer and checked for accuracy and completeness by a second reviewer. Any disagreements were resolved through discussion with the clinical leaders.

Data analysis was based on a published methodological review [21]. The primary outcome is accuracy of the screening test (i.e., sensitivity, specificity, positive and/or negative predictive values with corresponding 95% confidence intervals using standard formulas) [22]. For each individual study, we reconstructed a standard 2×2 table and if multiple studies had used the same index test and gold standard weighted averages of the sensitivities, specificities or predictive values were computed.

Results

The literature search revealed 5,989 references of which 256 were screened for inclusion. As shown in Figure 1 this resulted in 25 studies that satisfied all inclusion criteria.

Study Characteristics

The studies examined a range of bacterium types and assessed the accuracy of several combinations of diagnostic tests. Detailed characteristics of each study appear in Tables S1 and S2. These studies were published between 1986 and 2007 from 12 different countries. The majority of included studies originated from higher income countries (Australia, Italy, Spain, France, United States, Switzerland, Japan, and Finland), as defined by The World Bank, with 7 studies from the middle to low income category (China/Taiwan, Argentina, Brazil, and Bangladesh) [23]. All subjects were children between the ages of one month and 17 years, with a mean age of 6.56 years (based on 14 studies reporting a mean or median age). Gender was evenly distributed as specified in 12 of 25 studies (52.3% male). The majority of the studies collected patient data prospectively (21/25) from a single site (24/25). Eleven studies examined atypical species of bacterial pneumonia, six looked at typical bacteria, and seven combined both atypical and typical varieties. One study defined what they studied only as 'bacterial pneumonia'.

To be included in our review studies needed to clearly describe both the index and gold standards used. A specific gold standard was not defined *a priori*, therefore all combinations of index tests and gold standards were included, provided the studies met all inclusion criteria. We broadly categorized the types of diagnostic tests (both gold and index) as radiographic, hematologic, immunologic, microbiologic, virologic, or clinical variables (signs/symptoms) for ease of comparison. From the 25 included articles, we ended up with 23 distinct combinations of these categories. As a result of the wide range of testing modalities it was not possible to combine studies or compute weighted accuracy data (see Table S3 for individual study tests and data). Therefore we conducted a qualitative review of this literature and non-numerically summarized the major findings. Results for each of the studies can be found in Table S3. All 25 articles were assessed using the QUADAS tool and the scores ranged from 8 to 14, with an average score of 10.44 (see Table S4 for quality assessment of individual studies).

Categorization of Gold Standards

Eleven different gold standards were studied in the 25 included studies. The most common gold standard utilized was blood

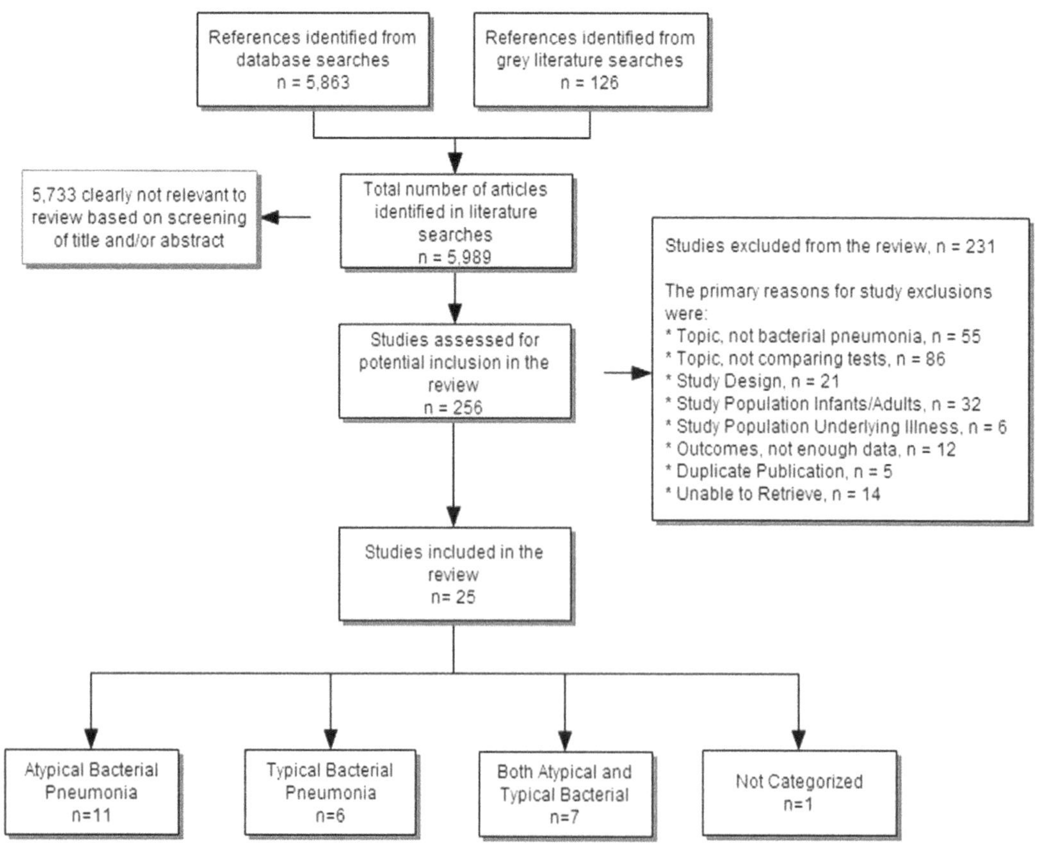

Figure 1. PRISMA flowchart of study selection, retrieval, and inclusion.

culture tests used in six studies [24–29]. These studies measured the criterion validity of nine different index tests, including the measurement of signs/symptoms, hematologic, chest radiograph, nested Polymerase Chain Reaction (PCR), procalcitonin (PCT), CRP, latex agglutination, immunochromatographic membrane assay, and lung aspirate. Sensitivities ranged from 10% for the lung aspirate as an index test to 100% with urine latex agglutination for Hib as an index test. Specificities ranged from 63.2% for the chest radiograph as an index test to100% with nested PCR as an index test.

Five studies [25,30–33] used a chest radiograph either alone or with other variables as the gold standard, measuring the validity of seven index tests. These index tests included: PCT with three cutoff points, WBC count, CRP, serology by complement fixation in 2 studies, latex particle agglutination, and nested PCR. With the chest radiograph as the gold standard, sensitivities ranged from 14.3% (radiograph exhibited air trapping) to 77.8% (PCT>0.5 ng/ml) and specificities ranged from 34.8% (PCT>0.5 ng/ml) to 100% (nested PCR).

The one study [28] that used pleural fluid cultures as the gold standard revealed that the immunochromatographic membrane assay for urinary pneumococcal antigen detection had a sensitivity of 90.9% and a specificity of 68.8%. Other gold standards utilized in the studies included: hematologic [34], microbiologic [35–39], hematologic/immunologic [40], serology [41,42], immunologic [43–46], and clinical signs and symptoms [47].

Categorization of Index Tests

Fourteen different tests were measured as index tests. PCT was the most common measured in five studies [26,30,36,42,46], each with a different gold standard. There were as many as four separate cutoff points set for the PCT levels utilized. The sensitivity of PCT ranged from 40% when 0.5 ng/dl was set as the cutoff point and chest radiography was used as a gold standard to 95.4% in two studies with a cutoff above 0.5 ng/dl when blood cultures were used as the gold standard. For all studies its sensitivity decreased and its specificity increased as the cutoff points were raised.

An additional four studies used clinical variables, PCR, and CRP as their index tests. PCR was used as the index test [25,34,44,45] with six different gold standards. Sensitivities ranged from 36.4% with complement fixation (Mycoplasma pneumonia) to 95.7% with Mycoplasma serology. Specificities ranged from 79.7% with mycoplasma serology to 100% with positive blood cultures or clinical and radiological evidence of pneumonia.

Clinical variables [24,39–41] and CRP [36,39,46,48] each demonstrated broad ranges in sensitivities and specificities for the array of clinical variables and the different cutoff points for CRP measured. The chest radiograph's accuracy was measured as an index test in four [24,35,40,47] of the studies. Its sensitivity peaked at 75% with a range of 0–75% depending on the radiological definition assigned while its specificity ranged from 50 to 100%. Four studies [24,39,42,48] utilized the total WBC count as an index test with three ranges being utilized. Sensitivities ranged from 20% to 65.1% and specificities ranged from 53.1% to79.3% when the total WBC count was above 15 000 ($x10^6/l$).

Other index tests utilized in the studies included: interleukin-6 at 3 different levels [36,42,46], immunologic [28,36–38], microbiologic [27,31–33,38], virologic [32,43], hematologic [39], and lung aspirate [29].

Discussion

Diagnostic testing provides physicians with information about the likelihood of certain diseases. Ideally these diagnostic tests have been validated against an agreed-upon gold/reference standard. The objective of the Standards for Reporting of Diagnostic Accuracy (STARD) initiative [49] is to improve the accuracy and completeness of reporting of studies of diagnostic accuracy. They defined the gold/reference standard to be "the best available method for establishing the presence or absence of the condition of interest." They further add that "the reference standard can be a single method, or a combination of methods, to establish the presence of the target condition. It can include laboratory tests, imaging tests, and pathology, but also dedicated clinical follow-up of subjects." This systematic review has demonstrated that diagnostic tests used for pediatric pneumonia have not been truly validated and there is little agreement as to what tests should be used as a gold standard. It is, therefore, difficult to recommend any of the reference standards used in the reviewed studies as "the best available method" given these limitations.

This review underscores the fundamental problem with diagnosing pneumonia in children when there is no proven and accurate gold standard. Since the standards used to define pneumonia are variable and inconsistent it is difficult to know whether the criterion validity of these diagnostic tests is accurate or not. A problem of 'circularity' exists for which there is no easy solution.

An additional problem is that the included studies did not all focus on the same type of bacterial disease. Eleven studies dealt with atypical pneumonia, six with typical pneumonia, and seven studied both typical and atypical pneumonia. And even within those studies which focused on the same type of bacterial etiology (e.g. pneumococcal pneumonia), each study defined the disease differently. For example, a patient with a positive blood culture for pneumococcus is likely clinically different from a patient with a negative blood culture.

One challenging aspect is that most of the studies were performed in high income countries with only seven studies performed in low income countries. This is contrast to the disease burden, where most of the mortality from pneumonia happens in low income countries. Future research should try to redress this imbalance.

Categorization of Gold Standards

Of the eleven different gold standards utilized, the blood culture and the chest radiograph were the most common tests. Chest radiography was utilized in five studies as the gold standard while in three other studies it was measured as an index test. When it was employed as an index test its sensitivity was generally low while its specificity was generally high. This sub-par performance as an index test illustrates that the use of chest radiography as a gold standard is potentially flawed. The use of ten other gold standards for twenty of the studies highlights that there is much disagreement amongst researchers worldwide whether the chest radiograph should be utilized as a gold standard or an index test. In most academic emergency departments, a chest radiograph is considered the standard of care and is readily obtained for pediatric patients with the clinical suspicion of bacterial pneumonia. Clinically similar patients with potential ambulatory pneumonia presenting to a clinic or private office are less likely to undergo chest radiography.

From a clinical perspective, the blood culture is somewhat invasive and the results are generally not available for several hours. Further only a relatively small percentage of patients with bacterial pneumonia yield a positive blood culture (which results in low sensitivity), and now with the widespread use of conjugate pneumoococcal vaccine, the yield of blood cultures would be even less.

Criterion Validity of Index Tests

Fourteen different index tests' criterion validity was measured. The heterogeneity of the different studies was further illustrated when the results of the different index tests were compared. Though the overall criterion validity of PCR was reasonably consistent, most other index tests (e.g. clinical variables, total WBC count, interleukin-6 and CRP) had highly variable accuracy.

As an example, in one study of PCT used as an index test, Don [30] concluded, in contrast to other studies, that serum PCT could not reliably distinguish bacterial from non-bacterial pneumonia. However, Don et al. [30] utilized as gold standard a chest radiograph that was inconclusive in 34% of their patients. This example illustrates that, given the diversity of the diagnostic methods used, current evidence is potentially inaccurate and highly misleading.

There is a critical need for experts in childhood pneumonia to develop an accepted gold standard. While it would be optimal for such a test to be cheap and readily available to practicing clinicians, the development of a more complex gold standard for use in research studies would be a major advance. As suggested in the STARD initiative,[49] one approach for developing a more complex standard is to use a combination of methods including imaging tests, laboratory tests available both immediately and long after the fact, and clinical features obtained not only at presentation but on dedicated follow-up subjects. The problem then becomes how each of these individual items should be weighted relative to the others. Given the highly variable results we found for most reference tests, a fixed algorithmic approach to combining methods is not possible. Alternatively an expert panel could use standard consensus methods to weigh the results of chest x-ray, standard and specialized laboratory tests, bacterial and viral diagnostic tests and clinical course of patients to classify patients as bacterial or non-bacterial.[50–51] The development of such a gold standard would greatly enhance and aid the evaluation of diagnostic tests for their accuracy in the future.

Although we conducted a comprehensive electronic and hand search of the literature, as well as verification of all extracted data this review is not without limitations. The main limitation of this review is the inability to include Latin American databases such as the Latin American and Caribbean Health Sciences Literature (LILACS) and Scientific Electronic Library Online (SciELO) as part of the electronic search strategy. At the onset of this review we were unable to identify a clinical expert fluent in Spanish to participate in the identification of search terms and in the screening, inclusion/exclusion, and extraction phases of the systematic review. African and Asian databases were also not included for similar reasons. We acknowledge this as a limiting factor of this review but with the breadth of other databases searched we do not believe this has altered the results.

In conclusion, we have found that studies assessing the diagnostic accuracy of clinical, radiological, and laboratory tests for bacterial childhood pneumonia have used a heterogeneous group of gold standards, and found, at least in part because of this, that index tests have widely different accuracies. These findings highlight the need for identifying a widely accepted gold standard for diagnosis of bacterial pneumonia in children.

Supporting Information

Table S1 Study Characteristics.

Table S2 Participant Characteristics.

Table S3 Criterion Validity for the Diagnosis of Bacterial Pneumonia.

Table S4 Quality Assessment of Studies of Diagnostic Accuracy included in Systematic Reviews (QUADAS).

PRISMA Checklist S1 PRISMA Checklist of items to include when reporting a systematic review or meta-analysis (diagnostic review consisting of cohort studies).

Acknowledgments

Ethics approval was not required for the conduct of this systematic review. The authors would like to acknowledge the contributions of Yuanyuan Liang, PhD for statistical consultation, Donna Dryden, PhD, and Lisa Hartling, PhD for methodological expertise. The authors would also like to thank the Alberta Research Centre for Health Evidence (ARCHE) and Pediatric Emergency Research Canada (PERC) for their support.

Author Contributions

Conceived and designed the experiments: TL LB JDK MHO TK TD RL DWJ. Performed the experiments: TL LB JDK MHO TK TD RL DWJ. Analyzed the data: LB. Wrote the paper: TL LB JDK MHO TK TD RL DWJ.

References

1. Shann F, Steinhoff MC (1999) Vaccines for children in rich and poor countries. Lancet 354 Suppl 2: SII7–11.
2. McIntosh K (2002) Community-acquired pneumonia in children. N Engl J Med 346: 429–437.
3. Shoham Y, Dagan R, Givon-Lavi N, Liss Z, Shagan T, et al. (2005) Community-acquired pneumonia in children: quantifying the burden on patients and their families including decrease in quality of life. Pediatrics 115: 1213–1219.
4. Michelow IC, Olsen K, Lozano J, Rollins NK, Duffy LB, et al. (2004) Epidemiology and clinical characteristics of community-acquired pneumonia in hospitalized children. Pediatrics 113: 701–707.
5. McCracken GH, Jr. (2000) Diagnosis and management of pneumonia in children. Pediatr Infect Dis J 19: 924–928.
6. Ferwerda A, Moll HA, de Groot R (2001) Respiratory tract infections by Mycoplasma pneumoniae in children: a review of diagnostic and therapeutic measures. Eur J Pediatr 160: 483–491.
7. Lichenstein R, Suggs AH, Campbell J (2003) Pediatric pneumonia. Emerg Med Clin North Am 21: 437–451.
8. Coote N, McKenzie S (2000) Diagnosis and investigation of bacterial pneumonias. Paediatr Respir Rev 1: 8–13.
9. Churgay CA (1996) The diagnosis and management of bacterial pneumonias in infants and children. Prim Care 23: 821–835.
10. Benguigui Y, Antunano FJL, Schmunis G, Yunes J (1999) Respiratory infections in children. Pan American Health Organization. Pan American Sanitary Bureau, Regional Office of the World Health Organization.
11. Lynch T, Gouin S, Larson C, Patenaude Y (2004) Does the lateral chest radiograph help pediatric emergency physicians diagnose pneumonia? A randomized clinical trial. Acad Emerg Med 11: 625–629.
12. Wilkins TR, Wilkins RL (2005) Clinical and radiographic evidence of pneumonia. Radiol Technol 77: 106–110.
13. Sinaniotis CA (1999) Community-acquired pneumonia: diagnosis and treatment. Pediatr Pulmonol Suppl 18: 144–145.
14. Egger M, Davey Smith G, Altman DG, eds. Systematic reviews in health care: meta-analysis in context. London: BMJ Publishing.
15. Cochrane Reviewers' Handbook4.2.2. Alderson P, Green S, Higgens JPT, eds. (2008) www.cochrane.org.

16. Deville WL, Buntinx F, Bouter LM, Montori VM, de Vet HC, et al. (2002) Conducting systematic reviews of diagnostic studies: didactic guidelines. BMC Med Res Methodol 2: 9.
17. Khan KS (2005) Systematic reviews of diagnostic tests: a guide to methods and application. Best Pract Res Clin Obstet Gynaecol 19: 37–46.
18. Irwig L, Macaskill P, Glasziou P, Fahey M (1995) Meta-analytic methods for diagnostic test accuracy. J Clin Epidemiol 48: 119–130.
19. Whiting P, Rutjes AW, Reitsma JB, Bossuyt PM, Kleijnen N (2003) The development of QUADAS: a tool for the quality assessment of studies of diagnostic accuracy included in systematic reviews. BMC Med Res Methodol 3: 25.
20. Whiting PF, Weswood ME, Rutjes AW, Reitsma JB, Bossuyt, et al. (2006) Evaluation of QUADAS, a tool for the quality assessment of diagnostic accuracy studies. BMC Med Res Methodol 6: 9.
21. Deeks JJ (2001) Systematic reviews in health care: Systematic reviews of evaluations of diagnostic and screening tests. BMJ 323: 157–162.
22. Rosner B (1995) Fundamentals of biostatistics. Belmont: Duxbury Press.
23. The WorldBank. Data and Statistics: Country Classification (2009) The World Bank Group, editor. Available: http://web.worldbank.org/WBSITE/EXTERNAL/DATASTATISTICS/0,,contentMDK:20420458~menuPK:64133156~pagePK:64133150~piPK:64133175~theSitePK:239419,00.htm. Accessed 15 February 2009.
24. Bettenay FA, de Campo JF, McCrossin DB (1988) Differentiating bacterial from viral pneumonias in children. Pediatr Radiol 18: 453–454.
25. Mayoral C, Norona M, Baroni MR, Giani R, Zalazar F (2005) Evaluation of a nested-PCR assay for Streptococcus pneumoniae detection in pediatric patients with community-acquired pneumonia. Rev Argent Microbiol 37: 184–188.
26. Prat C, Dominguez J, Rodrigo C, Gimenez M, Azuara M, et al. (2003) Procalcitonin, C-reactive protein and leukocyte count in children with lower respiratory tract infection. Pediatr Infect Dis J 22: 963–968.
27. Saha SK, Baqui AH, El Areefin S, Qazi S, Billal DS, et al. (2006) Detection of antigenuria for diagnosis of invasive Haemophilus influenzae type b disease. Ann Trop Paediatr 26: 329–336.
28. Tzeng DH, Lee YL, Lin YH, Tsai CA, Shi ZY (2006) Diagnostic value of the Binax NOW assay for identifying a pneumococcal etiology in patients with respiratory tract infection. J Microbiol Immunol Infect 39: 39–44.
29. Vuori-Holopainen E, Salo E, Saxen H, Hedman K, Hyypia T, et al. (2000) Etiological diagnosis of childhood pneumonia by use of transthoracic needle aspiration and modern microbiological methods.[see comment]. Clin Infect Dis 34: 583–590.
30. Don M, Valent F, Korppi M, Falleti E, De Candia A, et al. (2007) Efficacy of serum procalcitonin in evaluating severity of community-acquired pneumonia in childhood. Scand J Infect Dis 39: 129–137.
31. Jimenez AJ, Esteban RE, Girones IG, Sanchez PG, Orozco AL, et al. (1997) Usefulness of etiologic studies in pediatric inpatients with pneumonia. An Esp Pediatr 47: 493–498.
32. Esteban RE, Jimenez AM, Orozco AL, Girones IG, Sanchez PG, et al. (1996) Etiology of acute respiratory infections in 87 hospitalized children. Rev Clin Esp 196: 82–86.
33. Nunes AA, Camargos PA, Costa PR, Campos MT (2004) Antigen detection for the diagnosis of pneumonia. Pediatr Pulmonol 38: 135–139.
34. Blackmore TK, Reznikov M, Gordon DL (1995) Clinical utility of the polymerase chain reaction to diagnose Mycoplasma pneumoniae infection. Pathology (Phila) 27: 177–181.
35. Castriota-Scanderbeg A, Popolizio T, Sacco M, Coppi M, Scarale MG, et al. (1995) Diagnosis of mycoplasma pneumonia in children: which is the role of thoracic radiography? Radiol Med 89: 782–786.
36. Gendrel D, Moulin F, Lorrot M, Marc E, Gueren S, et al. (2002) Procalcitonin and markers of infection in community-acquired pneumonia of children. Medecine et Maladies Infectieuses Editions Scientifiques et Medicales Elsevier SAS, Paris, France 32: 88–97.
37. Nagayama Y, Sakurai N, Yamamoto K, Honda A, Makuta M, et al. (1988) Isolation of Mycoplasma pneumoniae from children with lower-respiratory-tract infections. J Infect Dis 157: 911–917.
38. Requejo HI (2007) Community-acquired pneumonia in the childhood: analysis of the diagnostic methods. Braz J Infect Dis 11: 246–248.
39. Tsai M, Huang Y, Chen C, Lin P, Chang LY, et al. (2005) Chlamydial pneumonia in children requiring hospitalization: effect of mixed infection on clinical outcome. Journal of Microbiology, Immunology and Infection Scientific Communications International Limited, Hong Kong, China 38: 117–122.
40. Esposito S, Bosis S, Cavagna R, Faelli N, Begliatti E, et al. (2002) Characteristics of Streptococcus pneumoniae and atypical bacterial infections in children 2–5 years of age with community-acquired pneumonia. Clin Infect Dis 35: 1345–1352.
41. Gambert C, Werner E, de KM, Monginet F, Bruel H, et al. (1993) Mycoplasma pneumoniae pneumopathies in children: clinical, biological and radiological study. Pediatrie 48: 241–247.
42. Moulin F, Raymond J, Lorrot M, Marc E, Coste J, et al. (2001) Procalcitonin in children admitted to hospital with community acquired pneumonia. Arch Dis Child 84: 332–336.
43. Hardy RD, Michelow IC, Rios AM, Olsen K, Lozano J, et al. (2003) Comparison of nasopharyngeal and oropharyngeal PCR for the diagnosis of mycoplasma pneumonia in children. 43rd ICAAC Abstracts (Abstract D-1859). pp 187.
44. Liu FC, Chen PY, Huang F, Tsai CR, Lee CY, et al. (2007) Rapid diagnosis of Mycoplasma pneumoniae infection in children by polymerase chain reaction. J Microbiol Immunol Infect 40: 507–512.
45. Nadal D, Bossart W, Zucol F, Berger C, Lips R, et al. (1999) Mycoplasma pneumoniae pneumonia in children and its etiologic diagnosis. Abstr Intersci Conf Antimicrob Agents Chemother Intersci Conf Antimicrob Agents Chemother 39: 701.
46. Toikka P, Irjala K, Juven T, Virkki R, Mertsola J, et al. (2000) Serum procalcitonin, C-reactive protein and interleukin-6 for distinguishing bacterial and viral pneumonia in children. Pediatr Infect Dis J 19: 598–602.
47. Swischuk LE, Hayden CK, Jr. (1986) Viral vs. bacterial pulmonary infections in children (is roentgenographic differentiation possible?). Pediatr Radiol 16: 278–284.
48. Virkki R, Juven T, Rikalainen H, Svedstrom E, Mertsola J, et al. (2002) Differentiation of bacterial and viral pneumonia in children. Thorax 57: 438–441.
49. Bossuyt PM, Reitsma JB, Bruns DE, for the STARD Group (2003) Towards complete and accurate reporting of studies of diagnostic accuracy: The STARD Initiative. Ann Intern Med 138: 40–44.
50. Jones J, Hunter D (1995) Consensus methods for medical and health services research. BMJ 311(7001): 376–80.
51. Alessandrini EA, Alpern ER, Chamberlain JM, Shea JA, Gorelick MH (2010) A new diagnosis grouping system for child emergency department visits. Acad Emerg Med 17(2): 204–13.

12

Recurrent *Plasmodium falciparum* Malaria Infections in Kenyan Children Diminish T-Cell Immunity to Epstein Barr Virus Lytic but not Latent Antigens

Cynthia J. Snider[1], Stephen R. Cole[1], Kiprotich Chelimo[2], Peter Odada Sumba[2], Pia D. M. MacDonald[1], Chandy C. John[3], Steven R. Meshnick[1], Ann M. Moormann[4,5]*

1 Department of Epidemiology, Gillings School of Global Public Health, University of North Carolina, Chapel Hill, North Carolina, United States of America, **2** Center for Global Health Research, Kenya Medical Research Institute, Kisumu, Kenya, **3** Departments of Pediatrics and Medicine, University of Minnesota Medical School, Minneapolis, Minnesota, United States of America, **4** Center for Global Health and Diseases, Case Western Reserve University, Cleveland, Ohio, United States of America, **5** Departments of Pediatrics and Quantitative Health Services, University of Massachusetts Medical School, Worcester, Massachusetts, United States of America

Abstract

Plasmodium falciparum malaria (*Pf*-malaria) and Epstein Barr Virus (EBV) infections coexist in children at risk for endemic Burkitt's lymphoma (eBL); yet studies have only glimpsed the cumulative effect of *Pf*-malaria on EBV-specific immunity. Using pooled EBV lytic and latent CD8+ T-cell epitope-peptides, IFN-γ ELISPOT responses were surveyed three times among children (10 months to 15 years) in Kenya from 2002–2004. Prevalence ratios (PR) and 95% confidence intervals (CI) were estimated in association with *Pf*-malaria exposure, defined at the district-level (Kisumu: holoendemic; Nandi: hypoendemic) and the individual-level. We observed a 46% decrease in positive EBV lytic antigen IFN-γ responses among 5–9 year olds residing in Kisumu compared to Nandi (PR: 0.54; 95% CI: 0.30–0.99). Individual-level analysis in Kisumu revealed further impairment of EBV lytic antigen responses among 5–9 year olds consistently infected with *Pf*-malaria compared to those never infected. There were no observed district- or individual-level differences between *Pf*-malaria exposure and EBV latent antigen IFN-γ response. The gradual decrease of EBV lytic antigen but not latent antigen IFN-γ responses after primary infection suggests a specific loss in immunological control over the lytic cycle in children residing in malaria holoendemic areas, further refining our understanding of eBL etiology.

Editor: Maria G. Masucci, Karolinska Institutet, Sweden

Funding: This work was supported by the Infectious Disease Epidemiology Training Program from the National Institutes of Health [5-T32-AI070114-03 to CJS]. The original study was supported by the National Institutes of Health [K08 AI51565, CA134051, AI01572, and AI056270]. The funders had no role in study design, data collection and analysis, decision to publish, or preparation of the manuscript.

Competing Interests: The authors have declared that no competing interests exist.

* E-mail: ann.moormann@umassmed.edu

Introduction

Plasmodium falciparum (*Pf*) malaria and Epstein Barr Virus (EBV) have been identified as co-factors in the pathogenesis of endemic Burkitt's lymphoma (eBL) [1] which is estimated to account for 70% of cancers among children in equatorial Africa [2,3]. In areas with intense perennial malaria transmission (holoendemic), the highest incidence of eBL is in children aged 4–8 years [4,5,6,7,8,9], in contrast to areas with low malaria transmission (hypoendemic) where eBL is rarely reported [7,10,11].

It has been hypothesized that *Pf*-malaria infections promote eBL in two mutually-compatible ways. In developing countries, most children experience primary EBV infection by 3 years of age, followed by life-long infection in memory B-lymphocytes [12,13]. *P. falciparum* induces polyclonal B-cell expansion and lytic EBV reactivation [14], thus increasing the number of latently-infected B-cells. In otherwise healthy individuals, interferon-gamma (IFN-γ) secreting cytotoxic CD8+ T-cells mediate immunosurveillance of EBV [5,12,15,16,17,18]. Repeated *Pf*-malaria infections could hence lead to exhaustion or hypo-responsiveness of EBV latent or lytic antigen CD8+ T-cells, thus increasing the chance for this EBV-associated malignancy to arise.

Limited evidence supports an impaired EBV-specific T-cell response in association with *Pf*-malaria. Using an in vitro regression assay as a measure of cytotoxicity, children with acute *Pf*-malaria demonstrated a transient loss of control over B-cell outgrowth [19,20,21]. Furthermore, case-control studies comparing acutely *Pf*-malaria infected individuals with healthy adults came to the same conclusion [22,23]. However, the cumulative effect of repeated often asymptomatic *Pf*-malaria infections on EBV persistence has not been thoroughly studied [1,6,24,25]. Two ecological studies provide the minimum understanding we have on the relationship. A study among adults found a loss of EBV-specific T-cell control among those exposed to holoendemic compared to hypoendemic malaria [26]. A second study only found significantly lower EBV latent and lytic antigen IFN-γ responses in children 5–9 years old residing in the holoendemic area compared to other age groups and children from a hypoendemic area [16].

The objective of this study was to examine the influence of cumulative *Pf*-malaria on EBV latent and lytic antigen CD8+ T-cell IFN-γ ELISPOT responses in children over a two-year period.

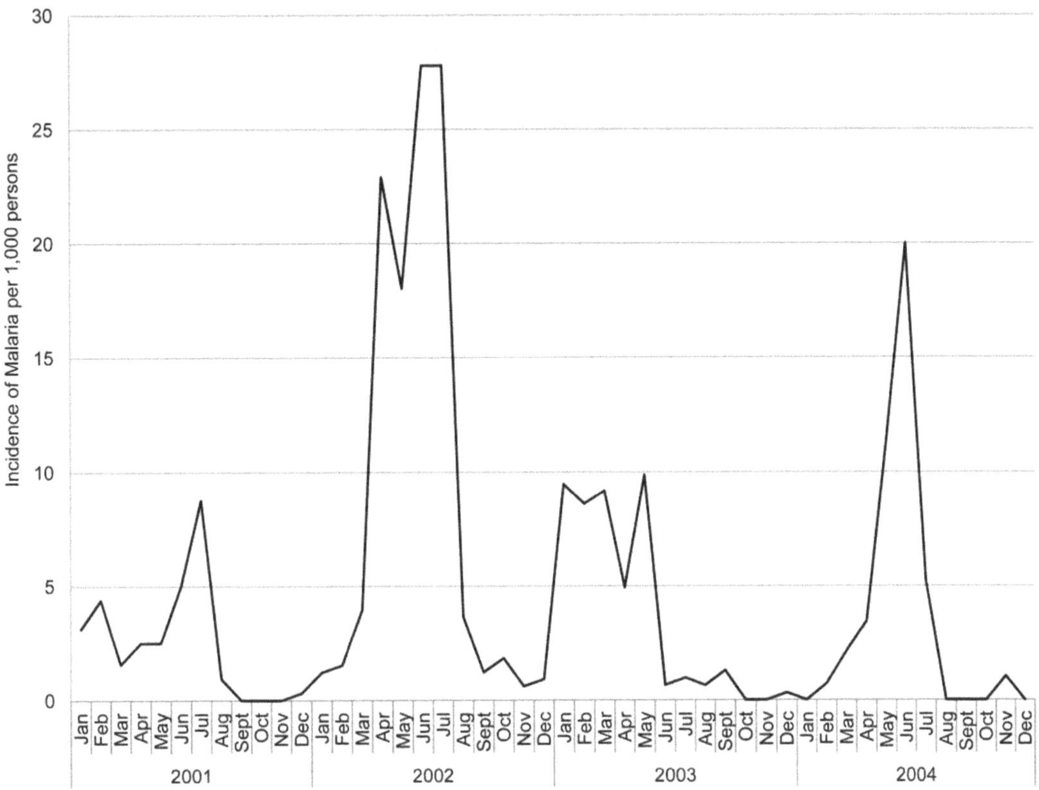

Figure 1. Malaria incidence in the highland area of Kipsamoite, 2001–2004.

Results

Participant summary

Of the 236 children enrolled, 230 (97.5%) were seropositive for EBV [27]. Our weighted analysis included 149 children who participated in all surveys and had interpretable EBV-specific T-cell responses (Table 1). The age and sex distribution between the districts were not significantly different ($P=.11$ and $P=.30$, respectively). Children in Kisumu experienced more *Pf*-malaria infections than children in Nandi ($P<.001$); only 3% of Kisumu children were never infected compared to 78% in Nandi. This was despite a classically defined malaria outbreak in Nandi during the survey periods (Figure 1).

The magnitude of EBV-specific IFN-γ responses did not differ significantly by malaria endemicity. The proportion of positive IFN-γ responses to PHA (positive control) demonstrates that children from both districts were equally able to elicit an IFN-γ response indicating no global signs of immune dysfunction (Table 2). There were no significant differences in median values of EBV lytic or latent CD8+ T-cell IFN-γ responses between children of similar age groups across districts. Therefore, *Pf*-malaria exposure does not appear to influence the magnitude of EBV-specific IFN-γ responses.

Table 1. Summary of participants in the Kisumu/Nandi cohort, Kenya 2002–2004[a].

	Site				Total
	Kisumu (holoendemic)		Nandi (hypoendemic)		
	n	%	*n*	%	
Sex					
Male	39	59.1	38	45.8	77
Female	27	40.9	45	54.2	72
Age (in years)					
0–4	16	24.2	30	36.1	46
5–9	33	50.0	35	42.2	68
≥10	17	25.8	18	21.7	35
Malaria infections					
All surveys	38	57.6	0	0	38
Two surveys	20	30.3	4	4.8	24
One survey	6	9.1	14	16.9	20
Never	2	3.0	65	78.3	67
Total	66		83		149

n, number; %, percentage.
[a]Data in the table are weighted according to the 149 children who participated in all surveys and had interpretable Epstein-Barr virus (EBV) specific CD8+ T-cell IFN-γ response.

Pf-malaria exposure (district-level) and EBV-specific T-cell IFN-γ responses

EBV lytic antigen CD8+ T-cell IFN-γ responses. We observed a few intriguing patterns in the prevalence of positive EBV lytic antigen CD8+ T-cell IFN-γ response when children were stratified into age groups by their baseline age (age group cohorts) (Figure 2A,C). In Kisumu, the prevalence of positive

Table 2. EBV-specific CD8+ T-cell IFN-γ Response by Residence and Age Group[a].

	EBV lytic antigens			EBV latent antigens			PHA[b]	
	n	%	Median[c] (range)	*n*	%	Median[c] (range)	*n*	%
Baseline (July–August 2002)								
Kisumu								
0–4 years	7/16	43.8	96 (14–166)	8/16	50.0	43 (20–98)	13/16	81.3
5–9 years	8/33	24.2	67 (18–170)	6/33	18.2	47 (16–448)	31/33	93.9
≥10 years	5/17	29.4	150 (20–350)	5/17	29.4	46 (16–404)	15/17	88.2
Nandi								
0–4 years	12/30	34.3	98 (28–836)	8/30	26.7	70 (18–146)	28/30	93.3
5–9 years	15/35	42.9	50 (22–792)	11/35	31.4	84 (42–668)	33/35	94.3
≥10 years	8/18	22.9	53 (36–304)	8/18	44.4	88 (26–1322)	18/18	100
First follow-up (February–March 2003)								
Kisumu								
0–4 years	4/16	25.0	46 (40–128)	2/16	12.5	55 (32–78)	16/16	100
5–9 years	1/33	3.0	20 (20)	6/33	18.2	15 (14–132)	31/33	93.9
≥10 years	5/17	29.4	30 (18–162)	2/17	11.8	23 (18–28)	16/17	94.1
Nandi								
0–4 years	6/30	20.0	98 (24–744)	4/30	13.3	77 (32–128)	26/30	86.7
5–9 years	8/35	22.9	82 (16–1742)	8/35	22.9	58 (20–248)	34/35	97.1
≥10 years	5/18	27.8	54 (32–382)	3/18	16.7	54 (14–354)	18/18	100
Second follow-up (July–August 2004)								
Kisumu								
0–4 years	5/16	31.3	76 (30–84)	2/16	12.5	106 (64–148)	15/16	93.8
5–9 years	3/33	9.1	60 (56–150)	3/33	9.1	42 (24–74)	33/33	100
≥10 years	3/17	17.7	250 (40–288)	1/17	5.9	16 (16)	17/17	100
Nandi								
0–4 years	8/30	26.7	50 (14–384)	2/30	6.7	69 (58–80)	25/30	83.3
5–9 years	7/35	20.0	76 (14–278)	6/35	17.1	59 (14–214)	31/35	88.6
≥10 years	5/18	27.8	26 (14–130)	5/18	27.8	56 (22–122)	18/18	100

n, number; %, percentage; EBV, Epstein-Barr Virus; PHA, Phytohemagglutinin.
[a]Data in the table are weighted according to the 149 children who participated in all surveys and had interpretable Epstein-Barr Virus (EBV) specific CD8+ T-cell IFN-γ response.
[b]Phytohemagglutinin (PHA) was used as a positive control.
[c]Median EBV-specific CD8+ T-cell IFN-γ responses were calculated among children with positive responses and is expressed as spot forming units (SFU) per 1×10^6 peripheral blood mononuclear cells (PBMC).

responses in the 0–4 year and 5–9 year cohorts decreased from baseline to first follow-up, but remained unchanged in the ≥10 year cohort. By the second follow-up, responses increased among the 0–4 and 5–9 year cohorts while responses decreased in ≥10 year cohort. However, children in the 5–9 year cohort had the lowest prevalence at each survey period. In Nandi, responses declined in all age group cohorts from baseline to first follow-up and remained almost unchanged in the 5–9 year and ≥10 year cohorts by the second follow-up. In the 0–4 year cohort, however, responses increased. The patterns and prevalence of responses among the age group cohorts were similar at all survey periods, varying <10%.

Using the district-level definition of *Pf*-malaria and the weighted model, we estimated the prevalence of positive responses in Kisumu was 0.70 (95% CI: 0.45–1.08) times the prevalence in Nandi although this 30% difference was not significant. In Kisumu, there were no significant differences in positive responses in children 0–4 years (PR: 1.39, 95% CI: 0.60–3.20) and 5–9 years (PR: 0.74, 95% CI: 0.37–1.48) when compared to children ≥10 years (Figure 3A). Likewise in Nandi, the prevalence of positive responses in children 0–4 years (PR: 1.10, 95% CI: 0.60–2.02) and 5–9 years (PR: 1.04, 95% CI: 0.61–1.76) did not differ significantly from children ≥10 years. When similar age groups were compared between districts, we detected a significant difference in children 5–9 years where the prevalence of positive responses in Kisumu was 0.54 (95% CI: 0.30–0.99) that of children in Nandi (Figure 3A). No other differences by age group were found.

EBV latent antigen CD8+ T-cell IFN-γ responses. Examining the patterns in the prevalence of positive EBV latent antigen CD8+ T-cell IFN-γ response by age group cohorts, there was variation within and between districts (Figure 2B,D). In Kisumu, the prevalence at baseline was highest among the 0–4 year cohort but then decreased to nearly the same prevalence as the other age group cohorts. In Nandi, there was a decreasing trend from baseline to second follow-up for the

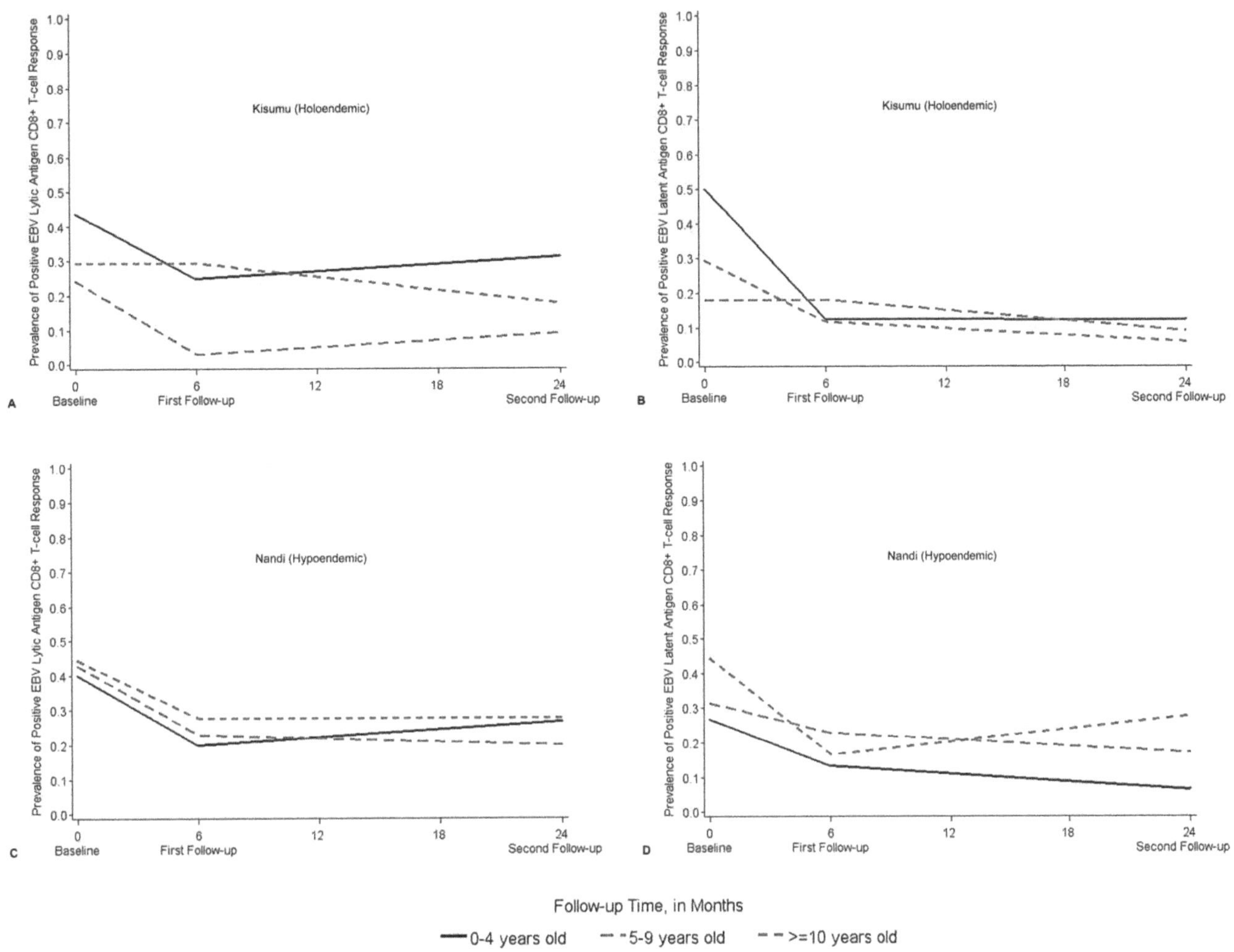

Figure 2. Change in prevalence of EBV-specific CD8+ T-cell IFNγ responses with age. Changes in prevalence of positive EBV lytic (A and C) and latent (B and D) antigen CD8+ T-cell IFNγ response from 2002–2004. Age group at each survey period is based on age at baseline. In Kisumu: 16 (0–4 years), 33 (5–9 years) and 17 (≥10 years). In Nandi: 30 (0–4 years), 35 (5–9 years) and 18 (≥10 years). Solid black line: 0–4 year olds; hash-mark green line: 5–9 year olds; and dotted blue line: ≥10 year old children.

0–4 year and 5–9 year cohorts. However, the ≥10 years cohort had the highest prevalence of response at baseline that decreased by the first follow-up but rebounded by the second follow-up.

From our weighted model, we observed the prevalence of positive responses in Kisumu was 0.80 (95% CI: 0.51–1.25) times the prevalence in Nandi, although not significant. In Kisumu, the prevalence of positive responses in children 0–4 years (PR: 1.93, 95% CI: 0.91–4.13) and 5–9 years (PR: 1.22, 95% CI: 0.61–2.45) was not significantly different from children ≥10 years, although there was a decrease in prevalence with increasing age group (Figure 3B). Similarly in Nandi, responses among children 0–4 years (PR: 0.72, 95% CI: 0.35–1.48) and 5–9 years (PR: 0.84, 95% CI: 0.47–1.49) did not differ significantly from children ≥10 years old, although there was a slight increase in response with increasing age. Despite these interesting trends, there were no significant differences in the prevalence of positive responses when similar age groups were compared between districts.

Pf-malaria infection (individual-level) and EBV-specific T-cell IFN-γ responses

EBV lytic antigen CD8+ T-cell IFN-γ responses. Using the individual-level definition of *Pf*-malaria in our weighted model, we found the association between recurrent *Pf*-malaria infections and EBV lytic antigen CD8+ T-cell IFN-γ response varied by age group and survey period. We therefore used two weighted models. In the first model, we stratified results by age group, while adjusting for sex and survey period. Similarly in the second model, we stratified by survey period while adjusting for sex and age group.

We noted three observations from our analysis. First, the PR of recurrent *Pf*-malaria infections and positive IFN-γ responses among Kisumu children were consistently lower than Nandi children for all age groups and survey periods (Table 3). In general, there is a two-fold difference in the PR between Kisumu and Nandi although not significant ($P = .32$). Secondly, the association between recurrent *Pf*-malaria infections and IFN-γ responses varied by age group. In both Kisumu and Nandi, the prevalence of positive responses among children 0–4 years with recurrent *Pf*-malaria infections was higher than that of similarly aged children never infected. In Nandi, the difference was statistically significant. Finally, the PR of recurrent *Pf*-malaria infections and IFN-γ responses to EBV lytic antigens varied by survey period in both districts. At baseline, for both districts, the PR of positive responses among children with recurrent *Pf*-malaria

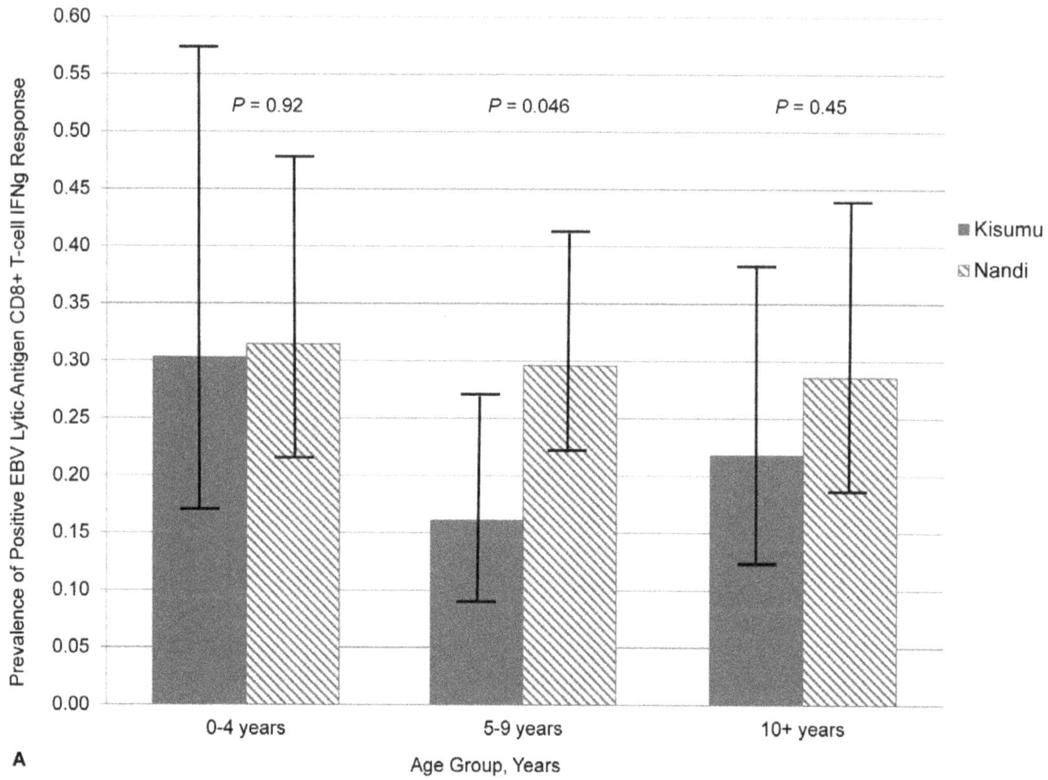

Figure 3. Prevalence of EBV-specific CD8+ T-cell IFNγ response by age group and residence. Prevalence of positive EBV lytic (A) and latent (B) antigen CD8+ T-cell IFNγ response by age group and site of residence, Kenya 2002–2004. Age group was classified as a time-varying factor. For both graphs, the number of observations for children in each age group in Kisumu was: 33 (0–4 years), 87 (5–9 years) and 78 (≥10 years). The number of observations for children in each age group in Nandi was: 54 (0–4 years), 125 (5–9 years) and 70 (≥10 years). *P* values for differences between areas of residence by age group are indicated.

infections was greater compared to children never infected; this result was statistically significant in Nandi, but not Kisumu. However, the PR decreased at subsequent study periods; the prevalence of positive responses among children with recurrent *Pf*-malaria infection diminished over time compared to children never infected. This could reflect functional diminishment of responsive EBV lytic antigen T-cells under continuous pressure from *Pf*-malaria.

Table 3. Prevalence Ratios for EBV Lytic Antigen CD8+ T-cell IFN-γ Response.

	Kisumu		Nandi	
	Constant *Pf*-malaria infection versus no infection		Constant *Pf*-malaria infection versus no infection	
	PR	95% CI	PR	95% CI
Unadjusted	0.64	0.23–1.77	1.43	0.73–2.81
Age groups[a]				
0–4 years	1.31	0.28–6.18	3.00	1.72–5.23
5–9 years	0.53	0.15–1.88	1.16	0.39–3.45
≥10 years	0.78	0.16–3.53	0.98	0.33–2.95
Survey periods[b]				
Baseline	1.24	0.49–3.11	1.76	1.07–2.91
Six months	0.29	0.05–1.62	0.73	0.17–3.22
Two years	0.21	0.05–0.92	0.22	0.02–3.23

Pf-malaria, *Plasmodium falciparum* malaria; EBV, Epstein-Barr virus; PR, prevalence ratio; CI, confidence interval; Ref, referent group.

[a]Adjusted for sex and survey period. Unstratified estimates for constant *Pf*-malaria infections compared to never infected in Kisumu ($P = 0.72$) and Nandi ($P = 0.97$) were not significant. Specific details on the number and prevalence of positive responses for each age group are included in Table 2.

[b]Adjusted for sex and age group. Unstratified estimates for constant *Pf*-malaria infections compared to never infected was not significant in Kisumu ($P = 0.65$) but significant in Nandi ($P = 0.03$). The number of children in Kisumu for each survey period was 66 and the number of children in Nandi was 83.

Table 4. Prevalence Ratio for EBV Latent Antigen CD8+ T-cell IFN-γ Response.

	Kisumu		Nandi	
	Constant Pf-malaria infection versus no infection		Constant Pf-malaria infection versus no infection	
	PR	95% CI	PR	95% CI
Unadjusted	1.60	0.37–6.92	1.54	0.71–3.35
Age groups[a]				
0–4 years	2.10	0.22–19.65	0.51	0.08–3.37
5–9 years	1.14	0.26–4.99	1.47	0.58–3.63
≥10 years	2.68	0.38–18.73	1.82	0.83–3.99

Pf-malaria, *Plasmodium falciparum* malaria; EBV, Epstein - Barr virus; PR, prevalence ratio; CI, confidence interval.
[a]Adjusted for sex and survey period. Unstratified estimates for constant *Pf*-malaria infections compared to never infected in Kisumu ($P = 0.32$) and Nandi ($P = 0.13$) were not significant. Specific details on the number and prevalence of positive responses for each age group are included in Table 2.

EBV latent antigen CD8+ T-cell IFN-γ responses. Using our weighted model, we did not observe any variation by age group (Table 4) or survey period (data not shown). In Kisumu, for all age groups, the adjusted prevalence of positive EBV latent antigen CD8+ T-cell IFN-γ response was higher among children with recurrent *Pf*-malaria infections compared to those never infected (Table 4). There was a two-fold difference in the PR for children 0–4 years and >10 years with recurrent *Pf*-malaria infections than children 5–9 years. In Nandi, children 0–4 years with recurrent *Pf*-malaria infections had fewer positive responses than children never infected, and a PR that was three-fold lower than older children. However, children in older age groups with recurrent *Pf*-malaria infections had higher positive responses than similarly aged children never infected. Despite estimates for Kisumu and Nandi being imprecise and not statistically significant, the observations suggest that children 5–9 years in Kisumu are unable to mount the type of T-cell response as younger and older children. Meanwhile, in Nandi, the increasing PR with age may reflect how a maturing immune system, not continuously exposed to *Pf*-malaria, is able to induce a T-cell response to latent antigens even when co-infected with *Pf*-malaria.

Discussion

Our study demonstrates that the prevalence of positive EBV lytic- but not latent-antigen CD8+ T-cell IFN-γ responses decreases in a malaria holoendemic area and not a hypoendemic area. This suggests that children repeatedly infected with *Pf*-malaria eventually lose functional IFN-γ producing CD8+ T-cells in response to EBV lytic antigens. In an effort to control viral replication induced by recurrent *Pf*-malaria infections [14], we hypothesize that EBV lytic antigen CD8+ T-cells have become exhausted and unable to produce IFN-γ or alternatively these cells were culled through apoptosis. As a result of the loss of responsive EBV lytic antigen CD8+ T-cells, more B-lymphocytes could become latently infected by EBV, and thus gradually increasing the risk of eBL. These findings are consistent with previous studies of this cohort, which detected significantly higher median EBV viral load and EBV-specific IgG antibodies to EBV lytic and latent antigens in the holoendemic compared to hypoendemic area [27,28].

Furthermore, the association between *Pf*-malaria infections and positive EBV lytic antigen CD8+ T-cell IFN-γ responses varied by age group. The EBV lytic antigen deficiency was most pronounced among children 5–9 years old in the malaria holoendemic area and was further potentiated in those recurrently infected with *Pf*-malaria. In our individual-level analysis, these children had the lowest PR of positive responses while this same age group in the hypoendemic area appeared to be affected little. Additionally, the patterns observed in the age group cohorts clearly showed that the 5–9 year cohort in Kisumu had the lowest prevalence of positive responses among all age group cohorts, in both districts, at each survey period. The sustained inability to produce an effective EBV lytic antigen CD8+ T-cell IFN-γ response among 5–9 year olds may be an etiologically relevant event in eBL development since eBL is most often diagnosed in this age group. Finally, the inconsistency of patterns between age group cohorts within a district suggests there is an age-dependent interaction between *Pf*-malaria and EBV-specific T-cell response. Studies of immune mechanisms that induce exhaustion or deletion are needed to understand maintenance of EBV-specific T-cell immunity, especially in children. In support of this premise is the observation that the ELISPOT responses in both groups of children were lower than those described for healthy adults [29] and our Kenyan adult controls (data not shown). To our knowledge there have been no studies of EBV-specific T-cell immunity in healthy children from non-malaria endemic countries. However our studies of malaria-specific immunity also demonstrate an age-associated instability in cytokine recall responses more pronounced in children compared to adults [30,31].

This study is an important early step to understanding the cumulative effect of *Pf*-malaria infections on EBV-specific T-cell immunity over time. Availability of data over two-years permitted identification of potentially important biological and environmental mechanisms that only became apparent over time. For example, the association between *Pf*-malaria infection and positive EBV lytic antigen CD8+ T-cell IFN-γ responses varied by age group and survey period. The variation noted with age group is expected because there is an age-dependent increase in T-cell immunity as children develop protection against *Pf*-malaria after repeated infections [32]. Children in malaria holoendemic areas acquire immunity to *Pf*-malaria and EBV during the first years of life, and ongoing studies will compare the development of *Pf*-malaria to EBV-specific T-cell memory. An impairment of EBV-specific T-cell control with progressive EBV reactivation has been described in HIV-infected individuals [33], lending support to a sequential series of events in the etiology of eBL.

Using data, collected during a two-year period, also allowed us to use an individual-level definition for *Pf*-malaria infections. Unlike other studies, our definition accounted for the cumulative effect of *Pf*-malaria infection which has been hypothesized to be critical in the pathogenesis of eBL, rather than the transient effect typically observed with acute *Pf*-malaria infection [1]. However, our definition was vulnerable to misclassification because *Pf*-malaria infection was assessed only twice during the two-year follow-up. Therefore, we may not have captured participants' malaria histories accurately. This misclassification was likely to be differential because children in the holoendemic area were exposed to *Pf*-malaria parasites at a higher frequency, averaging two malaria infections per year, than children in the hypoendemic area [34]. Therefore, we may have underestimated or overestimated the PR for *Pf*-malaria infections and EBV-specific T-cell responses in the holoendemic area.

A strength of our study was the use of two definitions for *Pf*-malaria: 1) district-level according to malaria transmission intensity, and 2) individual-level based on measured *Pf*-malaria infection. Although our findings of EBV lytic antigen CD8+ T-cell IFN-γ responses were consistent with both definitions, our findings of EBV latent antigen CD8+ T-cell IFN-γ responses were inconsistent. This may have been due to the limited power or an underestimation of the influence of *Pf*-malaria infections in hypoendemic areas. However, it also highlights the potential pitfall in attributing district-level results to the individual, also known as the ecological fallacy. The inconsistency may have been due to other factors that differed between the districts and unrelated to malaria transmission intensities. Therefore, we conclude that the use of malaria transmission intensity as a surrogate for malaria infection has been informative yet future studies should endeavor to prospectively collect *Pf*-malaria and EBV co-infections information from individuals to more accurately describe this complex relationship.

There were several potential confounders that were not captured in our study, specifically HIV status, nutritional status, schistosomiasis infection, and socioeconomic status. However, we do not believe the absence of these confounders materially affected our findings. When data were collected in western Kenya from 2002–2004, HIV testing in infants was conducted only when medically warranted. All children enrolled in this study were examined by a clinician and had no obvious signs of illness or malnourishment, and no deaths were reported as of 2009. Therefore, even though it was possible that an underlying HIV infection might influence the rate of malaria parasitaemia [35] the likelihood that a significant number of undiagnosed children remained in this study was low. Schistosomiasis infection was unmeasured yet an examination of the *Pf*-malaria and EBV response relationship indicated adjusting for schistosomiasis infection would have biased our analysis. Finally, is socioeconomic status had been measures, participants and their families would likely have been classified as low socioeconomic status because the main occupation was fishing (Kisumu) and farming (Nandi) in both rural study areas with homes constructed of locally available materials.

Our findings on EBV lytic antigen CD8+ T-cell IFN-γ responses were consistent with the studies that have used residence area (malaria transmission intensity) to explore the cumulative effect of *Pf*-malaria infections on EBV-specific T-cell response. We observed fewer positive EBV lytic antigen CD8+ T-cell IFN-γ responses among 5–9 year old than older children [16]. We also identified a reduction in EBV-specific T-cell response among children living in a holoendemic compared a hypoendemic area [26]. The consistency of our findings with previous studies is important given our limited sample size and precision. Meanwhile, our analysis of EBV lytic antigen CD8+ T-cell IFN-γ response at the individual-level supports findings from previous studies that used residence area as a surrogate for *Pf*-malaria infection.

However, we did not detect the same statistically significant district-level difference in positive EBV latent antigen CD8+ T-cell IFN-γ responses among 5–9 year olds as a previous study [16]. This discrepancy may be due to the limited power of our study. Furthermore, the difference between our individual-level analysis and the previous study may also be due to the use of a surrogate definition of *Pf*-malaria.

This study design marks a step toward examining the individual-level association of *Pf*-malaria infections and EBV-specific T-cell IFN-γ responses and identifies a potential difference between children recurrently infected with *Pf*-malaria compared to children never infected. To adequately quantify this effect, a longitudinal study should be considered which could accurately measure *Pf*-malaria infection and changes in *Pf*-malaria and EBV-specific T-cell immunity over time. The temporal aspects of future studies will be vital to elucidating the precise mechanism by which repeated *Pf*-malaria infections affect EBV persistence and immunity.

Materials and Methods

The Kisumu/Nandi cohort has been previously described [27]. In brief, the cohort consists of 236 children, randomly selected and between 10 months and 15 years at enrollment, from two districts in western Kenya with disparate *Pf*-malaria transmission intensities: Kisumu is characterized as holoendemic and Nandi as hypoendemic. Due to the age-related incidence of eBL, an equal distribution of children by age and sex were enrolled from each area: children 0–4 years have an elevated risk of eBL whereas 5–9 year olds are at highest risk and ≥10 years old have the lowest risk. Data were collected from 2002–2004 using a standardized survey. Three face-to-face interviews were conducted at baseline (July–August 2002), six month follow-up (February–March 2003), and two-year follow-up (July–August 2004). Blood was also collected for malaria and EBV testing.

Pf-malaria infection was confirmed on thick and thin blood smears by microscopy. Testing of EBV-specific T-cell response by IFN-γ ELISPOT has been previously described [16]. Lytic (BRLF1, BZLF1, and BMLF1) and latent (Epstein-Barr nuclear antigen [EBNA] 3A, EBNA 3B, and EBNA3C) antigens were selected and pooled for testing. One positive control (mitogen phytohemmagglutinin [PHA]) was used to stimulate wells and a negative control (phosphate buffer saline [PBS]) was used to measure background IFN-γ response in unstimulated wells. Assays were condensed into a three-week period using the same reagents and personnel to minimize inter-assay variability. Cytotoxic T-lymphocyte (CTL) ImmunoSpot scanning and imaging software (version 4; Cellular Technology Ltd, Shaker Heights, OH) was used to count the number of spot-forming units (SFU) per well; results were expressed as SFU per million peripheral blood mononuclear cells (PBMC). Using a two-sided Fisher's exact test ($P<.05$), EBV lytic and latent epitope-peptide CD8+ T-cell IFN-γ responses were categorized as positive or negative. A positive response was recorded if the proportion of SFUs in the stimulated well was significantly different from the proportion of SFU in the unstimulated well. The magnitude of response was calculated by subtracting the SFU in PBS wells (negative control) from the SFU in the stimulated wells. The median value for the negative control wells was 4 SFU per million PBMCs (range 0 to 772 SFU/million PBMC). Median values were calculated among positive responders only.

Analyses were restricted to EBV seropositive children at baseline [27]. We used two definitions of cumulative *Pf*-malaria. First, *Pf*-malaria exposure was defined according to the malaria transmission intensity of the district (district-level definition): Kisumu (holoendemic) or Nandi (hypoendemic). Next, *Pf*-malaria infection was defined as the cumulative average of *P. falciparum* infection (parasitemia) in a participant over the three survey periods (individual-level definition). The value ranged from 0 (never infected) to 1 (always infected); results and discussion focus on children who were always infected (referred to as recurrent) and never infected. With the individual-level definition, we also included the covariates age group, district, sex, and when the survey was conducted (referred to as survey period) in the analysis. We first examined covariates as potential effect measure modifiers using an a priori cutoff of $P = .20$. In the absence of evidence of effect measure modification, we included covariates in the model as potential confounders.

For descriptive analyses, we used the Chi-square statistic to measure associations between categorical exposures and outcomes. We used the two-sided Wilcoxon rank sum (Mann-Whitney *U*)/ Kruskal Wallis test for continuous outcomes. For multivariable analyses, we used weighted log-binomial regression with robust variances to estimate the prevalence ratios (PR) and corresponding 95% confidence intervals (CI). We used generalized estimating equations (GEE) with robust variance estimators to account for correlation due to repeated measurements. A weighted model with inverse probability weights (IPWs) was used to address missing observations due to children not participating in all surveys. When using IPW, observations are assumed to be missing at random; missing data are dependent on observed data but independent of unobserved data [36]. To calculate IPWs, the probability of participation was modeled using available predictor variables. The inverse of the predicted probabilities were calculated and assigned to each individual with complete data. Individuals with complete data were weighted to represent individuals with similar characteristics who have missing data.

To calculate the predicted probabilities for our study, we used logistic regression with first order interaction terms using the following equation:

$$
\begin{aligned}
Log\left[\frac{pi}{1-pi}\right] = {} & \beta 0 + \beta 1(sex) + \beta 2(age\ group\ 0-4\ years) \\
& + \beta 3(age\ group\ 5-9\ years) \\
& + \beta 4(site\ of\ residence) \\
& + \beta 5(sex \times age\ group\ 0-4\ years) \\
& + \beta 6(sex \times age\ group\ 5-9\ years) \\
& + \beta 7(sex \times site\ of\ residence) \\
& + \beta 8(age\ group\ 0-4\ years \times site\ of\ residence) \\
& + \beta 9(age\ group\ 5-9\ years \times site\ of\ residence)
\end{aligned}
$$

Where p_i was the probability of child i ($i = 1,2,3\ldots n$) participating in all surveys. Taking the inverse of the predicted probabilities, the mean IPW was 1.44 and ranged from 1.14–1.92. Children who participated in all three surveys were assigned the mean IPW value whereas children with missing observations were assigned an IPW of 0. We also conducted complete case analyses and found no differences in the PR or 95% CI; therefore we report results from the weighted analyses. Data were analyzed in SAS 9.1.3 (Cary, NC).

Written informed consent was obtained from a parent or guardian of the participant. This study was approved by the Institutional Review Boards at the University Hospitals of Cleveland, Case Western Reserve University where Dr. Moormann was affiliated at the time this study was done and also obtained from the Ethical Review Committee for the Kenya Medical Research Institute. It was deemed exempt by the Institutional Review Board at the University of North Carolina at Chapel Hill.

Acknowledgments

We are grateful to the Kenya Medical Research Institute staff for organizing blood sample collection and processing. We thank Nancy Raab-Trab for reviewing early versions of the manuscript. Special thanks to John Oyombe, John Ogone and Fred Opinya for recruiting and retaining study participants. We are also grateful to the parents/guardians of the study participants and the children that participated in the study. These data are published with the approval of the Director of the Kenya Medical Research Institute.

Author Contributions

Conceived and designed the experiments: CJS KC POS AMM. Performed the experiments: CJS KC POS AMM. Analyzed the data: CJS SRC PDMM CCJ SRM AMM. Contributed reagents/materials/analysis tools: SRC PDMM CCJ SRM AMM. Wrote the paper: CJS SRC KC POS PDMM CCJ SRM AMM.

References

1. Klein G (1982) Epstein-Barr virus, malaria and Burkitt's lymphoma. Scand J Infect Dis Suppl 36: 15–23.
2. Donati D, Espmark E, Kironde F, Mbidde EK, Kamya M, et al. (2006) Clearance of circulating Epstein-Barr virus DNA in children with acute malaria after antimalaria treatment. J Infect Dis 193: 971–977.
3. Roberts DE, Quincey E (1985) Epstein-Barr virus serology and malaria exposure in a small group of Liberian children with splenomegaly. J Trop Pediatr 31: 209–212.
4. Brady G, Macarthur GJ, Farrell PJ (2008) Epstein-Barr virus and Burkitt lymphoma. Postgrad Med J 84: 372–377.
5. Facer CA, Playfair JH (1989) Malaria, Epstein-Barr virus, and the genesis of lymphomas. Adv Cancer Res 53: 33–72.
6. Kafuko GW, Burkitt DP (1970) Burkitt's lymphoma and malaria. Int J Cancer 6: 1–9.
7. Burkitt D, Wright D (1966) Geographical and tribal distribution of the African lymphoma in Uganda. Br Med J 1: 569–573.
8. De-The G (1979) The epidemiology of Burkitt's lymphoma: evidence for a causal association with Epstein-Barr virus. Epidemiol Rev 1: 32–54.
9. Rasti N, Falk KI, Donati D, Gyan BA, Goka BQ, et al. (2005) Circulating epstein-barr virus in children living in malaria-endemic areas. Scand J Immunol 61: 461–465.
10. Burkitt DP (1969) Etiology of Burkitt's lymphoma–an alternative hypothesis to a vectored virus. J Natl Cancer Inst 42: 19–28.
11. Kafuko GW, Baingana N, Knight EM, Tibemanya J (1969) Association of Burkitt's tumour and holoendemic malaria in West Nile District, Uganda: malaria as a possible aetiologic factor. East Afr Med J 46: 414–436.
12. Rochford R, Cannon MJ, Moormann AM (2005) Endemic Burkitt's lymphoma: a polymicrobial disease? Nat Rev Microbiol 3: 182–187.
13. Rickinson AB, Kieff E (2007) Epstein-Barr Virus. In: Knipe DM, Howley PM, eds. Fields Virology. Fifth ed. Philadelphia, PA: Lippincott Williams & Wilkins.
14. Chene A, Donati D, Guerreiro-Cacais AO, Levitsky V, Chen Q, et al. (2007) A molecular link between malaria and Epstein-Barr virus reactivation. PLoS Pathog 3: e80.
15. Moss DJ, Rickinson AB, Pope JH (1978) Long-term T-cell-mediated immunity to Epstein-Barr virus in man. I. Complete regression of virus-induced transformation in cultures of seropositive donor leukocytes. Int J Cancer 22: 662–668.
16. Moormann AM, Chelimo K, Sumba PO, Tisch DJ, Rochford R, et al. (2007) Exposure to holoendemic malaria results in suppression of Epstein-Barr virus-specific T cell immunosurveillance in Kenyan children. J Infect Dis 195: 799–808.

17. Young LS, Rickinson AB (2004) Epstein-Barr virus: 40 years on. Nat Rev Cancer 4: 757–768.
18. Munz C (2005) Immune Response and Evasion in the Host-EBV Interaction. In: Robertson ES, ed. Epstein-Barr Virus. Norfolk, England: Cister Academic Press. pp 197–231.
19. Lam KM, Syed N, Whittle H, Crawford DH (1991) Circulating Epstein-Barr virus-carrying B cells in acute malaria. Lancet 337: 876–878.
20. Whittle HC, Brown J, Marsh K, Blackman M, Jobe O, et al. (1990) The effects of Plasmodium falciparum malaria on immune control of B lymphocytes in Gambian children. Clin Exp Immunol 80: 213–218.
21. Whittle HC, Brown J, Marsh K, Greenwood BM, Seidelin P, et al. (1984) T-cell control of Epstein-Barr virus-infected B cells is lost during P. falciparum malaria. Nature 312: 449–450.
22. Gunapala DE, Facer CA, Davidson R, Weir WR (1990) In vitro analysis of Epstein-Barr virus: host balance in patients with acute Plasmodium falciparum malaria. I. Defective T-cell control. Parasitol Res 76: 531–535.
23. Njie R, Bell AI, Jia H, Croom-Carter D, Chaganti S, et al. (2009) The effects of acute malaria on Epstein-Barr virus (EBV) load and EBV-specific T cell immunity in Gambian children. J Infect Dis 199: 31–38.
24. Morrow RH, Gutensohn N, Smith PG (1976) Epstein-Barr virus-malaria interaction models for Burkitt's lymphoma: implications for preventive trials. Cancer Res 36: 667–669.
25. Morrow RH, Kisuule A, Pike MC, Smith PG (1976) Burkitt's lymphoma in the Mengo Districts of Uganda: epidemiologic features and their relationship to malaria. J Natl Cancer Inst 56: 479–483.
26. Moss DJ, Burrows SR, Castelino DJ, Kane RG, Pope JH, et al. (1983) A comparison of Epstein-Barr virus-specific T-cell immunity in malaria-endemic and -nonendemic regions of Papua New Guinea. Int J Cancer 31: 727–732.
27. Moormann AM, Chelimo K, Sumba OP, Lutzke ML, Ploutz-Snyder R, et al. (2005) Exposure to holoendemic malaria results in elevated Epstein-Barr virus loads in children. J Infect Dis 191: 1233–1238.
28. Piriou E, Kimmel R, Chelimo K, Middeldorp JM, Odada PS, et al. (2009) Serological evidence for long-term Epstein-Barr virus reactivation in children living in a holoendemic malaria region of Kenya. J Med Virol 81: 1088–1093.
29. Hislop AD, Annels NE, Gudgeon NH, Leese AM, Rickinson AB (2002) Epitope-specific evolution of human CD8(+) T cell responses from primary to persistent phases of Epstein-Barr virus infection. J Exp Med 195: 893–905.
30. Moormann AM, John CC, Sumba PO, Tisch D, Embury P, et al. (2006) Stability of interferon-gamma and interleukin-10 responses to Plasmodium falciparum liver stage antigen-1 and thrombospondin-related adhesive protein in residents of a malaria holoendemic area. Am J Trop Med Hyg 74: 585–590.
31. Moormann AM, Sumba PO, Tisch DJ, Embury P, King CH, et al. (2009) Stability of interferon-gamma and interleukin-10 responses to Plasmodium falciparum liver stage antigen 1 and thrombospondin-related adhesive protein immunodominant epitopes in a highland population from Western Kenya. Am J Trop Med Hyg 81: 489–495.
32. Moormann AM (2009) How might infant and paediatric immune responses influence malaria vaccine efficacy? Parasite Immunol 31: 547–559.
33. Legoff J, Amiel C, Calisonni O, Fromentin D, Rajoely B, et al. (2004) Early impairment of CD8+ T cells immune response against Epstein-Barr virus (EBV) antigens associated with high level of circulating mononuclear EBV DNA load in HIV infection. J Clin Immunol 24: 125–134.
34. Bloland PB, Boriga DA, Ruebush TK, McCormick JB, Roberts JM, et al. (1999) Longitudinal cohort study of the epidemiology of malaria infections in an area of intense malaria transmission II. Descriptive epidemiology of malaria infection and disease among children. Am J Trop Med Hyg 60: 641–648.
35. Abu-Raddad LJ, Patnaik P, Kublin JG (2006) Dual infection with HIV and malaria fuels the spread of both diseases in sub-Saharan Africa. Science 314: 1603–1606.
36. Singer JD, Willett JB (2003) Applied Longitudinal Data Analysis: Modeling Change and Event Occurrence. New York: Oxford University Press.

13

Age- Matched Comparison of Children Hospitalized for 2009 Pandemic H1N1 Influenza with those Hospitalized for Seasonal H1N1 and H3N2

Susan S. Chiu[1]*, Kwok-Hung Chan[2], Wilfred H. S. Wong[1], Eunice L. Y. Chan[1], J. S. M. Peiris[2,3]

1 Department of Paediatrics and Adolescent Medicine, The University of Hong Kong, Pokfulam, Hong Kong, **2** Department of Microbiology, The University of Hong Kong, Pokfulam, Hong Kong, **3** Hong Kong University Pasteur Research Centre, Pokfulam, Hong Kong

Abstract

Background: A wide spectrum of clinical manifestation ranging from deaths to a mild course of disease has been reported in children infected with the 2009 pandemic H1N1 (pH1N1) influenza.

Methodology/Major Findings: We conducted an age-matched control study comparing children hospitalized for pH1N1 with historic controls infected with seasonal H1N1 and H3N2 influenza to correct for the effect of age on disease susceptibility and clinical manifestations. We also compared children with pH1N1 to children concurrently admitted for seasonal influenza during the pandemic period to adjust for differences in health-seeking behavior during the pandemic or other potential bias associated with historic controls. There was no death or intensive care admission. Children with pH1N1 were more likely to have at least one risk condition for influenza, an underlying chronic pulmonary condition, more likely to have asthma exacerbation and to be treated with oseltamivir. There was no difference in other aspects of the clinical course or outcome.

Conclusion: Disease manifestation of children hospitalized for pH1N1 infection was mild in our patient population.

Editor: Jane Deng, University of California Los Angeles, United States of America

Funding: This work was supported by the Area of Excellence Scheme of the University Grants Committee (grant AoE/M-12/06). The funders had no role in study design, data collection and analaysis, decision to publish, or preparation of the manuscript.

Competing Interests: The authors have declared that no competing interests exist.

* E-mail: ssschiu@hkucc.hku.hk

Introduction

Pandemic H1N1 (pH1N1) influenza emerged in March 2009 in Mexico. [1,2] There have been case series reports of severe disease and deaths, including that in children. [1–9]. However, there are also reports of a wide spectrum of clinical manifestation including a mild course of disease. [10–15]. Recently, a few studies compared pH1N1 with seasonal influenza infection. One study showed that children with pH1N1 presented with more lower respiratory infections and gastrointestinal symptoms than children with seasonal influenza in the previous 2 years. [16]. Two studies using different cohorts for comparison showed that pH1N1 did not appear to cause more severe disease than seasonal influenza A in children. [17,18]. However, none of these studies were age-matched and children of different age groups might have different susceptibility and disease manifestations. We therefore sought to document the characteristics and manifestations of children admitted to Queen Mary Hospital, Hong Kong with laboratory-confirmed pH1N1 and compared them to age-matched historic controls admitted to the same hospital with seasonal influenza. We also compared children hospitalized with pH1N1 with those concurrently admitted for seasonal influenza to correct for altered health seeking behavior during a pandemic and other potential biases associated with historic controls.

Materials and Methods

Queen Mary Hospital is a tertiary-care public hospital and is the teaching hospital of The University of Hong Kong. The pediatric general ward and intensive care unit take admission from its emergency department as well as referrals from other hospitals and clinics. We have been routinely performing virologic testing on nasopharyngeal aspirate (NPA) samples on all children admitted with fever and signs of acute respiratory symptoms such as rhinitis, cough or sorethroat since 1995. We conducted a retrospective study by retrieving the medical record of all patients $<$18 years of age hospitalized for pH1N1 in the first 3 months of the pandemic from 1 July 2009 through 30 September 2009 and that of age- matched controls hospitalized in our hospital for seasonal influenza H1N1 and H3N2 in the preceding years in a 1:1 ratio. These age-matched controls were selected patients from the database in the Department of Microbiology according to admission dates closest to the study period, matched to the closest year of age. To overcome the potential bias of comparison with historic controls, we also performed comparisons of children admitted with pH1N1 with children admitted for seasonal influenza during the pandemic period. Parameters collected included underlying conditions deemed high risk of influenza complications, discharge diagnoses, duration of hospitalization, intensive care admission, death, height of fever, white blood count and chest x ray abnormalities and oseltamivir and antibiotic use.

The study protocol was approved by the joint institutional review board of the University of Hong Kong and Queen Mary Hospital (Hong Kong) which waived the written consent. Written consent was not felt to be needed since virologic testing was a routine diagnostic procedure and patient information saved at the study database was delinked from individual patient identification. From the emergence of the pandemic until the 1st of July, Hong Kong implemented a containment and mitigation strategy where all patients confirmed to be infected with pH1N1 were hospitalized and discharged according to isolation and infection control measures, regardless of clinical indication. Starting June 29, 2009, when pH1N1 became more widely circulating in the community, the Department of Health and the Hospital Authority of Hong Kong implemented an adjustment of policy to hospitalize patients on the basis of clinical need rather than recommend mandatory hospitalization of all infected individuals [19]. Therefore, patients for this study were recruited from the 1st July onwards to avoid patients admitted for public health containment purposes irrespective of clinical need. Children were hospitalized either because 1) their respiratory infection symptoms warranted admission through the Emergency Department or 2) their respiratory symptoms led to pH1N1 testing in the outpatient clinics and admitted when they tested positive. All hospitalized children with virologically diagnosed pH1N1 or seasonal influenza were included in the analysis.

NPA were tested for Influenza A and B by direct antigen detection and virus culture in all recruited patients. All the NPA samples were tested for influenza virus type A and B and subtyped as pH1N1, seasonal H3N2 and seasonal H1N1 viruses by RT-PCR as previously described [20–21,22].

Comparisons between children with pandemic influenza A H1N1, seasonal H1N1 and H3N2, as well as that between those with pH1N1 and concurrently admitted seasonal influenza cases during the pandemic period were made. Children with pH1N1 were also compared to all control children admitted for seasonal influenza. Paired t-test was used to detect the difference of continuous variables such as maximum temperature, length of hospital stay between pairs of observation. McNemar's test was used to detect the agreement of the paired proportion in categorical risk factors. Unpaired t-test was used for comparison when there was a missing continuous variable. Chi-square test was used to detect the association of abnormal chest xray, lymphocyte and neutrophil counts between groups when there were missing data in these variables. A p value less than 0.05 was considered statistically significant. Post-hoc analysis demonstrated that 80 subjects per group had 80% power of detecting a 5% difference with a significance level of 0.05.

Results

Ninety-nine children with a median age of 5.7 (0.4–17.4) years were hospitalized and confirmed to have pH1N1 infection in the 2 study months, with a male to female ratio of 1.25:1. Since these children were not admitted for mandatory isolation under the containment and early mitigation phases, only 19.2% were known to have pH1N1 on admission, the others were admitted for respiratory symptoms and diagnosed as pH1N1 after admission. During the same time, 37 children with a median age of 2.7 years (6 days to11 years) were hospitalized for seasonal influenza (4 with seasonal H1N1 and 33 with H3N2). The mean age of children with seasonal influenza were younger than those with pH1N1: mean age of 3.6±2.9 years compared to that of 6.6±4.8 years in those with pH1N1 ($p = 0.0005$).

Patients admitted for pH1N1 infection were more likely to have at least one high risk condition for influenza. (Table 1). There was no difference in clinical diagnosis between the 4 groups of patients with the exception that asthma exacerbation and acute otitis media were diagnosed more often in children admitted for pH1N1 than children with seasonal influenza. (Table 2). Pneumonia was diagnosed in 11.1% of patients infected with pH1N1, 10 % and 11% in age matched children with seasonal H1N1 or H3N2 respectively, and in 5.4% in concurrently admitted children with seasonal influenza (p = NS) and 5.1%, 0%, 3% and 0% of them respectively were thought to have bacterial pneumonia (p = NS). There was no death or intensive care admission in any child in this study.

The mean maximum recorded temperature of patients infected with pH1N1 was statistically significantly lower than those infected with seasonal H1N1 and H3N2. Although statistically significant, the clinical significance of mean maximal recorded temperatures of 39.5 vs. 39.7 may be questionable (Table 3) A significant proportion of children infected with any influenza A infection were lymphopenic with no significant difference between pandemic and seasonal influenza. Duration of hospitalization of children with pH1N1 (mean of 3.4±2.1 days) was no different to those concurrently admitted with seasonal influenza but was significantly longer than the 2.5±1.1 days of those in the age matched group with seasonal H1N1 ($p = 0.0002$). However, only 9.1% of patients with pH1N1 were still febrile at discharge, as compared to 23.2% of those with seasonal pH1N1 ($p = 0.0176$) and 21.2% with H3N2 ($p = 0.031$).

Almost half of the patients admitted for pH1N1 were treated with a full course of oseltamivir, significantly more so that those with seasonal influenza admitted concurrently or in the age matched control group (Table 3). The increased use of oseltamivir in pH1N1 infected children was influenced more by concerns and guidelines of clinical care arising as a result of the pandemic, i.e. patients with underlying health conditions should have antiviral therapy, in contrast to the practice in previous years. We compared pH1N1 infected children who received oseltamivir with similarly infected children who did not. pH1N1 infected children treated with oseltamivir were older with a mean age of 7.8±4.7 years vs. 5.3±4.7 years ($p = 0.0095$), had a longer duration of hospitalization of 4±2.4 days vs. 2.7±1.4 days ($p = 0.0014$), and were more likely to have pneumonia: 20.4% vs. 2% ($p = 0.0095$) when compared to those who did not receive oseltamivir. There was a trend that patients who received oseltamivir were more likely to have one or more high risk conditions. Three of 49 (6.1%) of children who received oseltamivir for pH1N1 had adverse events: one each with vomiting, urticaria and behavioral problems. The child with behavioral changes was a 6 year old boy with moderate asthma attack and discharged from our hospital on oseltamivir. After taking 4 doses of oseltamivir, he became irritable and exhibited some violent acts including pointing a knife at his own neck and hitting his mother. When brought back to the hospital he was alert and conscious but uncooperative for examination. Oseltamivir was withheld, his behavior became normal in the ward and he was discharged the next day.

When age-matched controls with seasonal H1N1 or H3N2 who did not receive oseltamivir were compared to the 49 children with pH1N1 who did not receive oseltamivir, there was no difference in underlying risk conditions or discharge diagnoses. Uncomplicated URI accounted for 63%, 49% and 55% of the diagnoses in children with pH1N1, seasonal H1N1 and H3N2, respectively. (p = NS) Children with pH1N1 had a lower maximum temperature recorded when compared to those with seasonal influenza H3N2.

Table 1. Comparisons of pre-existing high risk conditions of children hospitalized for influenza A pH1N1 with age- matched controls hospitalized for seasonal H1N1 and H3N2, and with children hospitalized for seasonal influenza concurrently during the study period, respectively.

	pH1N1 (n = 99)	H1N1 (n = 99)	H3N2 (n = 99)	Concurrent seasonal influenza (n = 37)	pH1N1 vs. H1N1 P value	pH1N1 vs. H3N2 P value	pH1N1 vs. concurrent seasonal influenza P value	pH1N1 (N = 99) vs all influenza (N = 235)
≥1 underlying condition	40 (40.4%)	23 (23.2%)	23 (23.2%)	7 (18.9%)	0.0125	0.0171	0.032	0.0014
Prematurity	5 (5.1%)	4 (4%)	7 (7.1%)	0	NS	NS	NS	NS
Pulmonary	20 (20%)	8 (8.1%)	10 (10.1%)	0	NS	NS	0.007	NS
Cardiac	2 (2.0%)	3 (3.0%)	1 (1.0%)	3 (8.1%)	NS	NS	NS	NS
Immunodeficiency	4 (4.0%)	4 (4.0%)	1 (1.0%)	1 (2.7%)	NS	NS	NS	NS
Malignancy	1 (1.0%)	0	2 (2.0%)	1 (2.7%)	-	NS	NS	NS
Neurologic	10 (10.1%)	5 (5.1%)	7 (7.1%)	2 (5.4%)	NS	NS	NS	NS
Renal	2 (2.0%)	2 (1.1%)	1 (1.0%)	0	NS	NS	NS	NS
Metabolic	2 (2%)	1 (0.5%)	1 (0.5%)	1 (2.7%)	NS	NS	NS	NS

Discussion

Disease manifestations seen in children hospitalized with pH1N1 in our patient population was mild. One Canadian study compared 58 children hospitalized with pH1N1 with 200 children infected with seasonal influenza. [17] They found that those with pH1N1 with a median age of 6.6 years were significantly older than those with seasonal influenza A with a median age of 3.3 years. Similar proportions of children required intensive care admission and intubation and the authors concluded that pH1N1 did not appear to cause more severe disease than seasonal influenza A.

There was no death or intensive care admission in any of the hospitalized children in the 4 groups. Only half of the children infected with pH1N1 were treated with oseltamivir. The general recommendation at the time was to offer treatment to all children hospitalized for pH1N1, but the final decision was still up to that of the attending pediatrician in discussion with the parents. Considering that uncomplicated upper respiratory tract infection was the most common single diagnosis, the decision to not treat mild disease is understandable. All except one pH1N1 patients with pneumonia were given oseltamivir and 62.5% of children with one or more high risk conditions were treated as well. The recommendation for any child hospitalized for influenza has now changed to that antiviral should be considered. [23]

In contrast to early reports in adults, gastrointestinal symptoms were not prominent in our group of children hospitalized for pH1N1, regardless of oseltamivir therapy.

Lymphopenia had been associated with pneumonia and respiratory failure in adults. [2,24] Relative lymphopenia with or without increased monocyte percentage has even been proposed as a surrogate marker of pH1N1 and lymphopenia is thought by some to be uncommon in children with influenza A. [25,26] However, lymphopenia $<1\times10^9$/ml was quite commonly seen in our children with uncomplicated pH1N1 infection as well as in children with seasonal influenza.

A significant proportion of children with seasonal H1N1 and H3N2 in years prior to the pandemic were discharged while still febrile in our hospital, likely contributable to the availability of rapid virus diagnosis which reassured parents and doctors of a clinical diagnosis. We have previously shown that availability of rapid virus diagnosis shortens the duration of hospitalization.[27] However, children with pH1N1 and children with seasonal influenza hospitalized during the pandemic period were significantly less likely to be discharged while still febrile, presumably due to a more conservative attitude of both health care workers and parents during a pandemic with an increased reluctance to discharge a child who was still febrile. This low proportion of febrile children at discharge coupled with a lack of difference in duration of fever before and during hospitalization between pH1N1 and seasonal influenza A likely demonstrate that the total duration of fever in children infected with pH1N1 may in fact be shorter than those infected with seasonal influenza.

Up to the end of the study period, that is, as of September 27, 2009, 26,548 people in Hong Kong were virologically confirmed to be infected. [28] Between May 1, 2009 and May 23, 2010, there

Table 2. Comparison of clinical diagnosis of children hospitalized for influenza A pH1N1 with age- matched controls hospitalized for seasonal H1N1 and H3N2, and with children hospitalized for seasonal influenza concurrently during the study period, respectively.

	pH1N1 (N=99)	H1N1 (N=99)	H3N2 (N=99)	Concurrent seasonal influenza (N=37)	pH1N1 vs. H1N1 P value	pH1N1 vs. H3N2 P value	pH1N1 vs. concurrent seasonal influenza P value	pH1N1 (N=99) vs all influenza (N=235)
Uncomplicated URI	54 (54.5%)	50 (50.5%)	52 (52.5%)	27 (73.0%)	NS	NS	NS	NS
Febrile seizure (6 months-5 years)	6/44 (14.0%)	10/44 (22.7%)	13/44 (29.5%)	4/23 (17.4%)	NS	NS	NS	NS
Convulsion	11 (11.1%)	12 (12.1%)	10 (10.1%)	1 (2.7%)	NS	NS	NS	NS
Encephalopathy/ encephalitis	1 (1.0%)	1 (1.0%)	0	0	NS	-	NS	NS
Stroke	1 (1.0%)	0	0	0	-	-	NS	-
Delirium/ confusion	0	1 (1.0%)	1 (1.0%)	0	-		-	-
Syncope	1 (1.0%)	1 (1.0%)	2 (2.0%)	0	NS	-	NS	NS
Pneumonia (all)	11 (11.1%)	10 (10.1)	11 (11.1%)	2 (5.4%)	NS	NS	NS	NS
Bacterial pneumonia	5 (5.1%)	0	3 (3.0%)	0	-	NS	NS	NS
Croup	2 (2.0%)	3 (3.0%)	1 (1.0%)	0	NS	NS	NS	NS
Asthma exacerbation	8 (8.1%)	1 (1.0%)	1 (1.0%)	0	0.0455	0.0455	-	0.0014
Acute bronchiolitis	0	1 (1.0%)	3 (3.0%)	0	-	-	-	NS
Acute otitis media	5 (5.1%)	0	0	2 (5.4%)	-	-	NS	0.0425
Tonsillitis/ pharyngitis	0	1 (1.0%)	1 (1.0%)	0	-	-	-	-
Gastroenteritis	1 (1.0%)	6 (6.1%)	2 (2.0%)	1 (2.7%)	NS	NS	NS	NS
Viral rash/ urticaria	0	1 (1.0%)	2 (2.0%)	0	-	-	-	-
Myositis	2 (2.0%)	1 (1.0%)	0	0	NS	-	NS	NS

were a total of 36,546 laboratory-confirmed pH1N1 cases reported to the Centre for Health Protection in Hong Kong. Children aged below 10 years had the highest incidence rate of 2424 cases/ 100,000 population. Seventeen percent of all laboratory-confirmed cases required hospitalization and children below 5 years of age accounted for 32.8% of these. Public hospitals (of which Queen Mary Hospital is one) cater for 72.5% of general pediatric hospitalizations and almost 100% of PICU hospitalizations in Hong Kong. There has been in place a computerized medical system of all the public hospitals for mandatory reporting of Avian/pandemic influenza admissions (eFlu) since November 2005 and revised in July 2006 [29].Only 13 reports of serious

Table 3. Comparison of duration of fever, investigation results and treatment of children hospitalized for influenza A pH1N1 with age- matched controls hospitalized for seasonal H1N1 and H3N2, and with children hospitalized for seasonal influenza concurrently during the study period, respectively.

	pH1N1 (N=99)	H1N1 (N=99)	H3N2 (N=99)	Concurrent Seasonal Influenza (N=37)	pH1N1 vs. H1N1 P value	pH1N1 vs. H3N2 P value	pH1N1 vs. concurrent seasonal influenza P value	pH1N1 (N=99) vs all influenza (N=235)
Mean days of fever at presentation	2.2±1.5	2.6±2.9	2.2±1.5	2.0±1.54	NS	NS	NS	NS
Mean days of fever before discharge	3.7±1.8	4.1±3.1	3.9±2.0	3.7±1.5	NS	NS	NS	NS
% febrile at discharge	9 (9.1%)	23 (23.2%)	21 (21.2%)	4 (10.8%)	0.0176	0.031	NS	0.0185
Mean T_{max} (°C)	39.51±0.59	39.73±0.62	39.85±0.66	39.72±0.65	0.011	0.002	NS	0.0004
Mean days of hospitalization	3.4±2.1	2.5±1.1	2.9±1.6	3.1±2.3	0.0002	NS	NS	NS
Abnormal CXR	31/83 (44.6%)	26/72 (36.1%)	39/77 (50.6%)	11/33 (33.3%)	NS	NS	NS	NS
Lymphocyte < 1.0×10^9/L	33/79 (41.8%)	36/85 (42.4%)	43/96 (44.8%)	13/33 (39.4%)	NS	NS	NS	NS
Neutrophil < 1×10^9/L	3/79 (3.8%)	3/85 (3.5%)	2/96 (2.1%)	3/33 (9.1%)	NS	NS	NS	NS
Neutrophil > 8.3×10^9/L	10/79 (12.7%)	13/85 (15.3%)	21/96 (21.9%)	1/33 (3.0%)	NS	NS	NS	NS
Full course of Oseltamivir	50 (50.5%)	0	0	3 (8.1%)	<0.0001	<0.0001	<0.0001	<0.0001
Full course of antibiotic	18 (18.2%)	14 (14.1%)	13 (13.1%)	5 (13.5%)	NS	NS	NS	NS

pH1N1 admissions in children <18 years were made in the 5 months of the pandemic which included 11 PICU admissions. There were only 3 pediatric death cases, 2 of these children had cerebral palsy and one child had congenital heart disease in the whole of Hong Kong SAR during that time. The manifestations of pH1N1 in children appeared mild in Hong Kong, and the low case fatality rate corroborated with the findings of this study.

There are strengths and limitations in this study. There is a potential bias of using historical controls for comparison. However this approach was chosen because it was important to age stratify the patients for meaningful clinical comparisons. Using patients with concurrent seasonal influenza does not provide an age matched group for comparison and previous studies using concurrent controls are open to criticism for this reason. Thus we used both age matched historical controls as well as concurrent controls with seasonal influenza for comparison. The observation that pH1N1 is not clinically different to seasonal influenza is supported by both age matched and concurrent control groups. Another potential problem is that the threshold for admission may be different during pandemic and inter-pandemic periods. There might be potential bias for admission to include less severely affected children during the pandemic period who would otherwise not be admitted. This may be true to some extent in Hong Kong as in other places, however, there was no death case or ICU admission in any group in the study. Moreover, the study period was chosen to avoid the period of attempted containment when patients with pH1N1 were admitted for infection control purposes, irrespective of clinical need. Over 80% of the children admitted for pH1N1 were admitted through the Emergency Department and diagnosed after admission. The study was conducted over a short period but it included the period at which pH1N1 peaked in late September and provided us with an adequate number of patients for analysis.

In conclusion, using both age- matched patients with seasonal influenza supplemented with concurrent admissions for seasonal influenza, we demonstrated that children hospitalized for pH1N1 did not have more severe disease when compared to their controls infected with seasonal H1N1 or H3N2, although they were more likely to have one or more conditions deemed at risk for severe influenza infection, a chronic pulmonary condition, more likely to have asthma exacerbation and they were more likely to receive oseltamivir, especially if they had pneumonia. Overall, disease manifestations of children hospitalized for pH1N1 infection in our patient population were mild.

Author Contributions

Conceived and designed the experiments: SSC JSMP. Performed the experiments: K-HC. Analyzed the data: ELYC WHSW. Wrote the paper: SSC JSMP.

References

1. Chowell G, Bertozzi SM, Colchero MA, Lopez-Gatell H, Alpuche-Aranda C, et al. (2009) Severe respiratory disease concurrent with the circulation of H1N1 influenza. N Engl J Med 361: 674–679.
2. Perez-Padilla R, de la Rosa-Zamboni D, Ponce de Leon S, Hernandez M, Quiñones-Falconi F, et al. (2009) Pneumonia and respiratory failure from swine-origin influenza A (H1N1) in Mexico. N Engl J Med 361: 680–689.
3. Lister P, Reynolds F, Parlsow R, Chan A, Cooper M, et al. (2009) Swine-origin influenza virus H1N1, seasonal influenza virus, and critical illness in children. Lancet 374: 605–607.
4. Centers for Disease Control and Prevention (CDC) (2009) Surveillance for Pediatric Deaths associated with 2009 pandemic Influenza A (H1N1) virus infection---United States, April-August 2009. MMWR Weekly Rep 58: 941–947.
5. Libster R, Bugna J, Coviello S, Hijano DR, Dunaiewsky M, et al. (2010) Pediatric hospitalizations associated with 2009 pandemic influenza A (H1N1) in Argentina. N Engl J Med 362: 45–55.
6. Farias JA, Fernandez A, Monteverde E, Vidal N, Montes MJ, et al. (2010) Critically ill infants and children with influenza A (H1N1) in pediatric intensive care units in Argentina. Intensive Care Med 36: 1015–1022.
7. von Zwol A, Witteveen R, Markhorst D, Geukers VGM (2010) Clinical features of a Dutch Cohort of critically ill children due to the 2009 New Influenza A H1N1 Pandemic. Clin Pediatr 50: 69–72.
8. Shin SY, Kim JH, Kim HS, Kang YA, Lee HG, et al. (2010) Clinical characteristics of Korean pediatrics patients critically ill with influenza A (H1N1) virus. Pediatr Pulmonol 45: 1014–1020.
9. Kumar S, Havens PL, Chusid MJ, Willoughby RE, Simpson P, et al. (2010) Clinical and epidemiologic characteristics of children hospitalized with 2009 pandemic H1N1 influenza A infection. Pediatr Infect Dis J 29: 591–594.
10. Hackett S, Hill L, Patel J, Ratnaraja N, Ifeyinwa A, et al. (2009) Clinical characteristics of paediatric H1N1 admissions in Birmingham, UK. Lancet 374: 605.
11. Larcombe PJ, Moloney SE, Schmidt PA (2011) Pandemic (H1N1) 2009: a clinical spectrum in the general paediatric population. Arch Dis Child 96: 96–98.
12. Miroballi Y, Baird JS, Zackai S, Cannon JM, Messina M, et al. (2010) Novel influenza A (H1N1) in a pediatric health care facility in New York City during the first wave of the 2009 pandemic. Arch Pediatr Adolesc Med 164: 24–30.
13. Calitri C, Gabiano C, Garazzino S, Pinon M, Zoppo M, et al. (2010) Clinical features of hospitalized children with 2009 H1N1 influenza virus infection. Eur J Pediatr 169: 1511–1515.
14. Bettinger JA, Sauve LJ, Scheifele DW, Moore D, Vaudry W, et al. (2010) Pandemic influenza in Canadian children: A summary of hospitalized pediatric cases. Vaccine 28: 3180–3184.
15. Halasa NB (2010) Update on the 2009 pandemic influenza A H1N1 in children. Curr Opin Pediatr 22: 83–87.
16. Gordon A, Saborio S, Videa E, Lopez R, Kuan G, et al. (2010) Clinical attack rate and presentation of pandemic H1N1 influenza versus seasonal A and B in a pediatric cohort in Nicaragua. Clin Infect Dis 50: 1462–1467.
17. O'Riordan S, Barton M, Yau Y, Read SE, Allen U, et al. (2010) Risk factors and outcomes among children admitted to hospital with pandemic H1N1 influenza. CMAJ 182: 39–44.
18. Belongia EA, Irving SA, Waring SC, Coleman LA, Meece JK, et al. (2010) Clinical Characteristics and 30-day outcomes for influenza A 2009 (H1N1), 2008-2009 (H1N1), and 2007-2008 (H2N2) infections. JAMA 304: 1091–1098.
19. The Government of the Hong Kong Special Administrative Region, Centre for Health Protection website: Control measures at HSI mitigation phase adjusted., Available at: http://www.chp.gov.hk/en/content/116/17649.html# Accessed 29 June.
20. Chan KH, Yam WC, Pang CM, Chan KM, Lam SY, et al. (2008) Comparison of the NucliSens easyMAG and Qiagen BioRobot 9604 nucleic acid extraction systems for detection of RNA and DNA respiratory viruses in nasopharyngeal aspirate samples. J Clin Microbiol 46: 2195–2199.
21. Chan KH, Peiris JS, Lim W, Nicholls JM, Chiu SS (2008) Comparison of nasopharyngeal flocked swabs and aspirates for rapid diagnosis of respiratory viruses in children. J Clin Virol 42: 65–69.
22. To KK, Chan KH, Li IW, Tsang TY, Tse H, et al. (2010) Viral load in patients infected with pandemic H1N1 2009 influenza A virus. J Med Virol 82: 1–7.
23. American Academy of Pediatrics, Committee on Infectious Diseases (2010) Policy statement recommendations for prevention and control of influenza in children, 2010-2011. Pediatr 126: 816–826.
24. Chien YS, Su CP, Tsai HT, Huang AS, Lien CE, et al. (2010) Predictors and outcomes of respiratory failure among hospitalized pneumonia patients with 2009 H1N1 influenza in Taiwan. J Infect 60: 168–174.
25. Cunha BA, Pherez FM, Schoch P (2009) Diagnostic importance of relative lymphopenia as a marker of swine influenza (H1N1) in adults. Clin Infect Dis 49: 1454–1456.
26. Coskun O, Avci IY, Sener K, Yaman H, Ogur R, et al. (2010) Relative lymphopenia and monocytosis may be considered as a surrogate marker of pandemic influenza a (H1N1) J Clin Virol 47: 388–389.
27. Woo PC, Chiu SS, Seto WH, Peiris M (1997) Cost-effectiveness of rapid diagnosis of viral respiratory tract infections in pediatric patients. J Clin Microbiol 35: 1579–1581.
28. The Government of the Hong Kong Special Administrative Region, Centre for Health Protection website: Communicable Diseases Watch 2010 vol 7 no. 11 week 20-21. Available at: http://www.chp.gov.hk/en/epidemiology/441/112/551.html Accessed 29 June 2011.
29. The Government of the Hong Kong Special Administrative Region, Hospital Authority website: Operational Plan of eflu. Available at: http://www3.ha.org.hk/idctc/document/no. 14_-_operational_plan_of_eflu.pdf Accessed 29 June 2011.

14

Factors Associated with HIV/AIDS Diagnostic Disclosure to HIV Infected Children Receiving HAART

Sibhatu Biadgilign[1]*, Amare Deribew[1], Alemayehu Amberbir[2], Horacio Ruiseñor Escudero[3], Kebede Deribe[4]

1 Department of Epidemiology and Biostatistics, College of Public Health and Medical Science, Jimma University, Jimma, Ethiopia, 2 Addis Ababa University, Addis Ababa, Ethiopia, 3 Department of International Health, Bloomberg School of Public Health, Johns Hopkins University, Baltimore, Maryland, United States of America, 4 Department of General Public Health, College of Public Health and Medical Science, Jimma University, Jimma, Ethiopia

Abstract

Background: Diagnostic disclosure of HIV/AIDS to a child is becoming an increasingly common issue in clinical practice. Nevertheless, some parents and health care professionals are reluctant to inform children about their HIV infection status. The objective of this study was to identify the proportion of children who have knowledge of their serostatus and factors associated with disclosure in HIV-infected children receiving HAART in Addis Ababa, Ethiopia.

Methods: A cross-sectional study was conducted in five hospitals in Addis Ababa from February 18, 2008–April 28, 2008. The study populations were parents/caretakers and children living with HIV/AIDS who were receiving Highly Active Antiretroviral Therapy (HAART) in selected hospitals in Addis Ababa. Univariate and multivariate logistic regression analysis were carried out using SPSS 12.0.1 statistical software.

Results: A total of 390 children/caretaker pairs were included in the study. Two hundred forty three children (62.3%) were between 6–9 years of age. HIV/AIDS status was known by 68 (17.4%) children, 93 (29%) caretakers reported knowing the child's serostatus two years prior to our survey, 180 (46.2%) respondents said that the child should be told about his/her HIV/AIDS status when he/she is older than 14 years of age. Children less than 9 years of age and those living with educated caregivers are less likely to know their results than their counterparts. Children referred from hospital's in-patient ward before attending the HIV clinic and private clinic were more likely to know their results than those from community clinic.

Conclusion: The proportion of disclosure of HIV/AIDS diagnosis to HIV-infected children is low. Strengthening referral linkage and health education tailored to educated caregivers are recommended to increase the rate of disclosure.

Editor: Jacqueline Ho, Penang Medical College, Malaysia

Funding: This study was funded by Jimma University. The university had no role in the study design, data collection and analysis, decision to publish, or preparation of the manuscript.

Competing Interests: The authors have declared that no competing interests exist.

* E-mail: sibhatu2005@yahoo.com

Introduction

HIV/AIDS is increasingly affecting the health and welfare of children and undermining hard-won gains in child survival in some highly affected countries [1]. Recent estimates from the Joint United Nations Programme on HIV/AIDS (UNAIDS) suggest that, globally, about 2.5 million children younger than 15 years of age are infected with HIV; 90% of whom live in sub-Saharan Africa [2]. As highly active antiretroviral therapy (HAART) becomes increasingly available in low-resource settings, children affected by this disease are living longer [3], experience a less symptomatic early course of the disease and survive to older ages [4], with improved quality of life [3]. Given this scenario, the question of disclosure of HIV status to infected children is becoming increasingly important. Knowledge of HIV status may affect compliance with antiretroviral therapies and influence children's participation in healthcare decision-making [3]. The American Academy of Pediatrics guidelines on disclosure of HIV illness states that all adolescents should know their HIV status, while disclosure should be considered for school-age children [5]. In Ethiopia, it is recommended that adolescents 14 years of age old and older should know their HIV status [6].

Caregivers and healthcare workers are presented with an array of challenges around disclosure, including deciding on what is in the child's best interest and when, why and how information about his/her HIV status should be shared with him/her [7]. Disclosure of a child's HIV/AIDS is becoming an increasingly common clinical issue. Nevertheless, some parents and health care professionals are reluctant to inform the affected children about it. Data from several sites in other countries indicates that between 25% and 90% of school-age children with HIV infection/AIDS have not been told that they are infected [8–10].

Consequently, preparing family members for the emotional impact of disclosure is a major task facing providers. Also, disclosure takes on new significance, both within and outside the family, as sexuality becomes a dominant developmental issue during adolescence [11]. In the context of HAART, disclosure may have an important impact on disease progression and clinical management [12]. However, in one study, interviewed caregivers reported low disclosure rates (9%) [13] and healthcare providers reported low levels of direct involvement in disclosure to HIV-infected children (18%) [14]. Despite the importance of HIV disclosure, there has been limited research addressing pediatric HIV/AIDS disclosure, particularly in sub-Saharan Africa.

Methods

Clinical setting and Sample

In Ethiopia, the health system is arranged as a four-tier system, which includes: facility, district, city (region/zone/sub) and federal which should be appropriately linked, equitably distributed and managed in a decentralized, participatory and efficient manner. The Government of Ethiopia launched fee-based antiretroviral treatment in 2003 and free HAART in 2005. As of July 2010, about 97,000 adults and 4,800 children are accessing HAART services in the country. Guidelines from the Ethiopian National Pediatric HIV/AIDS Care and Treatment Guideline recommend HAART initiation in infants <12 months of age, as well as for all infants under 12 months of age with confirmed HIV infection, irrespective of clinical or immunological stage. For children 12 months of age or older, the World Health Organization (WHO) Paediatric Clinical Stage 4 disease (irrespective of CD4), WHO Paediatric Clinical Stage 3 disease (irrespective of CD4), WHO Paediatric Clinical Stage 2 disease and CD4 value at or below threshold. WHO Paediatric Clinical Stage 1 disease and CD4 value at or below threshold, and HIV antibody positive infants <18 months of age where virologic testing is not available to confirm HIV infection should be considered for HAART if they have clinically diagnosed severe HIV disease.

The study was carried out in selected antiretroviral therapy units of 5 tertiary level general hospitals in Addis Ababa, Ethiopia (Black Lion, Saint Peter, Yekatit 12, Zewditu, and ALERT) which serve as the major referral and reference hospitals in Ethiopia. According to the report obtained from registration records, at the time of the study, about 1,624 children were registered for HAART in the selected hospitals.

Of 1624 patients on HAART, 390 (100%) scheduled to present for care or pharmacy pick-ups between February 18 and April 18, 2008 fulfilled the inclusion criteria and were offered to participate. In this study most of the patients/caregivers use bus or taxi to attend the clinics.

The study design was a facility based cross-sectional study. This study was nested as part of a large Multicenter Pediatrics Cross-Sectional study that is published elsewhere [15].

Children who fulfilled the following criteria were included in the study: 1) Receiving continuous antiretroviral therapy for the past 12 weeks before the study in the selected hospitals; and 2) caregivers who had been previously counseled on the importance of drug adherence and on how to recognize common adverse drug reactions associated with antiretroviral drugs.

The study and survey instrument were approved by the Institutional Ethical Review Committee of Jimma University and Research Ethics Committee of Addis Ababa Health Bureau. Official letters of co-operation from the above organization and Federal Ministry of Health (FMOH) were given to respective hospitals. Only caregivers gave written consent for participation in the study. Data were collected by five trained HIV counselors, who were trained on how to interview caregivers with sensitivity, empathy and without expressing judgment. Interviews were carried out privately in a separate room in the Hospital where participants were recruited. In order to ensure participants' confidentiality, no names or personal identifiers were included in the written questionnaires. Identification of an informant was only possible through numerical codes.

Measurements

The outcome for this study was disclosure of HIV/AIDS serostatus to the participating children. Data was collected by structured questionnaire that had not been previously validated, which was originally developed in English and later translated to Amharic and retranslated back to English by a different person to check for consistency. The content of the questionnaire included: socio-demographic and socio-economic characteristics, medication related factors, health care delivery system related factors, which included access to care, quality of services, and diagnosis related items, referral and treatment, medication administration. Three days intensive training was given for all supervisors and data collectors. Data entry and analyses was carried out using SPSS version 12.0.1 statistical packages. One trained data clerk entered and cleaned the data. Stepwise logistic regression was done to identify factors associated with disclosure. Variables that showed statistical significance below or equal to $p \leq 0.05$ where retained for the final model.

Results

Socio-demographic and economic characteristics

Out of 390 children ages 1–14 (mean = 8.52, standard deviation [SD] = 2.97] years), 243 (62.3%) children were between 6–9 years of age, 215 (55.1%) were girls and 297 (76.2%) caregivers reported being Ethiopian Orthodox Christian. Of the 390 (100%) caregivers, 176 (45.1%) had primary school education; 174 (44.6%) caregivers were married. Two hundred and seventy seven (71.7%) caregivers mentioned that no one had helped the child financially for their treatment needs, while 6.4% biological fathers and 6.4% local Non-governmental Organizations (NGO's) were reported as being responsible for offering financial support to some of the children. The baseline socio-demographic and economic characteristics are presented in Table 1.

HIV infection, diagnosis, and treatment

Out of the 390 respondents, 210 (53.8%) had someone else living with HIV in their home. One hundred seventy seven of the individuals (84.3%) were taking HAART during the survey period, of which 59 (33.3%) were receiving HAART services in the same facility as the child and 27 (15.25%) had the same day appointment as the child. When asked about the time of the child's diagnosis, 320 (82.1%) caregivers knew it, 114 (29%) caregivers said that they had known about the child's HIV serostatus 2 years prior to the survey. Almost half, 191 (49%) children were referred for HIV screening from the hospital's in-patient ward and 131 (33.6%) from the community clinic.

Nutritional support including Ready-to-use Therapeutic Food (RUTF) provision was provided to 260 (66.7%) children from the hospital. Out of our total sample, 343 (88%) caregivers knew when the child had started HAART. From the 390 (100%) children/caretakers surveyed, 186 (54.4%) had started treatment 2 years before the survey was implemented. Of the children who were taking medication other than ARVs, cotrimoxazole, anti-Tuberculosis medication, as well as multi-vitamins were the most frequently used with 360 (92.3%), 68 (17.8%) and 20 (5%) children taking them, respectively.

Table 1. Disclosure status of children on HAART in Addis Ababa, Ethiopia in 2008, by demographic and social characteristics.

Variable	Disclosure status n (%)		P-value
	Not disclosed	Disclosed	
Age of the child (N = 390)			0.001
0–5 years (n = 58)	54(18.8)	4(5.9)	
6–9 years (n = 243)	215(66.8)	28(41.2)	
10–14years (n = 89)	53(16.5)	36(52.9)	
Sex of the child(N = 390)			0.349
Boy(n = 175)	141(43.8)	34(50.0)	
Girl(n = 215)	181(56.2)	34(50.0)	
Religion (N = 390)			0.07
Orthodox(n = 297)	239(74.2)	58(85.3)	
Others [1](n = 93)	83(25.8)	10(14.7)	
Caregiver's educational status (N = 390)			0.001
Unable to read and write(n = 94)	64(19.9)	30(44.1)	
Primary (1–8)(n = 176)	155(48.1)	21(30.9)	
Secondary (9–12)(n = 68)	58(18.0)	10(14.7)	
Diploma and above(n = 52)	45(14.0)	7(10.3)	
Marital status of the caregiver(N = 390)			0.049
Single(n = 38)	30(9.3)	8(11.8)	
Married(n = 174)	150(46.6)	24(35.3)	
Divorced(n = 40)	30(9.3)	10(14.7)	
Widowed(n = 138)	112(34.8)	26(38.2)	
Family income (USD per month) (N = 390)			0.026
<11(n = 277)	220(68.3)	57(83.8)	
11 -<16(n = 50)	43(13.4)	7(10.3)	
≥16 (n = 63)	59(18.3)	4(5.9)	
Relation of child-caregiver(N = 390)			0.162
Mother (n = 62)	54(87.0)	8(16.8)	
Grandmother/father (n = 112)	99(88.4)	13(30.7)	
Uncle/aunt (n = 54)	38(70.4)	16(11.8)	
Others [2](n = 162)	131(80.9)	31(40.7)	
Offering financial aid/support for the child(N = 390)			0.499
No one(n = 277)	231(71.7)	46(67.6)	
Others [3](n = 113)	91(28.3)	22(32.4)	
Preferred age of disclosure by the caregivers (years) (N = 390)			0.09
<12(n = 53)	49(15.2)	4(5.9)	
13(n = 157)	126(39.1)	31(45.6)	
>14(n-180)	147(45.7)	33(48.5)	
Do you know any other children in your community who has HIV?(N = 389)			0.816
Yes(n = 119)	99(30.8)	20(29.4)	
No(n = 270)	222(69.2)	48(70.6)	
Received child care grant(n = 390)			0.003
Yes(n = 85)	61(18.9)	24(35.3)	
No(n = 305)	261(81.1)	44(64.7	

[1] *Catholic, Protestant and Muslim.*
[2] *by himself/herself, Sister, Brother, Father, Both (mother/father) and Foster parents.*
[3] *Father, Local NGO, Uncle, Relatives and Family, Exchange rate 1 USD = 9.6 Ethiopian Birr (ETB).*

Social Support, Disclosure and Perceived Stigma and Discrimination

Three hundred and twenty-two (82.6%) of the children who participated in the study did not know their HIV serostatus. For none disclosures, 104 (32.3%) caregivers reported that their children were told that they had Tuberculosis (TB) and that their children assumed they were being taken to the health facility for TB appointments. Ninety-four (24.1%) of the caregivers had been attending a support group for caregivers of children with HIV and 89 (94.7%) attended a community organization for social support.

When caregivers were asked about the age at which the child should know about his/her serostatus, 180 (46.2%) respondents said that the child should be told about his/her HIV status when he/she was older than 14 years of age, while 54 (13.8%) pointed out that disclosure should be made at the age of 14. When caregivers were asked about who should have the responsibility of disclosing HIV serostatus to the child, 193 (60%) believed that the doctor should be responsible. A total of 270 (69.2%) respondents reported that they knew other children with HIV in the community (Table 2).

A total of 78 (20%) children reported being discriminated by their neighbors. Out of the 78 (20%) children that reported discrimination, 10 (13%) were from the HIV disclosed group and 68 (87%) were from the HIV non-disclosed group. One hundred and ninety-five (50%) of the caregivers reported as children or families affected by HIV/AIDS, including orphans are sometimes verbally mistreated.

HIV/AIDS disclosure predictors

After controlling for the effects of other variables in the multivariate logistic regression analysis, four characteristics were associated with disclosure of HIV status to children. Comparing children in the 10–14 years age group to children in the 0–5 age group and to those in the 6–9 years of age group, we observed that the last two groups are statistically significant less likely to be informed of their HIV status [(aOR = 0.11; 95% CI = 0.03–0.34 and (aOR = 0.19 ; 95% CI = 0.10–0.37, respectively)]. Perceived awareness of a child of caregiver's illness was also found to be associated with disclosure status. Children who were perceived to know their caregivers health problem were statistically significant more likely to be informed about their HIV status than their counterparts (aOR = 2.20; 95% CI: 1.14–4.28). Educational status of the caregivers was also statistically significant associated with disclosure. Children with caregivers that have education at or above primary level are statistically significant less likely to be informed of their result than those with illiterate caregivers (aOR = 0.28; 95% CI: 0.13–0 .54, aOR = 0.33; 95% CI: 0 .13–0.84 and aOR = 0.32; 95% CI: 0.12–0.86 comparing caregiver with no education vs. primary education, secondary education and diploma and above, respectively). Level of referral for HIV screening was associated with disclosure. Compared to children referred from community clinic, those children referred from hospitals (aOR = 2.87; 95% CI: 1.26–6.51) and private practitioners/NGOs (aOR = 3.88; 95% CI: 1.57–9.58) were more likely to be informed about their HIV test results (Table 3).

Table 2. Patterns of disclosure characteristics of caregivers and children in Addis Ababa, Ethiopia [N = 390], April 2008.

Variable	n (%)
Child know his/her HIV status	
Yes	68(17.4)
No	322(82.6)
People who know child's HIV status	
Father	111(28.5)
Mother	124(31.8)
Sibling	60(15.4)
Grandmother	108(27.7)
Aunt	146(37.4)
Uncle	94(24.1)
Others@	111(28.5)
Who do you think should be the person responsible for disclosure of HIV status? *	
Family (father/mother)	99(30.7)
Health worker (doctor/councilor)	193(60)
Child supporter	30(9.3)

@Teacher/school, Cousins, Neighbors and Grandfather.
*Total does not add up to 390 caregivers given that 68 were already aware of their HIV status. Some percentages don't add to 100% due to rounding.

Discussion

In this study only 68 (17.4%) children knew their serostatus. This is lower than the 33% reported in a study conducted in Uganda [16] but comparable with other studies conducted in Europe [17,18]. Generally, the prevalence of disclosure varies widely across studies and settings, from less than 50% to about 75% of children and youths [19,20]. The lower prevalence of disclosure in our study might be due to fear of stigma and discrimination by the family members that are not aware or/and caregiver's perceived lack of emotional preparedness of the children and if the child is told he/she will reveal to others leading to stigma and discrimination to the family.

In our study, most caregivers prefer to delay disclosure up to older ages (above 14), this being consistent with previous findings [21,22]. In addition, it has been documented that parents view children over the age of 12 as emotionally mature for disclosure of HIV status [22–26]. In many studies, older children was found to be a determinant factor for the children's' knowledge about their HIV status. Bor *et.al* reported 100% disclosure in children 16 years of age and older [27] and likewise; Cohen *et.al* reported that 95% of children older than 10 years of age were aware of their HIV status in Massachusetts [28]. Similar findings were also documented elsewhere [15,16]. This could be due to the caregivers' belief that at early age, the child is lacking the emotional and cognitive maturity needed to understand the disease and implications [19,24,29,30]. The perception that adolescence is the optimal period for disclosure may relate to the idea that at this life stage, children are now able to cope with this type of information and address any concerns that they may have as they become sexually active (e.g. HIV transmission) [22]. In our analysis we included children less than 3 years old to explore the disclosure status for all pediatric age groups. Their inclusion might reduce the disclosure rate; however they do not represent a significant proportion of the participants so we do not expect that the relationship is significantly affected due to their inclusion.

The relationship between HIV disclosure and educational level has been documented elsewhere [31,32]. Wiener *et al.* [30] found that more children who knew their HIV status came from families with a higher socio-economic status and as education is a proxy indicator of higher social economic status. In our study, illiterate caregivers were more likely to disclose the child's HIV status than

Table 3. Final Logistic Regression Model for Predictors of Disclosure of HIV/AIDS diagnosis to HIV-infected children in Addis Ababa, Ethiopia, April, 2008.

Variables	Disclosure status		Crude OR** (95%CI)	P-value	Adjusted OR (95%CI)	P-value
	Yes n (%)	No n (%)				
Age of the child (years)				0.001		0.001
0–5	4(5.9)	54(16.8)	0.11(0.03–0.32)		0.11(0.03–0.34)	
6–9	28(41.2)	215(66.8)	0.19(0.10–0.34)		0.19(0.10–0.37)	
10–14	36(52.9)	53(16.5)	1.00		1.00	
Child perceived to know health status of caregiver				0.037		0.019
Yes	24(35.3)	59(18.3)	2.43(1.37–4.30)		2.20(1.14–4.28)	
No	44(64.7)	263(81.7)	1.00		1.00	
Educational level of caregiver				0.004		0.002
Unable to read and write	30(44.1)	64(19.9)	1.00		1.00	
Primary (1–8 grade)	21(30.9)	155(48.1)	0.29(0.15–0.54)		0.28(0.13–0 .54)	
Secondary (8–12 grade)	10(14.7)	58(18.0)	0.37(0.17–0.82)		0.33(0 .13–0.84)	
Diploma and above	7(10.3)	45(14.0)	0.33(0.13–0.82)		0.32(0.12–0.86)	
Place of referral for HIV screening				0.019		0.011
From community clinic	10(14.7)	98(30.4)	1.00		1.00	
Hospital in-patients ward	35(51.5)	155(48.1)	2.20(1.05–4.67)		2.87(1.26–6.51)	
PMTCT programme	1(1.5)	19(5.9)	0.52(0.06–4.27)		0.58(0.07–5.03)	
Private practitioner/NGO*	22(32.4)	50(15.5)	4.31(1.89–9.80)		3.88(1.57–9.58)	

*-Non Governmental Organization.
**OR = Odds Ratio.

caregivers with a higher educational level. Again, those caregivers who didn't pay for their child's medication before HAART intake were 62% less likely to disclose the child's serostatus. Similar findings were reported by Wiener *et al.* in which more children who knew their HIV status came from families with a higher socio-economic status [30] but opposite to the study found in Thailand, as more children whose caregivers reported having financial problems knew their diagnosis than those whose care givers did not report to have any financial problems [26]. In the Ethiopian context, affluent families might want to keep their family's status quo by avoiding disclosure.

In practical terms, it is difficult for caregivers to handle the psychological adjustments of their HIV infected children. If the child is aware of the health problem of his/her caretaker, disclosure is more likely to occur. A mother's disclosure of any chronic or life-threatening illness to her child is often accompanied by some level of hesitation and/or anxiety regarding the child's reaction [33,34]. Similarly, mothers with HIV/AIDS might be particularly worried about their children learning of their illness given the stigma associated with the disease, as well as the methods of transmission [21,35,36]. In some cases, caretakers feel relieved of the burden of keeping the secret, and less anxious about medical visits and the possibility of accidental disclosure [9,37]. Once the caregiver's senses that the child has known the caregivers health problem, it might be easier to disclose the HIV status [38]. According to Murphy *et al.* [39] children's' knowledge of maternal HIV/AIDS status is associated with an increase in child psychosocial adjustment, including enhanced self-esteem among children who know of their mother's HIV infection.

The strength of our study is the large sample size, which represents an important amount of caregivers and their children receiving HAART in Ethiopia in multiple treatment sites, which represent the major HAART reference hospitals in Addis Ababa. Some of the limitations that we identified were the following: first, our sample is limited to urban settings, which might curb any extrapolation of our finding to other settings in Ethiopia. We could not outline whether the differences in disclosure status are associated with cultural factors or other characteristics that were not included in this study. In addition, we acknowledge the possibility of potential selection bias in our study; we investigated only HIV disclosure among people living with HIV/AIDS (PLWHAs) under HAART, but HAART may have a confounding impact on disclosure. Finally, the selection of continuous therapy for 12 weeks and previous counseling on adherence and adverse drug reactions-may bias the results of the study.

In conclusion, the rate of disclosure of pediatric HIV positive status was low in children in Addis Ababa. Given that there is no published research found in the country, this finding will provide evidence regarding pediatric HIV serostatus disclosure. To increase disclosure rate, it is important to target children from higher socioeconomic classes and educated caregivers, children referred from community clinics and younger children. In addition, encouraging disclosure of caregivers' health problems might facilitate disclosure. Intensified information education and communication to de-stigmatize the disease might have far reaching impact. Caregivers and health providers should have a co-responsibility to decide on the proper time to disclose. Finally, as more information is known regarding HIV infection in children and young adults who will become sexually active and who might potentially engage in high risk behavior for HIV infection and other sexually transmitted diseases as well as blood borne diseases (Hepatitis C Virus), we need to be aware that current and future guidelines that consider HIV disclosure need to be flexible, so new information can be included with the ultimate goal of improving the life of children living with HIV and of their caregivers.

Acknowledgments

We are also very grateful to extend our gratitude to the study participants and data collectors.

Author Contributions

Conceived and designed the experiments: SB AD AA KD. Performed the experiments: SB AD AA KD. Analyzed the data: SB AD AA KD HRE. Contributed reagents/materials/analysis tools: SB AD AA KD HRE. Wrote the manuscript: SB AD AA KD HRE.

References

1. World Health Organization and UNICEF (2008) Scale up of HIV-related prevention, diagnosis, care and treatment for infants and children: A Programming Framework. Geneva, World Health Organization and UNICEF (http://www.who.int/hiv/pub/paediatric/paediatric_programme_fmwk2008.pdf. Accessed 05 June 2009).
2. UNAIDS. Global AIDS epidemic update report(2010) Geneva, UNAIDS, (http://www.unaids.org/en/KnowledgeCentre/HIVData/GlobalReport/2008/2010_Global_report.asp, accessed December 15, 2010.
3. Lesch A, Swartz L, Kagee A, Moodley K, Kafaar Z, et al. (2007) Paediatric HIV/AIDS disclosure: towards a Developmental and process-oriented approach. AIDS care 19(6): 811–6.
4. Butler AM, Williams PL, Howland LC, Storm D, Hutton N, Seage GR, 3rd, Team (2009) Impact of disclosure of HIV infection on health-related quality of life among children and adolescents with HIV infection. Pediatrics 123(3): 935–43.
5. American Academy of Pediatrics Committee on Pediatrics AIDS (1999) Disclosure of illness status to children and adolescents with HIV infection. Pediatrics 103(1): 164–166.
6. Ministry of Health Ethiopia & Federal HIV/AIDS Prevention and Control Office (2008) Guidelines for Paediatric HIV/AIDS Care and Treatment in Ethiopia. July.
7. Brown LK, Lourie KJ, Pao M (2000) Children and adolescents living with HIV and AIDS: A review. Journal of Child Psychology and Psychiatry 41(1): 81–96.
8. Lipson M (1994) Disclosure of diagnosis to children with human immunodeficiency virus or acquired immunodeficiency syndrome. J Dev Behav Pediatr 15: 61–65.
9. Grubman S, Gross E, Lerner-Weiss N, et al. (1995) Older children and adolescents living with perinatally acquired human immunodeficiency virus infection. Pediatrics 95: 657–663.
10. Walsh ME, Bibace R (1991) Children's conceptions of AIDS: a developmental analysis. J Pediatr Psychol 16: 273–285.
11. Nishi EA, Cincotta N, Childs J, Salisbury K, Edwards W, et al. (2004) Disclosure in a new context: HIV infected children aging into adolescence. International Conference on AIDS Jul 11–16; 15: abstract no D10681.
12. Ferris M, Burau K, Schweitzer AM, Mihale S, Murray N, et al. (2007) The influence of disclosure of HIV diagnosis on time to disease progression in a cohort of Romanian children and teens. AIDS Care 19(9): 1088–94.
13. Moodley K, Myer L, Michaels D, Cotton M (2006) Paediatric HIV Disclosure in South Africa: Caregivers Perspectives on discussing HIV with infected children. South African Medical Journal 96(3): 201–202.
14. Myer L, Moodley K, Hendricks F, Cotton M (2006) Health care providers' perspectives on discussing HIV status with infected children. J Trop Pediatr 52(4): 293–295.
15. Biadgilign S, Deribew A, Amberbir A, Kebede D (2008) Adherence to highly active antiretroviral therapy and its correlates among HIV infected pediatric patients in Ethiopia. BMC Pediatrics 8: 53.
16. Bikaako-Kajura W, Luyirika E, Purcell D, et al. (2006) Disclosure of HIV status and adherence to daily drug regimens among HIV-infected children in Uganda. AIDS and Behavior 10: 85–93.
17. Thorne C, Newell ML, Peckham CS (2000) Disclosure of diagnosis and planning for the future in HIV-affected families in Europe. Child Care Health Dev 26: 29–40.
18. Lee CL, Johann-Liang R (1999) Disclosure of the diagnosis of HIV/AIDS to children born of HIV-infected mothers. AIDS Patient Care 13: 41–45.
19. Lester P, Chesney M, Cooke M, Whalley P, Perez B, et al. (2002) Diagnostic disclosure to HIV-infected children: How parents decide when and what to tell. Clinical Child Psychology and Psychiatry 7(1): 85–99.
20. Thorne C, Newell ML, Botet FA, et al. (2002) Older children and adolescents surviving with vertically acquired HIV infection. J Acquir Immune Defic Syndr 29: 396–401.
21. Armistead L, Tannenbaum L, Forehand R, et al. (2001) Disclosing HIV status: are mothers telling their children? J Pediatr Psychol 26: 11–20.
22. Funck-Brentano I, Costagliola D, Seibel N, et al. (1997) Patterns of disclosure and perceptions of the immunodeficiency virus in elementary school aged children. Arch Pediatr Adolesc Med 151: 978–985.
23. Mellins CA, Brackis-Cott E, Dolezal C, et al. (2002) Patterns of status disclosure to perinatally HIV-infected children and subsequent mental health outcomes. Clin Child Psychol Psychiatry 7: 101–114.
24. Flanagan-Klygis E, Ross LF, Lantos J, Frader J, Yogev R (2002) Disclosing the diagnosis of HIV in pediatrics. AIDS and Public Policy Journal 17(1): 3–12.
25. Blasini I, Chantry C, Cruz C, Ortiz L, Salabarría I, et al. (2004) Disclosure model for pediatric patients living with HIV in Puerto Rico: Design, implementation, and evaluation. Journal of Developmental and Behavioral Pediatrics 25: 181–189.
26. Oberdorfer P, Puthanakit T, Louthrenoo O, Charnsil C, Sirisanthana V, et al. (2006) Disclosure of HIV/AIDS diagnosis to HIV-infected children in Thailand. Journal of Paediatrics and Child Health 42(5): 283–8.
27. Bor R (1996) Disclosure (Vancouver conference review). AIDS Care 9: 49–53.
28. Cohen J, Reddington C, Jacobs D, et al. (1997) School-related issues among HIV infected children. Pediatrics 100: 1 p. e8.
29. Ledlie SW (1999) Diagnosis disclosure by family caregivers to children who have perinatally acquired HIV disease: When the time comes. Nursing Research 48(3): 141–9.
30. Weiner LS, Battles HB, Heilman N, Sigelman CK, Pizzo PA (1996) Factors associated with disclosure of diagnosis to children with HIV/AIDS. Pediatr AIDS HIV Infect 7(5): 310–324.
31. Landau G, York AS (2004) Keeping and disclosing a secret among people with HIV in Israel. Health and Social Work 29: 2 pp 116–126.
32. Peretti-Watel P, Spire B, Pierret J, Lert F, Obadia Y, VESPA Group (2006) Management of HIV-related stigma and adherence to HAART: evidence from a large representative sample of outpatients attending French hospitals (ANRS-EN12-VESPA 2003). AIDS Care 18(3): 254–61.
33. Tompkins TL, Henker B, Whalen CK, Axelrod J, Comer LK (1999) Motherhood in the context of HIV infection: Reading between the numbers. Cultural Diversity and Ethnic Minority Psychology 5: 197–208.
34. Semple SJ, Patterson TL, Temoshok LR, McCutchan JA, Straits-Troster KA, et al. (1993) Identification of psychobiological stressors among HIV positive women. Women and Health 20: 15–36.
35. Herek GM (1999) AIDS and stigma. American Behavioral Scientist 42: 1106–1116.
36. Kirshenbaum SB, Nevid JS (2002) The specificity of maternal disclosure of HIV/AIDS in relation to children's adjustment. AIDS Education and Prevention 14: 1–16.
37. Lipson M (1993) Disclosure within families. AIDS Clinical Care 5: 43–44.
38. Naeem-Sheik A, GrayGlenda (2005) HIV disclosure in children. The Southern African Journal of HIV Medicine 21: 46–48.
39. Murphy DA, Steers WN, Stritto ME (2001) Maternal disclosure of mothers' HIV serostatus to their young children. Journal of Family Psychology 15: 441–450.

15

Children Who Acquire HIV Infection Perinatally are at Higher Risk of Early Death than those Acquiring Infection through Breastmilk

Renaud Becquet[1,2]*, Milly Marston[3], François Dabis[1,2], Lawrence H. Moulton[4], Glenda Gray[5], Hoosen M. Coovadia[6], Max Essex[7], Didier K. Ekouevi[8], Debra Jackson[9], Anna Coutsoudis[10], Charles Kilewo[11], Valériane Leroy[1,2], Stefan Z. Wiktor[12], Ruth Nduati[13], Philippe Msellati[14], Basia Zaba[3], Peter D. Ghys[15], Marie-Louise Newell[16,17], the UNAIDS Child survival group¶

1 Institut National de la Santé et de la Recherche Médicale (INSERM), Unité 897, Centre de Recherche "Epidémiologie et Biostatistique", Bordeaux, France, **2** Institut de Santé Publique Epidémiologie Développement (ISPED), Université Victor Segalen Bordeaux 2, Bordeaux, France, **3** London School of Hygiene and Tropical Medicine, London, United Kingdom, **4** Department of International Health, Johns Hopkins Bloomberg School of Public Health, Baltimore, Maryland, United States of America, **5** Perinatal HIV Research Unit (PHRU), University of the Witwatersrand, Soweto, South Africa, **6** HIV Management, Maternal, Adolescent and Child Unit, University of the Witwatersrand, Soweto, South Africa, **7** Department of Immunology and Infectious Diseases, Harvard School of Public Health AIDS Initiative, Boston, Massachusetts, United States of America, **8** PAC-CI program, ANRS site in Côte d'Ivoire, Abidjan, Côte d'Ivoire, **9** School of Public Health, University of the Western Cape, Cape Town, South Africa, **10** Department of Paediatrics and Child Health, University of KwaZulu-Natal, South Africa, **11** Muhimbili University of Health and Allied Sciences, Dar es Salaam, Tanzania, **12** RETRO-CI project, Centers for Disease Control and Prevention, Global HIV/AIDS Program, Abidjan, Côte d'Ivoire, **13** Department of Pediatrics, University of Nairobi, Nairobi, Kenya, **14** Service de Pédiatrie, CHU Sourô Sanou, Bobo Dioulasso, Burkina Faso, **15** UNAIDS, Epidemiology and Analysis Division, Geneva, Switzerland, **16** Africa Centre for Health and Population Studies, University of KwaZulu-Natal, Somkhele, South Africa, **17** Centre for Paediatric Epidemiology and Biostatistics, University College London, Institute of Child Health, London, United Kingdom

Abstract

Background: Assumptions about survival of HIV-infected children in Africa without antiretroviral therapy need to be updated to inform ongoing UNAIDS modelling of paediatric HIV epidemics among children. Improved estimates of infant survival by timing of HIV-infection (perinatally or postnatally) are thus needed.

Methodology/Principal Findings: A pooled analysis was conducted of individual data of all available intervention cohorts and randomized trials on prevention of HIV mother-to-child transmission in Africa. Studies were right-censored at the time of infant antiretroviral initiation. Overall mortality rate per 1000 child-years of follow-up was calculated by selected maternal and infant characteristics. The Kaplan-Meier method was used to estimate survival curves by child's HIV infection status and timing of HIV infection. Individual data from 12 studies were pooled, with 12,112 children of HIV-infected women. Mortality rates per 1,000 child-years follow-up were 39.3 and 381.6 for HIV-uninfected and infected children respectively. One year after acquisition of HIV infection, an estimated 26% postnatally and 52% perinatally infected children would have died; and 4% uninfected children by age 1 year. Mortality was independently associated with maternal death (adjusted hazard ratio 2.2, 95%CI 1.6–3.0), maternal CD4<350 cells/ml (1.4, 1.1–1.7), postnatal (3.1, 2.1–4.1) or peri-partum HIV-infection (12.4, 10.1–15.3).

Conclusions/Results: These results update previous work and inform future UNAIDS modelling by providing survival estimates for HIV-infected untreated African children by timing of infection. We highlight the urgent need for the prevention of peri-partum and postnatal transmission and timely assessment of HIV infection in infants to initiate antiretroviral care and support for HIV-infected children.

Editor: Zulfiqar A. Bhutta, Aga Khan University, Pakistan

Funding: This pooled analysis was funded by the Epidemiology and Analysis Division of UNAIDS (Geneva, Switzerland). The funders had no role in study design, data collection and analysis, decision to publish, or preparation of the manuscript.

Competing Interests: Co-author Marie-Louise Newell is an Academic Editor for PLoS ONE. This does not alter the authors' adherence to all the PLoS ONE policies on sharing data and materials..

* E-mail: Renaud.Becquet@isped.u-bordeaux2.fr

¶ See the Acknowledgments section for the detailed constitution of the group.

Introduction

Sub-Saharan Africa remains the region most heavily affected by HIV. In 2008, an estimated 1,800,000 HIV-infected children under 15 years were living in sub-Saharan Africa, and this continent accounted for 91% of new HIV infections among children [1]. While it is important to have accurate estimates of survival when children are treated with antiretroviral therapy, assumptions about survival of HIV-infected children in Africa in the absence of treatment [2,3] need to be updated and refined to inform ongoing UNAIDS modelling of HIV epidemiology among children. For this purpose, UNAIDS convened a working group to attempt to pool data from all available clinical trials on mother-to-child HIV transmission prevention conducted in sub-Saharan Africa over the last 15 years, to reliably assess mortality rates in HIV-infected children.

More specifically, precise estimates of infant survival by timing of HIV-infection (perinatally or postnatally through breastfeeding) are urgently needed. Such estimates will provide benchmarks for assessing the impacts of paediatric HIV treatment whilst allowing for the effect of background mortality on survival post-infection of children. We here present the results based on data with consistent information on timing of acquisition of infection, both before or during delivery, and postnatally to reliably estimate infant survival by timing of HIV-infection. We update the previously conducted individual patient meta-analysis on survival in HIV-exposed children [3] which had limited statistical power especially on the timing of acquisition of infection.

Methods

Studies eligible for this pooled analysis were clinical trials or cohort studies in sub-Saharan African countries that investigated the effect of antiretroviral-based and/or infant feeding interventions in risk reduction of HIV vertical transmission with paediatric follow-up for 18–24 months and information about infant feeding. Overall, 18 trials and cohort studies aimed at the prevention of mother-to-child transmission of HIV in African settings were eligible for this pooled analysis and contacted (Figure 1). Of these, four teams did not want to participate or could not share the data at the time of the analysis [4,5,6,7], two datasets were excluded (missing key variables) [8,9], and 12 provided the necessary data [10,11,12,13,14,15,16,17,18,19,20,21]. The PRISMA checklist is available as supporting information; see Checklist S1.

Paediatric HIV infection was defined as a positive plasma HIV-1 DNA/RNA PCR at any age. Children with a positive HIV-1 diagnostic test result before 4–6 weeks of age (depending on the timing of collection of blood samples in each study) were considered to be HIV-infected in peri-partum [22,23]. This includes infants infected in utero and DNA/RNA positive on the day of birth. Children with a negative DNA/RNA PCR from a sample obtained at or after 4–6 weeks of age who subsequently acquired infection were considered to be HIV-infected postnatally [22,23]. Children with positive test results at or after 4–6 weeks of age but with either no previous negative test result, or last negative test result before 4–6 weeks were considered infected with unknown timing of infection [22,23].

Antiretroviral treatment became available to children in the Mashi trial on the first of October 2002, so follow-up was rightly censored at this point. Infant antiretroviral treatment was not available during the time of the other trials. Maternal antiretroviral treatment was available in the Mitra Plus study only.

Baseline characteristics were described for each study included in the pooled analysis. Overall mortality as a rate per 1000 child-years of follow-up was calculated by selected maternal and infant characteristics. The Kaplan-Meier method was used to estimate survival curves among HIV-infected children: children infected in peri-partum, infected in postnatal, and infected with unknown timing of infection. Estimated time of diagnosis of HIV-infection for those infected postnatally was taken as mid-way between the last HIV-negative test and the first HIV-positive test. The survival of children infected peri-partum or with unknown timing was estimated from birth. Studies were right-censored at the time of infant antiretroviral initiation. We used random-effects Weibull regression models to estimate mortality hazard ratios accounting for heterogeneity between trials and cohorts. Adjusted hazard ratios were obtained, both overall and for HIV-uninfected and HIV-infected children separately. The multivariable models included the following variables: region of origin (South Africa, East Africa, West Africa), sex (boys, girls, unknown), maternal vital status (time-varying: alive, dead), antenatal maternal CD4 count in cells/ml (≥350, <350, unknown), breastfeeding practice in the first year of life (ever, never), and child HIV-infection status (uninfected, determined infected in peri-partum, infected postnatally, infected with unknown timing). Age at time of infection was allowed for in the model.

Results

The characteristics of the datasets included in the first step analysis are detailed in Table 1 and Table 2. Overall 12,112 infants born to HIV-infected mothers were included. Children with unknown HIV status were excluded from the analysis (n = 639). Analysis was therefore conducted among uninfected children (n = 8,964) and HIV-infected (n = 2,509, HIV infection acquired perinatally, through breastfeeding, or with unknown timing).

Overall, 1,363 children acquired infection perinatally with median time of first positive DNA/RNA test at 19 days (interquartile range: 1–42 days), 581 children were negative at or after 4 weeks of age and acquired infection through breastfeeding at a median 24 weeks of age (interquartile range: 7–39 weeks), and 565 children were infected with unknown timing of infection and had a first positive DNA/RNA test at 80 days in median (interquartile range: 51–168 days).

Crude mortality rates per 1,000 child-years of follow-up were 39.3 and 381.6 for HIV-uninfected and HIV-infected children, respectively. Mortality rate per 1000 child-years of follow-up by selected maternal and infant characteristics are detailed in Table 3.

Mortality was estimated for HIV-infected children by timing of transmission; initial time was the estimated date of acquisition of HIV-infection (Figure 2). Overall, 12 months post-acquisition of infection, an estimated 52% of children with peripartum infection (95% confidence interval [CI]: 49–55%) and 26% (95% CI: 22–31%) of those with postnatal infection died. Among children with unknown timing, an estimated 38% (95% CI: 22–31%) died compared with an estimated 4% of uninfected children who died by age 1 year. Detailed probabilities are available as supporting information; see Table S1.

Adjusted mortality hazard ratios (aHR) with 95% CI by selected characteristics were estimated in regression analyses among HIV-infected and uninfected children (n = 11,473). With South Africa as reference, mortality was significantly higher in East Africa, aHR 1.41 (1.14–1.74), but not West Africa, aHR 1.20 (0.88–1.63). Mortality did not differ significantly by sex: with boys as reference, aHR in girls was 1.02 (0.76–1.36). When the mother died during follow-up, children were more than twice likely to die (aHR 2.21 (1.63–3.00)) than when mothers survived. With mothers with CD4≥350 cells/ml as reference, children born to women with CD4<350 (aHR 1.36 (1.08–1.71)) or to women with unknown CD4 (aHR 1.30 (0.72–2.37)) were at significantly increased risk of dying. Children who had never been breastfed were at more than double the risk of dying than ever breastfed children (aHR 2.21 (1.62–3.01)). Mortality was substantially and significantly associated with child HIV infection status: compared to uninfected children, the aHRs were 12.45 (10.15–15.27) for perinatally infected children, 3.08 (2.29–4.14) for children infected through breastfeeding and 7.21 (5.53–9.39) for children with unknown timing of infection.

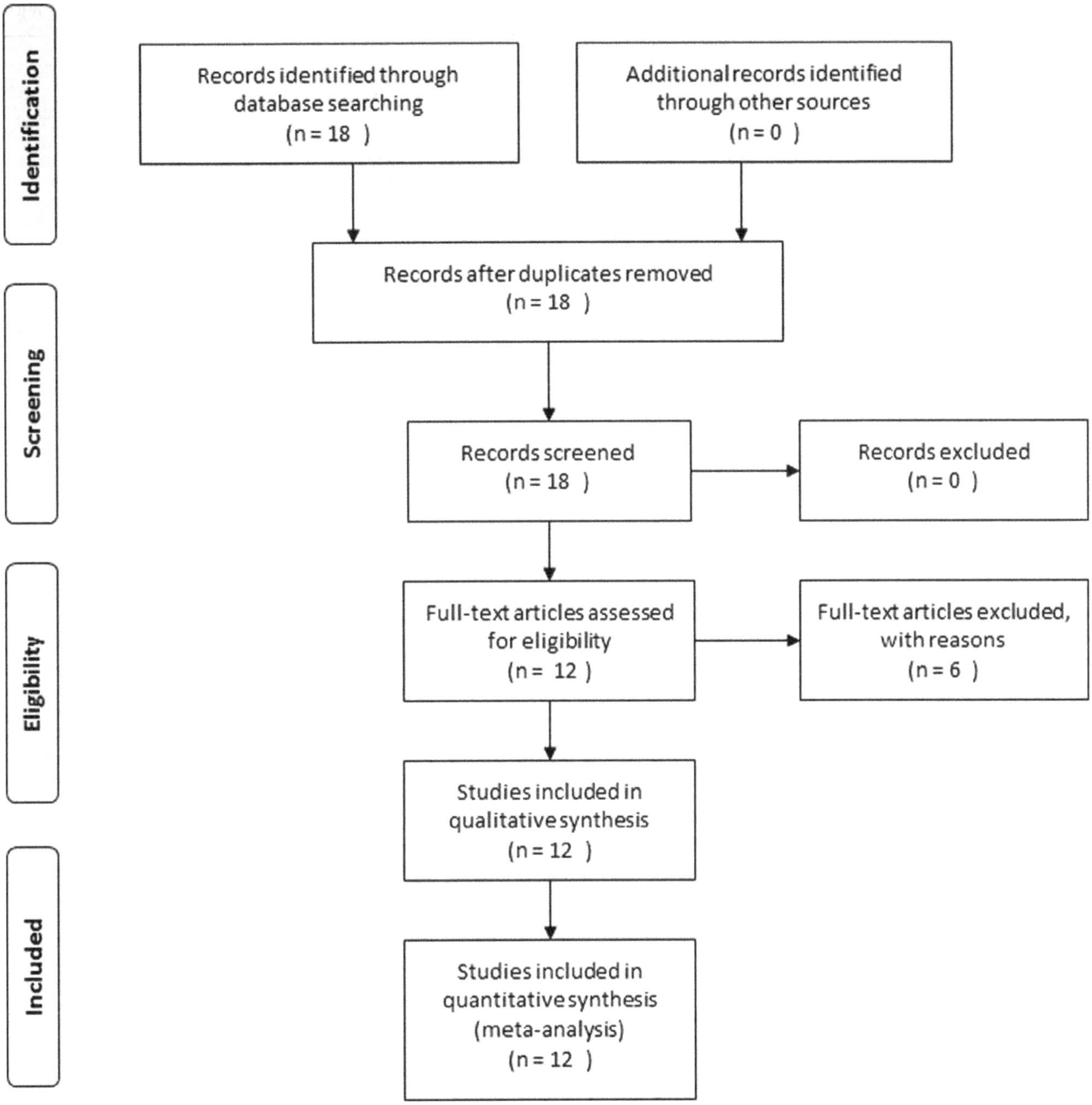

Figure 1. The PRISMA flow chart showing the progress of trials through the review.

Discussion

Mortality of children born to HIV-infected mothers was assessed on a large dataset from three different regions in sub-Saharan Africa. Overall mortality of HIV-infected children was dramatically elevated, irrespective of timing of acquisition of infection. However, among HIV-infected children, survival from acquisition of infection in postnatally infected children was higher than in those with infection acquired around delivery: the 18-month post-infection mortality risks were 36% (30%–42%) and 60% (57%–63%), respectively. Most these children had been included in research studies offering relatively high standard of care compared to less supported field areas; a closed clinical follow-up adapted to the child's age with free provision of care was provided to these children. Hence, we assume the survival estimates presented here were higher than what would be expected in more operational field settings. Our results are in accordance with previous findings of high mortality in vertically-infected children [24]: more than half of these children will have died by age two years. While the previously conducted meta-analysis on the subject had limited statistical power to assess infant mortality according to the timing of acquisition of HIV infection, we here present more reliable estimates on this matter.

Our analysis strategy implied that the survival was assessed from the estimated timing of infection in order to assess survival after infection for perinatally and postnatally infected children. This

Table 1. Characteristics of the mother-infant pairs included in the pooled analysis (first generation studies, before year 2000).

	ANRSa Ditrame Trial, *Côte d'Ivoire, Burkina Faso* **(Dabis Lancet 99)**	**ANRSb Ditrame Trial,** *Burkina Faso, Côte d'Ivoire* **(Msellati Sex Transm Infect 99)**	**Nairobi Trial,** *Kenya* **(Nduati Lancet 01)**	**Petra Trial,** *Tanzania, South Africa, Uganda* **(Petra Group Lancet 02)**	**Retro-CI Trial,** *Côte d'Ivoire* **(Wiktor Lancet 99)**	**Vitamin A Trial,** *South Africa* **(Coutsoudis Lancet 99)**
Mother-infant pairs	401	104	197	1458	261	660
Follow-up (days), median (IQR)	550 (303–639)	542 (293–589)	729 (332–849)	548 (388–554)	730 (290–1008)	300 (128–456)
Maternal Age (years), mean (SD)	25.6 (5.3)	24.5 (5.0)	23.9 (4.4)	27.0 (8.1)	26.4 (5.2)	26.2 (4.7)
Antenatal maternal CD4, median (IQR)	541 (359–741)	524 (384–768)	392 (262–530)	449 (295–630)	549 (354–726)	440 (311–597)
Maternal death, n (%)	18 (4.5)	9 (8.7)	17 (8.6)	61 (4.2)	9 (3.4)	5 (0.8)
Child age at maternal death (days), median (IQR)	274 (80–561)	342 (97–379)	240 (171–413)	341 (234–441)	142 (128–319)	229 (13–232)
Male child, n (%)	207 (51.6)	49 (47.2)	96 (48.7)	726 (49.9)	131(50.2)	317 (50.3)
Birthweight<2.5 kg, n (%)	62 (15.5)	18 (17.3)	13 (6.6)	96 (6.6)	27 (10.3)	74 (11.2)
Child ever breastfed, n (%)	401 (100.0)	104 (100.0)	197 (100.0)	1397 (95.8)	261 (100.0)	452 (68.5)
Breastfeeding duration (days), median (IQR)	274 (183–295)	342 (231–484)	398 (152–548)	212 (69–420)	458 (336–559)	90 (30–278)
Child death, n (%)	88 (22.0)	26 (25.0)	45 (22.8)	184 (12.6)	39 (14.9)	49 (7.4)
Child age at death (days), median (IQR)	202 (88–429)	175 (54–505)	247 (122–366)	171 (82–293)	101 (4–339)	86 (36–153)
HIV-infected child, n (%)	89 (24.0)	14 (16.5)	59 (30.9)	253 (18.1)	68 (27.2)	143 (22.8)
Peri-partum HIV infection, n	*38*	*1*	*27*	*110*	*41*	*111*
Postnatal HIVinfection, n	*22*	*5*	*19*	*87*	*23*	*22*
Unknown timing of HIV infection, n	*29*	*8*	*13*	*56*	*4*	*10*

Table 2. Characteristics of the mother-infant pairs included in the pooled analysis (second generation studies, after year 2000).

	VTS Cohort, *South Africa* **(Coovadia Lancet 07)**	**Zvitambo Trial,** *Zimbabwe* **(Humphrey JID 06)**	**ANRS Ditrame Plus Cohort,** *Côte d'Ivoire* **(Becquet PloS Med 07)**	**Good Start Cohort,** *South Africa* **(Doherty AIDS 07)**	**Mashi Trial,** *Botswana* **(Thior JAMA 06)**	**Mitra Plus Cohort,** *Tanzania* **(Kilewo JAIDS 09)**
Mother-infant pairs	1430	4548	747	665	1200	441
Follow-up (days), median (IQR)	583 (178–741)	456 (324–704)	730 (467–734)	252 (140–252)	1096 (725–1461)	730 (547–732)
Maternal Age (years), mean (SD)	25.5 (7.2)	25.0 (5.0)	27.1 (5.3)	25.4 (5.2)	27.6 (5.4)	27.0 (4.8)
Antenatal maternal CD4, median (IQR)	456 (313–626)	400 (259–570)	392 (251–561)	Not available	364 (234–514)	416 (267–579)
Maternal death, n (%)	71 (4.9)	246 (5.4)	13 (1.7)	20 (3.0)	39 (3.2)	9 (2.0)
Child age at maternal death (days), median (IQR)	473 (221–760)	285 (113–503)	291 (123–424)	141 (72–162)	472 (128–849)	354 (132–435)
Male child, n (%)	711 (50.4)	2235 (49.1)	378 (50.6)	328 (49.9)	554 (47.0)	225 (51.0)
Birthweight<2.5 kg, n (%)	157 (11.0)	776 (17.1)	94 (12.6)	96 (14.4)	94 (7.8)	59 (13.4)
Child ever breastfed, n (%)	1262 (88.2)	4186 (92.0)	434 (58.1)	259 (39.0)	592 (59.3)	441 (100.0)
Breastfeeding duration (days), median (IQR)	204 (109–279)	389 (274–528)	124 (96–204)	140 (112–168)	176 (118–183)	175 (140–182)
Child death, n (%)	201 (14.1)	885 (19.5)	79 (10.6)	67 (10.1)	114 (9.5)	35 (7.9)
Child age at death (days), median (IQR)	123 (62–305)	126 (80–301)	68 (1–204)	84 (35–140)	139 (28–284)	238 (175–361)
HIV-infected child, n (%)	249 (20.2)	1341 (30.1)	58 (7.8)	122 (24.8)	87 (7.4)	26 (5.9)
Peri-partum HIV infection, n	*127*	*728*	*40*	*68*	*56*	*16*
Postnatal HIV infection, n	*70*	*257*	*18*	*23*	*27*	*8*
Unknown timing of HIV infection, n	*52*	*356*	*0*	*31*	*4*	*2*

Table 3. Mortality rate per 1000 child-years of follow-up by selected maternal and infant characteristics (n = 12,112).

	Number (n = 12,112)	Deaths (n = 1,812)	Mortality rate per 1000 child-years of follow-up
Location			
Southern Africa	9270 (76.5)	1384	105.8
Eastern Africa	1329 (11.0)	196	100.1
Western Africa	1513 (12.5)	232	100.0
Maternal PMTCT ARV			
None	6634 (54.8)	1179	149.2
sdNVP	1657 (13.7)	223	99.3
2 or 3 drugs regimen	3821 (31.5)	410	56.8
Infant PMTCT ARV			
None	6892 (46.9)	1227	141.9
sdNVP +/− ZDV/3TC	5220 (53.1)	585	67.1
Maternal CD4 count			
<350	3973 (32.8)	796	135.2
≥350	6605 (54.5)	776	77.2
Unknown	1534 (12.7)	240	167.7
Maternal vital status			
Mothers known alive	11595 (95.7)	1598	95.6
Mothers known dead	517 (4.3)	214	332.3
Sex of the infant			
Girls	5957 (49.2)	883	103.5
Boys	6072 (50.1)	918	104.3
Unknown	83 (0.7)	11	-
Infant birthweight			
<2.5 kg	1566 (12.9)	445	232.4
≥2.5 kg	10372 (85.6)	1333	87.3
Unknown	174 (1.5)	34	-
Breastfeeding status			
Never	2126 (17.5)	310	113.9
Ever	9986 (82.5)	1502	102.6
Child infection status			
HIV-uninfected	8964 (74.0)	562	39.3
HIV-infected	2509 (20.7)	1096	381.6
Unknown	639 (5.3)	154	-

estimate would thus need to be interpreted in the light of the selection that occurs with children at risk of postnatal infection by definition being those who survived without infection the neonatal period which is one of high mortality risk. On the other hand, perinatally infected children will have to survive this risky period with the infection as an added exposure. However, there is no evidence of an increased neonatal mortality risk associated with perinatal infection [25]. Further, complementary analyses on the same dataset showed that differences seen in the survival of perinatally or postnatally infected children cannot be explained by differences in background mortality, which is much higher in the neonatal period [26]. We suggest that our findings are explained by the immunological immaturity, and thus reduced virological control, of the fetus and new-born at the time of acquisition of infection whereas postnatal acquisition of infection in infants who are more immunologically mature would be associated with a greater chance of survival [27].

We further also confirm the impact of both maternal health, as measured by her HIV immunological progression, and vital status on infant survival. Two-year infant mortality adjusted risk was one third higher among women with ante-partum CD4 count <350 cells/ml than among those with mothers a CD4 count above this threshold; and it was two times higher when the mother had died during the two years post-partum than when the mother was alive two years after birth. Lifelong antiretroviral treatment was not available to women followed-up in all studies selected for this pooled analysis but one. By lack of statistical power, it was therefore not possible to assess the impact of maternal antiretroviral treatment on the survival of children. Bearing in mind that maternal health is an important confounder of child survival, it would be crucial to investigate whether there is a positive impact of such a maternal treatment on infant survival. As maternal antiretroviral treatment keeps an infected mother alive, there would be an indirect effect of reducing child mortality in both her HIV-infected and uninfected children.

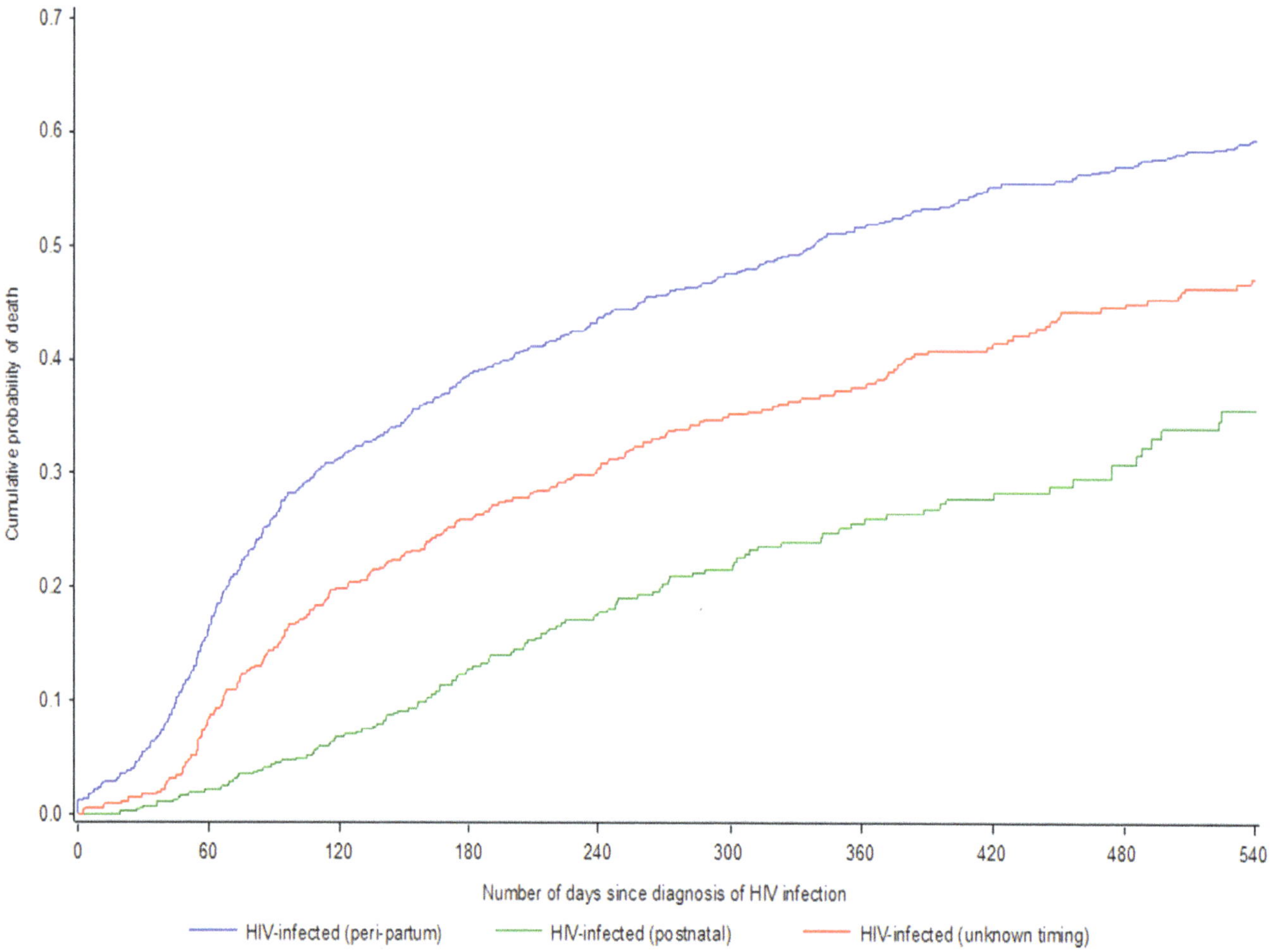

Figure 2. Estimated 18-month unadjusted mortality for HIV-infected children since acquisition of HIV infection (n = 2,509).

We present estimates of risk of mortality in children born to HIV-infected mothers in Africa, on the basis of a large dataset with wide variations in the characteristics of the patients included in the meta-analysis. The individual meta-analysis and adjustments in the model account for some of these effects. We acknowledge that there may have been confounding factors that had not been taken into account by our design, but we consider that the most important ones were controlled for. Additionally, the science in the prevention of mother-to-child transmission of HIV has changed since the time of the studies included in this meta-analysis. Expanding the indication of use of potent antiretroviral drug combinations to all pregnant, delivering, and breast-feeding HIV-infected women is now seen as an unprecedented opportunity to radically reduce the burden of paediatric AIDS [28]. The implication of this on the predicted trends in child mortality will need to be carefully assessed in future studies.

Our findings draw attention to the importance of comprehensive care for HIV-infected women. More specifically, our results stress the urgency of providing optimal antiretroviral treatment to women who need it for their own health (e.g. with ante-partum CD4 count <350 cell/ml according to the newly revised WHO guidelines [29]) to also improve survival of their (infected and uninfected) children. Maternal antiretroviral treatment will radically reduce the burden of paediatric HIV worldwide, and contribute to the improvement of survival of children born to HIV-infected women in improving maternal health and considerably lowering the risk of maternal death [30]. Moreover, there is still an urgent need for the effective prevention of mother-to-child transmission of HIV through breastfeeding: even postnatally infected children are three-times more likely to die than uninfected children. These findings also highlight the urgent need for the early assessment of HIV infection in HIV-exposed children to allow the timely initiation of antiretroviral care and support for HIV-infected children. Finally, these revised estimates of infant survival by timing of acquisition of HIV infection will now be used by UNAIDS to improve forecasts of the future of the HIV pandemic [31].

Acknowledgments

Composition of the UNAIDS Child survival group

Coordination. Renaud Becquet, François Dabis (INSERM, Unit 897, Bordeaux, France); Milly Marston, Basia Zaba (London School of Hygiene and Tropical Medicine, London, UK); Marie-Louise Newell (Africa Centre for Health and Population Studies, University of KwaZulu Natal, South Africa); Peter Ghys (UNAIDS, Epidemiology and Analysis Division, Geneva, Switzerland).

Data management. Sophie Karcher, Renaud Becquet (INSERM, Unit 897, Bordeaux, France).

Representatives of the participating studies. Larry Moulton (Zvitambo trial, Zimbabwe); Anna Coutsoudis (Vitamin A trial, South Africa); Glenda Gray (Petra trial, Tanzania-SA-Uganda); Charles Kilewo

(Mitra cohort, Tanzania); Jerry Coovadia (VTS cohort, South Africa); Valériane Leroy (ANRSa trial, Côte d'Ivoire); Max Essex (Mashi trial, Botswana); Stephan Wiktor (Retro-Ci trial, Côte d'Ivoire); Didier Ekouevi (Ditrame Plus cohort, Côte d'Ivoire); Ruth Nduati (Nairobi trial, Kenya); Debra Jackson (Good Start cohort, South Africa); Philippe Msellati (ANRSb trial, Burkina Faso).

Investigators and collaborators of the participating studies

ANRSa Trial, Côte d'Ivoire & Burkina Faso. *Investigators*: François Dabis, Philippe Msellati, Nicolas Meda, Christiane Welffens-Ekra, Bruno You, Olivier Manigart, Valériane Leroy, Arlette Simonon, Michel Cartoux, Patrice Combe, Amadou Ouangré, Rosa Ramon, Odette Ky-Zerbo, Crépin Montcho, Roger Salamon, Christine Rouzioux, Philippe Van de Perre, Laurent Mandelbrot.

Other investigators: L Dequae-Merchadou, R Lassalle (Bordeaux Coordination Unit); A Bazie, A M Cassel Beraud, B Dao, L Gautier-Charpentier, F D Ky, B Nacro, O Sanou, I Sombié, F Tall, S Tiendrebeogo, Y Traore, D Valea, S Yaro (Bobo-Dioulasso Centre); and D Bonnard, R Camara, M Dosso, N Elenga, G Gourvellec, J B Kottan, R Likikouet, V Noba, M Timité, I Viho.

ANRSb Trial, Burkina Faso & Côte d'Ivoire. *Biostatistics*: R Lassalle, V Leroy, R Salamon.

Epidemiology: M Cartoux, F Dabis (coordinator of the ANRS 049 trial/ DITRAME programme), N Meda (coordinator of Bobo-Dioulasso Center), P Msellati (coordinator of Abidjan Center), R Ramon.

Gynaecology-obstetrics: A Bazié, B Dao, R Likikouet, L Mandelbrot (principal investigator), C Welffens-Ekra (principal investigator).

Microbiology: D Bonard, P Combe, M Dosso, L Gautier-Charpentier, F D Ky, A Ouangré, T Ouassa, O Sanou, F Sylla-Koko, Y Traore, P Van de Perre.

Molecular biology: A M Cassel-Beraud, J B Kottan, OManigart, CMontcho, C Rouzioux, A Simonon, D Valea, B You.

Paediatrics: R Camara, N Elenga, B Nacro, F Tall, M Timité.

Trial monitoring: G Gourvellec, O Ky-Zerbo, V Noba, I Sombié, S Tiendrebeogo, I Viho, S Yaro.

Nairobi Trial, Kenya. Ruth Nduati, Barbra A Richardson, Grace John, Dorothy Mbori-Ngacha, Anthony Mwatha, Jeckoniah Ndinya-Achola, Job Bwayo, Francis E Onyango, Joan Kreiss.

Petra Trial, Tanzania - South Africa – Uganda. *Trial management committee*

J M A Lange (chair), J Saba (study coordinator), G Gray, J McIntyre, F Mmiro, Ch Ndugwa, J Moodley, H M Coovadia, D Moodley, Ch Kilewo, A Massawe, P Okong, P Kituuka, H von Briesen, J Goudsmit, G Biberfeld, F Mhalu, K Karlson, M Guliano, S Declich, S Clapp, G Haverkamp, G J Weverling, D Cooper, A Grulich, D Bray, J Perriens. Representatives of People Living with HIV: F Ngobeni, G Baguma, S Kyambadde.

Participating clinical centres

Uganda: Mulago Hospital, Mulago, Kampala (F Mmiro, Ch Ndugwa, P Musoke, C Nakabito, P Bakaki, I Kalyesbula, M Lutajumwa, S Mmiro, R Kato, R Byenkya, S Kabenge, R Mulira, R Bagenda, J Matavu, F Kikonyogo, E Kawuki, B Nkoyoyo, N Matovu, C Mukasa, C Dukar, M Mubiru, D Bagenda, K Khantaway); St Francis Hospital, Nsambya, Kampala (P Okong, P Kituuka, K Kayanja, S Kateera, B Sam, B Sabrina, M Ravera, E Omobono, M Magoni).

Tanzania: Muhimbili General Hospital, Dar es Salaam (Ch Kilewo, A Massawe, F Mhalu, E Urassa, F Kalokola, F Phillip, M Giattas, F Temu, K Kallanga, A Mkumbukwa, E Lugaiya, S Nyoni, S Haule, E Hilbayuded, N Kavugha, I Kayombo, E Lyamuya, E Mbena, V Msangi, C Lema, H Matimbwa, I Semali, K Karlsson).

South Africa: Chris Hani Baragwanath Hospital, Johannesburg (S Johnson, A Violari, L Connell, G Nelson, J Moetlo, A Makhofola, B Jivkov, F Ngobeni, M Kunene, G Ngakane, G Tshabalala, W Saba, P Khela, N Radebe); King Edward VII Hospital, Durban (J Moodley, H M Coovadia, D Moodley K Naidoo, M Adhikari, T Moniwa, D Moholo, I Mtshali, C Ngubane, A Mlaba, N Mkhize, C Sibiya, L Shozi, T Ngubane, V Mkhize, L Madurai, V Gopaul, L Thaver, G Swart, J Thomas).

Trial coordination, central data management and statistical analysis

Switzerland, Geneva, UNAIDS (J Saba, J Perriens); and International Antiviral Therapy Evaluation Center (J M A Lange, G Haverkamp, S Clapp, H Huisman, P Hollak, L Hendriks), and Department of Clinical Epidemiology and Biostatistics (G J Weverling), Academic Medical Centre, Amsterdam, Netherlands.

Laboratories

Germany, Frankfurt: Georg-Speyer-Haus (A de Amorim-Nink, H Klunker, L Kurunci, H von Briesen, A Simon). Sweden, Stockholm: Swedish Institute for Infectious Disease Control and Microbiology and Tumorbiology Center Karolinska Institute (G Biberfeld, K Karlsson, E Olausson Hansson, A Östborn). Netherlands, Amsterdam: Academic Medical Centre–Department of Human Retrovirology (J Goudsmit, S Jurriaans, E de Rooy, M Bakker, N Romp).

Retro-CI Trial, Côte d'Ivoire

Stefan Z Wiktor, Ehounou Ekpini, John M Karon, John Nkengasong, Chantal Maurice, Sibailly T Severin, Thierry H Roels, Moise K Kouassi, Eve M Lackritz, Issa-Malick Coulibaly, Alan E Greenberg.

Vitamin A Trial, South Africa

Investigators: Anna Coutsoudis, Kubendran Pillay, Louise Kuhn, Elizabeth Spooner, Wei-Yann Tsai and Hoosen M. Coovadia.

Additional members: Gill Sinclair, Anne Mburu, Nolwandle Mngqundaniso, Kerry Uebel, Ingrid Coetzee, Ken Annamalai, Trevor Doorasamy, Ugene Govender, Juana Willumsen, Nigel Rollins, Jagidesa Moodley and Daya Moodley.

VTS Cohort, South Africa

Study investigators: Ruth Bland, Hoosen Coovadia (principal investigator), Anna Coutsoudis, Marie-Louise Newell, Nigel Rollins.

Steering Committee: Janet Darbyshire (chair), Nono Simelela (South African National Department of Health), Victoria Sithole (Community Advisory Board) and the study investigators.

Data management: Cookie Govender, Londiwe Mthethwa and team.

Clinical team: Thembi Blose, Nqobile Mkhwanazi, Dumo Mkwanazi and team.

Field team: Zanele Fakude, Samukelisiwe Dube and team.

Laboratory team: Johannes Viljoen, Natalie Graham, Siva Davaviah and team.

Zvitambo Trial, Zimbabwe

Investigators: Peter J. Iliff, Ellen G. Piwoz, Naume V. Tavengwa, Clare D. Zunguzac, Edmore T. Marinda, Kusum J. Nathoo, Lawrence H. Moulton, Brian J. Ward, Jean H. Humphrey.

Additional members: Henry Chidawanyika, John Hargrove, Florence Majo, Kuda Mutasa, Mary Ndhlovu, Robert Ntozini and Phillipa Rambanepasi (ZVITAMBO); Agnes Mahomva (AIDS and TB Unit, Ministry of Health and Child Welfare, Zimbabwe); Lucie Malaba (Faculty of Science, University of Zimbabwe); Michael Mbizvo, Partson Zvandasara and Lynn Zijenah (University of Zimbabwe College of Health Sciences); Lidia Propper and Andrea Ruff (The Johns Hopkins Bloomberg School of Public Health, Department of International Health).

ANRS Ditrame Plus Cohort, Côte d'Ivoire

Principal Investigators: Francois Dabis, Valériane Leroy, Marguerite Timite-Konan, Christiane Welffens-Ekra.

Coordination in Abidjan: Laurence Bequet, Didier K. Ekouevi, Besigin Tonwe-Gold, Ida Viho.

Methodology, biostatistics and data management: Gérard Allou, Renaud Becquet, Katia Castetbon, Laurence Dequae-Merchadou, Charlotte Sakarovitch, Dominique Touchard.

Clinical team: Clarisse Amani-Bosse, Ignace Ayekoe, Gédéon Bedikou, Nacoumba Coulibaly, Christine Danel, Patricia Fassinou, Apollinaire Horo, Ruffin Likikouet, Hassan Toure. Laboratory team: André Inwoley, Francois Rouet, Ramata Touré.

Psycho-social team: Hortense Aka-Dago, Alphonse Sihé.

Social sciences team: Hélène Agbo, Hermann Brou, Annabel Desgrées-du-Lou , Annick Tijou-Traoré, Benjamin Zanou.

Good Start Cohort, South Africa

Mark Colvin, Mickey Chopra, Tanya Doherty, Debra Jackson, Jonathan Levin, Juana Willumsen, Ameena Goga, Pravi Moodley.

MASHI Trial, Botswana (Trial Registration: clinicaltrials.gov Identifier: NCT00197587).

Investigators: Ibou Thior, Shahin Lockman, Laura M. Smeaton, Roger L. Shapiro, Carolyn Wester, S. Jody Heymann, MD, Peter B. Gilbert, Lisa Stevens, Trevor Peter, PhD, Soyeon Kim, Erik van Widenfelt, Claire Moffat, Patrick Ndase, Peter Arimi, Poloko Kebaabetswe, Patson Mazonde, Joseph Makhema, Kenneth McIntosh, Vladimir Novitsky, Tun-Hou Lee, Richard Marlink, Stephen Lagakos, Max Essex.

Collaborators: Drs C. Anude and J. Chanda, study physicians; L. Makori, nursing diploma, study nurse; J. B. Moorad, T. A. Modise, T. Moyo, and M. Malamba, nursing and midwifery diplomas, study nurses; D. Arbi and K. Koloi, nursing diplomas, nurse recruiters; L. Dube and T. Mmolotsi, health education diplomas, health educators and recruiters; S. Babitseng and D. Mere, nursing diplomas, recruiters (Molepolole site); Dr J. Boyle, study physician; J. Magetse, V. Modikwa, and M. Tsuro, nursing and midwifery diplomas, study nurses; T. Sekoto, family nurse practitioner diploma, study nurse; L. Garebatho, nursing diploma, study nurse; M. Sesinyi and K. Kelebalekgosi, health educator diplomas, health educators and recruiters (Mochudi site); Dr Z. Tedla, study physician; G. Mayondi, K. Sebinang, J. Setswalo, nursing and midwifery diplomas, study nurses; N. Makubate, community health nursing and midwifery diploma, study nurse; L. Tsalaile, MSc nursing education, study nurse; B. Tsule, nursing diploma, study nurse; I. Thebeetsile, nursing diploma, nurse recruiter; I. Leteane and O. Makgabana, health education diplomas, health educators and recruiters (Lobatse Site); Drs. M. Mogodi, A. Owor, I. Hove, and A. Asmelash, study physicians; T. Kakhu, P. Ramalepa, and J. Lubinda, nursing and midwifery diplomas, study nurses; S. Ndebele, F. Modise, C. Bohule, K. Motshabi, and M. Ntshimane, nursing diplomas, nurse recruiters; (Gaborone site).

MITRA Plus Cohort, Tanzania

Investigators: Charles Kilewo, Katarina Karlsson, Matilda Ngarina, Augustine Massawe, Eligius Lyamuya, Andrew Swai, Rosina Lipyoga, Fred Mhalu, Gunnel Biberfeld.

Physicians: G. Msemo, B. Mohamed, J. Method, J. Yuda, E. Naburi.

Nurses: A. Mkumbukwa, E. Rugaiya, N. Makundi, A. Temu.

Laboratory Technologists: E. Mbena, D. Kalovya, V. Msangi, E Olausson-Hansson and A. Östborn.

Secretary: C. Lema.

Author Contributions

Conceived and designed the experiments: RB FD LM GG HMC ME DKE DJ AC CK VL SZW RN PM M-LN. Performed the experiments: RB FD LM GG HMC ME DKE DJ AC CK VL SZW RN PM M-LN. Analyzed the data: RB MM FD BZ PDG M-LN. Contributed reagents/materials/analysis tools: RB MM FD BZ PDG M-LN.

References

1. UNAIDS (2009) AIDS epidemic update (UNAIDS website. Available: http://www.unaids.org/en/dataanalysis/epidemiology/2009aidsepidemicupdate. Accessed 2011 December 7).
2. Marinda E, Humphrey JH, Iliff PJ, Mutasa K, Nathoo KJ, et al. (2007) Child mortality according to maternal and infant HIV status in Zimbabwe. Pediatr Infect Dis J 26: 519–526.
3. Newell ML, Coovadia H, Cortina-Borja M, Rollins N, Gaillard P, et al. (2004) Mortality of infected and uninfected infants born to HIV-infected mothers in Africa: a pooled analysis. Lancet 364: 1236–1243.
4. Kuhn L, Aldrovandi GM, Sinkala M, Kankasa C, Semrau K, et al. (2008) Effects of Early, Abrupt Weaning for HIV-free Survival of Children in Zambia. N Engl J Med 359: 130–141.
5. Six Week Extended-Dose Nevirapine (SWEN) Study Team (2008) Extended-dose nevirapine to 6 weeks of age for infants to prevent HIV transmission via breastfeeding in Ethiopia, India, and Uganda: an analysis of three randomised controlled trials. Lancet 372: 300–313.
6. Taha TE, Kumwenda NI, Gibbons A, Broadhead RL, Fiscus S, et al. (2003) Short postexposure prophylaxis in newborn babies to reduce mother-to-child transmission of HIV-1: NVAZ randomised clinical trial. Lancet 362: 1171–1177.
7. Thomas TK, Masaba R, Borkowf CB, Ndivo R, Zeh C, et al. (2011) Triple-antiretroviral prophylaxis to prevent mother-to-child HIV transmission through breastfeeding–the Kisumu Breastfeeding Study, Kenya: a clinical trial. PLoS Med 8: e1001015.
8. Gaillard P, Mwanyumba F, Verhofstede C, Claeys P, Chohan V, et al. (2001) Vaginal lavage with chlorhexidine during labour to reduce mother-to-child HIV transmission: clinical trial in Mombasa, Kenya. Aids 15: 389–396.
9. Moodley D, Moodley J, Coovadia H, Gray G, McIntyre J, et al. (2003) A Multicenter Randomized Controlled Trial of Nevirapine Versus a Combination of Zidovudine and Lamivudine to Reduce Intrapartum and Early Postpartum Mother-to-Child Transmission of Human Immunodeficiency Virus Type 1. J Infect Dis 187: 725–735.
10. Becquet R, Bequet L, Ekouevi DK, Viho I, Sakarovitch C, et al. (2007) Two-year morbidity–mortality and alternatives to prolonged breast-feeding among children born to HIV-infected mothers in Côte d'Ivoire. PLoS Medicine 4: e17.
11. Coovadia HM, Rollins NC, Bland RM, Little K, Coutsoudis A, et al. (2007) Mother-to-child transmission of HIV-1 infection during exclusive breastfeeding: the first six months of life. Lancet 369: 1607–1616.
12. Coutsoudis A, Pillay K, Spooner E, Kuhn L, Coovadia HM (1999) Influence of infant-feeding patterns on early mother-to-child transmission of HIV-1 in Durban, South Africa: a prospective cohort study. South African Vitamin A Study Group. Lancet 354: 471–476.
13. Dabis F, Msellati P, Meda N, Welffens-Ekra C, You B, et al. (1999) 6-month efficacy, tolerance, and acceptability of a short regimen of oral zidovudine to reduce vertical transmission of HIV in breastfed children in Cote d'Ivoire and Burkina Faso: a double-blind placebo-controlled multicentre trial. DITRAME Study Group. DIminution de la Transmission Mere-Enfant. Lancet 353: 786–792.
14. Humphrey JH, Iliff PJ, Marinda ET, Mutasa K, Moulton LH, et al. (2006) Effects of a single large dose of vitamin A, given during the postpartum period to HIV-positive women and their infants, on child HIV infection, HIV-free survival, and mortality. J Infect Dis 193: 860–871.
15. Jackson DJ, Chopra M, Doherty TM, Colvin MS, Levin JB, et al. (2007) Operational effectiveness and 36 week HIV-free survival in the South African programme to prevent mother-to-child transmission of HIV-1. Aids 21: 509–516.
16. Kilewo C, Karlsson K, Ngarina M, Massawe A, Lyamuya E, et al. (2009) Prevention of mother-to-child transmission of HIV-1 through breastfeeding by treating mothers with triple antiretroviral therapy in Dar es Salaam, Tanzania: the Mitra Plus study. J Acquir Immune Defic Syndr 52: 406–416.
17. Msellati P, Meda N, Leroy V, Likikouet R, Van de Perre P, et al. (1999) Safety and acceptability of vaginal disinfection with benzalkonium chloride in HIV infected pregnant women in west Africa: ANRS 049b phase II randomized, double blinded placebo controlled trial. DITRAME Study Group. Sex Transm Infect 75: 420–425.
18. Nduati R, John G, Mbori-Ngacha D, Richardson B, Overbaugh J, et al. (2000) Effect of breastfeeding and formula feeding on transmission of HIV-1: a randomized clinical trial. Jama 283: 1167–1174.
19. Petra study team (2002) Efficacy of three short-course regimens of zidovudine and lamivudine in preventing early and late transmission of HIV-1 from mother to child in Tanzania, South Africa, and Uganda (Petra study): a randomised, double-blind, placebo-controlled trial. Lancet 359: 1178–1186.
20. Thior I, Lockman S, Smeaton LM, Shapiro RL, Wester C, et al. (2006) Breastfeeding plus infant zidovudine prophylaxis for 6 months vs formula feeding plus infant zidovudine for 1 month to reduce mother-to-child HIV transmission in Botswana: a randomized trial: the Mashi Study. Jama 296: 794–805.
21. Wiktor SZ, Ekpini E, Karon JM, Nkengasong J, Maurice C, et al. (1999) Short-course oral zidovudine for prevention of mother-to-child transmission of HIV-1 in Abidjan, Cote d'Ivoire: a randomised trial. Lancet 353: 781–785.
22. Alioum A, Cortina-Borja M, Dabis F, Dequae-Merchadou L, Haverkamp G, et al. (2003) Estimating the efficacy of interventions to prevent mother-to-child transmission of human immunodeficiency virus in breastfeeding populations: comparing statistical methods. Am J Epidemiol 158: 596–605.
23. Alioum A, Dabis F, Dequae-Merchadou L, Haverkamp G, Hudgens M, et al. (2001) Estimating the efficacy of interventions to prevent mother-to-child transmission of HIV in breast-feeding populations: development of a consensus methodology. Stat Med 20: 3539–3556.
24. Newell ML, Brahmbhatt H, Ghys PD (2004) Child mortality and HIV infection in Africa: a review. AIDS 18: S27–S34.
25. Rollins NC, Coovadia HM, Bland RM, Coutsoudis A, Bennish ML, et al. (2007) Pregnancy outcomes in HIV-infected and uninfected women in rural and urban South Africa. J Acquir Immune Defic Syndr 44: 321–328.
26. Marston M, Becquet R, Zaba B, Moulton LH, Gray G, et al. (2011) Net survival of perinatally and postnatally HIV-infected children: a pooled analysis of individual data from sub-Saharan Africa. Int J Epidemiol.
27. Chakraborty R (2005) HIV-1 infection in children: a clinical and immunologic overview. Curr HIV Res 3: 31–41.
28. Becquet R, Ekouevi DK, Arrive E, Stringer J, Meda N, et al. (2009) Universal antiretroviral therapy for pregnant and breast-feeding HIV-infected women: towards the elimination of mother-to-child transmission of HIV-1 in resource-limited settings. Clin Infect Dis 49: 1936–1945.
29. WHO (2010) Recommendations for Use of Antiretroviral Drugs for Treating Pregnant Women and Preventing HIV Infection in Infants. Guidelines on Care, Treatment and Support for Women Living with HIV/AIDS and their Children in Resource-Constrained Settings (WHO website. Available: http://www.who.int/hiv/pub/mtct/guidelines/en/. Accessed 2011 December 7).
30. Ndirangu J, Newell ML, Tanser F, Herbst AJ, Bland R (2010) Decline in early life mortality in a high HIV prevalence rural area of South Africa: evidence of HIV prevention or treatment impact? Aids 24: 593–602.
31. Stover J, Johnson P, Hallett T, Marston M, Becquet R, et al. (2010) The Spectrum projection package: improvements in estimating incidence by age and sex, mother-to-child transmission, HIV progression in children and double orphans. Sex Transm Infect 86 Suppl 2: ii16–21.

16

Interethnic Differences in Antigen-Presenting Cell Activation and TLR Responses in Malian Children during *Plasmodium falciparum* Malaria

Charles Arama[1,2*☯], Pablo Giusti[1☯], Stéphanie Boström[1], Victor Dara[2], Boubacar Traore[2], Amagana Dolo[2], Ogobara Doumbo[2], Stefania Varani[1,3,4] , Marita Troye-Blomberg[1]

1 Department of Immunology, Wenner-Gren Institute, Stockholm University, Stockholm, Sweden, **2** Malaria Research and Training Centre, Faculty of Medicine, Pharmacy and Dentistry, University of Bamako, Bamako, Mali, **3** Department of Laboratory Medicine, Division of Clinical Microbiology, Karolinska University Hospital, Huddinge, Sweden, **4** Department of Haematology and Clinical Oncology, "L. and A. Seragnoli", University of Bologna, Bologna, Italy

Abstract

The Fulani ethnic group from West Africa is relatively better protected against *Plasmodium falciparum* malaria as compared to other sympatric ethnic groups, such as the Dogon. However, the mechanisms behind this lower susceptibility to malaria are largely unknown, particularly those concerning innate immunity. Antigen-presenting cells (APCs), and in particular dendritic cells (DCs) are important components of the innate and adaptive immune systems. Therefore, in this study we investigated whether APCs obtained from Fulani and Dogon children exhibited differences in terms of activation status and toll-like receptor (TLR) responses during malaria infection. Lower frequency and increased activation was observed in circulating plasmacytoid DCs and BDCA-3^{+} myeloid DCs of infected Fulani as compared to their uninfected counterparts. Conversely, a higher frequency and reduced activation was observed in the same DC subsets obtained from peripheral blood of *P. falciparum*-infected Dogon children as compared to their uninfected peers. Moreover, infected individuals of both ethnic groups exhibited higher percentages of both classical and inflammatory monocytes that were less activated as compared to their non-infected counterparts. In line with APC impairment during malaria infection, TLR4, TLR7 and TLR9 responses were strongly inhibited by *P. falciparum* infection in Dogon children, while no such TLR inhibition was observed in the Fulani children. Strikingly, the TLR-induced IFN-γ release was completely abolished in the Dogon undergoing infection while no difference was seen within infected and non-infected Fulani. Thus, *P. falciparum* infection is associated with altered activation status of important APC subsets and strongly inhibited TLR responses in peripheral blood of Dogon children. In contrast, *P. falciparum* induces DC activation and does not affect the innate response to specific TLR ligands in Fulani children. These findings suggest that DCs and TLR signalling may be of importance for the protective immunity against malaria observed in the Fulani.

Editor: Francesco Dieli, University of Palermo, Italy

Funding: This work was supported by grants from the Swedish Agency for Research and Development with Developing Countries, http://www.sida.se (Sida/SAREC SWE 1995-117), the European and Developing Countries Clinical Partnership's grant, http://www.edctp.org (EDCTP CG-TA 05 40204_003), as well as a grant within the BioMalPar European Network of Excellence, http://www.biomalpar.org (LSHP-CT-2004-503578) and from the European Community's Seventh Framework Programme, http://www.evimalar.org/ (FP7/2007-2013) under grant agreement N°242095. The funders had no role in study design, data collection and analysis, decision to publish, or preparation of the manuscript.

Competing Interests: The authors have declared that no competing interests exist.

* E-mail: charles.arama@wgi.su.se

☯ These authors contributed equally to this work.

¶ These authors also contributed equally to this work.

Introduction

Half of the world's population remains at risk of contracting malaria. During 2008 malaria was estimated to be responsible for 767.000 deaths in Africa alone, mostly in children below the age of 5 [1]. Previous studies performed in a rural area in Mali have shown different susceptibility to *Plasmodium falciparum* (*P. falciparum*) infection between two ethnic groups; the Fulani and the Dogon. These populations live under similar social, cultural and geographic conditions and are exposed to identical malaria pressure [2]. However, the Fulani show less clinical symptoms of malaria, and parasites are less frequently detected in their blood [3,4]. In addition, they exhibit higher titres of *P. falciparum*-specific IgG subclasses [3], and IgM antibodies [4,5]. Recent evidence shows lower numbers of regulatory T cells [6] and more potent early IFN-γ responses against the parasite [7] in Fulani as compared to other sympatric ethnic groups, suggesting that these immunological phenomena can lead to more robust anti-malarial immunity. Nevertheless, little is known about the functionality of innate immunity in Fulani and sympatric ethnic groups and how this branch of immunity influences susceptibility to malaria infection.

Innate immunity has two important functions in the defence against the parasite. First, it acts to inhibit rapid parasite growth thereby limiting the onset of malaria pathology. Second, it is crucial for the development of parasite-specific adaptive immunity

[8]. Antigen-presenting cells (APCs), and in particular dendritic cells (DCs) are important components of the innate and adaptive branches of the immune system. In humans, two main populations of DCs have been described in peripheral blood; the CD11c$^-$, CD123$^+$, blood dendritic cell antigen (BDCA)-2$^+$ plasmacytoid DCs (pDCs) and the CD11c$^+$, CD123$^-$ myeloid DCs (mDCs). The latter can be further divided into three subtypes; the BDCA-1$^+$ DCs, the BDCA-3$^+$ DCs and the CD16$^+$ DCs [9–11].

It has been shown that monocyte/macrophage- and mDC functions are impaired *in vitro* by the malaria parasite or by products derived from infection [12–14]. Another study has shown that HLA-DR levels are decreased on circulating DCs of *P. falciparum*-infected children as compared to healthy controls [15]. In addition, higher numbers of circulating BDCA-3$^+$ mDCs have been detected in the blood of severely infected children combined with reduced immunostimulatory ability. This indicates that malaria may impair mDC functionality and suggests that the BDCA-3$^+$ DC subset may play a crucial role in the immune response against the parasite in humans [16,17].

P. falciparum also modulates pDC responses *in vitro* by inducing increased secretion of interferon (IFN)-α [18]. Daily injection of this cytokine protects against severe malaria caused by *P. berghei* in mice [19] and higher plasma levels of IFN-α have been associated with milder *P. falciparum* malaria episodes in humans [20]. However, while mDCs are crucial in triggering an effective T-cell response during malaria infection, pDCs are not required for the induction of malaria parasite-specific responses as recently shown in murine models of experimental infection [21,22].

Evidence demonstrates a fundamental role for monocytes in activation of NK cells [23] and in differentiation of regulatory T cells [24] upon *P. falciparum* stimulation *in vitro*. Nevertheless, the role of this cell subset during the infection in the natural host is only partially understood. Monocytes can trigger adaptive immune responses and contribute to parasite clearance through antibody-dependent cellular inhibition and phagocytosis [25]. Two major monocyte subpopulations have been described [26]; one classical (CD14$^+$CD16$^-$) and one inflammatory (CD14$^+$CD16$^+$) [27]; the latter has been found to be increased during acute uncomplicated malaria [28,29]. A recent study reported that the levels of CD16/Fcγ receptor IIIA on CD16$^+$ monocytes were higher in children with severe *P. falciparum* anaemia, which could enhance erythrophagocytosis and TNF-α production in this cell subset [30].

APCs interact with pathogens through specialized receptors termed pattern-recognition receptors (PRRs) that have evolved to detect danger signals such as pathogen-associated molecular patterns (PAMPs) [31]. A well-studied family of PRRs are the toll-like receptors (TLRs) [32], which are expressed differently in different APC populations. The monocyte and mDC subsets express mainly TLR1 through TLR6, while TLR7 and TLR9 are expressed in pDCs [33,34]. Recent evidence suggests that TLRs are central mediators of pro-inflammatory responses during malaria [35–37]. For example, it is known that *Plasmodium* DNA bound to either malaria pigment [37] or protein components [38], activates the TLR9 pathway and that *P. falciparum* glycosylphosphatidylinositol (GPI) activates TLR2 [39]. However, the role of TLRs in the development of immunity to malaria and in the pathology of malaria is not well understood.

In this study, we evaluated the activation status of different DC and monocyte subpopulations in peripheral blood of Fulani and Dogon children with or without *P. falciparum* malaria infection in an endemic area of Mali. In addition, the impact of *P. falciparum* on the activation of APCs was examined by stimulating peripheral blood mononuclear cells (PBMCs) with specific TLR ligands. LPS was employed to activate TLR4 on monocytes and mDC subsets while imiquimod and CpG-A ODN were used to selectively stimulate TLR7 and TLR9, respectively, which are expressed in pDCs [9,10,40].

Results

Study subject characteristics

The mean age of the Dogon children was 6.36 years for uninfected and 6.70 years for the infected ones. In the Fulani children, the mean age was 6.44 years for uninfected and 4.50 years for the infected ones. The infected Fulani were younger than the infected Dogon (Table 1). During *P. falciparum* infection, the mean temperature was significantly higher in the infected Dogon (37.74°C) as compared to infected Fulani (36.71°C, $p \leq 0.05$). The mean parasite density was 18758 [150-122000] asexual parasites/µl for Fulani and 13845 [575-48625] asexual parasites/µl for the Dogon.

Interethnic and intraethnic differences in the frequency and immunophenotype of blood DCs during *P. falciparum* infection

Circulating DCs are defined as leukocyte lineage negative and HLA-DR positive mononuclear cells [41]. Blood DCs were divided into four different subsets by employing monoclonal antibodies against the surface markers BDCA-1, BDCA-2, BDCA-3 and CD16 after gating lineage negative PBMCs. The activation status of each subset was assessed by measuring HLA-DR and CD86 levels.

The infected Dogon exhibited significantly higher frequency of circulating BDCA-2$^+$ ($p = 0.034$) and BDCA-3$^+$ ($p = 0.016$) DCs than their uninfected peers (Figure 1A). Conversely, the infected Fulani had a slightly reduced frequency of BDCA-2$^+$ ($p = 0.060$) and BDCA-3$^+$ ($p = 0.038$) DCs as compared to their uninfected peers. When comparing only the infected children from each ethnic group, the percentage of circulating BDCA-2$^+$ and BDCA-3$^+$ DCs was significantly lower in Fulani as compared to Dogon ($p = 0.04$ and $p = 0.01$, respectively). No interethnic differences were observed between the uninfected children from each group. A similar trend was observed when evaluating absolute numbers of BDCA-2$^+$ and BDCA-3$^+$ DCs/ml of blood although differences were not significant (data not shown). The percentage and absolute numbers of circulating CD16$^+$ and BDCA-1$^+$ DCs did not show any inter- or intra-ethnic difference (Figure 1A and data not shown).

When examining DC-activation status, we observed that expression levels of the activation marker HLA-DR was significantly lower on all examined DC subsets in the infected Dogon as compared to uninfected peers (Figure 1B). In addition, the Dogon children undergoing infection had a decreased expression of CD86 on BDCA-2$^+$ DCs (Figure 1C) as compared to their uninfected peers ($p = 0.0003$). Conversely, the infected Fulani children exhibited significantly increased levels of HLA-DR on pDCs ($p = 0.009$) and slightly increased levels of HLA-DR on BDCA-3$^+$ mDCs ($p = 0.057$) as compared to uninfected peers. In addition, expression levels of HLA-DR were reduced on CD16$^+$ mDCs of both Dogon and Fulani children undergoing infection as compared to their uninfected peers.

When comparing children undergoing infection from each ethnic group, the Fulani exhibited higher levels of HLA-DR and CD86 on the BDCA-1$^+$, BDCA-2$^+$ and BDCA-3$^+$ DCs but not on CD16$^+$ DCs as compared to the infected Dogon children. Thus, interethnic differences were observed in terms of blood DC activation status upon malaria and all circulating DC subpopulations excluding

Table 1. Baseline characteristics of the study population.

n = 77	Mean age (Year)	Mean Hb level (g/dL)	Mean body weight (Kg)	Parasitaemia Mean [min-max] (parasites/μL)	Mean axillary temperature (°C)
Uninfected Dogon	6.36	10.36	19.25	-	36.43
Infected Dogon	6.70	9.80	20.15	13845 [575-48625]	37.74
Uninfected Fulani	6.44	9.78	17	-	36.71
Infected Fulani	4.50	9.36	12.93	18758 [150-122000]	36.81
P values	*DI-FI *F-FI	NS	*DI-FI *F-FI	NS	*D-DI *DI-FI

Note. D: Uninfected Dogon; DI: Infected Dogon; F: Uninfected Fulani; FI: Infected Fulani;
*p value≤0.05 Fisher exact test (Anova); NS: not significant.

CD16$^+$ DCs were significantly more mature in Fulani than in Dogon children during *P. falciparum* infection. In order to evaluate if these differences could be dependent on parasite burdens, we correlated levels of parasitaemia with HLA-DR expression levels on the affected DC subpopulations from each study participant. No significant correlation was observed in Dogon and Fulani children undergoing *P. falciparum* infection. For BDCA-1$^+$ DCs the results of the correlation tests were Rho = −0.38 (p = 0.106) for Dogon children and Rho = 0.20 (p = 0.72) for Fulani children. For BDCA-2$^+$ DCs the results were Rho = −0.16 (p = 0.49) for Dogon children and Rho = 0.20 (p = 0.72) for Fulani children. For BDCA-3$^+$ DCs the results were Rho = −0.28 (p = 0.22) for infected Dogon children and Rho = −0.40 (p = 0.48) for infected Fulani children. This suggests that the differences observed in the DC subpopulations could not be correlated to the differences in parasite burden between the populations.

Interethnic and intraethnic differences in monocyte frequency and activation status during *P. falciparum* infection

Given the importance of monocytes in inflammation and clearance of parasites, we investigated the classical (CD14$^+$CD16$^-$) and inflammatory (CD14$^+$CD16$^+$) monocytic subsets during *P. falciparum* infection in the children participating in the study.

A significantly increased proportion of both classical (p = 0.02) and inflammatory (p = 0.02) monocytes was observed in Dogon children undergoing infection as compared to their uninfected peers. A similar trend, although not significant, was found between infected and non-infected Fulani (Figure 2A).

When examining the activation status of circulating monocytes, a significantly decreased expression of HLA-DR was observed on classical monocytes from both Dogon and Fulani groups undergoing infection as compared to their uninfected peers (p = 0.0001 and p = 0.004, respectively; Figure 2B). A decreased expression of HLA-DR was also observed in inflammatory monocytes of Fulani (p = 0.02) but not of Dogon children (p = 0.41) undergoing infection as compared to their uninfected peers. Finally, in infected Dogon children the expression of the co-stimulatory marker CD86 was also significantly impaired on classical and inflammatory monocytes as compared to uninfected peers (Figure 2C). When comparing children undergoing infection from each ethnic group, the Fulani exhibited higher levels of HLA-DR and CD86 on classical but not on inflammatory monocytes as compared to Dogon children. Thus, interethnic differences were observed in classical monocytes during malaria infection and these cells were significantly more activated in infected Fulani than in infected Dogon children.

P. falciparum infection impairs cytokine responses upon TLR stimulation in Dogon but not in Fulani children

The ability of APCs to secrete cytokines upon TLR stimulation was investigated by stimulating PBMCs with ligands for TLR4, TLR7 and TLR9, i.e. LPS, imiquimod and CpG-A, respectively.

In Dogon, the TLR4 pathway was strongly impaired during *P. falciparum* infection, as shown by inhibited production of IL-1β, IL-6, IL-10, TNF-α and IFN-γ by PBMCs upon LPS stimulation (Figure 3). Similarly, release of IL-1β, IL-6, IL-10, TNF-α, IFN-α and IFN-γ was inhibited in infected Dogon as compared to uninfected peers when PBMCs were treated with a TLR9 ligand. Also TLR7 responses were impaired upon *P. falciparum* infection in Dogon children and IFN-α and TNF-α levels were lower in PBMCs stimulated with imiquimod in infected Dogon as compared to their uninfected peers.

Conversely, no differences were observed in cytokine release between PBMCs obtained from infected and uninfected Fulani upon TLR4, TLR7 and TLR9 stimulation (Figure 3). As compared to infected Dogon children, the infected Fulani secreted significantly higher levels of IL-1β, IL-6, IL-10, TNF-α and IFN-γ upon TLR4 stimulation and higher levels of IL-6, IFN-α, TNF-α and IFN-γ when PBMCs were stimulated with TLR7 or TLR9 ligands.

Taken together, these results indicate that *P. falciparum* infection impaired TLR4-, TLR7-, and TLR9-induced cytokine responses in the Dogon children, while such responses were unaffected in the Fulani children. As a consequence, the levels of most cytokines that were released upon TLR stimulation were higher in Fulani than Dogon children undergoing *P. falciparum* infection.

To further analyse the clinical relevance of the cytokines secreted by the PBMCs from Dogon and Fulani children when exposed to *P. falciparum* infection, the ratios of TNF-α/IL10 and IFN-γ/IL-10 were calculated. The TNF-α/IL10 ratio was significantly decreased upon *P. falciparum* infection in Dogon children when PBMCs were stimulated with TLR7 (p = 0.02) and TLR9 (p = 0.01) ligands, indicating an impaired pro-inflammatory activity in these specific TLR pathways upon *P. falciparum* infection in this ethnic group (Figure 4A). Conversely, the TNF-α/IL10 ratio was slightly increased upon *P. falciparum* infection in Dogon children when PBMCs were stimulated with LPS (p = 0.08). This might indicate that the TLR4 signalling pathway may be less affected than the TLR7 and TLR9 signalling in Dogon undergoing infection. This ratio was not affected in infected Fulani as compared to uninfected peers upon TLR4, TLR7 and TLR9 stimulation. When comparing children undergoing infection from each ethnic group, the TNF-α/IL-10 ratio was higher in Fulani than Dogon children when cells were stimulated with TLR9 ligands (p = 0.04), suggesting a significantly higher proinflammatory activity induced by TLR9

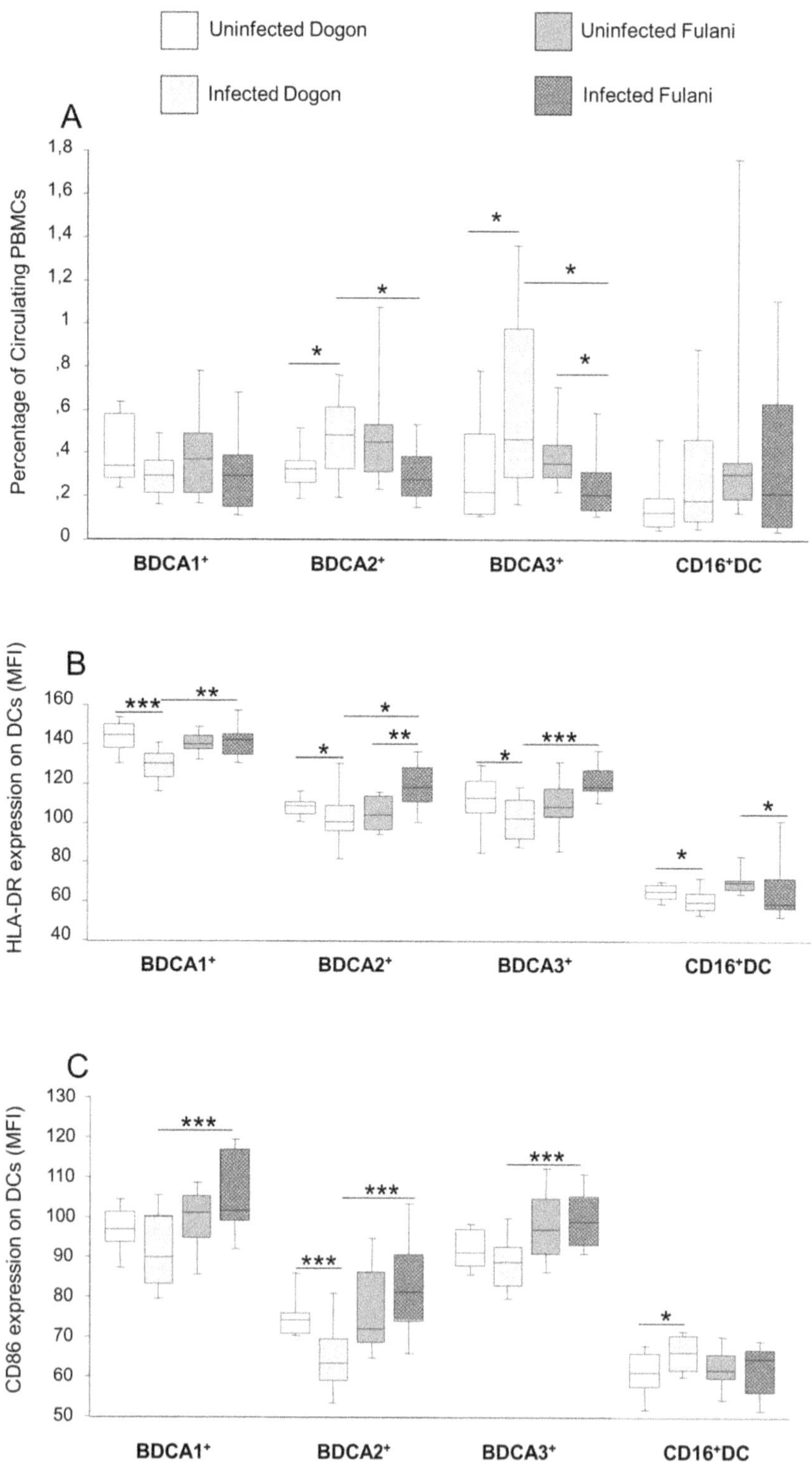

Figure 1. Interethnic and intraethnic differences in the frequency and activation markers of blood DCs. PBMCs from the study participants were stained with monoclonal antibodies for subsequent flow cytometric analysis using a FACSCalibur. The samples were categorised as uninfected Dogon (n = 20), infected Dogon (n = 20), uninfected Fulani (n = 13) and infected Fulani (n = 10). An increase was observed of BDCA2$^+$ and BDCA3$^+$ cells in the circulation of infected Dogon whereas the opposite was seen for the Fulani (Figure 1A). The expression of activation marker HLA-DR (Figure 1B) and CD86 (Figure 1C) was lower in BDCA2$^+$ and BDCA3$^+$ cells of the Dogon when undergoing infection while it was increased in the Fulani. It is known that DCs travel to the lymph nodes upon activation. Therefore, it is possible that the lower numbers seen in the infected Fulani is a consequence of activation. The boxplots illustrate the medians and the 25th and 75th quartile and the whiskers represent the 10% and 90% percentiles. Data were analyzed by Mann-Whitney rank sum test. *; $p \leq 0.05$. **;$p < 0.01$. ***; $p < 0.001$.

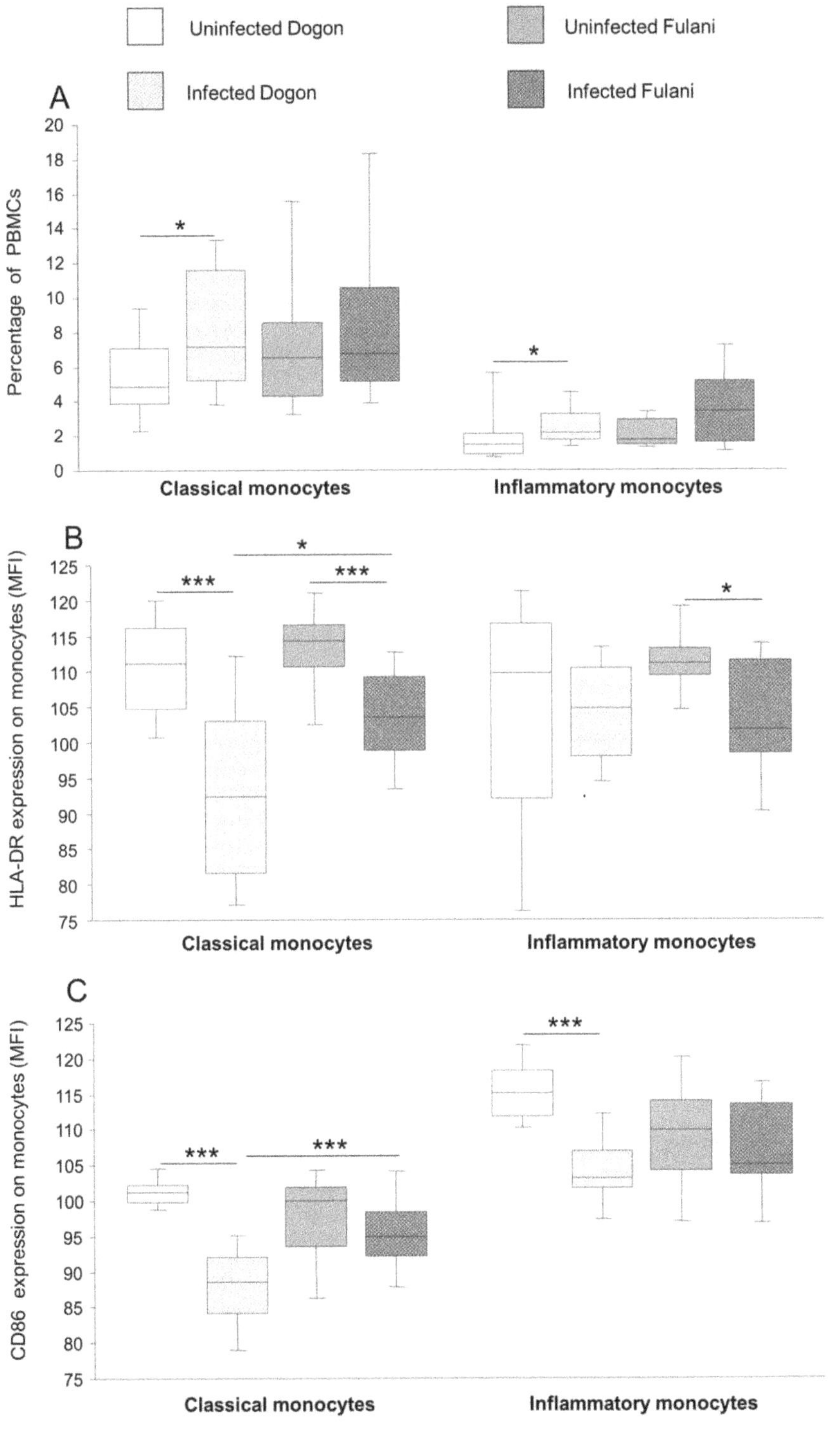

Figure 2. Interethnic and intraethnic differences in the frequency and activation markers of circulating monocytes. PBMCs were stained with monoclonal antibodies and subsequently analyzed using FACSCalibur. The samples were categorized as uninfected Dogon (n = 20), infected Dogon (n = 20), uninfected Fulani (n = 13) and infected Fulani (n = 10). An increase of circulating monocytes was observed for both groups although only statistically significant for the Dogon (Figure 2A). There was a decreased expression of HLA-DR (Figure 2B) in classical monocytes for both ethnic groups. The levels of HLA-DR were also suppressed in the inflammatory monocytes although not statistically significant for the Dogon. The expression of CD86 (Figure 2C) was decreased on both monocytic subsets although only statistically significant for the Dogon classical monocytes from both Dogon and Fulani. Although the levels of activation markers seem similarly regulated in both groups the classical monocytes of the Fulani exhibit a pattern of higher activation when undergoing infection than the Dogon when infected. The boxplots illustrate the medians and the 25th and 75th quartile and the whiskers represent the 10% and 90% percentiles. Data were analyzed by Mann-Whitney rank sum test. *; $p \leq 0.05$. ***; $p < 0.001$.

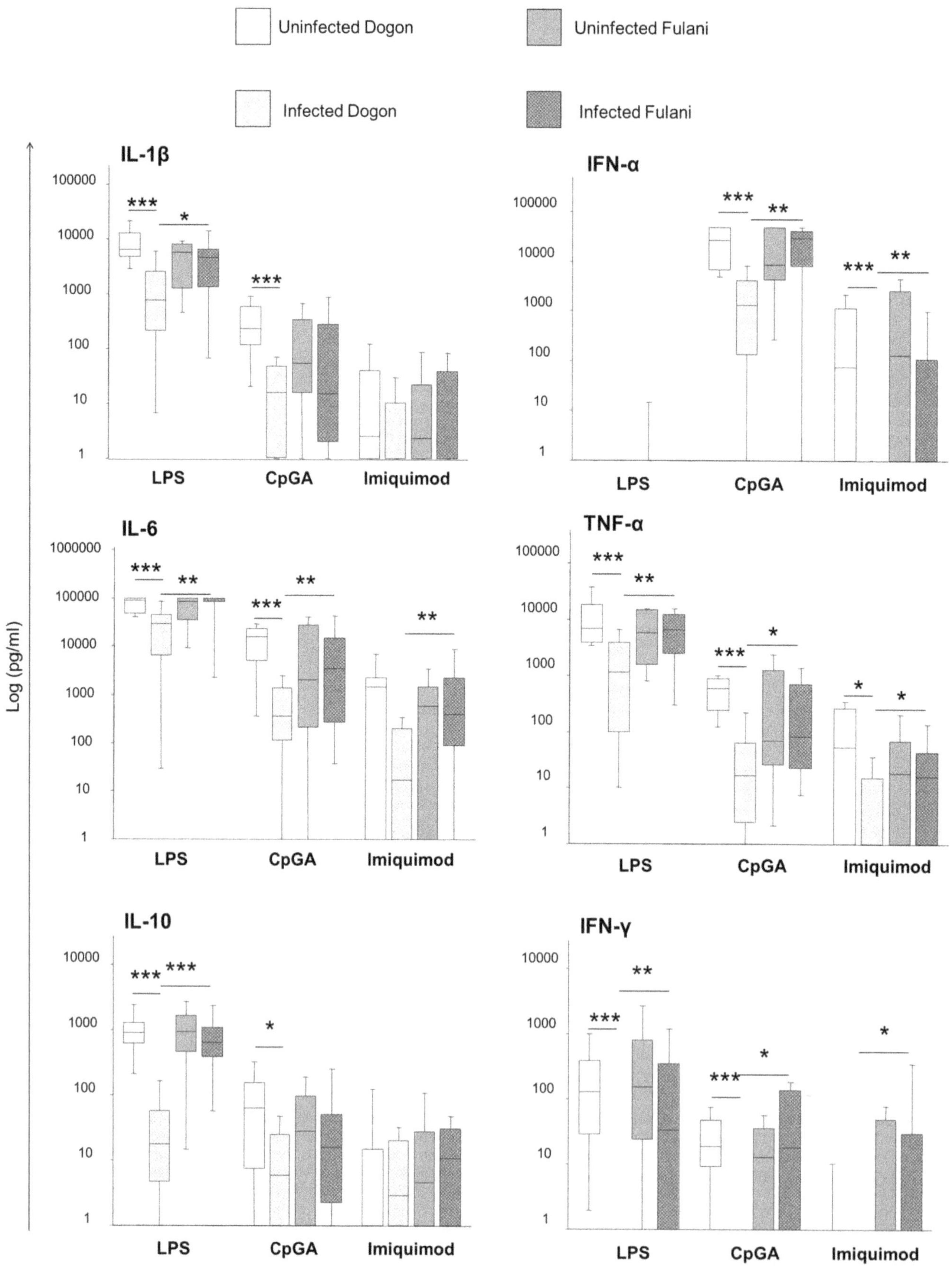
Uninfected Dogon
Uninfected Fulani
Infected Dogon
Infected Fulani
Log (pg/ml)
IL-1β
IFN-α
IL-6
TNF-α
IL-10
IFN-γ
LPS
CpGA
Imiquimod

Figure 3. TLR-induced cytokine responses in PBMCs from Dogon and Fulani children with or without *P. falciparum* infection. PBMCs (1 million/ml) were stimulated or not with LPS (100 ng/ml), CpG-A (3 μg/ml) or imiquimod (1 μg/ml). After 16 hours, supernatants were collected and analysed for the presence of cytokines. The samples were categorized as uninfected Dogon (n = 20), infected Dogon (n = 20), uninfected Fulani (n = 14) and infected Fulani (n = 23). The levels of IL-1β, IL-6, IL-10, TNF-α and INF-γ were severely supressed in the infected Dogon as compared to their uninfected peers when the cells had been stimulated with either LPS or CpGA. As a result, the levels of the infected Fulani were higher than infected Dogon for all cytokines except for IFN-α when stimulated with LPS and except for IL-1β and IL-10 when stimulated with CpG. Similarly, when stimulated with imiquimod cells of the infected Fulani secreted higher levels of IL-6, IFN-α, TNF-α and INF-γ than the infected Dogon due to the suppressed secretion of Dogon when undergoing infection. Data presented as box plots illustrate the medians and the 25th and 75th quartile and the whiskers represent the 10% and 90% percentiles. Data were analyzed using Mann-Whitney rank sum test. *; $p \leq 0.05$. **; $p<0.01$. ***; $p<0.001$.

ligation in Fulani than Dogon children undergoing *P. falciparum* infection. Similarly, the ratio of IFN-γ/IL-10 was decreased in the infected Dogon children as compared to their uninfected peers upon stimulation with TLR4 ($p<0.0001$) and TLR9 ($p<0.0001$; Figure 4B). When comparing PBMCs obtained from children undergoing infection from each ethnic group, the IFN-γ/IL-10 ratio was significantly higher in Fulani than in Dogon upon stimulation with TLR4 and TLR9 ligands ($p = 0.002$ and $p = 0.0051$; respectively). The same patterns were observed for cells stimulated with TLR7 although the data did not reach statistical significance. Thus, these data confirm that, during *P. falciparum* malaria infection, PBMCs from Fulani children exhibit a higher pro-inflammatory profile upon TLR stimulation as compared to the Dogon children.

Discussion

In this study, we investigated certain aspects of the innate immunity to malaria in children from two different ethnic groups that live in a malaria endemic area in Mali and exhibit different susceptibility to *P. falciparum* infection. The impact of ethnicity on allele and genotype frequency for innate soluble factors, such as IL-4 and IL-10, has been previously established in asymptomatic individuals belonging to Dogon and Fulani's groups in Mali [42]. However, functional studies focusing on the role of *P. falciparum* in affecting innate responses in these two ethnic groups are lacking.

Our findings indicate that *P. falciparum* infection inhibited the expression of HLA-DR in mDCs and pDCs in Dogon children. These results are in line with previous findings showing reduced expression of HLA-DR on mDCs of Kenyan children during acute malaria [15]. HLA class II expression on DCs is fundamental for presenting antigens to T cells and inducing their activation [43]. Higher numbers of circulating BDCA-3$^+$ mDCs have been detected in blood of severely infected children [16]. Similarly, we observed that the frequency of this mDC subset was increased in peripheral blood of Dogon children undergoing malaria infection as compared to uninfected peers. It has also been previously shown that APCs from children with severe malaria exhibit lower immunostimulatory abilities than those of healthy children [16]. Thus, the reduced expression of HLA-DR on the surface of DCs in Dogon children undergoing malaria infection may indicate impaired DC functionality, which in turn, may contribute to impaired cell-mediated responses.

Conversely, higher activation levels were observed in blood pDCs and BDCA-3$^+$ mDCs of infected Fulani as compared to uninfected children belonging to the same ethnic group. It is known that DC activation is coupled to increased cell migration to lymphoid organs [41]. Therefore, activation of these DC subsets may trigger their migration to the spleen and other lymphoid organs and thereby account for the lower frequency of pDCs, and BDCA-3$^+$ mDCs observed in the peripheral blood of infected Fulani. However, the absolute numbers of circulating DCs were only slightly affected by malaria infection in Fulani. Therefore, the reduced frequency of these DC subsets in infected subjects may also be explained by a relative increase in some other leukocyte population. In fact, it is known that the Fulani have a higher spleen rate than other sympatric ethnic groups [2,5,44,45] that could be coupled to an increased number of T- and B-cell subsets in circulation. Thus, it is possible that circulating BDCA-3$^+$ mDCs and pDCs become activated and migrate to secondary lymphoid organs such as the spleen to a higher extent in the Fulani than in the Dogon during malaria infection.

Recent evidence suggests that BDCA-3$^+$ DCs in humans exhibit superior capacity in stimulating cytotoxic T-cell (CTL) responses. These cells may be the counterpart of murine CD8-α$^+$ DCs [11,46], which are known to cross-present parasite antigens and mediate effective CTL responses against blood stage *P. berghei* in a murine model of malaria [47]. In addition, pDCs are known to play a crucial role in triggering humoral immunity against viruses [48,49]. Thus, the specific activation of these DC subsets observed in the Fulani, but not in the Dogon, during *P. falciparum* infection may contribute to more robust anti-malarial cellular IFN-γ responses [7] and antibody responses [3,5,44,50] that have been observed in the Fulani as compared to other sympatric ethnic groups.

The frequencies of both classical and inflammatory monocytes were increased both in Dogon and Fulani children upon *P. falciparum* infection. These results are in accordance with previous findings in Thai-Burmese patients where patients with acute malaria exhibited a higher frequency of inflammatory monocytes in peripheral blood [28]. We also found that *P. falciparum* infection impaired monocyte immunophenotypes, as reflected by the reduced expression of activation markers on classical and inflammatory monocytes in both Fulani and Dogon children, suggesting that *P. falciparum* alters the functionality of these cells in both ethnic groups. However, interethnic differences were observed during malaria infection as classical monocytes were significantly more activated in infected Fulani than in infected Dogon children.

To further evaluate the innate response in the Fulani and Dogon children during malaria infection, we investigated cytokine release by PBMCs after stimulation with specific TLR ligands. Cytokines are crucial in the pathogenesis of malaria and the balance between pro- and anti- inflammatory cytokines plays a central role in the clinical outcome of this infection [51,52]. In this context, we report that, in Dogon children, TLR4, TLR7 and TLR9 pathways were impaired by *P. falciparum* infection while such TLR inhibition was not observed in the Fulani children. This is in line with the impairment of DC phenotype that was observed in Dogon but not Fulani children upon malaria infection. In humans, TLR7 and TLR9 are mainly expressed in pDCs and it has been established that TLR9 is involved in recognition of malarial products [37,38,53]. It is also known that TLR7 and TLR9 signalling mediates robust induction of type I IFNs, increased cross presentation of antigens and strong CTL responses [54,55]. In our study, impairment has been specifically observed in the pro-inflammatory activity of these two TLR pathways upon *P. falciparum* infection in Dogon children, but not in the Fulani ethnic group.

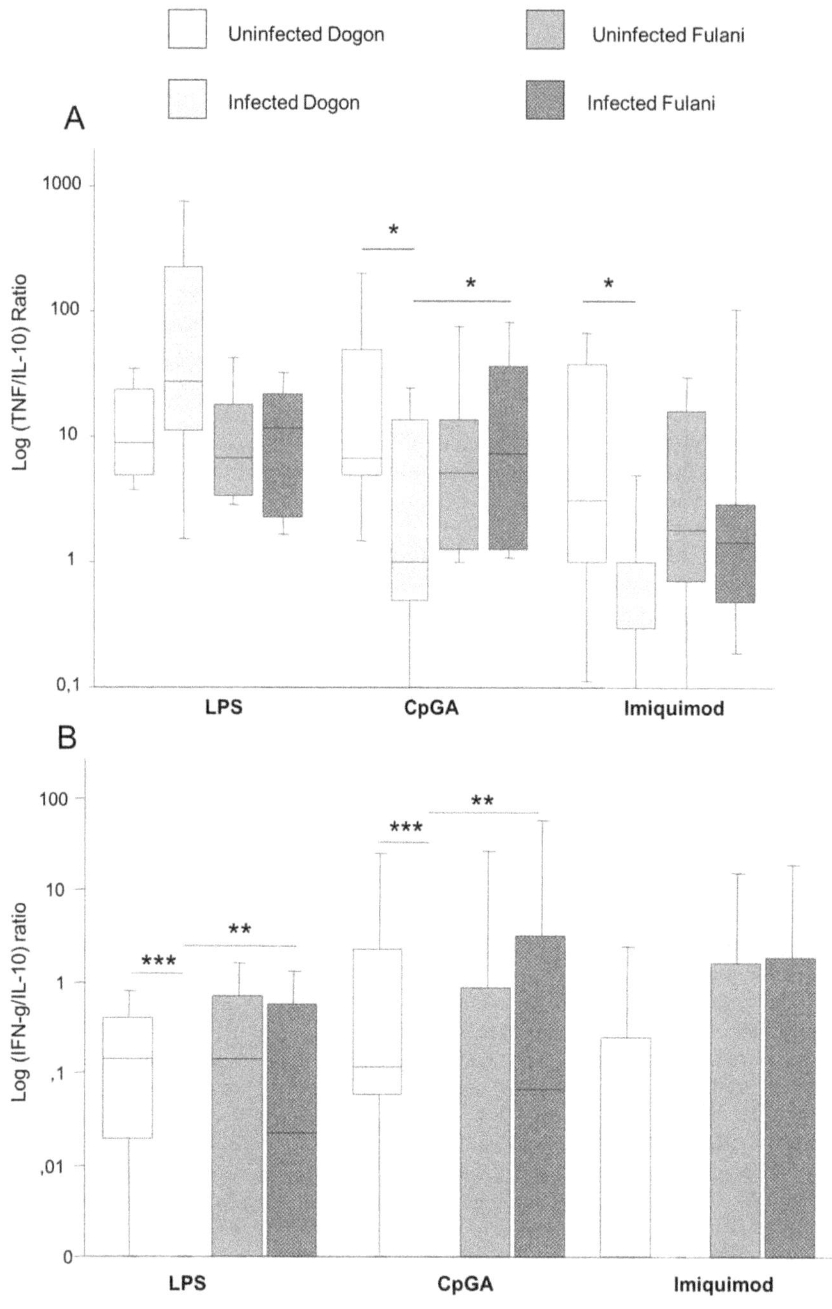

Figure 4. Interethnic and intraethnic differences in the TNF-α/IL-10 and IFN-γ/IL-10 ratios upon TLR stimulation of PBMCs. PBMCs (1 million/ml) were stimulated or not with LPS (100 ng/ml), CpG-A (3 μg/ml) or imiquimod (1 μg/ml). After 16 hours, supernatants were collected, cytokine levels were analyzed and the TNF-α/IL-10 (Figure 4A) and IFN-γ/IL-10 (Figure 4B) ratios were calculated. The samples from 77 children were categorized as uninfected Dogon (n = 20), infected Dogon (n = 20), uninfected Fulani (n = 23) and infected Fulani (n = 14). The TNF-α/IL-10 ratio (Figure 4A) was significantly lower in the infected Dogon as compared to their uninfected peers when stimulated with CpG or imiquimod. This resulted in significantly higher TNF-α/IL-10 ratio of infected Fulani as compared to the infected Dogon. Due to the severe suppression of IFN-γ the IFN-γ/IL-10 ratios (Figure 4B) were severely suppressed in the LPS and CpG stimulated cells of the Dogon and therefore higher in the infected Fulani than in the infected Dogon. The boxplots illustrate the medians and the 25th and 75th quartile and the whiskers represent the 10% and 90% percentiles. Data were analyzed using Mann-Whitney rank sum test. *; $p \leq 0.05$. **; $p < 0.01$. ***; $p < 0.001$.

In general, the importance of TLRs in malaria is underlined by the fact that TLR4 polymorphisms can predispose to severe malaria [56] and that polymorphisms in both TLR4 and TLR9 may play a role in the severity of pregnancy associated malaria [57]. Contradictory findings however, have been reported about the effect of malaria infection on TLR signalling. Enhanced pro-inflammatory cytokine production has been shown in response to TLR1/2, TLR4, TLR7/8 and TLR9 stimulation in PBMCs obtained from volunteers undergoing experimental malaria [58] or patients with natural infection [59], while others have suggested that malaria has a suppressive effect on TLR signalling, possibly through cross-tolerance following recognition of *Plasmodium* antigens by TLRs [60]. In partial agreement with the latter study, we observed that *P. falciparum* infection suppresses TLR responses in Dogon children while no effects were observed in the Fulani children. There may be several reasons for the discrepancies seen in these studies. Firstly, both the studies by McCall et *al.* and Franklin et *al.* were performed in adults while, in our study, only children were included. Secondly, these studies were performed in malaria naïve adults at the earliest stages of *P. falciparum* infection [58] and in an area with low transmission of malaria [61], respectively. Conversely, our study area is mesoendemic with high transmission during rainy seasons. As this work was performed at the end of the rainy season, the children included in our study should have experienced at least 2 episodes of *P. falciparum* infection during the same season as estimated by previous observations in the same area (Arama C. unpublished results). Thus, malaria infection may have a biphasic influence on the innate immune system, initially inducing TLR priming and then, in case of frequent exposure to the parasite, tolerance will ensue. Interestingly, such a suppressive phase was observed in Dogon but not in the children belonging to the Fulani ethnic group.

Moreover, we observed higher release of IFN-γ by PBMCs of infected Fulani children as compared to infected Dogon upon TLR stimulation. This is in line with recent findings indicating that PBMCs from Fulani specifically stimulated with *P. falciparum in vitro* release higher amount of IFN-γ than Dogon [7]. Studies in both humans and mice indicate that the magnitude of an early IFN-γ response is a crucial determinant of the outcome of malaria infection [23,62]. Our findings suggest that the impaired innate IFN-γ responses upon TLR stimulation in infected Dogon as compared to infected Fulani may be one of the underlying causes for the relative susceptibility to malaria in the Dogon ethnic group as compared to the Fulani.

It is possible that APC dysfunction could be dependent on the levels of parasitaemia in an infected individual. This suggests that the APC alteration observed in Dogon individuals upon *P. falciparum* infection merely depends on differences in parasitaemias in this ethnic group as compared to Fulani. However, we did not observe any significant correlation between parasitaemia and HLA-DR expression levels on distinct APC subsets in infected children. Therefore, differences in levels of parasitaemia do not appear to account for the APC dysfunction observed in Dogon children as compared to Fulani in our cohort.

In conclusion, in this study we found that *P. falciparum* infection impairs the phenotype of blood DCs and alters TLR responses of PBMCs from Dogon but not Fulani children. In particular, malaria infection induces differential innate IFN-γ release in the two ethnic groups. These findings suggest that activation of certain DC subsets and additional mechanisms triggering cytokine release by APCs through TLR activation may represent immunological correlates of protection against *P. falciparum* malaria. However, the prospective evaluation of a larger cohort of patients is required to confirm our results and to analyze the potential occurrence of distinct TLR polymorphisms in these two ethnic groups. The understanding of innate immune responses to *P. falciparum* in naturally exposed children may yield important insights in the development of immunity to malaria with particular regard to rational vaccine development.

Materials and Methods

Ethics statement

Ethical approval was obtained from the institutional review boards of the University of Bamako, Mali (N°08_64/FMPOS) and by the Swedish ethical research committee (03-536). Before the inclusion of each child in the study, the community leaders' permission and individual consent form were obtained from the parents of each child.

Study population

The study was conducted in a rural area of the Dogon valley of Mali where malaria is mesoendemic with intense transmission during the rainy season. The study area and the study population have been described in details elsewhere [2]. Children between 2 and 10 years of age belonging to either the Fulani or the Dogon ethnic group were included in the study. Forty children from the Dogon population and 37 from the Fulani were recruited. The study included healthy children and infected children that were classified as uncomplicated malaria. A thick blood smear was performed in all subjects included in the study. The slides were stained in 3% Giemsa and examined for the presence of *P. falciparum* parasites. Presence of malaria infection was defined as a positive thick smear with or without any malaria symptom. Among the Dogon, 20 children were undergoing malaria infection and 20 children were healthy, while among Fulani 14 children were suffering from malaria and 23 were uninfected. Unfortunately not all slides could be recovered from the field study so we only have parasitaemias for eight of the Fulani and nineteen of the Dogon children.

Blood collection and cell preparation

Venous whole blood samples were collected from healthy and infected children of both ethnicities. From each volunteer, 6 ml of peripheral blood was collected in heparin tubes (BD Vacutainer® Plasma Tube, Franklin Lakes, NJ, USA) and were transported to the Malaria Research and Training Centre Laboratory in Bandiagara, north-east of Mali, for further experiments. PBMCs were isolated by density gradient centrifugation using Ficoll-Paque (GE Healthcare, Uppsala, Sweden) and used for APC immunophenotyping and TLR stimulation.

Immunophenotype

Purified PBMCs were fixed and frozen immediately after purification as previously described [63]. Briefly, cells were resuspended in PBS to a concentration of 2 million cells/ml and treated with DNAse (Sigma-Aldrich®, Steinheim, Germany) for 5 minutes at 37°C at a concentration of 666 units/ml. Cells were then washed and resuspended in 3 ml of prewarmed (37°C) 4% paraformaldehyde (PFA) (Sigma-Aldrich®, Steinheim, Germany), incubated for 5 minutes and then washed in cold PBS +1% foetal bovine serum (FBS, Gibco, Paisley, UK) Finally, cells were resuspended in 1 ml PBS +10% DMSO and frozen at −80°C. For staining, cells were thawed and resuspended in PBS 5 mM EDTA 2% FBS. FcR blocking reagent and mouse monoclonal antibodies conjugated with fluorescein isothiocyanate (FITC) or phycoerythrin (PE), peridinin chlorophyll protein (PerCP) or allophycocyanin were added. Antibodies used for cell-surface staining included those recognizing BDCA-1 (clone AD5-8E7), BDCA-2 (clone AC144), BDCA-3 (clone AD5-14H12), CD3 (BW264/56), CD14 (clone TUK4), CD19 (clone LT19), and mouse isotype controls IgG1 and IgG2a (Miltenyi Biotec, GmbH, Germany) and CD16 (clone B73.1), CD56 (clone NCAM16.2), CD86 (clone 2331 FUN-1), HLA-DR (clone L243 G46-6; Pharmingen, San Diego, CA, USA). The cells were finally resuspended in PBS 1% PFA, acquired and analysed using a FACSCalibur (BD Biosciences, San Diego, CA, USA) and the BD CellQuest™Pro version 5.2.1 software.

PBMCs stimulation with TLR ligands

PBMCs were resuspended in RPMI supplemented with 10% FCS, 200 mM L-Glutamine, 100 µg/ml streptomycin and 100 U/ml penicillin to a final concentration of 1 million cells/ml. Two hundred μl of cell suspension were distributed into 5 different wells of 96-well flat bottom plate for cell cultures (Sarstedt Inc. Newton, NC, USA). Cells were stimulated with LPS (Sigma-Aldrich® Steinheim, Germany) (100 ng/ml), CpG-A (Metabion, Martinsried, Germany) (3 μg/ml), imiquimod (InvivoGen, San Diego, USA) (1 μg/ml) and unstimulated control. The plates were incubated for 16 hrs at 37°C + 5% CO2 and then the cells and supernatants were collected and stored at −80°C for subsequent cytokine analysis.

Determination of cytokines in supernatants by cytometric bead array

Levels of IL-1β, IL-6, IL-8, IL-10, IL-12 (p70) and TNF-α in supernatants obtained from stimulated PBMCs were determined by cytometric-bead array (CBA) technology (BD Biosciences, San Diego, CA, USA) and the fluorescent signals were detected by Flow Cytometry according to the manufacturer's recommendation. This sensitive technique allows detection by flow cytometry of multiple cytokines in small quantities of samples. All samples were diluted 1:10 in Assay Diluent (BD Biosciences, San Diego, CA, USA). Data were acquired with fluorescent activated cell sorter (FACS) Calibur (BD Biosciences, San Diego, CA, USA) and analyzed using CellQuest and FCAP Array software. The lower detection limit for the various cytokines was 4.8, 4.7, 3.2, 3.8, 3.7 and 4.9 pg/ml for IL-1β, IL-6, IL-8, IL-10, IL-12 (p70) and TNF-α, respectively.

Determination of cytokine levels in supernatants by ELISA

Levels of IFN-α and IFN-γ were measured by conventional sandwich enzyme-linked immunosorbent assay (ELISA) kits using pairs of capture and detection antibodies (Mabtech, Nacka, Sweden). All samples were tested in duplicates according to the manufacturer's recommendation. The optical densities were measured at 405 nm in an ELISA plate reader (VmaxTM Kinetic Microplate Reader, Menlo Park, CA, USA). The assay sensitivity was 2 pg/ml for IFN-α and 7 pg/ml for IFN-γ, respectively.

Statistical analysis

Statistical significance was determined using non-parametric tests. A Kruskal-Wallis test was employed to analyze the results when more than two groups were involved. The Mann-Whitney U-test was employed to evaluate significance between two unpaired groups when the Kruskal-Wallis test showed a significant difference between the four groups. Linear regression analysis (Spearman rank correlation test) was employed when analysing possible correlations. For all tests $p \leq 0.05$ was considered significant and no correction was made for using multiple tests. The data were analyzed using the StatView software.

Acknowledgments

We sincerely thank the participants and the residents of Manteourou and surrounding villages in Mali for their ongoing support of this study.

Author Contributions

Conceived and designed the experiments: CA PG SB VD BT AD OD SV MT-B. Analyzed the data: CA PG SV. Contributed reagents/materials/analysis tools: MT-B SV BT AD OD. Wrote the paper: CA PG SV MT-B. Provided medical care for study participants and collected clinical data at the field site: CA VD AD. Processed biological specimens and performed clinical assays: CA PG SB.

References

1. World Health Organization (2009) World malaria report 2009.
2. Dolo A, Modiano D, Maiga B, Daou M, Dolo G, et al. (2005) Difference in susceptibility to malaria between two sympatric ethnic groups in Mali. Am J Trop Med Hyg 72(3): 243–248.
3. Israelsson E, Vafa M, Maiga B, Lysen A, Iriemenam NC, et al. (2008) Differences in fcgamma receptor IIa genotypes and IgG subclass pattern of anti-malarial antibodies between sympatric ethnic groups in Mali. Malar J 7: 175.
4. Bolad A, Farouk SE, Israelsson E, Dolo A, Doumbo OK, et al. (2005) Distinct interethnic differences in immunoglobulin G class/subclass and immunoglobulin M antibody responses to malaria antigens but not in immunoglobulin G responses to nonmalarial antigens in sympatric tribes living in west Africa. Scand J Immunol 61(4): 380–386.
5. Farouk SE, Dolo A, Bereczky S, Kouriba B, Maiga B, et al. (2005) Different antibody- and cytokine-mediated responses to *Plasmodium falciparum* parasite in two sympatric ethnic tribes living in Mali. Microbes Infect 7(1): 110–117.
6. Torcia MG, Santarlasci V, Cosmi L, Clemente A, Maggi L, et al. (2008) Functional deficit of T regulatory cells in Fulani, an ethnic group with low susceptibility to *Plasmodium falciparum* malaria. Proc Natl Acad Sci U S A 105(2): 646–651.
7. McCall MB, Hopman J, Daou M, Maiga B, Dara V, et al. (2010) Early interferon-gamma response against *Plasmodium falciparum* correlates with interethnic differences in susceptibility to parasitemia between sympatric Fulani and Dogon in Mali. J Infect Dis 201(1): 142–152.
8. Stevenson MM, Riley EM (2004) Innate immunity to malaria. Nat Rev Immunol 4(3): 169–180.
9. Piccioli D, Tavarini S, Borgogni E, Steri V, Nuti S, et al. (2007) Functional specialization of human circulating CD16 and CD1c myeloid dendritic-cell subsets. Blood 109(12): 5371–5379.
10. Lindstedt M, Lundberg K, Borrebaeck CA (2005) Gene family clustering identifies functionally associated subsets of human *in vivo* blood and tonsillar dendritic cells. J Immunol 175(8): 4839–4846.
11. Jongbloed SL, Kassianos AJ, McDonald KJ, Clark GJ, Ju X, et al. (2010) Human CD141+ (BDCA-3)+ dendritic cells (DCs) represent a unique myeloid DC subset that cross-presents necrotic cell antigens. J Exp Med 207(6): 1247–1260.
12. Urban BC, Ferguson DJ, Pain A, Willcox N, Plebanski M, et al. (1999) *Plasmodium falciparum*-infected erythrocytes modulate the maturation of dendritic cells. Nature 400(6739): 73–77.
13. Urban BC, Roberts DJ (2002) Malaria, monocytes, macrophages and myeloid dendritic cells: Sticking of infected erythrocytes switches off host cells. Curr Opin Immunol 14(4): 458–465.
14. Skorokhod OA, Alessio M, Mordmuller B, Arese P, Schwarzer E (2004) Hemozoin (malarial pigment) inhibits differentiation and maturation of human monocyte-derived dendritic cells: A peroxisome proliferator-activated receptor-gamma-mediated effect. J Immunol 173(6): 4066–4074.
15. Urban BC, Mwangi T, Ross A, Kinyanjui S, Mosobo M, et al. (2001) Peripheral blood dendritic cells in children with acute *Plasmodium falciparum* malaria. Blood 98(9): 2859–2861.
16. Urban BC, Cordery D, Shafi MJ, Bull PC, Newbold CI, et al. (2006) The frequency of BDCA3-positive dendritic cells is increased in the peripheral circulation of Kenyan children with severe malaria. Infect Immun 74(12): 6700–6706.
17. Todryk SM, Urban BC (2008) Dendritic cells in *Plasmodium* infection. Future Microbiol 3: 279–286.
18. Pichyangkul S, Yongvanitchit K, Kum-arb U, Hemmi H, Akira S, et al. (2004) Malaria blood stage parasites activate human plasmacytoid dendritic cells and murine dendritic cells through a toll-like receptor 9-dependent pathway. J Immunol 172(8): 4926–4933.
19. Vigario AM, Belnoue E, Gruner AC, Mauduit M, Kayibanda M, et al. (2007) Recombinant human IFN-alpha inhibits cerebral malaria and reduces parasite burden in mice. J Immunol 178(10): 6416–6425.
20. Luty AJ, Perkins DJ, Lell B, Schmidt-Ott R, Lehman LG, et al. (2000) Low interleukin-12 activity in severe *Plasmodium falciparum* malaria. Infect Immun 68(7): 3909–3915.
21. deWalick S, Amante FH, McSweeney KA, Randall LM, Stanley AC, et al. (2007) Cutting edge: Conventional dendritic cells are the critical APC required for the induction of experimental cerebral malaria. J Immunol 178(10): 6033–6037.
22. Voisine C, Mastelic B, Sponaas AM, Langhorne J (2010) Classical CD11c+ dendritic cells, not plasmacytoid dendritic cells, induce T cell responses to *Plasmodium chabaudi* malaria. Int J Parasitol 40(6): 711–719.
23. Newman KC, Korbel DS, Hafalla JC, Riley EM (2006) Cross-talk with myeloid accessory cells regulates human natural killer cell interferon-gamma responses to malaria. PLoS Pathog 2(12): e118.
24. Scholzen A, Mittag D, Rogerson SJ, Cooke BM, Plebanski M (2009) *Plasmodium falciparum*-mediated induction of human CD25Foxp3 CD4 T cells is independent of direct TCR stimulation and requires IL-2, IL-10 and TGFbeta. PLoS Pathog 5(8): e1000543.
25. Bouharoun-Tayoun H, Druilhe P (1992) *Plasmodium falciparum* malaria: Evidence for an isotype imbalance which may be responsible for delayed acquisition of protective immunity. Infect Immun 60(4): 1473–1481.

26. Passlick B, Flieger D, Ziegler-Heitbrock HW (1989) Identification and characterization of a novel monocyte subpopulation in human peripheral blood. Blood 74(7): 2527–2534.
27. Ziegler-Heitbrock L (2007) The CD14+ CD16+ blood monocytes: Their role in infection and inflammation. J Leukoc Biol 81(3): 584–592.
28. Chimma P, Roussilhon C, Sratongno P, Ruangveerayuth R, Pattanapanyasat K, et al. (2009) A distinct peripheral blood monocyte phenotype is associated with parasite inhibitory activity in acute uncomplicated *Plasmodium falciparum* malaria. PLoS Pathog 5(10): e1000631.
29. Jaworowski A, Kamwendo DD, Ellery P, Sonza S, Mwapasa V, et al. (2007) CD16+ monocyte subset preferentially harbors HIV-1 and is expanded in pregnant Malawian women with *Plasmodium falciparum* malaria and HIV-1 infection. J Infect Dis 196(1): 38–42.
30. Ogonda LA, Orago AS, Otieno MF, Adhiambo C, Otieno W, et al. (2010) The levels of CD16/Fc gamma receptor IIIA on CD14+ CD16+ monocytes are higher in children with severe *Plasmodium falciparum* anemia than in children with cerebral or uncomplicated malaria. Infect Immun 78(5): 2173–2181.
31. Jin MS, Lee JO (2008) Structures of the toll-like receptor family and its ligand complexes. Immunity 29(2): 182–191.
32. Kawai T, Akira S (2010) The role of pattern-recognition receptors in innate immunity: Update on toll-like receptors. Nat Immunol 11(5): 373–384.
33. Kadowaki N, Ho S, Antonenko S, Malefyt RW, Kastelein RA, et al. (2001) Subsets of human dendritic cell precursors express different toll-like receptors and respond to different microbial antigens. J Exp Med 194(6): 863–869.
34. Muzio M, Bosisio D, Polentarutti N, D'amico G, Stoppacciaro A, et al. (2000) Differential expression and regulation of toll-like receptors (TLR) in human leukocytes: Selective expression of TLR3 in dendritic cells. J Immunol 164(11): 5998–6004.
35. Coban C, Ishii KJ, Uematsu S, Arisue N, Sato S, et al. (2007) Pathological role of toll-like receptor signaling in cerebral malaria. Int Immunol 19(1): 67–79.
36. Franklin BS, Rodrigues SO, Antonelli LR, Oliveira RV, Goncalves AM, et al. (2007) MyD88-dependent activation of dendritic cells and CD4(+) T lymphocytes mediates symptoms, but is not required for the immunological control of parasites during rodent malaria. Microbes Infect 9(7): 881–890.
37. Parroche P, Lauw FN, Goutagny N, Latz E, Monks BG, et al. (2007) Malaria hemozoin is immunologically inert but radically enhances innate responses by presenting malaria DNA to toll-like receptor 9. Proc Natl Acad Sci U S A 104(6): 1919–1924.
38. Wu X, Gowda NM, Kumar S, Gowda DC (2010) Protein-DNA complex is the exclusive malaria parasite component that activates dendritic cells and triggers innate immune responses. J Immunol 184(8): 4338–4348.
39. Krishnegowda G, Hajjar AM, Zhu J, Douglass EJ, Uematsu S, et al. (2005) Induction of proinflammatory responses in macrophages by the glycosylphosphatidylinositols of *Plasmodium falciparum*: Cell signaling receptors, glycosylphosphatidylinositol (GPI) structural requirement, and regulation of GPI activity. J Biol Chem 280(9): 8606–8616.
40. Krug A, Rothenfusser S, Hornung V, Jahrsdorfer B, Blackwell S, et al. (2001) Identification of CpG oligonucleotide sequences with high induction of IFN-alpha/beta in plasmacytoid dendritic cells. Eur J Immunol 31(7): 2154–2163.
41. Banchereau J, Briere F, Caux C, Davoust J, Lebecque S, et al. (2000) Immunobiology of dendritic cells. Annu Rev Immunol 18: 767–811.
42. Vafa M, Maiga B, Berzins K, Hayano M, Bereczky S, et al. (2007) Associations between the IL-4 -590 T allele and *Plasmodium falciparum* infection prevalence in asymptomatic Fulani of Mali. Microbes Infect 9(9): 1043–1048.
43. Banchereau J, Steinman RM (1998) Dendritic cells and the control of immunity. Nature 392(6673): 245–252.
44. Vafa M, Israelsson E, Maiga B, Dolo A, Doumbo OK, et al. (2009) Relationship between immunoglobulin isotype response to *Plasmodium falciparum* blood stage antigens and parasitological indexes as well as splenomegaly in sympatric ethnic groups living in Mali. Acta Trop 109(1): 12–16.
45. Bereczky S, Dolo A, Maiga B, Hayano M, Granath F, et al. (2006) Spleen enlargement and genetic diversity of *Plasmodium falciparum* infection in two ethnic groups with different malaria susceptibility in Mali, west Africa. Trans R Soc Trop Med Hyg 100(3): 248–257.
46. Poulin LF, Salio M, Griessinger E, Anjos-Afonso F, Craciun L, et al. (2010) Characterization of human DNGR-1+ BDCA3+ leukocytes as putative equivalents of mouse CD8alpha+ dendritic cells. J Exp Med 207(6): 1261–1271.
47. Lundie RJ, de Koning-Ward TF, Davey GM, Nie CQ, Hansen DS, et al. (2008) Blood-stage *Plasmodium* infection induces CD8+ T lymphocytes to parasite-expressed antigens, largely regulated by CD8alpha+ dendritic cells. Proc Natl Acad Sci U S A 105(38): 14509–14514.
48. Jego G, Palucka AK, Blanck JP, Chalouni C, Pascual V, et al. (2003) Plasmacytoid dendritic cells induce plasma cell differentiation through type I interferon and interleukin 6. Immunity 19(2): 225–234.
49. Varani S, Cederarv M, Feld S, Tammik C, Frascaroli G, et al. (2007) Human cytomegalovirus differentially controls B cell and T cell responses through effects on plasmacytoid dendritic cells. J Immunol 179(11): 7767–7776.
50. Luoni G, Verra F, Arca B, Sirima BS, Troye-Blomberg M, et al. (2001) Antimalarial antibody levels and IL4 polymorphism in the Fulani of west Africa. Genes Immun 2(7): 411–414.
51. Clark IA, Budd AC, Alleva LM, Cowden WB (2006) Human malarial disease: A consequence of inflammatory cytokine release. Malar J 5: 85.
52. Walther M, Woodruff J, Edele F, Jeffries D, Tongren JE, et al. (2006) Innate immune responses to human malaria: Heterogeneous cytokine responses to blood-stage *Plasmodium falciparum* correlate with parasitological and clinical outcomes. J Immunol 177(8): 5736–5745.
53. Coban C, Ishii KJ, Kawai T, Hemmi H, Sato S, et al. (2005) Toll-like receptor 9 mediates innate immune activation by the malaria pigment hemozoin. J Exp Med 201(1): 19–25.
54. Liu YJ (2005) IPC: Professional type 1 interferon-producing cells and plasmacytoid dendritic cell precursors. Annu Rev Immunol 23: 275–306.
55. Pulendran B, Ahmed R (2006) Translating innate immunity into immunological memory: Implications for vaccine development. Cell 124(4): 849–863.
56. Mockenhaupt FP, Cramer JP, Hamann L, Stegemann MS, Eckert J, et al. (2006) Toll-like receptor (TLR) polymorphisms in African children: Common TLR-4 variants predispose to severe malaria. Proc Natl Acad Sci U S A 103(1): 177–182.
57. Mockenhaupt FP, Hamann L, von Gaertner C, Bedu-Addo G, von Kleinsorgen C, et al. (2006) Common polymorphisms of toll-like receptors 4 and 9 are associated with the clinical manifestation of malaria during pregnancy. J Infect Dis 194(2): 184–188.
58. McCall MB, Netea MG, Hermsen CC, Jansen T, Jacobs L, et al. (2007) *Plasmodium falciparum* infection causes proinflammatory priming of human TLR responses. J Immunol 179(1): 162–171.
59. Franklin BS, Parroche P, Ataide MA, Lauw F, Ropert C, et al. (2009) Malaria primes the innate immune response due to interferon-gamma induced enhancement of toll-like receptor expression and function. Proc Natl Acad Sci U S A 106(14): 5789–5794.
60. Boutlis CS, Yeo TW, Anstey NM (2006) Malaria tolerance–for whom the cell tolls? Trends Parasitol 22(8): 371–377.
61. Hay SI, Okiro EA, Gething PW, Patil AP, Tatem AJ, et al. (2010) Estimating the global clinical burden of *Plasmodium falciparum* malaria in 2007. PLoS Med 7(6): e1000290.
62. De Souza JB, Williamson KH, Otani T, Playfair JH (1997) Early gamma interferon responses in lethal and nonlethal murine blood-stage malaria. Infect Immun 65(5): 1593–1598.
63. Pinto LA, Trivett MT, Wallace D, Higgins J, Baseler M, et al. (2005) Fixation and cryopreservation of whole blood and isolated mononuclear cells: Influence of different procedures on lymphocyte subset analysis by flow cytometry. Cytometry B Clin Cytom 63(1): 47–55.

17

Risk Factors and Characterization of Plasmodium Vivax-Associated Admissions to Pediatric Intensive Care Units in the Brazilian Amazon

Ellen Fátima Caetano Lança[1,5], Belisa Maria Lopes Magalhães[1,4], Sheila Vitor-Silva[1,4], André Machado Siqueira[1,2,4], Silvana Gomes Benzecry[1], Márcia Almeida Araújo Alexandre[1,2,3], Connor O'Brien[6], Quique Bassat[7], Marcus Vinícius Guimarães Lacerda[1,2,3,4]*

1 Universidade do Estado do Amazonas, Manaus, Amazonas, Brazil, **2** Fundação de Medicina Tropical Dr. Heitor Vieira Dourado, Manaus, Amazonas, Brazil, **3** Universidade Nilton Lins, Manaus, Amazonas, Brazil, **4** National Institute of Science and Technology for Innovation in Neglected Diseases, Rio de Janeiro, Brazil, **5** Universidade Federal do Amazonas, Manaus, Amazonas, Brazil, **6** Columbia University Medical Center, New York, New York, United States of America, **7** Centre de Recerca en Salut Internacional de Barcelona (CRESIB)/Hospital Clínic, Universitat de Barcelona, Barcelona, Spain

Abstract

Background: *Plasmodium vivax* is responsible for a significant proportion of malaria cases worldwide and is increasingly reported as a cause of severe disease. The objective of this study was to characterize severe vivax disease among children hospitalized in intensive care units (ICUs) in the Western Brazilian Amazon, and to identify risk factors associated with disease severity.

Methods and Findings: In this retrospective study, clinical records of 34 children, 0–14 years of age hospitalized in the 11 public pediatric and neonatal ICUs of the Manaus area, were reviewed. *P. falciparum* monoinfection or *P. falciparum/P. vivax* mixed infection was diagnosed by microscopy in 10 cases, while *P. vivax* monoinfection was confirmed in the remaining 24 cases. Two of the 24 patients with *P. vivax* monoinfection died. Respiratory distress, shock and severe anemia were the most frequent complications associated with *P. vivax* infection. Ninety-one children hospitalized with *P. vivax* monoinfections but not requiring ICU were consecutively recruited in a tertiary care hospital for infectious diseases to serve as a reference population (comparators). Male sex ($p = 0.039$), age less than five years ($p = 0.028$), parasitemia greater than $500/mm^3$ ($p = 0.018$), and the presence of any acute ($p = 0.023$) or chronic ($p = 0.017$) co-morbidity were independently associated with ICU admission. At least one of the WHO severity criteria for malaria (formerly validated for *P. falciparum*) was present in 23/24 (95.8%) of the patients admitted to the ICU and in 17/91 (18.7%) of controls, making these criteria a good predictor of ICU admission ($p = 0.001$). The only investigated criterion not associated with ICU admission was hyperbilirubinemia ($p = 0.513$)].

Conclusions: Our study points to the importance of *P. vivax*-associated severe disease in children, causing 72.5% of the malaria admissions to pediatric ICUs. WHO severity criteria demonstrated good sensitivity in predicting severe *P. vivax* infection in this small case series.

Editor: Rick Edward Paul, Institut Pasteur, France

Funding: This work was supported by: PRONEX Malaria Network, funded by the Brazilian Ministry of Science and Technology (MCT), National Council for Scientific and Technological Development (CNPq), Brazilian Ministry of Health (DECIT/SCTIE/MS) and the Research Support Foundation from Amazonas (FAPEAM); Fundació Cellex; and the National Institute of Science and Technology for Innovation in Neglected Diseases (INCT-IDN). Dr. Lacerda is a level 2 productivity fellow from CNPq. The funders had no role in study design, data collection and analysis, decision to publish, or preparation of the manuscript.

Competing Interests: The authors have declared that no competing interests exist.

* E-mail: marcuslacerda.br@gmail.com

Introduction

Malaria is one of the most important public health problems in the world, with almost half of the world's population at risk of disease and an estimated 800.000 deaths annually, mainly in children under five years of age [1]. Of the various *Plasmodium* species affecting humans, *Plasmodium vivax* was previously considered a relatively benign infection. Recent reports, however, have linked *P. vivax* to severe disease [2,3].

Malaria in Brazil has been by and large attributed to *P. vivax* infection since the 1990's [4]. In 2009, Brazil reported 308,498 cases of malaria (257,571 of *P. vivax*), predominantly in the Amazon Region, representing 54.9% of all the malaria reported in the Americas [1]. In the last two decades, the city of Manaus (capital of the Amazonas State) has faced successive outbreaks of malaria due to intense immigration, deforestation and unplanned human settlements [5]. Today, with an estimated population of 2 million people, Manaus is one of three cities, which account for 25% of all reported malaria cases in Brazil. High case burdens persist despite a well-structured public health system with universal access to diagnosis (based on thick blood smear) and treatment.

Previously, *P. vivax* was considered a non-fatal infection. This perception, however, has changed in recent years, and vivax has become recognized as a cause of severe malarial disease. Severe clinical complications of *P. vivax* infection have been reported in Brazil for the past decade, especially in Manaus [6–12]. Despite being a significant source of morbidity, to date, no data on risk factors of severe *P. vivax* disease have been published in Latin America. The current data on predictors of clinical outcomes originates from regions where *P. falciparum* and *P. vivax* are equally prevalent, which could make the clinical tools inappropriate for use in managing vivax monoinfections [13]. This lack of prioritizing predictors of severity in *P. vivax* is due to the fact that fatalities related to this species remain uncommon. According to the official statistics, between 1998 and 2008, only 234 deaths related to *P. vivax* infection were reported in the Brazilian Amazon [4].

The first attempt to assemble the available knowledge on severe malaria was conducted at an informal technical meeting convened by the World Health Organization (WHO) in Kuala Lumpur, Malaysia in 1985 [14]. The document focused on *P. falciparum* infection, since, at that time, *P. vivax* was not thought to cause severe disease. Throughout the years, no effort has been made to validate or standardize specific severity criteria for vivax infections, and current definitions seem to be heterogeneous. This absence of consistency poses technical problems for literature review, meta-analyses and estimation of risk factors.

Alarmingly, the incidence of severe infection appears to be increasing [15]. Data from Manaus clearly demonstrate this increase in a setting where uniform study criteria are applied across time. The mechanism behind this increase remains poorly understood as are the clinical predictors of severity and outcome. The most robust endpoint for validating a criterion linked to severity is death, but in vivax infections in Brazil the number of deaths is small, which limits prognostic studies. Given this limitation a surrogate is required to replace death. Intensive care unit (ICU) admission could serve as this surrogate marker of severity, in combination with well-validated severity scoring systems that predict mortality in ICU patients. A uniform comparator is urgently needed to help establish management guidelines for vivax infections, especially for children under the age of 14, which accounted for 24.3% of all malaria infections in 2010 in Manaus (SIVEP, Malaria 2010).

This study aimed to characterize all children under 14 years of age admitted with a malaria diagnosis to an ICU in the Manaus area from 2004 to 2009, to assess potential risk factors associated with ICU admission (as proxy of clinical severity), and secondarily to address the applicability of WHO falciparum severity criteria to vivax infection, by comparing these cases to *P. vivax* hospitalized children not requiring intensive care.

Methods

Ethical considerations

The review of clinical files was approved by the Ethics Review Board (ERB) of the *Fundação de Medicina Tropical Dr. Heitor Vieira Dourado* (approval number 1980), as well as by the ERB of the Health Secretariat of Manaus and the Health Secretariat of the Amazonas State. All data analyzed were anonymized. Since data were obtained exclusively from clinical charts, the ERB gave a waiver of informed consent.

Study Sites and Patient Selection

The selection of cases was performed in the city of Manaus, capital of the Amazonas State, where *Anopheles darlingi* is the major malaria vector and the annual parasite index (API) was 11.5 cases/1,000 inhabitants, in 2009. The city has universal health assistance for citizens (*Sistema Único de Saúde - SUS*), and offers five public pediatric ICUs (44 total available beds) and six neonatal ICUs (50 total available beds) in 11 tertiary care pediatric hospitals and maternity wards. The infrastructure of all 11 hospitals is very similar and staff pediatricians are from the same cooperative society, which utilizes a single set of admission criteria and clinical management guidelines for ICU admission (severe compromise of respiratory and/or hemodynamic functions and/or coma). Since every febrile patient in Manaus is subject to a thick blood smear (TBS) and the symptoms of uncomplicated *P. vivax* and *P. falciparum* malaria are similar, treatment seeking bias seems unlikely. Since the access to tertiary care hospitals is relatively easy, we assume that all critically ill patients seeking health care were subsequently hospitalized in one of Manaus' ICUs. Patients in private ICUs in Manaus were excluded from this study because the patients are generally from non-malaria endemic areas. Patients infected with *P. vivax* that required an ICU admission were compared to children of the same age range infected with *P. vivax* not requiring an ICU admission but concurrently admitted to a tertiary care center for infectious diseases (*Fundação de Medicina Tropical Dr. Heitor Vieira Dourado*).

Study Design

This study is a retrospective review of clinical and laboratory records from hospital databases. Case files for children 0–14 years old admitted to any of the ICUs with a suspicion of malaria between January 2004 to December 2009 were reviewed for: (1) ICU logbooks (in which demographic data from each admitted patient, a presumptive diagnosis at admission and a final diagnosis at discharge are systematically registered), (2) hospital laboratory logbooks (in which the semi-quantitative results of TBSs performed in each hospital are systematically registered), and (3) SIVEP-Malaria (the National Malaria Information System available on-line, which registers results of TBSs performed in each reporting unit such as the hospitals of interest). Cases were included if there was evidence of malaria diagnosis by microscopy in any of the three information systems searched. The study enrolled only patients after 2004 because of better reliability of the National Malaria Information System (SIVEP-Malaria) and access to the clinical files, avoiding retrieval bias.

As comparators, clinical and laboratory data from children of the same age group admitted between January 2009 and July 2010 to the *Fundação de Medicina Tropical Dr. Heitor Vieira Dourado* with a diagnosis of malaria were retrieved electronically from the computerized hospital records system (iDoctor®) and reviewed. With the exception of automated full blood count, routinely requested for all these hospitalized children, more specific laboratory tests (such as biochemistry and arterial gas analysis) were requested only if clinical symptoms were suggestive of complications. As part of routine follow-up, all malaria admitted children were reassessed in the Outpatient Clinics seven days after discharge to guarantee adequate clinical and parasitological follow-up.

Diagnosis of Malaria and Quantification of Parasitemia

TBSs are routinely performed for the diagnosis of malaria in Brazil, prepared as recommended by the Walker technique [16] and evaluated by a local microscopist. The results of peripheral parasitemia are given using the following semi-quantitative system: ½+ (200–300 parasites/mm^3); 1+ (301–500 parasites/mm^3); 2+ (501–10,000 parasites/mm^3); 3+ (10,001–100,000 parasites/mm^3); and 4+ (>100,001 parasites/mm^3). The cut-off to define high parasitemia (in the final analysis) was based on the distribution of semi-quantitative parasitemia results. All positive slides and 10% of negative slides are routinely reviewed in a reference unit with experienced microscopists. In case of divergence, the reviewed result is updated in the on-line system. PCR diagnosis for malaria was not routinely performed in these patients. Only children with a positive TBS for *Plasmodium* spp. are treated according to the Brazilian Anti-Malarial Treatment Guidelines, which recommends chloroquine (25 mg/kg over 3 days)+primaquine (0.5 mg/kg/day over 7 days) for *P. vivax* infection and artemether/lumefantrine for 3 days for non-severe *P. falciparum* infection. Severe *P. falciparum* infections are treated with parenteral artemether or artesunate for 7 days.

Data collection and definitions

Data for each admitted individual was systematically retrieved from the medical charts by the same member of the study team, and included the following variables: sex, age, malarial species, semi-quantitative parasitemia, duration of disease (in days) prior to the admission to the ICU or ward, outcome, presence of a given acute co-morbidity other than malaria or a chronic disease confirmed through a reliable diagnostic method, and presence of any WHO-defined severe malaria criteria [17]. Briefly, WHO criteria for severe falciparum malaria validated for adults and children include: (1) impaired consciousness or unrousable coma (Blantyre coma scale ≤ 2 or Glasgow coma scale ≤ 10); (2) prostration, i.e. generalized weakness such that the patient is unable to walk or sit up without assistance; (3) failure to feed; (4) multiple convulsions (greater than two episodes in 24 h); (5) respiratory distress defined as the presence of deep (acidotic) breathing or retractions; (6) circulatory collapse or shock, systolic blood pressure <50 mmHg (algid malaria) and/or need for vasopressor support; (7) clinical jaundice or total bilirubin >3 mg/dL; (8) hemoglobinuria (blackwater fever); (9) abnormal spontaneous bleeding (disseminated intravascular coagulation); (10) pulmonary edema (radiological); (11) hypoglycemia (blood glucose <40 mg/dL); (12) metabolic acidosis (plasma bicarbonate <15 mmol/L); (13) severe anemia (Hb<5 g/dL); (14) hyperlactatemia (lactate >5 mmol/L); or (15) acute renal failure (serum creatinine >3 mg/dL). Acute respiratory distress syndrome (ARDS) was defined as acute bilateral lung infiltrates in chest X-rays, and a PaO_2:FiO_2<200 mmHg. The data retrieved were reviewed by another member of the study team and discrepancies resolved by a third member if necessary.

In all ICUs, collection of venous blood samples for aerobic culture and arterial blood for gas analysis was routinely carried out on admission prior to administration of antibiotics. From all the patients hospitalized in the ICU, the Pediatric Index of Mortality (PIM) score was calculated with data from the first hour of admission, based on the systolic blood pressure, pupillary reactions to bright light, PaO_2, FiO_2, base excess in arterial blood, need for mechanical ventilation at any time during the first hour in ICU, elective admission, and presence of concomitant diagnoses [18]. Severity was defined in the presence of at least one of the aforementioned WHO severity criteria. As blood gas analysis samples were not systematically collected for patients not admitted to the ICU, hyperlactatemia and metabolic acidosis were not used to classify severity nor assessed as a risk factor associated with ICU admission. The disease was classified as being directly caused by plasmodial infection if no other cause was identified and no concurrent acute or chronic diseases were confirmed.

Statistical Analyses

Data were analyzed using SPSS® version 16.0 for Windows (SPSS Inc.® Chicago, IL, USA). Proportions of fatality were compared by Fisher exact test (corrected by Yates' test if necessary); differences were considered statistically significant for $p<0.05$. The crude *Odds Ratio* (OR) with its respective 95% Confidence Interval (95% CI) was determined considering the admission to ICU as the dependent variable. Logistic regression was used for the multivariate analyses and the adjusted *Odds Ratios* with 95% CI were also calculated. A multivariate logistic regression was performed with admission to the ICU as the outcome, using an automated backward and forward stepwise estimation. All variables that were associated with admission to the ICU at a significance level of $p<0.10$ in the univariate analysis were included in the multivariate analysis. Statistical significance was considered if $p<0.05$ in the Hosmer-Lemeshow goodness-of-fit test.

Results

According to the official reporting systems, during the period of 2004–2009, 64,032 children 0–14 years of age were diagnosed with malaria in Manaus (52,828 with vivax; 10,691 with falciparum and 513 with both species). The review of logbooks disclosed that 40 of these children were admitted with malaria to one of the 11 pediatric or neonatal ICUs in Manaus. Thirty-four clinical files were actually retrieved from these 40 cases (29 of which were due to *P. vivax* infections), as shown in Figure 1, and six cases were excluded because records could not be found. A rough estimation of the risk of ICU admission per species showed similar relative risks for *P. vivax* (4.7/10,000 cases) and *P. falciparum* (5.5/10,000 cases), but a much higher relative risk for mixed infections (116.9/10,000 cases).

Table 1 summarizes the clinical description of the 10 ICU cases in which *P. falciparum* was diagnosed (four cases as monoinfection, and six cases of *P. falciparum*/*P. vivax* mixed infection). Altogether, respiratory distress (7/10) and shock (7/10) were the most common clinical complications in these children and the case fatality rate was 30.0% (3/10) (only two with *P. falciparum* monoinfection). No other concurrent cause for ICU admission was found in 40.0% (4/10) of the children while in the other six children, acute and/or chronic conditions were probably acting synergistically to produce the complications. Only one concomitant bacterial infection was diagnosed (*Pseudomonas aeruginosa*) in a child with *P. falciparum* monoinfection. In all 10 patients, at least one of the WHO criteria for severe malaria was present.

Clinical and laboratory data from the 24 children with *P. vivax* monoinfection admitted to the ICU are presented in tables 2 and 3, respectively. Considering all the patients (admitted or not to the ICU), 46/108 (~42%) patients presented with semi-quantitative parasitemia $\geq$2+ (500–10,000 parasites/mm^3), and therefore 500 parasites/mm^3 (the lower bound of this range) was chosen as the cut-off to define high parasitemia in our analysis, enabling similar number of patients in both categories (low and high parasitemia). Respiratory distress (16/24) and shock (13/24) were also the most common complications associated with this species. Three out of 16 patients with respiratory distress had ARDS and 8/16 presented with simultaneous metabolic acidosis. No other apparent concurrent cause for ICU admission was found in 10/24 (41.6%) children, while in the remaining 14 children there was evidence of the participation of acute and/or chronic conditions in the occurrence of complications. All children were treated with chloroquine (through nasogastric catheter when the child was intubated), primaquine after discharge, and one or more empiric

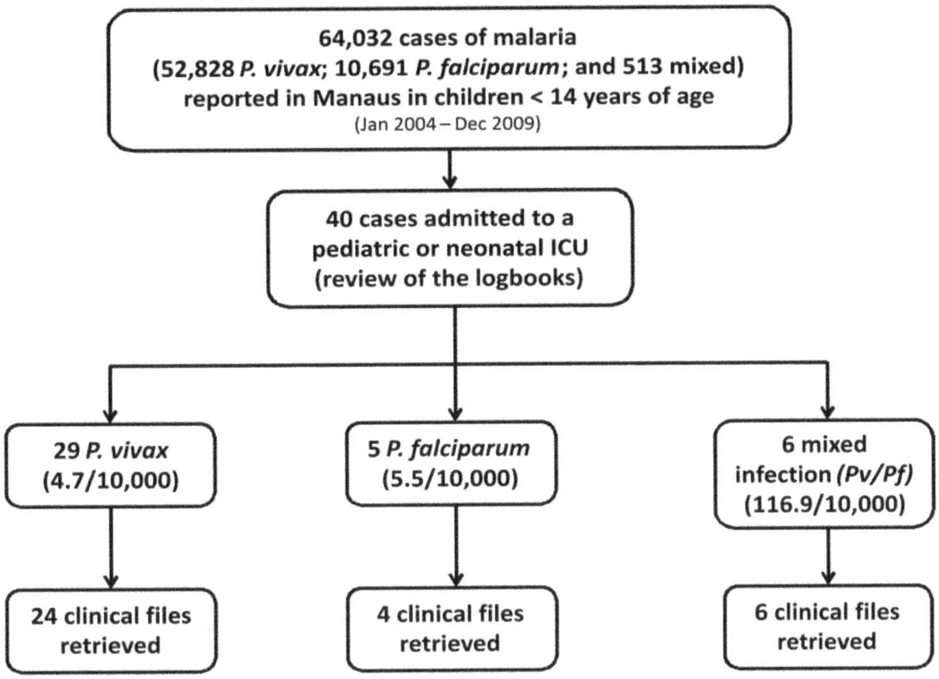

Figure 1. Flow diagram of patients admitted to ICUs enrolled in the analysis.

antibiotic regimens. Although, only two patients (one of which with dual infection) presented positive blood cultures during the admission (table 2). Two patients with confirmed glucose-6-phosphate dehydrogenase (G6PD) deficiency experienced severe hemolysis, hemoglobinuria and acute renal failure after the beginning of primaquine (all started with hemoglobinuria during the second or third day of treatment). All the patients who developed shock syndrome required administration of vasoactive amines. With the exception of one patient with a previous diagnosis of idiopathic thrombocytopenic purpura (ITP), who presented with moderate bleeding and was admitted to the ICU as a result, all remaining 23 patients had one or more WHO severity criteria for malaria. All the patients demonstrated a TBS negative for *Plasmodium* spp. following chloroquine treatment.

Table 4 summarizes the results of the univariate and multivariate logistic regression evaluating risk factors associated with ICU admission. Males [OR = 5.90 (95% CI = 1.28–34.25); (p = 0.039)], age <5 years [OR = 6.36 (95% CI = 2.67–13.63); (p = 0.028)], peripheral parasitemia greater than 500/mm^3 [OR = 4.94 (95% CI = 1.31–18.63); (p = 0.018)], the presence of acute [OR = 8.13 (95% CI = 1.33–49.81); (p = 0.023)] and/or chronic co-morbidities [OR = 6.02 (95% CI = 1.38–26.35); (p = 0.017)] were all independently associated with the risk of developing life-threatening *P. vivax* monoinfection requiring admission to an ICU. None of the children not admitted to the ICU developed severe disease after their discharge, as reviewed in their electronic files from follow-up visits in the outpatient clinics.

Table 5 compares ICU admitted *P. vivax* monoinfections with hospitalized *P. vivax* patients not requiring ICU admission. Of all variables assessed for both groups, the odds of being admitted to the ICU increased in patients fulfilling at least one WHO severity criterion, particularly in those with severe anemia or coma. The mean of the PIM, a validated score that parallels bad prognosis in pediatric ICUs, was higher in children with shock and coma. *P. falciparum* or *P. falciparum/P. vivax* infected children (30.0%) died more frequently than those infected with *P. vivax* monoinfection (8.3%), but this difference was not significant (Yate's corrected Fisher's exact test; p = 0.138). *P. falciparum* monoinfection showed higher fatality (2/4; 50.0%) when compared to *P. vivax* monoinfection (2/24; 8.6%), but this difference likewise was not significant (p = 0.086).

Discussion

This study showed that in Manaus most of the malaria-associated hospitalizations in ICUs were related to *P. vivax* during the period of study, confirming the public health impact of this infection [19–20]. Male sex, age less than five years, parasitemia greater than 500/mm^3, and the presence of any acute or chronic co-morbidity were independently associated with ICU admission. At least one of the WHO severity criteria for malaria (formerly validated for *P. falciparum* infection only) was present in most of the patients admitted to the ICU. WHO severity criteria may also serve as predictors of severity for *P. vivax* patients. Further studies, however, are needed to confirm this finding considering the small number of cases presented in our series.

A significant male sex predominance among children admitted to the ICU in our study contrasts with data from Indonesia and India, where the female sex was associated with severity in vivax infection [3,21]. One possible explanation of this difference is the heterogeneous age range of infected children in these continents.

Similar to what was observed by Tjitra and colleagues in Papua, Indonesia [3], respiratory distress, present in two-thirds of patients in our series, was the most frequent complication among patients admitted to the ICU with *P. vivax* infection, and had a particularly poor prognosis. In *P. falciparum* malaria, respiratory distress arises secondary to either primary pulmonary pathology mediated by sequestration of parasitized erythrocytes in the lung microvasculature or from the drive to compensate metabolic acidosis. For *P. vivax* malaria, however, the pathophysiology behind respiratory distress is not well understood. Studies performed in uncomplicated vivax patients suggest that progressive alveolar-capillary

Table 1. Clinical information from 10 children 0–14 years of age admitted to any of the pediatric or neonatal ICUs in Manaus, from January 2004 to December 2009, with parasitological diagnosis of *P. falciparum* or mixed infection (*P. falciparum/P. vivax*).

Patient	Species	Age/gender	Time of disease (days)	Associated acute comorbidity	Associated chronic comorbidity	Respiratory distress	Severe anemia	ARF	Coma	Jaundice	Shock	Metabolic acidosis	Low glucose	PIM score (%)	Outcome
1	*P.f.*	6 y/F	14	Rotavirus gastroenteritis*+Sepsis* (*Pseudomonas aeruginosa*)	Congenital cardiopathy*	+					+			84.7	Died
2	*P.f.*	7 y/F	5			+ (ARDS)	+		+					40.0	Recovered
3	*P.f.*	10 y/F	5					+	+	+	+	+	+	45.7	Died
4	*P.f.*	1 mo/M	7			+	+							10.6	Recovered
5	*P.f./P.v.*	7 mo/F	2	Rotavirus gastroenteritis		+					+			7.4	Recovered
6	*P.f./P.v.*	13 y/M	30		G6PD deficiency*		+	+**				+		1.3	Recovered
7	*P.f./P.v.*	5 mo/F	48		Malnutrition*	+				+	+			NA	Died
8	*P.f./P.v.*	3 y/M	7	Rotavirus gastroenteritis		+ (ARDS)					+			15.4	Recovered
9	*P.f./P.v.*	9 y/M	7		Sickle cell anemia* + Malnutrition		+			+	+			1.4	Recovered
10	*P.f./P.v.*	2 mo/M	2			+ (ARDS)					+			13.9	Recovered

Y: years; mo: months; d: days; NA: Non-available; ARDS: acute respiratory distress syndrome; ARF: acute renal failure; PIM: Pediatric Index of Mortality.
***Malnutrition** confirmed by body mass index (BMI) Z-score <-2; **rotavirus gastroenteritis** confirmed by immunochromatographic rapid test in the stool; **sepsis** confirmed by two positive blood cultures; **G6PD deficiency** confirmed by qualitative Brewer's test; **congenital cardiopathy** confirmed by echocardiogram; **sickle cell anemia** confirmed by electrophoresis; ARDS defined as acute bilateral lung infiltrates and a PaO_2:FiO_2<200 mmHg.
**Blackwater fever.

Table 2. Detailed clinical information from 24 children 0–14 years old, admitted to any of the pediatric or neonatal ICUs in Manaus, from 2004 to 2009, with parasitological diagnosis of *P. vivax*.

Patient	Age/gender	Time of disease (days)	Associated acute comorbidity	Associated chronic comorbidity	Respiratory distress	Severe anemia	Coma	Jaundice	Shock	Metabolic acidosis	Low glucose	Blackwater fever (ARF)	PIM score (%)	Outcome
1	6 y/M	7			+				+				1.9	Recovered
2	1 mo/M	7			+	+		+		+			24.8	Recovered
3	8 y/F	3	Viral encephalitis*				+		+				45.9	Died
4	1 y/F	4	Gastroenteritis	Malnutrition*	+				+	+			28.1	Recovered
5	3 y/M	4	Rotavirus gastroenteritis*	Cystic fibrosis*	+								1.6	Recovered
6	1 mo/M	3				+		+	+	+			9.1	Recovered
7	1 mo/M	1	Gastroenteritis and drug-induced hepatitis		+	+			+	+			21.1	Recovered
8	1 y/M	2		Neurological sequelae	+ (ARDS)		+		+	+	+		40.5	Recovered
9	2 y/F	25			+ (ARDS)								9.9	Recovered
10	11 y/M	7		Malnutrition	+			+	+	+			24.9	Recovered
11	7 mo/F	26	Rotavirus gastroenteritis+Sepsis (*Acinetobacter* sp.+*Klebsiella* sp.)*		+ (ARDS)				+				11.4	Recovered
12	8 y/M	10		G6PD deficiency*		+						+	4.0	Recovered
13	3 y/M	23			+				+	+			11.3	Recovered
14	3 y/M	7		G6PD deficiency		+					+	+	2.4	Recovered
15	2 y/M	2			+						+		8.4	Recovered
16	2 y/M	4	Bacterial pneumonia with lung empyema*		+				+	+			12.6	Recovered
17	8 mo/F	15			+				+				4.1	Recovered
18	2 mo/F	10	Urosepsis (*Klebsiella* sp.)*	Neurological sequelae		+	+						7.5	Recovered
19	3 y/M	7			+		+		+				55.7	Died
20	1 mo/M	8	Rotavirus gastroenteritis	Malnutrition		+				+			8.7	Recovered
21	2 y/F	3		ITP*									2.0	Recovered
22	1 y/M	31			+		+		+				36.6	Recovered
23	5 mo/M	6	Rotavirus gastroenteritis	Malnutrition	+					+			2.8	Recovered
24	18 d/M	5						+					1.2	Recovered

y years; mo: months; d: days; NA: Non-available; ARDS: Acute Respiratory Distress Syndrome; ARF: Acute Renal Failure; PIM: Pediatric Index of Mortality; ITP: Immune Trombocytopenic Purpura.
***Viral encephalitis** confirmed by autopsy; diagnosis of **malnutrition** confirmed by body mass index (BMI) Z-score <-2; **rotavirus gastroenteritis** confirmed by immunochromatographic rapid test in the stool; **cystic fibrosis** suggested by lung biopsy; **sepsis** confirmed by two positive blood cultures; **G6PD deficiency** confirmed by qualitative Brewer's test; **lung empyema** confirmed by computed tomography; **urosepsis** confirmed by both positive urine and blood culture; **ITP** confirmed by ASH criteria; ARDS defined as acute bilateral lung infiltrates and a PaO_2:FiO_2<200 mmHg.

Table 3. Detailed laboratorial information from 24 children 0–14 years old, at the moment of admission to any of the pediatric or neonatal ICUs in Manaus, from 2004 to 2009, with parasitological diagnosis of *P. vivax*.

Patient	Hb (g/dL)	Leukocyte/ mm^3	Platelets/mm^3	AST (mg/dL)	ALT (mg/dL)	Creatinin (mg/dL)	Total bilirubin (mg/dL)	Glucose (mg/dL)
1	9.1	18,600	49,000	286	253	0.7	0.9	90
2	2.8	25,600	34,000	160	111	0.6	4.3	55
3	8.5	6,400	161,000	23	15	0.6	0.6	70
4	8.5	19,300	180,000	73	22	1.9	0.3	304
5	10.4	9,000	378,000	20	30	1.0	1.0	199
6	2.5	28,600	13,000	83	48	0.6	8.3	59
7	5.0	22,500	16,000	961	1400	2.7	1.0	64
8	9.5	13,700	113,000	15	23	0.8	1.0	28
9	8.3	30,100	207,000	17	19	0.5	1.0	64
10	8.6	12,700	129,000	23	27	0.8	6.7	88
11	7.9	57,700	93,000	34	45	1.1	1.0	67
12	5.0	12,100	170,000	222	53	7.5	2.7	42
13	5.9	10,100	174,000	56	10	0.4	1.0	63
14	4.2	18,700	303,000	29	26	7.1	1.4	39
15	8.8	4,600	78,000	30	28	0.4	1.0	38
16	6.5	16,600	611,000	25	15	0.9	1.0	75
17	9.1	16,800	196,000	22	29	0.4	1.0	90
18	5.0	31,500	76,000	34	43	0.4	1.0	67
19	7.4	8,500	190,000	133	46	0.3	2.8	98
20	3.3	31,600	19,000	30	45	0.8	1.6	70
21	6.2	29,600	6,000	20	17	0.9	1.0	88
22	8.7	19,600	104,000	159	64	0.7	1.0	52
23	7.3	11,200	69,000	34	50	1.0	1.0	70
24	7.4	2,100	15,000	45	23	1.0	24.2	101

Hb: hemoglobin; ALT: alanine aminotransferase; AST: aspartate aminotrasferase.

dysfunction occurs after treatment, and this inflammatory response is proportional to initial parasite burden in *P. vivax* [22]. More recently, *ex vivo* adhesion of *P. vivax*-parasitized red blood cells to human lung endothelial cells was demonstrated for the first time [23], suggesting that cytoadhesion could play a role in the pathogenesis of this disease. Although, in a patient who died of ARDS, histopathological analysis did not show any evidence of cythoadhesion [24]. Patient outcomes in this series support the hypothesis of a primary pulmonary lesion driving the respiratory clinical manifestations, complicated by the presence of concomitant metabolic acidosis or severe anemia. Half of the 16 patients with respiratory distress had concomitant metabolic acidosis, but only 2 had severe anemia simultaneously. Pneumonia is another confounding diagnosis of respiratory distress, and in all the

Table 4. Univariate and multivariate (logistic regression) analysis of factors associated to the admission in the ICUs of children 0–14 years old with *P. vivax* infection, in Manaus, from 2004 to 2009.

	Cases admitted to the ICU n/N (%)	Patients not requiring admission to the ICU n/N (%)	Crude odds ratio (95% CI)	Adjusted odds ratio (95% CI)	p-value
Male sex	17/24 (70.8)	53/91 (58.2)	1.91 (0.92–5.71)	5.90 (1.28–34.25)	0.039
Age (<5 years)	20/24 (83.3)	25/91 (27.5)	4.64 (2.05–7.65)	6.36 (2.67–13.63)	0.028
Peripheral parasitemia (>500 parasites/ mm^3)	14/19 (73.6)	32/89 (36.0)	4.99 (1.65–15.12)	4.94 (1.31–18.63)	0.018
Time of acute disease prior to treatment (>7 days)	8/24 (33.3)	22/91 (24.2)	1.57 (0.60–4.16)	3.39 (0.81–14.10)	0.093
Presence of any chronic disease	10/24 (41.7)	9/91 (9.9)	6.50 (2.25–18.86)	6.02 (1.38–26.35)	0.017
Presence of any other acute co-morbidity	9/24 (37.5)	7/91 (7.7)	7.20 (2.33–22.30)	8.13 (1.33–49.81)	0.023

Table 5. Descriptive data and univariate analysis of *P. vivax* monoinfection cases admitted to the ICU versus patients not requiring ICU admission, according to the WHO type of severity.

	Cases admitted to the ICU n/N (%)	Patients not requiring ICU admission n/N (%)	Odds ratio (95% CI)	p-value	PIM Score (%) of cases (Mean ± SD)
WHO criteria for malaria severity	23/24 (95.8)	17/91 (18.7)	100.11 (12.60–793.60)	<0.001	16.2±15.6
Respiratory distress	16/24 (66.7)	0/91 (0.0)	-	-	18.4±15.7
Shock (algid malaria)	13/24 (54.2)	0/91 (0.0)	-	-	23.3±17.0
Metabolic acidosis	10/24 (41.6)	-	-	-	16.0±12.3
Severe anemia	7/24 (29.2)	5/91 (5.5)	7.08 (2.00–24.97)	0.003	11.0±8.5
Coma	5/24 (20.8)	2/91 (2.2)	11.71 (2.11–64.94)	<0.001	37.2±18.1
Hyperbilirrubinemia	4/24 (16.7)	11/91 (12.1)	1.45 (0.42–5.05)	0.513	15.0±11.8
Hypoglycemia	3/24 (12.5)	0/91 (0.0)	-	-	17.1±20.4
Acute renal failure (ARF) due to hemoglobinuria	2/24 (8.3)	0/91 (0.0)	-	-	3.2±1.1
Death	2/24 (8.3)	0/91 (0.0)	-	-	50.8±6.9

children in the present report antibiotics were prescribed empirically.

The occurrence of severe anemia also paralleled data from other endemic areas [25], and was consistent with previous data published from Manaus [11,26]. Further corroborating data from Indonesia [27], we observed that 5 out of 6 children under 3 months of age presented severe anemia, confirming *P. vivax* as a cause of severe morbidity in the early infancy. Severe anemia can also be seen, not triggered by the parasite itself, in patients with G6PD deficiency, as a complication of the use of primaquine for the radical cure of hypnozoites, as observed in three patients described here (two with pure *P. vivax* and one with mixed infection). If followed by acute renal failure (ARF), it constitutes the syndromic presentation of blackwater fever [28]. Acute renal failure was mostly related to acute hemolysis in patients with G6PD deficiency. The possibility of concomitant *P. malariae* infection, a species known to cause acute or delayed renal complications seems highly improbable, as this species is not detected in Manaus [33]. G6PD deficiency seems to be frequent in Brazilian malaria-endemic areas, where it is not routinely screened before the prescription of antimalarials. The prevalence of the A$^-$ variant among males has been estimated at 3% [29], and a number of hospitalizations due to this complication have been reported [30]. If G6PD deficiency is not ruled out in epidemiological studies focusing on vivax-related anemia, this complication triggered by the parasite per se could be falsely overestimated.

Circulatory collapse (algid malaria) associated with *P. vivax* infection was both frequent and severe, requiring the use of vasopressors, with or without a confirmed positive blood culture for aerobes. Even for *P. falciparum* malaria, the etiology of this complication is uncertain and the potential role of septic shock as a concomitant entity has been proposed [31]. In such cases therefore, blood cultures are mandatory to rule out bacterial co-infections, which may be related to severity and consequently to ICU hospitalization.

The presence of hyperbilirubinemia is becoming recognized recently as an inappropriate criterion of severe disease if found in isolation [32]. In our data this laboratory finding was not predictive of ICU hospitalization [OR = 1,45 (CI = 0,42–5,05), p = 0,513]. Jaundice detected on a routine physical exam, however, could still be used as a warning sign of severity, given that in 3/4 cases jaundice was accompanied by another severity criterion. As serology for the common viral hepatitis in this region was not requested, it is difficult to ascertain whether such episodes were primarily caused by *P. vivax per se* or resulted from a concomitant liver infection.

Coma was also reported in our series, but in 3 out of 5 children with coma, additional explanations other than cerebral malaria could be found, such as viral encephalitis in one, and decompensation of previous neurological sequelae in two. In one patient hypoglycemia could also be a superimposed factor. Cerebral vivax malaria actually seems to be more common in children [34], but the possibility of other infectious diseases of the central nervous system has to be taken into consideration given the low prevalence of cerebral malaria in vivax infection [35].

It is noteworthy that acute or chronic co-morbidities were detected in 58% (14/24) of the patients with *P. vivax*. This was also observed in an almost identical proportion (6/10) of *P. falciparum* patients, which leads to the conclusion that the presence of co-morbidities may contribute to or facilitate the appearance of complications in all malaria. Importantly, this aspect seems to have been specially underreported in prospective studies on vivax severity [3]. Recent data suggests that *P.vivax*-triggered anemia could be related to parvovirus B19 infection [36]. In our series, rotavirus infection was found among ICU-admitted *P. vivax* (4 cases) and *P. falciparum* (2 cases) children. Despite the lack of local data on rotavirus infection, the worldwide-recognized increased severity in those less than 5 years of age could in part explain the younger age of the ICU hospitalized children. Furthermore, in our children, septic shock with confirmed bacteremia was observed in three cases. In Mozambique, the systematic performance of blood cultures on hospital admissions showed that a positive culture for aerobes in children with malaria was associated with an increased risk of death [37]. Therefore, a predisposition to malarial infection in the setting of other bacterial infections may apply to all *Plasmodium* species. The finding of four malnourished children among vivax cases admitted to the ICU does not seem negligible, and should be taken into consideration as a potential confounding factor when severity frequencies are compared across the world [38]. Although *P. vivax* can surely independently cause severe or even life threatening episodes in adults and children, the relative importance of co-morbidities or other chronic existing conditions in accelerating the progression to a severe disease cannot be disregarded.

Despite the WHO recommendation to treat patients with severe *P. vivax* malaria as patients with severe *P. falciparum/P. vivax* malaria, due to the possibility of submicroscopic parasitemia of the first species, the Brazilian Guidelines for Antimalarial Treatment have only recently changed. During the study period of the present study, chloroquine was prescribed to all patients. Resistance to chloroquine was described for the first time in Latin America in Manaus [39], and more recent data suggest that *in vivo* resistance in this locality is estimated at 10% [40]. However the resistance does not seem to be disseminated throughout the country [41], and the first line treatment for *P. vivax* is still chloroquine. Ecological studies suggest that severity in vivax infection could be related to chloroquine-resistance [42]. These and previous data, however, show a good response to chloroquine in severe patients, and suggest that in the Brazilian Amazon this association is not well understood [11].

The fatality rate among *P. vivax* patients hospitalized in the ICU (8.3%) was not insignificant, even in the Brazilian scenario where diagnosis and treatment of malaria are free and universally available. These numbers could be far larger, however, if a reasonably established health system with tertiary care facilities is not in place. Our small sample was unable to show that *P. falciparum* children died more frequently than those infected with *P. vivax*. Actually data from other settings point to a similar fatality rate between the two species [21,43]. From our data it is possible to detect a high risk of ICU admission among children with mixed infections, however this finding needs to be confirmed in other similar settings in Latin America. PIM score predicted mortality relatively well and its use should be emphasized in future similar pediatric studies.

An important limitation of this study is its retrospective design, and all analyzed information is based on the available registration in clinical charts. Besides that, the absence of PCR confirmation of malarial infections is an additional limitation. Species-specific PCR increases the diagnostic accuracy and can detect submicroscopic infections that may have been disregarded only after standard microscopy. It is possible therefore, that some of our assumed *P. vivax* monoinfections may in fact be mixed cases. Although possible, this seems unlikely, as a preliminary analysis from our laboratory shows that only 5% of the positive TBSs for *P. vivax* identify mixed infections, based on real-time PCR (data not shown). Another limitation is the lack of information on total number of patients hospitalized due to malaria in Manaus in the period.

In the present study we showed that, in absolute numbers, *P. vivax* infection was responsible for most of the ICU admissions of children 0–14 years old due to severe malaria (despite of similar proportional numbers when compared to *P. falciparum* infections reported), and that the clinical complications were very similar to those seen in *P. falciparum* in this same endemic area. Despite the fact that peripheral parasitemia greater than 500/mm^3 was associated with ICU hospitalization, the positive predictive value of this cut-off for predicting need for ICU admission is extremely low, given the tiny fraction of malaria cases requiring ICU in the general population. Severe vivax patients should also trigger the routine screening of additional infectious diseases in the daily practice in the tropics. From the public health perspective, decision-makers from national malaria programs should re-orientate clinical management algorithms in order to improve treatment, diminish the burden of hospitalization, decrease costs and reduce malaria-associated mortality.

From the basic science perspective, pathogenesis studies in severe vivax should carefully rule out other diseases, which may alter the immune response [44]. Definitely respiratory distress, shock and anemia are major complications associated with *P. vivax* infection, for which mechanisms are poorly understood even in the case of severe *P. falciparum*. More studies are needed to evaluate the applicability of these findings in other age groups. Due to the fact that studies on the clinical aspects and biology of *P. vivax* have been neglected during most of the 20th century, the large knowledge gaps regarding this parasite [45] may pose challenges for future malaria eradication plans [46].

Acknowledgments

We thank all the directors of the ICUs for their support with data collection, the Health Secretariat of Manaus (SEMSA) and the Health Secretariat of the Amazonas State (SUSAM).

Author Contributions

Conceived and designed the experiments: EFCL MVGL. Performed the experiments: EFCL BMLM SVS SGB. Analyzed the data: AMS MAAA QB MVGL. Wrote the paper: EFCL CO QB MVGL.

References

1. World Health Organization (WHO) (2008) World malaria report 2008. Geneva.
2. Kochar DK, Saxena V, Singh N, Kochar SK, Kumar SV, et al. (2005) *Plasmodium vivax* malaria. Emerg Infect Dis 11: 132–134.
3. Tjitra E, Anstey NM, Sugiarto P, Warikar N, Kenangalem E, et al. (2008) Multidrug-Resistant *Plasmodium vivax* Associated with Severe and Fatal Malaria: A Prospective Study in Papua, Indonesia. PLoS Med 5: e128.
4. Oliveira-Ferreira J, Lacerda MV, Brasil P, Ladislau JL, Tauil PL, et al. (2010) Malaria in Brazil: an overview. Malar J 9: 115.
5. Saraiva MG, Amorim RD, Moura MA, Martinez-Espinosa FE, Barbosa MG (2009) Urban expansion and spatial distribution of malaria in the municipality of Manaus, State of Amazonas. Rev Soc Bras Med Trop 42: 515–522.
6. Lacerda MV, Alexandre MA, Santos PD, Arcanjo AR, Alecrim WD, et al. (2004) Idiopathic thrombocytopenic purpura due to vivax malaria in the Brazilian Amazon. Acta Trop 90: 187–190.
7. Lomar AV, Vidal JE, Lomar FP, Barbas CV, Matos GJ, et al. (2005) Acute respiratory distress syndrome due to vivax malaria: case report and literature review. Braz J Infect Dis 9: 425–430.
8. Lacerda MV, Hipolito JR, Passos LN (2008) Chronic *Plasmodium vivax* infection in a patient with splenomegaly and severe thrombocytopenia. Rev Soc Bras Med Trop 41: 522–523.
9. Lacerda MVG, Oliveira SL, Alecrim MGC (2007) Splenic hematoma in a patient with *Plasmodium vivax* malaria. Rev Soc Bras Med Trop 40: 96–97.
10. Siqueira AM, Alexandre MAA, Mourão MPG, Santos VS, Nagahashi-Marie SK, et al. (2010) Case Report: Severe Rhabdomyolysis from Vivax Malaria in the Brazilian Amazon. Am J Trop Med Hyg 83: 271–273.
11. Alexandre MA, Ferreira CO, Siqueira AM, Magalhaes BL, Mourao MPG, et al. (2010) Severe *Plasmodium vivax* Malaria, Brazilian Amazon. Emerg Infect Dis 16: 1611–1614.
12. Andrade BB, Reis-Filho A, Souza-Neto SM, Clarencio J, Camargo LM, et al. (2010) Severe *Plasmodium vivax* malaria exhibits marked inflammatory imbalance. Malar J 9: 13.
13. Maitland K, Williams TN, Bennett S, Newbold CI, Peto TE, et al. (1996) The interaction between *Plasmodium falciparum* and *P. vivax* in children on Espiritu Santo island, Vanuatu. Trans R Soc Trop Med Hyg 90: 614–620.
14. WHO (1986) Severe and complicated malaria. World Health Organization Malaria Action Programme. Trans R Soc Trop Med Hyg 80 Suppl: 3–50.
15. Santos-Ciminera PD, Roberts DR, Alecrim MG, Costa MR, Quinnan GV Jr (2007) Malaria diagnosis and hospitalization trends, Brazil. Emerg Infect Dis 13: 1597–1600.
16. WHO (2006) Microscopic diagnosis of Malaria. 4th edition ed. Geneva.
17. WHO (2010) Guidelines for the treatment of malaria. .
18. Shann F, Pearson G, Slater A, Wilkinson K (1997) Paediatric index of mortality (PIM): a mortality prediction model for children in intensive care. Intensive Care Med 23: 201–207.
19. Khoo KL, Tan WL, Eng P, Ong YY (1998) Malaria requiring intensive care. Ann Acad Med Singapore 27: 353–357.

20. Koh KH, Chew PH, Kiyu A (2004) A retrospective study of malaria infections in an intensive care unit of a general hospital in Malaysia. Singapore Med J 45: 28–36.
21. Kochar DK, Tanwar GS, Khatri PC, Kochar SK, Sengar GS, et al. (2010) Clinical features of children hospitalized with malaria-a study from Bikaner, northwest India. Am J Trop Med Hyg 83: 981–989.
22. Anstey NM, Handojo T, Pain MC, Kenangalem E, Tjitra E, et al. (2007) Lung injury in vivax malaria: pathophysiological evidence for pulmonary vascular sequestration and posttreatment alveolar-capillary inflammation. J Infect Dis 195: 589–596.
23. Carvalho BO, Lopes SC, Nogueira PA, Orlandi PP, Bargieri DY, et al. (2010) On the Cytoadhesion of *Plasmodium vivax*-Infected Erythrocytes. J Infect Dis 202: 638–647.
24. Valecha N, Pinto RG, Turner GD, Kumar A, Rodrigues S, et al. (2009) Histopathology of fatal respiratory distress caused by Plasmodium vivax malaria. Am J Trop Med Hyg 81: 758–762.
25. Mueller I, Namuigi P, Kundi J, Ivivi R, Tandrapah T, et al. (2005) Epidemic malaria in the highlands of Papua New Guinea. Am J Trop Med Hyg 72: 554–560.
26. Caicedo O, Ramirez O, Mourao MP, Ziadec J, Perez P, et al. (2009) Comparative hematologic analysis of uncomplicated malaria in uniquely different regions of unstable transmission in Brazil and Colombia. Am J Trop Med Hyg 80: 146–151.
27. Poespoprodjo JR, Fobia W, Kenangalem E, Lampah DA, Hasanuddin A, et al. (2009) Vivax Malaria: A Major Cause of Morbidity in Early Infancy. Clin Infect Dis.
28. Burgoine KL, Bancone G, Nosten F (2010) The reality of using primaquine. Malar J 9: 376.
29. Santana MS, Lacerda MVG, Barbosa MGV, Alecrim WD, Alecrim MGC (2009) Glucose-6-phosphate dehydrogenase deficiency in an endemic area for malaria in Manaus: a cross-sectional survey in the Brazilian Amazon. PLoS ONE 4: e5259.
30. Ramos Junior WM, Sardinha JF, Costa MR, Santana MS, Alecrim MG, et al. (2010) Clinical aspects of hemolysis in patients with *P. vivax* malaria treated with primaquine, in the Brazilian Amazon. Braz J Infect Dis 14: 410–412.
31. Lacerda MV, Mourao MP, Santos PJ, Alecrim MG (2009) Algid malaria: a syndromic diagnosis. Rev Soc Bras Med Trop 42: 79–81.
32. Anstey NM, Price RN (2007) Improving case definitions for severe malaria. PLoS Med 4: e267.
33. Costa MR, Vieira PP, Ferreira Cde O, Lacerda MV, Alecrim WD, et al. (2008) Molecular diagnosing of malaria in a tertiary care center in the Brazilian Amazon region. Rev Soc Bras Med Trop 41: 381–385.
34. Beg MA, Khan R, Baig SM, Gulzar Z, Hussain R, et al. (2002) Cerebral involvement in benign tertian malaria. Am J Trop Med Hyg 67: 230–232.
35. Lampah DA, Yeo TW, Hardianto SO, Tjitra E, Kenangalem E, et al. (2011) Coma associated with microscopy-diagnosed *Plasmodium vivax*: a prospective study in Papua, Indonesia. PLoS Negl Trop Dis 5: e1032.
36. Wildig J, Michon P, Siba P, Mellombo M, Ura A, et al. (2006) Parvovirus B19 infection contributes to severe anemia in young children in Papua New Guinea. J Infect Dis 194: 146–153.
37. Bassat Q, Guinovart C, Sigauque B, Mandomando I, Aide P, et al. (2009) Severe malaria and concomitant bacteraemia in children admitted to a rural Mozambican hospital. Trop Med Int Health 14: 1011–1019.
38. Caulfield LE, Richard SA, Black RE (2004) Undernutrition as an underlying cause of malaria morbidity and mortality in children less than five years old. Am J Trop Med Hyg 71: 55–63.
39. Alecrim MGC, Alecrim W, Macêdo V (1999) *Plasmodium vivax* resistance to chloroquine (R2) and mefloquine (R3) in Brazilian Amazon region. Rev Soc Bras Med Trop 32: 67–68.
40. Santana Filho FS, Arcanjo AR, Chehuan YM, Costa MR, Martinez-Espinosa FE, et al. (2007) Chloroquine-resistant *Plasmodium vivax*, Brazilian Amazon. Emerg Infect Dis 13: 1125–1126.
41. Orjuela-Sanchez P, da Silva NS, da Silva-Nunes M, Ferreira MU (2009) Recurrent parasitemias and population dynamics of Plasmodium vivax polymorphisms in rural Amazonia. Am J Trop Med Hyg 81: 961–968.
42. Price RN, Douglas NM, Anstey NM (2009) New developments in *Plasmodium vivax* malaria: severe disease and the rise of chloroquine resistance. Curr Opin Infect Dis 22: 430–435.
43. Barcus MJ, Basri H, Picarima H, Manyakori C, Sekartuti, et al. (2007) Demographic risk factors for severe and fatal vivax and falciparum malaria among hospital admissions in northeastern indonesian papua. Am J Trop Med Hyg 77: 984–991.
44. Bassat Q, Alonso PL (2011) Defying malaria: Fathoming severe *Plasmodium vivax* disease. Nat Med 17: 48–49.
45. Mueller I, Galinski MR, Baird JK, Carlton JM, Kochar DK, et al. (2009) Key gaps in the knowledge of *Plasmodium vivax*, a neglected human malaria parasite. Lancet Infect Dis 9: 555–566.
46. Alonso PL, Brown G, Arevalo-Herrera M, Binka F, Chitnis C, et al. (2011) A research agenda to underpin malaria eradication. PLoS Med 8: e1000406.

18

Infectious Events Prior to Chemotherapy Initiation in Children with Acute Myeloid Leukemia

Carol Portwine[1], David Mitchell[2], Donna Johnston[3], Biljana Gillmeister[4], Marie-Chantal Ethier[4], Rochelle Yanofsky[5], David Dix[6], Sonia Cellot[7], Victor Lewis[8], Victoria Price[9], Mariana Silva[10], Shayna Zelcer[11], Lynette Bowes[12], Bruno Michon[13], Kent Stobart[14], Josee Brossard[15], Joseph Beyene[4,16], Lillian Sung[4,17]*

1 Hematology/Oncology, McMaster Children's Hospital at Hamilton Health Sciences, Hamilton, Ontario, Canada, **2** Hematology/Oncology, Montreal Children's Hospital, Montreal, Québec, Canada, **3** Hematology/Oncology, Children's Hospital of Eastern Ontario, Ottawa, Ontario, Canada, **4** Child Health Evaluative Sciences, The Hospital for Sick Children, Toronto, Ontario, Canada, **5** Hematology/Oncology, CancerCare Manitoba, Winnipeg, Manitoba, Canada, **6** Pediatric Hematology/Oncology, British Columbia Children's Hospital, Vancouver, British Columbia, Canada, **7** Hematology/Oncology, Hospital Sainte-Justine, Montreal, Quebec, Canada, **8** Hematology/Oncology/Transplant Program, Alberta Children's Hospital, Calgary, Alberta, Canada, **9** Pediatrics, IWK Health Centre, Halifax, Nova Scotia, Canada, **10** Hematology/Oncology, Cancer Centre of Southeastern Ontario at Kingston, Kingston, Ontario, Canada, **11** Hematology/Oncology, London Health Sciences, London, Ontario, Canada, **12** Hematology/Oncology, Janeway Child Health Centre, St. John's, Newfoundland, Canada, **13** Pediatric Hematology/Oncology Centre, Hospitalier Universitaire de Quebec Centre, Quebec City, Quebec, Canada, **14** Stollery Children's Hospital, University of Alberta Hospital, Edmonton Clinic Health Academy (ECHA), Edmonton, Alberta, Canada, **15** Hematology/Oncology, Centre Hospitalier Universitaire de Sherbrooke, Sherbrooke, Quebec, Canada, **16** Population Genomics Program, Department of Clinical Epidemiology and Biostatistics, McMaster University, Hamilton, Ontario, Canada, **17** Division of Haematology/Oncology, The Hospital for Sick Children, Toronto, Ontario, Canada

Abstract

Background: The primary objective was to describe infectious complications in children with acute myeloid leukemia from presentation to the healthcare system to initiation of chemotherapy and to describe how these infections differ depending on neutropenia.

Methods: We conducted a retrospective, population-based cohort study that included children and adolescents with acute myeloid leukemia diagnosed and treated at 15 Canadian centers. We evaluated infections that occurred between presentation to the healthcare system (for symptoms that led to the diagnosis of acute myeloid leukemia) until initiation of chemotherapy.

Results: Among 328 children, 92 (28.0%) were neutropenic at presentation. Eleven (3.4%) had sterile-site microbiologically documented infection and four had bacteremia (only one Gram negative). Infection rate was not influenced by neutropenia. No child died from an infectious cause prior to chemotherapy initiation.

Conclusion: It may be reasonable to withhold empiric antibiotics in febrile non-neutropenic children with newly diagnosed acute myeloid leukemia until initiation of chemotherapy as long as they appear well without a clinical focus of infection. Future work could examine biomarkers or a clinical score to identify children presenting with leukemia and fever who are more likely to have an invasive infection.

Editor: Ray Borrow, Health Protection Agency, United Kingdom

Funding: This work was supported by the Canadian Cancer Society (grant number 019468) and the C17 Research Network. LS is supported by a New Investigator Award from the Canadian Institutes of Health Research. The funders had no role in study design, data collection and analysis, decision to publish, or preparation of the manuscript.

Competing Interests: The authors have declared that no competing interests exist.

* E-mail: lillian.sung@sickkids.ca

Introduction

Children with acute myeloid leukemia (AML) receive intensive chemotherapy and during treatment, they are at substantial risk of morbidity and mortality from invasive infections.[1] The management of fever with neutropenia is relatively straightforward in these children after they begin chemotherapy.[2] However, when children with acute leukemia initially enter the healthcare system, fever is a common presentation and neutropenia may also be present.[3] The optimal management of children with newly diagnosed leukemia with fever in the period preceding initiation of chemotherapy is uncertain, both for those with and without neutropenia. Cancer-specific fever and neutropenia guidelines do not provide recommendations for this scenario since the setting for guidelines is usually restricted to patients who are receiving treatments for cancer.[2,4] Furthermore, it would be useful to know if infection outcomes differed depending on the presence or absence of neutropenia in this setting since the presence of neutropenia is a major criterion that influences the decision to start antibiotics in febrile children receiving treatment for cancer.

Consequently, we conducted a population-based study of pediatric AML using a retrospective cohort design. The primary objective was to describe infectious complications in children with AML from presentation to the healthcare system to initiation of chemotherapy and to describe how these infections differ depending on neutropenia.

Materials and Methods

Ethics Statement

This study was approved by the Research Ethics Board at The Hospital for Sick Children and local Research Ethics Boards of the 14 other participating sites (McMaster University-Hamilton Health Sciences/Faculty of Health Sciences Research Ethics Board, Montreal Children's Hospital Research Ethics Board, Children's Hospital of Eastern Ontario Research Ethics Board, University of Winnipeg Research Ethics Board, University of British Columbia/Children's and Women's Health Centre of British Columbia Research Ethics Board, Centre Hospitalier Universitaire Sainte-Justine Research Ethics Board, University of Calgary Conjoint Health Research Ethics Board, IWK Research Ethics Board, Queen's University-Health Sciences Research Ethics Board, University of Western Ontario Research Ethics Board for Health Science Research Involving Human Subjects, Memorial University Human Investigation Committee, Centre Hospitalier Universitaire de Quebec Research Ethics Board, University of Alberta Health Research Ethics Board-Biomedical Panel, and Centre Hospitalier Universitaire de Sherbrooke Research Ethics Board). As this was a retrospective review study, the Research Ethics Board at The Hospital for Sick Children and those at the 14 other participating sites waived the need for written informed consent. All demographic information and information about the child's diagnosis and treatment were abstracted from the child's chart.

Study Sample

This manuscript is related to a large retrospective, population-based cohort study in which we included children and adolescents with AML diagnosed and treated in each Canadian province except Saskatchewan.[5] We included children and adolescents ≤18 years with *de novo* AML diagnosed between January 1, 1995 and December 31, 2004. Children with Down syndrome were also included. We excluded those with acute promyelocytic leukemia, secondary AML, and previous diagnosis of immunodeficiency.

Outcome Measures

We evaluated infections that occurred between presentation to the healthcare system (for symptoms that led to the diagnosis of AML) until initiation of chemotherapy. Data abstraction was conducted by trained clinical research associates who travelled to each site to abstract and code all data.

We described the occurrence of sterile site invasive infection[6], clinically documented infection and fever of unknown origin. Fever was defined as a single oral temperature of 38.3° C or a temperature of 38.0° C for 1 hour.[7] In this study, we did not distinguish between infections present at the time of admission and those acquired after admission but prior to initiation of treatment. Positive cultures with common contaminants such as coagulase negative *Staphylococcus* were only considered true infection if there were two or more positive cultures in the same episode or if the infection was associated with sepsis. In this study, sepsis was defined as systemic inflammatory response syndrome in the presence of suspected or proven infection and organ dysfunction.[8] Clinically documented infections were classified based upon the Centers for Disease Control and Prevention (CDC) definitions of nosocomial infections.[9] However, for our study, we did not require that clinically documented infections be not present or incubating at the time of admission to hospital. Fever of unknown origin was fever occurring in the absence of a positive microbiology result or clinical site of infection.

Potential Predictors

We compared baseline characteristics and infection outcomes depending upon if the patient was neutropenic (absolute neutrophil count (ANC)$<0.5\times10^9$/L) at presentation.

Characteristics evaluated were: gender, age, Down syndrome, body mass index percentile at diagnosis, peripheral blood counts at diagnosis and AML morphology. Obesity was defined as body mass index (BMI) ≥95th percentile and underweight was defined as BMI ≤10th percentile for age and gender according to the CDC for those at least 2 years of age.[10] BMI was evaluated as obesity previously has been associated with treatment-related mortality and infections in pediatric AML[11,12].

Statistics

Characteristics and infection outcomes were compared between those who were and were not neutropenic at presentation using the Wilcoxon rank sum test for continuous variables and Chi square or Fisher's exact test for categorical variables. All tests of significance were two-sided, and statistical significance was defined as $P<0.05$. Statistical analysis was performed using the SAS statistical program (SAS-PC, version 9·3; SAS Institute Inc., Cary, NC).

Results

There were 343 children with de novo AML who met eligibility criteria in the study time frame. Of these children, 15 began chemotherapy on the same day as presentation to the healthcare center and thus, there were 328 children with pre-chemotherapy information available. The median time between presentation and initiation of chemotherapy was 2 (range 0 to 274) days. There were two patients who had very lengthy delays between presentation and initiation of chemotherapy of 59 and 274 days.

Table S1 illustrates that 92 (28.0%) children were neutropenic at presentation. Gender and age were not significantly associated with neutropenia at presentation whereas children with Down syndrome were significantly less likely to present with neutropenia. Children with neutropenia had a significantly lower initial peripheral blast count and hemoglobin level compared to non-neutropenic children although the initial platelet count was similar between the two groups.

Table 1 and Table S2 illustrate the infection outcomes. Overall, there were 11/328 (3.4%) children who experienced 12 sterile site microbiologically documented infections; the risk did not significantly differ by the presence or absence of neutropenia. There were four episodes of bacteremia with viridans group streptococci (n = 3) and *Pseudomonas aeruginosa* (n = 1), all occurring in non-neutropenic children. Among the six episodes of urinary tract infection, the causative agents were: *Enterococcus* species (n = 2), *Escherichia coli* (n = 2), *P. aeruginosa* (n = 1) and *Candida albicans* (n = 1). The two other sterile site infections were *Staphylococcus aureus* from a peritoneal drain (see below) and a lymph node biopsy. Other than for the one *C. albicans* urinary tract infection, no other fungi from sterile or non-sterile sites were observed (data

Table 1. Infection outcomes before chemotherapy initiation by neutropenia at presentation.*

	Neutropenic at Presentation (N = 92)	Not Neutropenic at Presentation (N = 236)	P Value
Median days of fever (range)	1.0 (0.0–17.0)	1.0 (0.0–16.0)	0.794
Sterile site microbiologically documented infection (%)	2 (2.2)	9 (3.8)	0.734
Gram-positive sterile site infection (%)	1 (1.1)	6 (2.5)	0.678
Gram-negative sterile site infection (%)	1 (1.1)	3 (1.3)	1.000
Bacteremia (%)[a]	0	4 (1.7)	0.580
Invasive fungal infection (%)	1 (2.2)	0	0.281
Clinically documented infection (%)	12 (13.0)	31 (13.1)	1.000
Fever of unknown origin (%)	35 (38.0)	86 (36.4)	0.886
Median days intravenous antibiotics (range)	1.0 (0.0–16.0)	0.0 (0.0–25.0)	0.073
Sepsis (%)	1.0 (1.1)	0	0.281
Infection-related mortality (%)	0	0	NC

Abbreviation: NC–not calculable.
*Infection outcomes denote at least one occurrence during the pre-chemotherapy period.
[a]Bacteremias were viridans group streptococci (n = 3) and *Pseudomona aeruginosa* (n = 1).

not shown). One child experienced sepsis with concurrent pneumonia.

Three children died before initiation of chemotherapy. Two children died of hyperleukocytosis and pulmonary leukostasis. A third child presented with a 10 day history of fever and was found to have pneumonia on chest radiograph; the absolute neutrophil count was 0.2×10^9/L at presentation. The child was treated with broad-spectrum antibiotics and after 10 days of persistent fever, she was found to have *C. albicans* from urine and therefore, amphotericin B was initiated. Over the next four days, she developed acute respiratory distress and multi-organ failure; a peritoneal drain grew *S. aureus*. Autopsy failed to reveal an infectious cause of death and death was attributed to progressive AML.

Discussion

We conducted a comprehensive assessment of infections occurring before chemotherapy initiation in newly diagnosed pediatric AML. We found that sterile site infections were rare, Gram negative bacteremia occurred in only one child, and many infections were from a urinary site. Infection outcomes were similar between neutropenic and non-neutropenic children. Our findings suggest that it may be reasonable to withhold empiric antibiotics in febrile non-neutropenic children with newly diagnosed AML until initiation of chemotherapy as long as they appear well without a clinical focus of infection. Reducing antibiotic exposure is important given the relationship between greater antibiotic use and antibiotic resistance[13,14] and invasive fungal infection.[15] However, the safety of this approach has not yet been tested.

Although our analysis did not show a difference in outcomes by neutropenia at presentation, limited power for this comparison is an important consideration since only 28% of children were neutropenic. Patients with non-cancer related neutropenia may be at risk of invasive infection if the neutropenia is associated with profound immunosuppression.[16] Thus, we do not suggest withholding empiric antibiotics in this situation and suggest empiric antibiotics be initiated in a febrile neutropenic child with newly diagnosed AML. Our data also suggest that if empiric antibiotics are initiated (for example, because of neutropenia, unwell appearance or a clinical site of infection), broad-spectrum antibiotics with activity against *P.aeruginosa* are important.

Future work could examine biomarkers or a clinical score to identify children presenting with leukemia and fever who are more likely to have an invasive infection. This approach may allow antibiotic therapy to be tailored to children at higher risk of infection.

The strengths of our report are the multi-center nature of the study which allowed capture of a large number of children with AML. Further, the data are highly generalizable. However, there are important limitations to our study. Centers had different approaches to supportive care and urgency of chemotherapy initiation. Second, the retrospective design made it more difficult to appreciate the clinical status of the child at presentation.

In conclusion, we found that in children with AML, 28% will present with neutropenia. Sterile site infections were rare. It may be reasonable to withhold empiric antibiotics in febrile non-neutropenic children with newly diagnosed AML until initiation of chemotherapy as long as they appear well without a clinical focus of infection.

Acknowledgments

All authors contributed to data collection and manuscript writing. All authors have approved the final version of the manuscript.

CANADIAN INFECTIONS IN AML RESEARCH GROUP: David Dix (PI) and Nita Takeuchi (CRA) from British Columbia Children's Hospital; Kent Stobart (PI), Brenda Ennis (CRA) and Linda Churcher (CRA) from Stollery Children's Hospital; Victor Lewis (PI), Janice Hamilton (CRA) and Karen Mazil (CRA) from Alberta Children's Hospital; Sonia Cellot (PI), Dominique Lafreniere (CRA) and Catherine Desjean (CRA) from Hospital Sainte-Justine; Victoria Price (PI), Tina Bocking (CRA), Lynn Russell (CRA) and Emily Murray (CRA) from IWK Health Centre; Lynette Bowes (PI) and Gale Roberts (CRA) from Janeway Child Health Centre; Carol Portwine (PI) and Sabrina Siciliano (CRA) from McMaster Children's Hospital at Hamilton Health Sciences; Joseph Beyene (Collaborator) from McMaster University; Mariana Silva (PI) from Kingston General Hospital; Rochelle Yanofsky (PI), Rebekah Hiebert (CRA) and Krista Mueller (CRA) from CancerCare Manitoba; Shayna Zelcer (PI), Martha Rolland (CRA) and Julie Nichols (CRA) from London Health Sciences; Donna Johnston (PI) and Elaine Dollard (CRA) from

Children's Hospital of Eastern Ontario; David Mitchell (PI), Martine Nagy (CRA) and Margaret Hin Chan (CRA) from Montreal Children's Hospital; Bruno Michon (PI), Josee Legris (CRA) and Marie-Christine Gagnon (CRA) from Hospitalier Universitaire de Quebec; Josee Brossard (PI) and Lise Bilodeau (CRA) from Centre Hospitalier Universitaire de Sherbrooke; Lillian Sung (PI), Biljana Gillmeister (CRA), Marie-Chantal Ethier (CRA), Renee Freeman (Collaborator), Jeffrey Traubici (Collaborator), and Upton Allen (Collaborator) from The Hospital for Sick Children.

Author Contributions

Conceived and designed the experiments: BG MCE LS. Performed the experiments: CP DM DJ BG MCE RY DD SC VL VP MS SZ LB BM KS J. Brossard J. Beyene LS. Analyzed the data: J. Beyene LS. Contributed reagents/materials/analysis tools: LS. Wrote the paper: CP DM DJ BG MCE RY DD SC VL VP MS SZ LB BM KS J. Brossard J. Beyene LS.

References

1. Hann I, Viscoli C, Paesmans M, Gaya H, Glauser M (1997) A comparison of outcome from febrile neutropenic episodes in children compared with adults: results from four EORTC studies. International Antimicrobial Therapy Cooperative Group (IATCG) of the European Organization for Research and Treatment of Cancer (EORTC). Br J Haematol 99: 580–588.
2. Lehrnbecher T, Phillilps R, Alexander S, Alvaro F, Carlesse F, et al. (2012) Guidelines for the management of fever and neutropenia in children with cancer and/or undergoing hematopoietic stem cell transplantation. J Clin Oncol. In Press.
3. Fadoo Z, Mushtaq N, Alvi S, Ali M (2012) Acute myeloid leukaemia in children: experience at a tertiary care facility of Pakistan. J Pak Med Assoc 62: 125–128.
4. Freifeld AG, Bow EJ, Sepkowitz KA, Boeckh MJ, Ito JI, et al. (2011) Clinical practice guideline for the use of antimicrobial agents in neutropenic patients with cancer: 2010 update by the infectious diseases society of america. Clin Infect Dis 52: e56–93.
5. Dix D, Cellot S, Price V, Gillmeister B, Ethier MC, et al. (2012) Association between Corticosteroids and Infection, Sepsis and Infectious Death in Pediatric Acute Myeloid Leukemia: from the Canadian Infections in AML Research Group. Clin Infect Dis. In press.
6. Santolaya ME, Alvarez AM, Becker A, Cofre J, Enriquez N, et al. (2001) Prospective, multicenter evaluation of risk factors associated with invasive bacterial infection in children with cancer, neutropenia, and fever. J Clin Oncol 19: 3415–3421.
7. Hughes WT, Armstrong D, Bodey GP, Bow EJ, Brown AE, et al. (2002) 2002 guidelines for the use of antimicrobial agents in neutropenic patients with cancer. Clin Infect Dis 34: 730–751.
8. Goldstein B, Giroir B, Randolph A (2005) International pediatric sepsis consensus conference: definitions for sepsis and organ dysfunction in pediatrics. Pediatr Crit Care Med 6: 2–8.
9. Garner JS, Jarvis WR, Emori TG, Horan TC, Hughes JM (1996) CDC definitions for nosocomial infections. In: Olmsted RN, ed,: APIC Infection Control and Applied Epidemiology: Principles and Practice. St. Louis: Mosby.
10. Ogden CL, Kuczmarski RJ, Flegal KM, Mei Z, Guo S, et al. (2002) Centers for Disease Control and Prevention 2000 growth charts for the United States: improvements to the 1977 National Center for Health Statistics version. Pediatrics 109: 45–60.
11. Lange BJ, Gerbing RB, Feusner J, Skolnik J, Sacks N, et al. (2005) Mortality in overweight and underweight children with acute myeloid leukemia. JAMA 293: 203–211.
12. Sung L, Lange BJ, Gerbing RB, Alonzo TA, Feusner J (2007) Microbiologically documented infections and infection-related mortality in children with acute myeloid leukemia. Blood 110: 3532–3539.
13. Almyroudis NG, Lesse AJ, Hahn T, Samonis G, Hazamy PA, et al. (2011) Molecular epidemiology and risk factors for colonization by vancomycin-resistant Enterococcus in patients with hematologic malignancies. Infect Control Hosp Epidemiol 32: 490–496.
14. Rangaraj G, Granwehr BP, Jiang Y, Hachem R, Raad I (2010) Perils of quinolone exposure in cancer patients: breakthrough bacteremia with multidrug-resistant organisms. Cancer 116: 967–973.
15. Hu R, Jiang X, Wu Y (2012) Risk factors for invasive pulmonary fungal infection in patients with hematological malignancies not receiving hematopoietic stem cell transplant. Neoplasma 59: 669–675.
16. Sung L, Johnston DL (2007) Approach to febrile neutropenia in the general paediatric setting. Paediatr Child Health 12: 19–21.

Potential Role of *M. tuberculosis* Specific IFN-γ and IL-2 ELISPOT Assays in Discriminating Children with Active or Latent Tuberculosis

Elena Chiappini[1]*, Chiara Della Bella[2], Francesca Bonsignori[1], Sara Sollai[1], Amedeo Amedei[2], Luisa Galli[1], Elena Niccolai[2], Gianfranco Del Prete[2†], Mahavir Singh[3], Mario M. D'Elios[2], Maurizio de Martino[1]

1 Anna Meyer University Hospital, Department of Science for Woman and Child Health, University of Florence, Florence, Italy, **2** Department of Internal Medicine, University of Florence, Florence, Italy, **3** Lionex GmbH, Braunschweig, Germany

Abstract

Background: Although currently available IGRA have been reported to be promising markers for TB infection, they cannot distinguish active tuberculosis (TB) from latent infection (LTBI).

Objective: Children with LTBI, active TB disease or uninfected were prospectively evaluated by an in-house ELISPOT assay in order to investigate possible immunological markers for a differential diagnosis between LTBI and active TB.

Methods: Children at risk for TB infection prospectively enrolled in our infectious disease unit were evaluated by in-house IFN-γ and IL-2 based ELISPOT assays using a panel of *Mycobacterium tuberculosis* antigens.

Results: Twenty-nine children were classified as uninfected, 21 as LTBI and 25 as active TB cases (including 5 definite and 20 probable cases). Significantly higher IFN-γ ELISPOT responses were observed in infected *vs.* uninfected children for ESAT-6 ($p<0.0001$), CFP-10 ($p<0.0001$), TB 10.3 ($p=0.003$), and AlaDH ($p=0.001$), while differences were not significant considering Ag85B ($p=0.063$), PstS1 ($p=0.512$), and HspX (16 kDa) ($p=0.139$). IL-2 ELISPOT assay responses were different for ESAT-6 ($p<0.0001$), CFP-10 ($p<0.0001$), TB 10.3 ($p<0.0001$), HspX (16 kDa) ($p<0.0001$), PstS1 ($p<0.0001$) and AlaDH ($p=0.001$); but not for Ag85B ($p=0.063$). Comparing results between children with LTBI and those with TB disease differences were significant for IFN-γ ELISPOT only for AlaDH antigen ($p=0.021$) and for IL-2 ELISPOT assay for AlaDH ($p<0.0001$) and TB 10.3 antigen ($p=0.043$). ROC analyses demonstrated sensitivity of 100% and specificity of 81% of AlaDH-IL-2 ELISPOT assay in discriminating between latent and active TB using a cut off of 12.5 SCF per million PBMCs.

Conclusion: Our data suggest that IL-2 based ELISPOT with AlaDH antigen may be of help in discriminating children with active from those with latent TB.

Editor: Pere-Joan Cardona, Fundació Institut d'Investigació en Ciències de la Salut Germans Trias i Pujol. Universitat Autònoma de Barcelona. CIBERES, Spain

Funding: Financial support was given in part by Italian Health Ministry, Young Research Prize, 2007, and by European Union FP7 NOPERSIST research grants. The funders had no role in study design, data collection and analysis, decision to publish, or preparation of the manuscript.

Competing Interests: MS is the owner and director of commercial company Lionex GmbH, Braunschweig, Germany. Lionex has not provided any financial support for the research mentioned in the manuscript. This does not alter the authors' adherence to all the PLOS ONE policies on sharing data and materials. All other authors do not have a commercial or other association that might pose a conflict of interest.

* E-mail: echiappini@unifi.it

† Deceased.

Introduction

Substantial advances have been recently achieved in the immunological diagnosis of *Mycobacterium tuberculosis* infection [1]. Three *Mycobacterium tuberculosis* specific interferon-γ (INF-γ) release assays (IGRAs) are now commercially available. With respect of tuberculin skin test (TST), IGRAs have a number of advantages: they are minimally influenced by previous bacille Calmette-Guérin (BCG) vaccination or infection by non-tuberculosis mycobacteria, do not cause booster effect, do not necessitate of a double access to health care facility, and interpretation of results is not operator-dependent [2]. In adults IGRAs have been reported to be more specific and at least as sensitive as TST [3], and are currently included in diagnostic algorithms in adult guidelines [4]. However, reported IGRAs sensitivity and specificity largely vary among studies in paediatric populations and caution is recommended regarding their use in children [1,5,6,7]. Moreover, IGRAs do not distinguish LTBI from active tuberculosis (TB) patients [8]. This issue is fundamental for paediatricians since a definite diagnosis of active TB is rare in children. Paediatric TB disease is typically paucibacillary and most TB diagnoses are "probable "diseases, based on TST/IGRA results, clinical symptoms and signs, radiological findings, epidemiological data, and response to antitubercular therapy [1,5–8]. Therefore a test able to distinguish accurately LTBI from active TB would be valuable. IGRAs based on cytokines other than IFN- γ or exploring immune response to other mycobacterial antigens besides those included in the commercially available IGRAs are currently under investigations [8].

Previous observations suggest a possible role of IL-2- based ELISPOT assay in addition to the IFN-gamma-based assay in discriminating active from latent TB, as only cells from individuals with LTBI and not those from individuals with active TB has been found to secrete IL-2 after specific stimulation [9]. These results probably reflect the increased number of IL-2 secreting and IL-2/ IFN-gamma secreting central memory T cells and the reduced number of IFN-gamma effector T-cells in LTBI patients, associated with the low bacterial replication and low antigen load [10]. In the present study we prospectively evaluated the performances of in-house IFN-γ and IL-2 based ELISPOT assays by the use of a panel of *Mycobacterium tuberculosis* antigens in children consecutively referred to one paediatric infectious disease unit and at risk for TB infection with the aim of investigating possible immunological markers for a differential diagnosis between LTBI and active TB.

Materials and Methods

Study subjects

Children at risk for TB infection consecutively referred to our Infectious Disease Unit were prospectively enrolled between 1 st January 2009 and 31st April 2010. Study children were those with clinical suspicion of TB disease and/or in close contact with recently diagnosed cases of contagious TB disease and/or internationally adopted or recently immigrated children coming from countries with a high-prevalence of TB. Children with congenital or acquired immunodeficiency disorders (based on their medical history, clinical examination and/or laboratory tests) were excluded from the study. This study was approved by the ethical committee of the Anna Meyer University Hospital, Florence, Italy. All the parents/tutors of the study children gave written consent to the study.

Tuberculin skin test (TST)

TST was administered by trained nurses dedicated to our Infectious Disease Unit and was performed according to the Mantoux method by injecting intradermally 5 tuberculin units (in 0.1 mL) of purified protein derivative (Statens Serum Institute, Copenhagen, Denmark) into the volar surface of the forearm. The transversed skin induration was recorded (in mm) after 48–72 hours directly by a pediatrician of the Infectious Disease Unit. Following the American Academy of Pediatrics guidelines [7], a positive TST was defined as an induration size ≥5 mm for children in close contact with known or suspected contagious case of TB disease or for children suspected to have TB disease (based on clinical evidence and/or chest radiograph) and ≥10 mm for children born in countries with a high prevalence of TB and recently immigrated.

QuantiFERON Gold In tube test (QFT-G-IT)

The QFT-IT assay (Cellestis Inc., Australia) was performed according to the manufacturer's instructions as described previously. After subtracting the value from the negative control, the result was positive if, the antigen-dependent response was ≥0.35 IU, negative if the mitogen–induced response was ≥0.5 IU/mL and the antigen-dependent response was <0.35 IU/mL, and indeterminate if both mitogen-induced and antigen-dependent responses were below cut-off or mitogen-induced response >8 IU/mL.

ELISPOT Assay

In-house ELIPOT assay detecting IFN-gamma and IL-2 responses were performed using recombinant *M. tuberculosis* antigens (ESAT-6, CFP-10, TB 10.3, AlaDH, Ag85B, PstS1, HspX (16 kDa) protein), provided by Lionex Diagnostics & Therapeutics GmbH (Braunschweig, Germany), as previously reported [10,11]. Characteristics of the used antigens are summarized in Table 1. Briefly, peripheral blood mononuclear cells (PBMCs; 1×10^6 cells/mL) of each patients were stimulated with *M. tuberculosis* recombinant antigen (5 μg/mL), and seeded in triplicate in 96-well plates coated with anti–IFN-γ or anti–IL-2 antibody. Cells stimulated with medium alone served as negative controls. Cells stimulated with phytohemoagglutinin (PHA) served as positive controls. IFN-γ and IL-2 ELISPOT microplates were then incubated at 37°C in 5% CO_2 for 24 hours. At the end of the culture period, plates were washed and incubated for 3 hours with the appropriate biotinylated anti–IFN-γ or anti–IL-2 monoclonal antibody. Streptavidin-HRP complex was then added for 2 hours, followed by the substrate solution. Spot forming colonies (SFCs) were counted using an automated ELISPOT reader (Autoimmune Diagnostika GmbH) and results expressed as number of SFCs per million PBMCs, as described [12]. Laboratory workers were blind to the clinical status of participants.

Study design

Information regarding demographic data, prior TB exposure, and past medical history was obtained from each child's parents or tutors or from medical documentation and recorded into the study database. Children were considered vaccinated with BCG whether a clear documentation was available and/or a scar was present. All children underwent clinical evaluation, TST and venipuncture for IGRAs (QFT-G-IT and in-house ELISPOT assay) and results entered into a databse. Blood was taken during the first examination after the parent's or tutor's informed consent had been obtained and before starting any anti-tubercular treatment. Chest radiography was performed in all symptomatic children, in those with a positive TST, and in all contacts aged less than 5 years [7]. Children with suspected pulmonary TB had three sputum or early morning gastric aspirates samples collected for *Mycobacterium tuberculosis* detection (by means of microscopy, polymerase chain reaction and culture) [7]. Chest computed tomography (CT) scan was performed in selected cases at the paediatrician's discretion. No suspected or ascertained extra-pulmonary TB cases presented at the Infectious Disease Unit during the study period.

The study received approval from the Ethical Committee of Anna Meyer Children University Hospital.

Definition of study groups

Study children were classified as not-infected, LTBI cases, or active TB disease cases, following the American Academy Guidelines definition [7]. In the event of discordant TST/QFT-G-IT results, children were assigned to the corresponding group on the bases on the TST result [7]. In particular, asymptomatic children with negative TST were defined as uninfected. LTBI diagnosis was assigned to any child with a positive TST and no clinical or radiographic evidence of active TB [7]. Cases of active TB were defined according to two categories: 1) definite TB, children with *Mycobacterium tuberculosis* cultured or detected by microscopy or molecular methods from sputum or gastric aspirate culture; 2) probable TB: absence of microbiological confirmation but presence of all of the following criteria: (A) clinical symptoms and signs of active TB, (B) abnormal radiography and/or CT scan consistent with lung TB, (C) response to TB therapy plus, (D)

Table 1. Characteristics of the used antigens: all the used antigens were recombinant proteins (from Hoghart et al. [14], modified).

Protein	Gene Bank Accession number	Remarks	Putative function
ESAT-6	Rv3875	6 kDa early secreted antigen	Unknown
CFP-10	Rv3874	10 kDa culture filtrate antigen of *M. tuberculosis*	Unknown
Ag85B	Rv1886c	Secreted antigen, member of the immunodominant complex Antigen 85	Cell wall synthesis, fibronectin binding
PstS1 (38 kDa)	Rv0934	Periplasmic phosphate binding protein	Protein mediated phosphate transport
TB10.3	Rv3019c	Secreted ESAT6-like protein	Unknown
HspX (16 kDa;Acr)	Rv2031c	Heat shock protein. It has been identified as a major protein expressed in dormant state	Stress protein induced by anoxia. It has a role in manteinance of long-term viability during latent asymptomatic infection and a proposed role in replication during initial infection
AlaDH	Rv2780	Secreted L-alanine deydrogenase of *M. tuberculosis*	May play a role in cell wall synthesis (as L-alanine in an important constituent of the peptidoglycan layer) ; crystal structure varies in the phase of active disease with respect to the state of latent infection in "open" and "closed" ternary forms

either a history of TB contact or travel to a TB-endemic country within the last 24 months [13]. No suspected or ascertained extra-pulmonary TB cases presented at the Infectious Disease Unit during the study period.

Statistical Analysis

Categorical data were compared using the Chi-squared test (or Fisher's exact test, when expected cell sizes were smaller than five). The Wilcoxon-Mann-Whitney test was used for continuous measurements to test relationships in unpaired analysis, when assumed that the dependent variable is a not normally distributed interval variable. Test concordance was assessed by Cohen's κ-statistics with agreement considered slight'for $k \leq 0.2$, 'fair' for $0.2 < k \leq 0.4$, 'moderate'for $0.4 < k \leq 0.6$, 'substantial'for $0.6 < k \leq 0.8$ and 'optimal'for $0.8 < k \leq 1.0$. Receiver operating characteristic (ROC) curve analysis was conducted to determine the best IL-2 and IFN-γ ELISPOT result thresholds in discriminating between children with active or latent TB, relatively to a specific *M. tuberculosis* antigen, and correspondent sensitivity and specificity were reported. The area under the ROC curve (AUC) and 95% confidence interval (CI) were also calculated. Statistical analysis was performed using the statistical software SPSS for Windows, version 14.0. $P < 0.05$ was considered statistically significant.

Results

Seventy five children were included in the study. Twenty-none children were classified as uninfected, 21 as LTBI and 25 as active TB cases (including 5 definite and 20 probable cases). Characteristics of the study children are summarized in Table 2.

Discordant TST/QFT-G-IT result was obtained in four children (one child with definite TB, positive QFT-G-IT and negative TST and three children with probable TB, negative QFT-G-IT and positive TST). The overall agreement between QFT-G-IT and the TST was substantial with a *k* value of 0.679.

IFN-γ and IL-2 ELISpot results

ELISPOT assay results are summarized in Table 3. Significantly higher median values were evidenced in infected *vs.* uninfected children considering IFN-γ ELISPOT responses to ESAT-6 ($p < 0.0001$), CFP-10 ($p < 0.0001$), TB 10.3 ($p = 0.003$), and AlaDH ($p = 0.001$), while differences were not significant considering Ag85B ($p = 0.063$), PstS1 ($p = 0.512$), and HspX (16 kDa) protein ($p = 0.139$). Considering IL-2 ELISPOT results significantly different responses were evidenced for ESAT-6 ($p < 0.0001$), CFP-10 ($p < 0.0001$), TB 10.3 ($p < 0.0001$), HspX (16 kDa) ($p < 0.0001$), PstS1 ($p < 0.0001$) and AlaDH ($p = 0.001$); but not for Ag85B ($p = 0.063$). Comparing results between children with LTBI and those with TB disease (probable plus definite disease) differences were significant for IFN-γ ELISPOTt only for AlaDH antigen ($p = 0.021$) (Table 3). With regard to IL-2 ELISPOT assay, significant differences were observed for AlaDH ($p < 0.0001$) and TB 10.3 antigen ($p = 0.043$), while no difference was evidenced considering other antigens. ROC analyses demonstrated sensitivity of 100% and specificity of 81%, in discriminating between latent and active TB, considering response to AlaDH by IL-2 ELISPOT assay for a cut off of 12.5 SCF per million PBMCs. For IFN-γ ELISPOT assay the performance was much poorer: for the best threshold of 42.0 SCF per million PBMCs sensitivity was 88% and specificity 56% (Figure 1).

Discussion

In the present study we evaluated the performances of IFN-γ and IL-2 based ELISPOT assays in children at risk for TB using an array of *M. tuberculosis* specific antigens. We observed significantly different responses between infected and not-infected children with respect to antigens included in the commercially available IGRAs (ESAT-6 and CFP-10), as well as to other mycobacterial antigens (TB 10.3, AlaDH for IFN-gamma and IL-2; HspX and PstS1 only for IL-2 based ELISPOT), but not for Ag86B. This latter result was in contrast to what we expected,

Table 2. Characteristic of the 75 study children, according to their final diagnosis.

	Uninfected	Latent TB	Probable TB disease	Definite TB disease
	n = 29	n = 21	n = 20	n = 5
	n (%)	n (%)	n (%)	n (%)
Age, months (median and IQR)	77 (28–101)	86 (61–101)	52(27–82)	47 (8–97)
Immigrated	21 (72.4)	15 (71.4)	18 (90)	4 (80.0)
BCG vaccinated	5 (17.2)	7 (33.3)	1 (5.0)	0 (0.0)
TST (mm)				
<5	28 (96.5)	0 (0.0)	0 (0.0)	1 (20.0)
≥5 and <10	1 (3.5)	1 (4.8)	2 (10.0)	0 (0.0)
≥10 and <15	0 (0.0)	5 (23.1)	1 (5.0)	1 (20.0)
≥15	0 (0.0)	15 (71.5)	17 (85.0)	3 (60.0)
QFT-G-IT result				
negative	29 (100.0)	5 (23.1)	3 (15.0)	5 (100.0)
positive	0 (0.0)	15 (71.5)	17 (85.0)	0 (0.0)
indeterminate	0 (0.0)	1 (4.8)	0 (0.0)	0 (0.0)

Note. TB: tuberculosis; BCG: Bacille Calmette-Guérin vaccine; TST = tuberculin skin test; QFT-G-IT: QuantiFERON-Gold In Tube test.

considering that Ag85B has been described to elicit a robust immune response in TB patients and it is a candidate protein to be included in new antitubercular vaccines [14]. Indeed Ag85B is one of the most dominant protein antigens secreted from all mycobacteria species, showing extensive cross-reactivity between different species [15]. Thus, exposure to enviromental mycobacteria might sustain an immune response to this antigen in children not-infected by *M. tuberculosis*.

No difference in responses to ESAT-6, CFP-10 and other mycobacterial antigens (Ag85B, PstS1, HpsX) was found between children with latent and active tuberculosis, while significant differences were found in responses to TB 10.3 and AlaDH antigens. TB 10.3 is a member of the large 23 protein ESAT-6 gene family and contains several unique T-cell epitopes strongly recognised by TB patients [13]. The recognition of a number of unique epitopes on TB10.3 suggests that this protein is highly

Table 3. ELISPOT assay results from 75 study children according to final diagnosis.

	Uninfected	Latent TB	Probable TB disease	Definite TB disease	P	P
	(n = 29)	(n = 21)	n = 20	n = 5	Uninfected vs. infected children	Latent vs. overt disease
IFN-γ ELISpot result*						
- ESAT-6	35 (1–102)	320 (157–520)	292 (170–631)	330 (190–1575)	<0.0001	0.724
- CFP-10	40 (1–120)	305 (130–625)	280 (76–986)	875 (200–3532)	<0.0001	0.691
- Ag85B	65 (12–152)	150 (47–322)	107 (46–192)	90 (27–1517)	0.063	0.724
- TB 10.3	100 (27–292)	270 (135–465)	252 (80–395)	570 (225–1742)	0.003	0.487
- AlaDH	35 (12.5–110)	85 (17–180)	147 (71–303)	280 (115–1565)	<0.001	0.021
- PstS1	40 (1–122)	50 (1–197)	60 (11–241)	95 (18–982)	0.0512	0.504
- HspX - 16KD	10 (1–162)	85 (1–300)	42 (1–307)	40 (13–1345)	0.139	0.720
IL-2 ELISpot result*						
- ESAT-6	10 (1–35)	220 (35–410)	110 (60–402)	420 (155–1365)	<0.0001	0.791
- CFP-10	10 (1–20)	210 (85–710)	160 (100–637)	510 (355–1735)	<0.0001	0.574
- Ag85B	20 (10–75)	40 (10–140)	45 (17–195)	200 (135–1485)	0.063	0.188
- TB 10.3	1 (1–30)	50 (12.5–210)	130 (52–402)	390 (220–1695)	<0.0001	0.043
- AlaDH	1 (1–20)	1 (1–10)	75 (36–130)	340 (110–1365)	0.001	<0.0001
- PstS1	10 (1–50)	20 (1–75)	20 (10–95)	10 (5–155)	<0.0001	0.755
- HspX- 16 KD	1 (1–10)	60 (20–280)	45 (1–155)	240 (45–920)	<0.0001	0.626

Note.
*Results are expressed as median and interquartile range of spot forming colonies per million PBMCs; TB:tuberculosis.

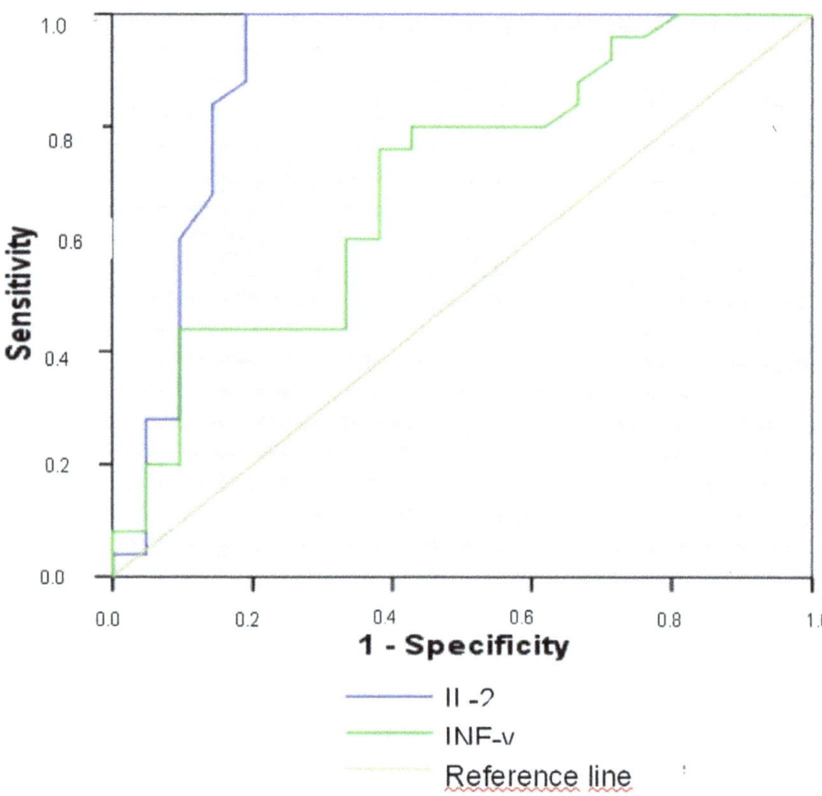

Figure 1. A receiver operator characteristic (ROC) plot is shown, illustrating sensitivity and specificity of AlaDH IFN-γ and IL-2 ELISpot results in discriminating children with latent (n = 21) and overt (n = 25) tuberculosis. Area under the ROC curve was 0.700 (95%IC: 0.547-0.853; p = 0.021 *vs.* the identity - diagonal - line) considering IFN-γ ELISpot and 0,896 (95%IC: 0.785–1.008; p<0.0001 *vs.* the identity - diagonal - line) for IL-2 ELISPOT.

expressed by the bacteria during active TB infection, potentially explaining our finding [16]. To our knowledge this is the first report on a potential role of TB 10.3 to differentiate between LTBI and active TB, deserving further investigations.

Considering AlaDH antigen, the differences observed in children with LTBI and active TB may have a biological explanation. Differently from the other antigens included in our study, AlaDH is the only whose conformation is modified in latent with respect to active TB [17]. It has been demonstrated that AlaDH shows altered expression profile upon adaptation to dormancy: a condition that may be related to the state of latent infection. Though an obligatory aerobic organism, *M. tuberculosis* is able to adapt to and survive in the hypoxic and hostile environment of host macrophages undergoing a dramatic change in gene transcription during a latent infection [8]. AlaDH is an enzyme involved in nitrogen metabolism and has been implicated in the adaptation of mycobacteria to the anaerobic dormant state. The crystal structure varies in the phase of active disease with respect to the state of latent infection in "open" and "closed" ternary forms, thus explaining a possible different host immune response according to the infectious status [17]. We observed that different responses between children with LTBI and active TB were more pronounced with the IL-2 based than with the IFN-γ based ELISPOT. ROC analyses demonstrated that, for a cut off of 12,5 SCF per million PBMC, the sensitivity in discriminating children with LTBI and active TB reached 100% while specificity was 81% by the use of IL-2 based ELISpot assay. The performance of the IFN-γ ELISpot assay was poor, especially due to its low specificity. These findings suggest that IL-2 based ELISPOT assay with AlaDH antigen may be of help in discriminating children with active from those with latent TB. The finding that the differences in response to AlaDH were more pronounced considering IL-2 instead of IFN-γ based ELISPOT assays are not clearly explainable. In contrast with our findings, in adults studies, ESAT-6 and CFP-10 IFN-γ ELISPOT assays were more likely to be positive in recently infected patients, while IL-2 a positive ELISPOT was related to ancient exposure, since this test better explores the central memory T-cell response [9,18]. A higher production of IL-2 in latently infected people after 72 h incubation has been documented. Thus a prolonged incubation period seems to be essential to reveal increased number of central memory T-cells in LTBI adults [9]. However, it should be remembered that the T_H1 response may be immature and peculiar in children. In this population IL-2 based IGRAs have been reported to show higher performance than IFN-γ based assays, explaining, at least partially, our results [19]. Further pediatric studies prolonging the culture up to 3 days could provide further information in children. Further pediatric studies prolonging the culture up to 3 days could provide further information in children. We did not observe any difference between children with active or latent diseases when exploring response to HspX (16 kDa) antigen. This antigen has been depicted as one of the most prominent latency proteins [20], and a strong response to HspX, largely restricted to latently infected individuals, has been previously reported by Demissie and colleagues in adults [20]. Discrepancies between our and previous findings at this regard may be due to the limited datasets, or to actual differences in the immune response between adult and paediatric populations.

Our study has several limitations. Definition of study groups was based on TST results and not on QFT-G-IT results according to the most recent US guidelines in children [7]. However, children could have been classified according to their QFT-G-IT instead of TST results and three of our study children with discordant TST+/QFT-G-IT would have assigned to a different group. We repeated the analyses after excluding these children and results were substantially unchanged. Moreover, similarly to the majority of paediatric studies most of the overt TB cases were probable and not definite diseases and in general our dataset is small. Thus even if intriguing, our findings should be confirmed in larger paediatric populations.

Conclusion

Our data suggest that IL-2 and IFN-gamma based ELISPOT with AlaDH antigen may be of help in discriminating children with active from those with latent TB.

Author Contributions

Performed the experiments: MdM CDB MMD AA EN MS. Analyzed the data: EC FB LG. Contributed reagents/materials/analysis tools: MdM CDB MMD. Wrote the paper: EC MMD MdM FB. Performed data collection, analysis and wrote the draft: EC GFDP CDB MdM. Supervised the project: MdM. Performed data collection and analysis: LG FB SS. Commented on and approved the final draft: EC CDB FB SS AA LG EN GFDP MS MMD MdM.

References

1. Machingaidze S, Wiysonge CS, Gonzalez-Angulo Y, Hatherill M, Moyo S, et al. (2011) The utility of an interferon gamma release assay for diagnosis of latent tuberculosis infection and disease in children: a systematic review and meta-analysis. Pediatr Infect Dis J 30:694–700.
2. Chiappini E, Fossi F, Bonsignori F, Sollai S, Galli L, et al. (2012) Utility of Interferon-γ Release Assay Results to Monitor Anti-Tubercular Treatment in Adults and Children. Clin Ther. 2012 Apr 16. [Epub ahead of print]
3. Pai M, Zwerling A, Menzies D (2008) Systematic review: T-cell-based assays for the diagnosis of latent tuberculosis infection: an update. Ann Intern Med. 149:177–84.
4. Mazurek GH, Jereb J, Vernon A, LoBue P, Goldberg S, et al. (2010) IGRA Expert Committee; Centers for Disease Control and Prevention (CDC).Updated guidelines for using Interferon Gamma Release Assays to detect Mycobacterium tuberculosis infection - United States, 2010.MMWR Recomm Rep 59:1–25.
5. Sun L, Xiao J, Miao Q, Feng WX, Wu XR, et al. (2011) Interferon gamma release assay in diagnosis of pediatric tuberculosis: a meta-analysis. FEMS Immunol Med Microbiol. 63:165–73
6. Mandalakas AM, Detjen AK, Hesseling AC, Benedetti A, Menzies D (2011) Interferon-gamma release assays and childhood tuberculosis: systematic review and meta-analysis. Int J Tuberc Lung Dis 15:1018–32.
7. American Academy of Pediatrics. (2009) [Tuberculosis]. In: Pickering LK, Baker CJ, Kimberlin DW, Long SS, eds. Red Book: 2009 Report of the Committee on Infectious Diseases. 28th ed. Elk Grove Village, IL: American Academy of Pediatrics; 680–701.
8. Amanatidou V, Syridou G, Mavrikou M, Tsolia MN (2012) Latent tuberculosis infection in children: diagnostic approaches. Eur J Clin Microbiol Infect Dis. 2012 Jan 4. [Epub ahead of print]
9. Biselli R, Mariotti S, Sargentini V, Sauzullo I, Lastilla M, et al. (2010) Detection of interleukin-2 in addition to interferon-gamma discriminates active tuberculosis patients, latently infected individuals, and controls. Clin Microbiol Infect 16:1282–4.
10. Millington KA, Fortune SM, Low J, Garces A, Hingley-Wilson SM (2011) Rv3615c is a highly immunodominant RD1 (Region of Difference 1)-dependent secreted antigen specific for Mycobacterium tuberculosis infection.. Proc Natl Acad Sci U S A. 108:5730–5.
11. Vilaplana C, Ruiz-Manzano J, Gil O, Cuchillo F, Montané E, et al. (2008) The tuberculin skin test increases the responses measured by T cell interferon-gamma release assays. Scand J Immunol 67:610–7.
12. Benagiano M, Munari F, Ciervo A, Amedei A, Paccani SR, et al. (2012) Chlamydophila pneumoniae phospholipase D (CpPLD) drives Th17 inflammation in human atherosclerosis. Proc Natl Acad Sci U S A. 109:1222–7.
13. Kampmann B, Whittaker E, Williams A, Walters S, Gordon A, et al. (2009) Martinez-Alier N, Williams B, Crook AM, Hutton AM, Anderson ST. Interferon-gamma release assays do not identify more children with active tuberculosis than the tuberculin skin test. Eur Respir J 33:1374–82
14. Hogarth PJ, Logan KE, Ferraz JC, Hewinson RG, Chambers MA (2006) Protective efficacy induced by Mycobacterium bovis bacille Calmette-Guèrin can be augmented in an antigen independent manner by use of non-coding plasmid DNA. Vaccine. 24:95–101
15. Takamura S, Matsuo K, Takebe Y, Yasutomi Y (2005) Ag85B of mycobacteria elicits effective CTL responses through activation of robust Th1 immunity as a novel adjuvant in DNA vaccine. J Immunol175:2541–7.
16. Skjøt RL, Brock I, Arend SM, Munk ME, Theisen M, et al. (2002) Epitope mapping of the immunodominant antigen TB10.4 and the two homologous proteins TB10.3and TB12.9, which constitute a subfamily of the esat-6 gene family. Infect Immun 70:5446–53.
17. Agren D, Stehr M, Berthold CL, Kapoor S, Oehlmann W, et al. (2008) Singh M, Schneider G.Three-dimensional structures of apo- and holo-L-alanine dehydrogenase from Mycobacterium tuberculosis reveal conformational changes upon coenzyme binding. J Mol Biol 377:1161–73.
18. Krummel B, Strassburg A, Ernst M, Reiling N, Eker B, et al. (2010) Potential role for IL-2 ELISpot in differentiating recent and remote infection in tuberculosis contact tracing. PLoS One. 5:e11670.
19. Mori T (2009) Usefulness of interferon-gamma release assays for diagnosing TB infection and problems with these assays. J Infect Chemother. 15:143–55
20. Demissie A, Leyten EM, Abebe M, Wassie L, Aseffa A, et al. (2006) VACSEL Study Group. Recognition of stage-specific mycobacterial antigens differentiates between acute and latent infections with Mycobacteriumtuberculosis.Clin Vaccine Immunol. 13:179–86.

20

Five Years Experience of *Clostridium difficile* Infection in Children at a UK Tertiary Hospital: Proposed Criteria for Diagnosis and Management

Sumita Pai[1], Sani Hussaini Aliyu[1], David Andrew Enoch[2], Johannis Andreas Karas[1]*

1 Clinical Microbiology & Public Health Laboratory, Health Protection Agency, Addenbrookes Hospital, Cambridge, United Kingdom, 2 Peterborough & Stamford Hospitals NHS Foundation Trust, Peterborough City Hospital, Bretton Gate, Peterborough, United Kingdom

Abstract

Background: *Clostridium difficile* infection (CDI) is associated with significant morbidity and mortality in adults. There is increasing evidence of the pathogenic role of *C. difficile* in the paediatric population. We sought to ascertain the clinical presentation and severity of CDI in children at our institution and develop criteria to aid management.

Methods: Clinical data was retrospectively collected from all children (0–16 yrs) with a positive *C. difficile* toxin result over a 5-year period. National adult guidelines were used to assess the severity and management of CDI.

Results: Seventy-five patients were included with a mean age of 2.97 years. Forty-nine were hospital onset, 22 community onset and 4 healthcare-associated. The most common co-morbidity among the hospital onset infections was malignancy. Gastrointestinal conditions were most common among community onset infections. Fifty-five cases (73.3%) had received antibiotics in the preceding month, 7 (9.3%) had cow's milk intolerance and 9 (12%) had co-infection with another gut pathogen. According to national adult guidelines 57 cases (76%) were categorised as severe. Thirty cases received oral metronidazole, two patients required intensive care and one patient had a sub-total colectomy for pseudomembranous colitis. No mortality was observed.

Discussion: We confirm the association of paediatric CDI with co-morbidities such as haematological and solid organ malignancies, recent antibiotic use and hospitalisation. We observed an association between cows milk protein intolerance and *C. difficile.* The use of adult criteria overestimated severity of disease in this cohort, as most cases experienced a mild course of illness with low morbidity and no mortality. This indicates that adult scoring criteria are not useful in guiding management and we propose specific criteria for children.

Editor: Dongsheng Zhou, Beijing Institute of Microbiology and Epidemiology, China

Funding: This work was part of an official hospital audit and was supported by Cambridge University Hospitals NHS Foundation Trust. The funders had no role in study design, data collection and analysis, decision to publish, or preparation of the manuscript.

Competing Interests: The authors have declared that no competing interests exist.

* E-mail: karasja@gmail.com

Introduction

Clostridium difficile (*C. difficile*) is the commonest cause of hospital acquired diarrhoea in adults and is associated with significant mortality and morbidity. [1] The role of *C. difficile* in children is less certain. The convention is to regard *C. difficile* in stools in children less than two years of age to represent colonisation (i.e. not a cause of diarrhoea), although severe disease does occur. The mandatory surveillance in England and Wales does not include children less than two years of age and many laboratories do not test samples from children. Numerous surveys and studies looking at the significance of isolating *C. difficile* in children show increasing evidence for a potential pathogenic role in the paediatric population. [2–4] *C. difficile* is also becoming increasingly recognised as a significant co-morbid factor in prominent paediatric inpatient populations such as oncology [5–8] and with patients with gastrointestinal disorders. [9,10] Community onset *C. difficile* infection (CDI) without previous direct or indirect contact with a hospital environment remains rare compared with hospital onset CDI. Nevertheless, it has been reported in populations that were previously thought to be at low risk, such as young individuals and pregnant women [11].

A recently published literature review looking at colonisation and disease in children with *C. difficile* showed that *C. difficile* is frequently isolated from children of all ages and colonisation appears to occur soon after birth and rises to high levels at one year. High carriage rates are associated with hospitalisation. CDI was strongly linked to antibiotic associated diarrhoea in children but symptoms were more likely to be severe in the presence of co-morbidities such as malignancy and immunosuppression [12].

The current UK Department of Health (DH) & Health Protection Agency (HPA) guidelines for clinical diagnosis has an adult focus and prompts testing for *C. difficile* when there is a history of abdominal pain, profuse, foul-smelling, soft stools, and fever. [13] These features are not specific but should be taken into context with recent antibiotic use and/or stay in hospital. [11] It has been suggested that leucocytosis is particularly prominent in CDI, but again this alone is inadequate for diagnosis. Radiological imaging of the abdomen is non-specific. [13] Management is based on severity of infection with oral metronidazole as the recommended first line treatment in mild to moderate cases and vancomycin used or added in severe cases. Colectomy is considered in life-threatening disease [13].

The aim of this study was to ascertain the clinical presentation and severity of disease in children with a positive *C. difficile* toxin result over a 5 year period at our institution and to develop criteria to aid diagnosis and management.

Methods

Addenbrooke's Hospital is a tertiary centre covering both rural and urban populations. Paediatric care includes neonatal and paediatric intensive care units (ICU), general medical and surgical beds and a specific haematology/oncology ward. Addenbrooke's has 81 paediatric beds and in 2010 it treated 3,442 paediatric day cases and 3,844 paediatric inpatients.

We performed a retrospective descriptive study of all patients with a positive *C. difficile* toxin result over a 5-year period, from 1st January 2005 to 31st December 2009. The study was identified as a service evaluation and approval to carry out the study was obtained from the trust's audit committee. Research ethics was not required.

We followed the UK HPA Steering Group on Healthcare Associated Infection (2008) guidance for testing *C. difficile* in laboratories. [13] These guidelines recommend diarrhoea to be defined as stool loose enough to take the shape of the container, or as Bristol Stool Chart types 5–7. [14] All samples from patients ≥2 years of age were routinely tested for *C. difficile* toxin. Patients under two were tested only on the specific request of paediatricians and following discussion with the laboratory. Samples classified as Bristol Stool Chart type 1–4 were tested only after discussion between the paediatricians and the laboratory on an individual basis. *C. difficile* testing was performed by EIA (VIDAS, BioMerieux, Basingstoke, UK) followed by confirmation with cell cytotoxin assay (Vero cell line). Samples were not retested within 28 days of a positive result. A positive *C. difficile* toxin test ≥28 days after the initial positive assay was defined as a recurrence in line with DH criteria. [13] Samples were also tested at the same time for bacteriology (*Campylobacter, Salmonella, Shigella, E. coli* 0157) using HPA methodology, parasitology (*Cryptosporidium*) by immunofluorescent staining and viruses.

Hospital onset infection was defined as a positive test after two days of hospital admission. Community onset was defined as a positive test within two days of admission and healthcare-associated if patients came from nursing homes or palliative care facilities.

Information that was collected for each patient included demographics, past medical history, risk factors, laboratory diagnosis, severity score, clinical management and outcome at 3 months. Clinical data were obtained from medical, nursing, pharmacy and microbiology records and laboratory data was obtained from the laboratory information management system. *P*-values were calculated for the following – age distribution and co-morbidities (gastro-intestinal, haematology, immunosuppression and solid organ malignancy) using chi-squared test the via online GraphPad software.

Disease severity was classified using the Department of Health criteria of mild, moderate, severe and life-threatening infection. [13] Mild CDI was defined as typically associated with <3 stools of types 5–7 on the Bristol Stool Chart per day with a normal WCC, moderate CDI is associated with a raised WCC that is <15 x109/L and typically associated with 3–5 stools per day, severe CDI is associated with a WCC >15 x109/L, or an acute rising serum creatinine (i.e. >50% increase above baseline), a temperature of >38.5°C or evidence of severe colitis (abdominal or radiological signs), whilst features of life-threatening CDI included hypotension, partial or complete ileus or toxic megacolon, or CT evidence of severe disease. These guidelines also recommend treating according to severity, daily monitoring using the Bristol Stool Chart and multidisciplinary clinical review of cases.

Results

Eighty nine patients had a positive *C. difficile* toxin result over the 5 years. Data could not be found on 14 patients and were excluded, leaving 75 patients for analysis. There were 27 cases in 2005, 15 in 2006, 20 in 2007, 9 in 2008 and 4 in 2009. The mean age was 2.97 years and the median age was 2 years (range 2 days to 14 years). Thirty-six (48%) patients were below the age of 2 years. Thirty-seven (49.3%) patients were female. Of the 75 cases, 49 (65.3%) were hospital onset, 22 (29.3%) community onset and four (5.3%) were healthcare-associated. The mean in-patient days prior to *C. difficile* being isolated from stools was 27.2 days with a median of 10 days (range 0 to 213 days) for the hospital onset cases. Thirty-one (58.5%) of the hospital onset cases had prior in-patient days of >1 month in the preceding year before isolation of *C. difficile* from stools. Detailed results comparing hospital and community onset cases are presented in table 1.

Sixty-eight patients (90.7%) had significant co-morbidities (table 1). Among the haematology patients, 7 had acute lymphoblastic leukaemia, three had acute myeloid leukaemia and two had non-Hodgkins lymphoma. Seven patients (9.3%) were diagnosed with possible cows milk protein allergy.

Four patients had previous CDI prior to 2005 and two patients had recurrences. Both recurrences occurred in haematology patients with prolonged stay in hospital.

Twenty patients (26%) had no exposure to antibiotics in the preceding month. Six patients had ≥2 antibiotics in the preceding month. Antibiotics most frequently implicated included 3rd generation cephalosporins (30) and fluoroquinolones (19), but also included flucloxacillin, piperacillin-tazobactam, meropenem, vancomycin and gentamicin (table 1). Five (7%) patients were on PPIs prior to the onset of symptoms and 19 (25%) had recently received H_2 receptor antagonists. Other risk factors are shown in table 2.

Virology tests were performed for 51 cases; three were co-infected with adenovirus, three with norovirus, two with rotavirus and one with enterovirus. No additional bacterial infection was found in any of the cases.

Nine patients were considered to have mild infection, 8 moderate, 57 severe and one patient had life-threatening disease according to adult parameters devised by the DH/HPA.13 The findings of blood parameters and symptoms of infections are summarised in table 3.

Seven patients (9.3%) were tested with a sample consistent with Bristol stool chart of 1–4.Treatment was deemed unnecessary in a further 33 patients (44%) by their respective clinical teams. Thirty (40%) cases were treated with metronidazole alone and two received probiotic treatment only. No patient received cholestyramine. Metronidazole usage led to symptom resolution in a mean of two days. Escalation of treatment was required in three cases with oral vancomycin being added to metronidazole.

In nine patients preceding broad spectrum antibiotics were continued despite ongoing diarrhoea. Laxatives were not stopped

Table 1. Results comparing hospital onset with community onset cases.

		Hospital associated (%)(N = 53)	Community associated (%) (N = 22)	Total (%)(N = 75)	p- values
Age (yrs)	<2 years	16 (30.2)	20 (90)	36 (48)	0.0001
	2–5 years	26 (49)	1 (4.5)	27 (36)	
	>6 years	11 (20.7)	1 (4.5)	12 (16)	
Gender	Male	25 (47.2%)	12 (54.5%)	37 (49.4%)	
Year	2005	14	13	27	
	2006	11	4	15	
	2007	15	5	20	
	2008	9	0	9	
	2009	4	0	4	
Co-morbidities*	Cardiovascular	3 (5.7)	0	3 (4)	
	Neuromuscular	3 (5.7)	1 (4.5)	4 (5.3)	
	Gastrointestinal	3 (5.6)	5 (22.7)	8 (10.7)	<0.0001
	Haematology + immunosuppression	11 (20.7)	1 (4.5)	12 (16)	0.0001
	Malignancy (solid organ)	20 (37.7)	0	20 (26.7)	0.0001
	Renal+Metabolic	3 (5.6)	0	3 (4)	
	Cows milk allergy	1 (1.8)	6 (11.3)	7 (9.3)	<0.0001
	Respiratory	1 (1.8)	1 (4.5)	2 (2.7)	
	Others	7 (13)	3 (13.6)	10 (13.3)	
Antibiotic history	Penicillins (Amoxicillin & Co-amoxiclav)	5 (9.4)	5 (22)	10 (13.4)	
	Cephalosporins	27 (50.9)	3 (13.6)	30 (40)	
	Quinolones (Ciprofloxacin)	19 (35.8)	0	19 (25)	
	Others	5 (9.4)	2 (9)	7 (9.3)	
	No antibiotics	7 (13.2)	13 (59)	20 (26.7)	
Co-infections	Bacterial	0	0	0	
	Viral	6 (11.3)	3 (13.6)	9 (12)	
Other risk factors	Intensive Care stay	12 (22.6)	0	12 (16)	
	Surgery**	14 (26.4)	4 (18)	18 (24)	
Severity score***	Mild	7 (13.2)	2 (9)	9 (12)	
	Moderate	6 (11.3)	2 (9)	8 (10.7)	
	Severe	39 (73.6)	18 (81.8)	57 (76)	
	Life threatening	1 (1.9)	0	1 (1.4)	
Treatment	Not required	27 (51)	13 (59)	40 (53.4)	
	Metronidazole	22 (41.5)	8 (36.4)	30 (40)	
	Escalation of treatment to Vancomycin	3 (5.7)	0	3 (4)	
	Probiotics	1 (1.9)	1 (4.5)	2 (2.7)	
Outcome	Alive at 3 months	45 (81)	19 (81.8)	64 (81.4)	
	ICU requirement	2 (2.8)	0	2 (2.7)	
	Colectomy	1 (1.8)	0	1 (1.3)	
	Crude mortality	2 (3.8)	2 (9)	4 (5.4)	
	Missing notes	2	1	3	
	Transferred	3	1	4 (5.4)	

*Note some patients had more than one risk factor.
**Of the 18 surgeries 9 were gastrointestinal surgeries (Resection of abdominal mass, appendicectomy).
***Severity scoring criteria as recommended by Department of Health and Health Protection Agency.

in 6 patients. A stool chart was kept only in 26 (34.7%) cases throughout the symptomatic period.

Outcome data are shown in table 1. One case developed pseudomembranous colitis (diagnosed endoscopically) and required a sub-total colectomy. Thirty-five (46.7%) cases required admission or prolongation of their hospital stay due to CDI. Four patients died (5.3%). One was thought to be due to a combination

Table 2. Blood parameters and symptoms of infection for symptomatic patients (n = 68).

Parameter		Number of patients (%)
Blood parameters at CDT date	WCC (>15×10^9)	28 (41.2)
	Rising Creatinine	2 (2.9)
	Falling Albumin (<25 g/L)	10 (14.7)
	CRP (>25 mg/L)	40 (58.8)
	Hb (<10 g/L)	28 (41.2)
Fever ≥38.5°C		34 (50)
Abdominal pain, tenderness, distension		17 (25)
Diarrhoea >5 times a day		50 (73.5)
Pseudomembranous colitis		2 probable* 1 definite
Surgery required		1

*In two cases the endoscopy results was unable to discriminate between typhlitis and pseudomembranous colitis.
Key: WCC - white cell count; CRP - C-reactive protein; Hb - haemoglobin; CDT - *Clostridium difficile* toxin.

of significant bacteraemia along with ongoing diarrhoea and the other three died due to their underlying disease.

Using our proposed criteria (table 3), of the 68 symptomatic cases in our study, 54 fulfilled the diagnosis of likely CDI. Of these 54; 26 (48%) would have been categorised as having mild disease (versus 9 using adult criteria), 23 (42.6%) moderate disease (versus 8), 5 (9%) severe disease (versus 57) and none with life-threatening disease (versus one). The severity numbers are lower and befitting the observations from our study.

Discussion

We describe the presentation and severity of *Clostridium difficile* in children. We found that a significant number of patients did not require treatment and the overall morbidity and mortality rates were low, despite most being categorised as "severe" by the UK DH adult standards. The majority (49.3%) of cases were hospital onset, most had received antibiotics and most (59.6%) were undergoing or had already received chemotherapy for haematological or solid organ malignancies. Of the community onset cases, most had a past history of gastrointestinal conditions including cow's milk protein allergy, gastro-oesophageal reflux disease or recent gastrointestinal surgery. We found a reduction in the total number of cases from 2005 to 2009. This was similar to observed trends in adult patients with CDI in our centre and likely reflects enhanced infection control measures including early isolation of patients, enhanced environmental cleaning and antibiotic stewardship. There was no change in laboratory test methods during this period.

Table 3. Proposed revised criteria for severity of *Clostridium difficile* infection in children.

Criteria	Point
Diarrhoea >5 times a day	1
Abdominal pain and discomfort	1
Rising white cell count	1
Raised C-reactive protein	1
Pyrexia >38°C	1
Evidence of pseudomembranous colitis	2
Intensive care unit requirement	2

Score
1–2 = mild disease.
3–4 = moderate disease.
≥5 = severe disease.

Over the 5-year period to 2006, a large US study by Kim and colleagues reported a steady increase in the annual incidence of CDI amongst paediatric inpatients, from 2.6 to 4 cases per 1000 admissions. The median age of children with CDI was 4 years. They also noted an increase in CDI cases in the 5–17 year age groups over this time period. [15] In contrast, our study demonstrated a younger median age of 2 years (mean was 2.97 years) and there was no increase in cases in the 5–17 year age groups.

Seven of our cases were asymptomatic, but were tested on special request and therefore did not fit the DH criteria [13] for diagnosis of CDI; colonisation was thought to be more likely among these patients.

CDI appears to be strongly linked to the presence of co-morbidities such as haematological malignancies, immunosuppression and bowel disorders. [7,10,16–19] In our study, among the 68 patients with significant co-morbidities 12 (17.6%) had haematological malignancies and 20 (29%) had solid organ tumours. Both groups of patients were receiving or had previously received chemotherapy. These groups also had the highest rate (59.5%, p value of 0.0001) of hospital onset *C. difficile*. Other studies have similarly found increased rates of CDI in these patient groups. [7,18,20] Haematology/oncology patients are recognised as a frequent source of *C. difficile* in hospitals amongst the paediatric population. [5,6,16,17,19] This could be due to a combination of factors such as frequent hospital encounters, prolonged antibiotic usage (these patients had the most number of antibiotic prescriptions) and immunosuppression (62.5% were neutropenic). Neutrophils have been implicated as playing a pivotal role in the pathophysiology of CDI [19].

Gastrointestinal co-morbidities were more common in community onset CDI (45%; p value of <0.0001). Seven out of the ten cases were being investigated for cow's milk protein allergy (CMA) along with multiple food allergies. Only one of these 7 cases had prior exposure to antibiotics (amoxicillin) and had loose stools prior to starting antibiotics. An association has been described between gut colonisation with *Clostridium difficile* and allergy in children [21].

Antibiotic usage is a widely recognised major risk factor for development of CDI. [16,22,23,24,25] In our study, 55 patients (74%, p value 0.0001) had received antibiotics in the previous month, of which 50 (91%) were symptomatic with profuse diarrhoea (more than 5 times a day). Cephalosporins were the most commonly used antibiotics but this may reflect greater use in children overall. Ciprofloxacin was the second most frequently used antibiotic, mainly in the haematology and oncology patients.

Exposure to stomach acid-reducing agents, such as H_2 receptor antagonists and PPIs, remains a controversial risk factor, and has been associated with CDI in some studies [22] but not in others. [11,26] Only five (7%) of our patients were on PPIs prior to the onset of symptoms and 19 (25%) had recently received H_2 receptor antagonists.

To date, the significance of co-infection with another gut pathogen is uncertain. In our study, nine patients had evidence of co-infection; three of these had community onset diarrhoea (two rotavirus and one norovirus) and the other six were hospital onset (three adenovirus, one enterovirus and two norovirus). Two of the three cases with norovirus co-infection were symptomatic and settled eventually after four days without treatment. Lukkarinen and colleagues hypothesized in two cases that norovirus may affect epithelial homeostasis of intestine and exacerbate the effects of toxins produced by *C. difficile* ribotype 027 [27].

All patients were reviewed on a daily basis by their respective clinical teams. In the majority of cases the clinical teams did not classify patients according to severity of disease. In ten cases (13.3%) the clinical teams judged the infection to be severe; 7 improved with metronidazole alone whilst the remaining three received additional vancomycin due to non-resolution of symptoms. Of the three cases that received dual antibiotic therapy, two required ICU admission for monitoring of their renal function and another had disease severe enough to require a subtotal colectomy. In contrast, using national DH/HPA adult criteria an additional 47 cases would have fallen into the severe category of disease. Examining these 47 cases, 18 spontaneously recovered without active treatment and two received probiotic treatment alone. The remaining 27 cases received metronidazole with three requiring additional vancomycin and ICU input in two cases. The commonest symptoms and signs among our cohort were diarrhoea, a rising CRP, white cell count $>15\times109/L$ and pyrexia $>38.5°C$. These signs and symptoms are included in the DH description of severe CDI. The DH/HPA adult guidance recommends treatment of severe disease with oral vancomycin initially and adding IV metronidazole if no improvement is observed, which differs to the treatment received by our patients.

The majority of the patients in our study had a favourable outcome. The primary outcome was all-cause 3-month mortality rate. There was no *C. difficile* related death in our cohort and morbidity was low. From published studies the mortality and morbidity data due to CDI in children is low [15,16,25].

The above findings highlight three important observations of CDI in children. Firstly, children appear to have a mild course of disease despite having an acute response physiologically to infection. This would explain the discrepancy between the observed course of disease and that predicted by the DH/HPA adult severity scoring system (which uses acute response as a predictor for disease prognosis). Secondly, most of our cases had an overall good outcome with either no treatment or oral metronidazole. Lastly, the intuitive clinical triaging used by the teams in our study appears to be more relevant to the paediatric population in grading patient severity.

Based on the results of our study, we propose the following guidance for CDI in children in an attempt to help differentiate between *C. difficile* colonisation and infection and secondly, a scoring system to accurately grade severity and guide appropriate treatment.

Proposed Diagnostic Criteria

1. Fulfils likely diagnosis of CDI if – Diarrhoea (Bristol stool chart 5–7) **and** one or more of the following:

- Significant co-morbidities – Haematology/oncology, Gastrointestinal disease
- Stay in hospital for >2 days
- Antibiotic use in the last 1 month (especially ciprofloxacin and cephalosporins)

Our revised criteria for severity of infection are described in table 3.

Proposed Medical Management

Mild disease. No need to treat if symptoms settle within 24 hours but consider oral metronidazole for 10–14 days if symptoms persist beyond 24 hours.

Moderate disease. Oral metronidazole for 10–14 days and consider escalation by changing to oral vancomycin if non-resolution of symptoms or decline in severity score.

Severe disease. Oral vancomycin and IV metronidazole. Colectomy should be considered if there if evidence of caecal dilatation.

Our intention is to carry out a prospective study using our proposed criteria to see whether it provides a consistent and beneficial tool towards the management of CDI in children.

In conclusion, from our study we found that applying the adult DH/HPA *C. difficile* severity scoring criteria overestimates the number of severe cases and is not a reliable guide for management in children. Most children in our study had a self-limiting course of illness regardless of treatment. We confirmed the association of CDI with co-morbidities such as haematology/oncology malignancies, recent antibiotic use and hospitalisation. We also observed a possible link between gastrointestinal disorders like cows milk protein intolerance and *C. difficile* but this area requires further investigation. We have proposed a diagnostic and severity scoring system to guide appropriate management.

Author Contributions

Conceived and designed the experiments: JAK DE. Performed the experiments: SP SA JAK DE. Analyzed the data: SP SA JAK DE. Contributed reagents/materials/analysis tools: SP SA JAK DE. Wrote the paper: SP SA JAK DE.

References

1. Karas JA, Enoch DA, Aliyu SH (2010) A review of mortality due to *Clostridium difficile* infection. J Infect 61(1): 1–8.
2. Murrell WG, Stewart BJ, O'Neill C, Siarakas S, Kariks S (1993) Enterotoxigenic bacteria in the sudden infant death syndrome. J Med Microbiol 39(2): 114–27.
3. Viscidi R, Laughon BE, Yolken R, Bo-Linn P, Moench T, et al. (1983) Serum antibody response to toxins A and B of *Clostridium difficile*. J Infect Dis. 148(1): 93–100.
4. Zwiener RJ, Belknap WM, Quan R (1989) Severe pseudomembranous enterocolitis in a child: case report and literature review. Pediatr Infect Dis J. 8(12): 876–82.

5. Burgner DP, Rfidah H, Beattie TJ, Seal DV (1993) *Clostridium difficile* after haemolytic uraemic syndrome. Arch Dis Child. 69(2): 239–40.
6. Simon A, Fleischhack G, Hasan C, Bode U, Engelhart S, et al. (2000) Surveillance for nosocomial and central line related infections among pediatric hematology- oncology patients. Infect Control Hosp Epidemiol. 21(9): 592–6.
7. Schuller I, Saha V, Lin L, Kingston J, Eden T, et al. (1995) Investigation and management of *Clostridium difficile* colonisation in a paediatric oncology unit. Arch Dis Child. 72(3): 219–22.
8. Brunetto AL, Pearson AD, Craft AW, Pedler SJ (1988) *Clostridium difficile* in an oncology unit. Arch Dis Child. 63(8): 979–81.
9. Thomas DF, Fernie DS, Bayston R, Spitz L, Nixon HH (1986) Enterocolitis in Hirschsprung's disease: a controlled study of the etiologic role of *Clostridium difficile.* J Pediatr Surg. 21(1): 22–5.
10. Wultanska D, Banaszkiewicz A, Radzikowski A, Obuch-Woszczatynski P, Mlynarczyk G, et al. (2010) *Clostridium difficile* infection in Polish pediatric outpatients with inflammatory bowel disease. Eur J Clin Microbiol Infect Dis. 29(10): 1265–70.
11. Wilcox MH, Mooney L, Bendall R, Settle CD, Fawley WN (2008) A case-control study of community-associated *Clostridium difficile* infection. J Antimicrob Chemother. 62(2): 388–96.
12. Enoch DA, Butler MJ, Pai S, Aliyu SH, Karas JA (2011) *Clostridium difficile* in children: Colonisation and disease. J. Infect. 63: 105–113.
13. Department of Health and Health Protection Agency (2008) *Clostridium difficile:* How to deal with the problem. Best practice guidance. Available: http://www.hpa.org.uk/webc/HPAwebFile/HPAweb_C/1232006607827. Accessed 2009 April 1.
14. Lewis SJ, Heaton KW (1997) Stool Form Scale as a Useful Guide to Intestinal Transit Time. Scandinavian Journal of Gastroenterology. 32(9): 920–924.
15. Kim J, Smathers SA, Prasad P, Leckerman KH, Coffin S, et al. (2008) Epidemiological features of *Clostridium difficile* - associated disease among inpatients at children's hospitals in the United States, 2001–2006. Pediatrics. 122(6): 1266–70.
16. Morinville V, McDonald J (2005) *Clostridium difficile* - associated diarrhea in 200 Canadian children. Can J Gastroenterol 19(8): 497–501.
17. Simon A, Ammann RA, Bode U, Fleischhack G, Wenchel HM, et al. (2008) Healthcare-associated infections in pediatric cancer patients: results of a prospective surveillance study from university hospitals in Germany and Switzerland. BMC Infect Dis 8: 70.
18. El-Mahallawy HA, El-Din NH, Salah F, El-Arousy M, El-Naga SA (2004) Epidemiologic profile of symptomatic gastroenteritis in pediatric oncology patients receiving chemotherapy. Pediatr Blood Cancer 42(4): 338–42.
19. Castagnola E, Battaglia T, Bandettini R, Caviglia I, Baldelli I, et al. (2009) *Clostridium difficile* - associated disease in children with solid tumors. Support Care Cancer 17(3): 321–4.
20. Wolfhagen MJ, Meijer K, Fluit AC, Torensma R, Bruinsma RA, et al. (1994) Clinical significance of *Clostridium difficile* and its toxins in faeces of immunocompromised children. Gut 35(11): 1608–12.
21. Penders J, Thijs C, Van den Brandt PA, Kummeling I, Snijders B, et al. (2007) Gut microbiota composition and development of atopic manifestations in infancy: the KOALA Birth Cohort Study. Gut 56: 661–7.
22. Spivack JG, Eppes SC, Klein JD (2003) *Clostridium difficile* associated diarrhea in a pediatric hospital. Clin Pediatr (Phila) 42(4): 347–52.
23. Oguz F, Uysal G, Dasdemir S, Oskovi H, Vidinlisan S (2001) The role of *Clostridium difficile* in childhood nosocomial diarrhea. Scand J Infect Dis 33(10): 731–3.
24. Klein EJ, Boster DR, Stapp JR, Wells JG, Qin X, et al. (2006) Diarrhea etiology in a Children's Hospital Emergency Department: a prospective cohort study. Clin Infect Dis 43(7): 807–13.
25. Ellis ME, Mandal BK, Dunbar EM, Bundell KR (1984) *Clostridium difficile* and its cytotoxin in infants admitted to hospital with infectious gastroenteritis. Br Med J (Clin Res Ed) 288(6416): 524–6.
26. Rupnik M, Wilcox MH, Gerding DN (2009) *Clostridium difficile* infection: new developments in epidemiology and pathogenesis. Nature 7: 526–36.
27. Lukkarinen H, Eerola E, Ruohola A, Vainionpaa R, Jalava J, et al. (2009) *Clostridium difficile* ribotype 027-associated disease in children with norovirus infection. Pediatr Infect Dis J 28(9): 847–8.

Increased Gastric IL-1β Concentration and Iron Deficiency Parameters in *H. pylori* Infected Children

Dulciene Maria Magalhaes Queiroz[1*❡], Andreia Maria Camargos Rocha[1], Fabricio Freire Melo[1], Gifone Aguiar Rocha[1], Kádima Nayara Teixeira[1], Simone Diniz Carvalho[2], Paulo Fernando Souto Bittencourt[2], Lucia Porto Fonseca Castro[3], Jean E. Crabtree[4❡]

1 Laboratory of Research in Bacteriology, Faculdade de Medicina, Universidade Federal de Minas Gerais, Belo Horizonte, Brazil, **2** Endoscopy Service, University Hospital, Universidade Federal de Minas Gerais, Belo Horizonte, Brazil, **3** Department of Pathology, Faculdade de Medicina, Universidade Federal de Minas Gerais, Belo Horizonte, Brazil, **4** Leeds Institute of Molecular Medicine, University of Leeds, Leeds, United Kingdom

Abstract

Association between *H. pylori* infection, iron deficiency and iron deficiency anaemia has been described, but the mechanisms involved have not been established. We hypothesized that in *H. pylori* infected children increased gastric concentrations of IL-1β and/or TNF-α, both potent inhibitors of gastric acid secretion that is essential for iron absorption, are predictors for low blood concentrations of ferritin and haemoglobin, markers of early depletion of iron stores and anaemia, respectively. We evaluated 125 children undergoing endoscopy to clarify the origin of gastrointestinal symptoms. Gastric specimens were obtained for *H. pylori* status and cytokine evaluation and blood samples for determination of iron deficiency/iron deficiency anaemia parameters and *IL1* cluster and *TNFA* polymorphisms that are associated with increased cytokine secretions. Higher IL-1β and TNF-α gastric concentrations were observed in *H. pylori*-positive (n = 47) than in -negative (n = 78) children. Multiple linear regression models revealed gastric IL-1β, but not TNF-α, as a significant predictor of low ferritin and haemoglobin concentrations; results were reproduced in young children in whom *IL1RN* polymorphic genotypes associated with higher gastric IL-1β expression and lower blood ferritin and haemoglobin concentrations. In conclusion, high gastric levels of IL-1β can be the link between *H. pylori* infection and iron deficiency/iron deficiency anaemia in childhood.

Editor: Valli De Re, Centro di Riferimento Oncologico, IRCCS National Cancer Institute, Italy

Funding: The study was supported by the Sixth Framework Programme of the European Union, Project CONTENT (INCO-DEV-3-032136); Conselho Nacional de Desenvolvimento Científico e Tecnológico (CNPq/Brazil); Coordenação de Aperfeiçoamento de Pessoal de Nível Superior (CAPES/Brazil) and Instituto de Biomedicina do Semi-Árido (INCT-IBISAB/Brazil). The funders had no role in study design, data collection and analysis, decision to publish, or preparation of the manuscript.

Competing Interests: The authors have declared that no competing interest exist.

* E-mail: dqueiroz@medicina.ufmg.br

❡ These authors contributed equally to this work.

Introduction

Anaemia is a major public health problem in developing countries and approximately half of all cases are due to iron deficiency (ID) [1,2]. Iron deficiency anaemia (IDA) is the final stage in the spectrum of a persistent negative iron balance, being preceded by an iron-restricted erythropoiesis characterized by low iron stores. The greater demand for iron due to growth, expansion of red cell mass and menstrual blood loss in female adolescents favors the development of ID/IDA in childhood/adolescence [2]. Factors which contribute to the high frequency of ID/IDA in developing countries include poor iron intake, low dietary iron bioavailability and blood loss due to gastrointestinal parasitic infections [2,3].

Helicobacter pylori colonizes the stomach of more than a half of the world's population. Concomitant high prevalence of *H. pylori* infection and ID/IDA in some areas, particularly in developing countries, has led to the hypothesis that *H. pylori* may contribute to ID/IDA. Potential mechanisms proposed include increased blood loss due to *H. pylori*-induced gastric lesions [4], iron uptake by *H. pylori* [5], deficient iron absorption due to decreased gastric acidity [6,7], that isessential for the reduction and solubilization of non-heme iron, and reduced gastric juice ascorbic acid concentrations [6].

The acute phase of *H. pylori* infection is accompanied by transient hypochlorydria of variable duration [8–10]. Similar perturbations in gastric acid secretion occur in animals following infection with gastric *Helicobacter* species [11] or *H. pylori* [12]. In the latter study, reversal of the hypochlorhydria induced by *H. pylori* infection in gerbils by treatment with recombinant IL-1 receptor antagonist implicated the *IL-1B* gene cluster in hypochlorhydric response to *H. pylori*. As *H. pylori* infection is mainly acquired in childhood [13], it is biologically plausible that infected children are at increased risk of developing ID/IDA as a consequence of hypochlorhydria.

Concentrations of IL-1β and TNF-α, potent inhibitors of gastric acid secretion [14], are increased in the gastric mucosa of *H. pylori* infected adults and children [15–17]. As both cytokines are capable of directly inhibiting gastric acid secretion by parietal cells, they might be one of the links between ID and *H. pylori* infection in childhood [13]. Furthermore, *H. pylori* infected adults with functional polymorphisms in the *IL1* gene cluster associated with over expression of IL-1β have increased hypochlorydria [17] that could, theoretically, interfere with intestinal iron absorption leading to ID.

We hypothesized that in *H. pylori* infected children without the known common causes of ID, increased gastric concentrations of IL-1β and/or TNF-α could be predictors for low blood concentrations of ferritin and haemoglobin, markers of early depletion of iron stores and anaemia, respectively.

Patients and Methods

This study was approved by the Ethics Committee of the Universidade Federal de Minas Gerais, Belo Horizonte, Brazil and the National Ethics Committee on Research from the Health Ministry of Brazil. Signed informed consent to participate was obtained from the children (whenever possible) and adolescents and their parents.

Patients

Between June 2007 and July 2010 125 children and adolescents (74 girls and 51 boys, mean age 11.1±2.9 years, range 4–16 years) undergoing gastrointestinal endoscopy to clarify the origin of symptoms related to the upper gastrointestinal tract were prospectively studied. All the patients were from Minas Gerais state, localized in the Southeast Brazil. To avoid confounding factors which can modify the gastritis classification and the diagnosis of *H. pylori* infection, or which independently can modify iron stores, rigorous exclusion criteria were used. Exclusions included children who had received antimicrobial drugs, anticholinergic and steroidal and non-steroidal anti-inflammatory agents for at least 30 days, or proton pump inhibitors for at least 15 days before endoscopy; children with peptic ulcer disease, coeliac disease and intestinal parasitic infections; children with gastrooesophageal varices, coagulation disorders, acquired or congenital immunosuppression, inflammatory diseases, renal failure, hematological disorders and neoplasias. Following endoscopy, additional exclusion criteria were previously undiagnosed coeliac disease or any histological non-specific duodenal inflammation in the absence of duodenal gastric metaplasia. From each female adolescent data was obtained on age of menarche, interval between the menses, duration and amount of monthly flow. Those with heavy menstrual blood loss were not included in the study. The menstrual cycle was considered normal when the interval between flows was 25–31 days and duration between 3 and 5 days [18].

Biopsy specimens were obtained from the antral and corpus gastric mucosa for evaluation of *H. pylori* status, histological parameters and cytokine concentrations. Duodenal biopsies were taken for histological analysis and the exclusion of coeliac disease and tropical enteropathy. In addition, stool samples were obtained for parasitology and *H. pylori* monoclonal stool antigen assay (HpSA Plus; Meridian Bioscience, Cincinnati, OH).

Blood samples were collected to determine the haemoglobin concentration, haematocrit value, *IL1B, IL1RN* and *TNFA* polymorphisms and serum ferritin concentration.

H. pylori Status

H. pylori status was evaluated by culture, preformed urease test, carbolfuchsin-stained histological section, polymerase chain reaction (PCR) for *ure*A, monoclonal HpSA and ^{13}C-urea breath test as previously described [19,20]. Patients were considered *H. pylori*-positive when culture was positive or at least two of the other tests were positive and *H. pylori*-negative when the results of all tests were negative.

Histology

Endoscopic biopsy specimens were fixed in 10% formalin and embedded in paraffin wax, and 4-µm-thick histological sections were stained with haematoxylin and eosin for histological analysis according to the revised Sydney System [21] and with carbolfuchsin for detection of spiraled organisms. Mononuclear (MN) and polymorphonuclear (PMN) cell infiltrations as well as intestinal metaplasia and atrophy were graded as absent (0), mild (1), moderate (2), or marked (3).

Blood Haemoglobin, Haematocrit and Ferritin Values

Blood haemoglobin concentration and haematocrit values were determined by using an automated electronic counter, Sysmex XT 1800i (Sysmex Corporation, Kobe, Japan). The serum ferritin concentration was determined by a chemiluminescence method employing the ADVIA Centaur® Immunoassay CP System (Siemens Healthcare, Erlangen, Germany).

Gastric Cytokine Levels

IL-1β and TNF-α gastric concentrations were evaluated separately in biopsies from the lesser curvature of the antrum and from the greater curvature of the corpus by ELISA and were expressed as picogram of cytokine per milligram of protein (pg/mg protein) as previously described [14].

IL1B-31T/C, IL1RN VNTR and *TNFA*-307G/A Genotyping

As *IL1B/IL1RN* and *TNFA* polymorphisms might affect transcript levels of *IL1B* and *TNFA*, respectively, they were investigated in blood DNA extracted by the QIAamp DNA mini kit (QIAGEN, GmbH, Hilden, Germany). *IL1B-31T/C* genotypes were determined with Taqman double-stranded SNP ID: rs4986790 (Applied Biosystems, Foster City, CA). *IL1RN* penta-allelic variable number tandem repeats (VNTR) was genotyped according to Mansfield *et al* [22]. The alleles 1, 3, 4 and 5 were classified into long and the allele 2 into short categories [22]. The *TNFA*-307G/A genotypes were investigated by PCR-restriction length polymorphism (RFLP) [22].

Statistical Analysis

Data were analysed with SPSS statistical software package version 17.0 (SPSS Inc., Chicago, IL). Hardy-Weinberg equilibrium of alleles at individual loci was tested by $\chi 2$-test with Yate's correction or Fisher's exact text. The Kolmogorov-Smirnov goodness-of-fit was used to assess the normality of the data. When significant departures from normality were detected, the data were log-transformed. The histopathological scores in binary variables were transformed by combining absent/mild and moderate/severe scores to compare histopathological data with IL-1β and TNF-α gastric concentrations. The degree of gastric chronic (mononuclear) and active (polymorphonuclear) in *H. pylori*-positive and -negative children was compared by the two-tailed Mann Whitney U test. Correlations were evaluated by the Pearsons correlation (continuous normally distributed data) or Spearmans correlation (scores). The comparisons between antral and corpus cytokine concentrations were undertaken by two-tailed paired Student's t test or Wilcoxon test. The level of significance was set at $p \leq 0.05$. Multiple linear regression analyses ("enter option") were used in order to quantify the simultaneous and mutually independent contribution, of selected relevant predictor candidates, e.g. IL-1β and TNF-α gastric concentrations, for low ferritin and haemoglobin blood concentration (dependent variables) while controlling for confounders such as gender and age. Variables with p values ≤0.20 in the univariate analyses were selected for the multivariate analyses. The optimum sample size, based on a significant level of 0.05 and a statistical power of 0.80 (type II error 0.02) is 125 cases, even when only a small effect size (f = 0.10) is expected.

Results

Among the 125 children, 47 (37.6%) were *H. pylori*-positive (mean age 11.7±2.7 years; 29 girls) and 78 (62.4%) were *H. pylori*-negative (mean age 10.7±2.9 years, 45 girls).

Gastric Cytokine Concentrations

A 17.2-fold increase in corpus and antral gastric concentration of IL-1β as well as a 7.0-fold increase in corpus and 57.7-fold increase in antral gastric TNF-α concentrations were observed in infected children when compared with non-infected children ($p<0.001$). Comparisons between *H. pylori*-negative and -positive children are shown in Figure 1A and 1B. The concentrations of IL-1β were higher in the corpus than in the antral gastric mucosa (2.5-fold increase) in both *H. pylori*-positive ($p<0.001$) and *H. pylori*-negative ($p = 0.02$) children. Conversely, the TNF-α concentration was higher in the antral than in the corpus gastric mucosa in *H. pylori*-positive children (2.5-fold increase, $p<0.001$) (Figure 1A and 1B).

Blood IDA Parameters and Gastric Cytokine Concentrations

The multiple regression analyses revealed the gastric concentration of IL-1β, but not TNF-α, as a significant independent predictor for low serum ferritin and haemoglobin concentrations (Table 1). In addition, the male gender was an independent predictor of ferritin increase and the age was an independent predictor of haemoglobin increase. As *H. pylori* infection is mainly acquired by young children and we have previously observed differences in the inflammatory and immune response between children younger and older than 10–12 years [23], we stratified children by age: 12 years old or younger, and those older than 12 years of age. IL-1β remained a predictor of low ferritin concentration and was a stronger predictor of low haemoglobin concentration in the younger age group. The male gender was an independent predictor of ferritin increasing (Table1).

When *H. pylori*-positive and -negative children were separately analyzed, significant correlations were observed only in the *H. pylori*-positive group [ferritin ($r = -0.42$, $p = 0.004$) and haemoglobin ($r = -0.35$, $p = 0.02$)] (Figure 2). The values of haematocrit were also negatively correlated with gastric IL-1β concentrations ($r = -0.40$, $p = 0.007$]. In contrast, corpus and antral TNF-α concentrations neither correlated with serum ferritin ($p \geq 0.48$), nor with haemoglobin ($p \geq 0.74$) or haematocrit ($p \geq 0.40$) values.

Gastric Inflammation and Cytokine Concentrations

The degrees of antral and corpus chronic and active inflammation were significantly higher ($p<0.001$ for all) in *H. pylori*-positive than in -negative children (Table 2). In *H. pylori*-positive children, the corpus concentration of IL-1β was significantly higher in children with a mild/moderate degree of corpus chronic inflammation than in those without corpus inflammation (672.48±300.37 pg/mg vs. 504.39±28.81 pg/mg, respectively, $p = 0.002$). Furthermore, the corpus concentration of TNF-α was higher ($p<0.001$) in infected children with a mild/moderate degree of corpus active inflammation than in those without corpus PMN cell infiltration (369.2±75.3 pg/mg vs. 277.8±75.3 pg/mg).

IL1B, *IL1RN* and *TNFA* Polymorphisms

IL1B ($p = 0.45$), *IL1RN* ($p = 0.36$) and *TNFA* ($p = 0.78$) polymorphic genotypes did not associate with *H. pylori* status (Table 3). No association between *IL1B* and *TNFA* polymorphic alleles and blood ID/IDA parameters ($p \geq 0.17$) was observed.

In the *H. pylori*-positive group, carriers of the polymorphic *IL1RN* allele 2 had increased corpus inflammatory scores ($p = 0.02$) and significantly higher ($p = 0.01$ for both) IL-1β concentrations than the non-carriers (antrum 354.4±189.3 pg/mg vs. 253.5±74.3 pg/mg and corpus 873.4±466.6 pg/mg vs.

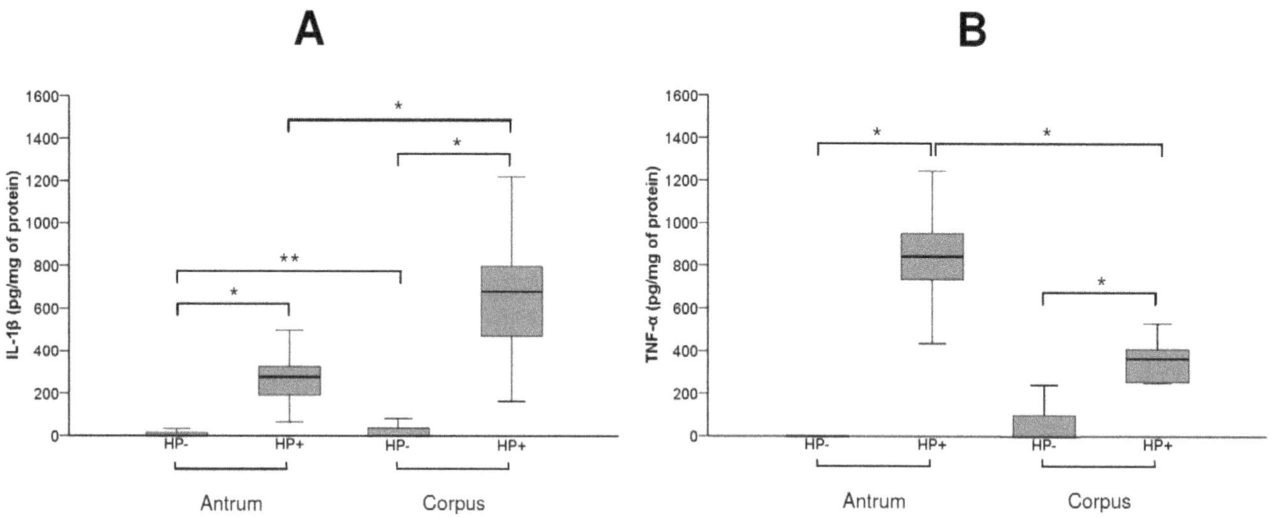

Figure 1. Box plots representing the comparison of gastric IL-1β (A) and TNF-α (B) concentrations (pg/mg of protein) between *H. pylori*-positive (HP+, n = 47) and -negative (HP-, n = 78) children, and between antral and corpus concentration in *H. pylori*-positive and -negative groups. The upper and lower limits of the boxes represent the 75th and 25th percentiles, respectively. The horizontal bar across the box indicates the median and the capped bars indicate the minimum and maximum data values. Statistical analysis by Student's t test after log transformation in the case of IL-1β; *$p<0.001$ and **$p = 0.02$.

Table 1. Multiple linear regression model including ferritin or haemoglobin as dependent variables and IL-1β and TNF-α gastric corpus concentrations, gender and age as independent variables.

	Univariate analysis		Multivariate analysis	
	Beta coefficient	P value	Beta coefficient	P value
FERRITIN				
Children of all ages (n = 125)				
age	0.119	0.19	0.126	0.15
male gender	0.280	0.002	0.279	0.02
IL-1β	−0.200	0.006	−0.205	0.04
TNF-α	−0.075	0.41	-	-
Children ≤12 years of age (n = 84)				
age	−0.040	0.32	-	-
male gender	0.208	0.20	0.229	0.02
IL-1β	−0.202	0.03	−0.219	0.02
TNF-α	−0.106	0.35	-	-
HAEMOGLOBIN				
Children of all ages (n = 125)				
age	0.285	0.001	0.301	0.001
male gender	0.151	0.09	0.158	0.07
IL-1β	−0.220	0.02	−0.244	0.03
TNF-α	−0.135	0.14	−0.001	0.99
Children ≤12 years of age (n = 84)				
age	0.145	0.19	0.112	0.28
male gender	−0.170	0.12	−0.094	0.37
IL-1β	−0.399	<0.001	−0.439	<0.001
TNF-α	−0.167	0.13	0.092	0.49

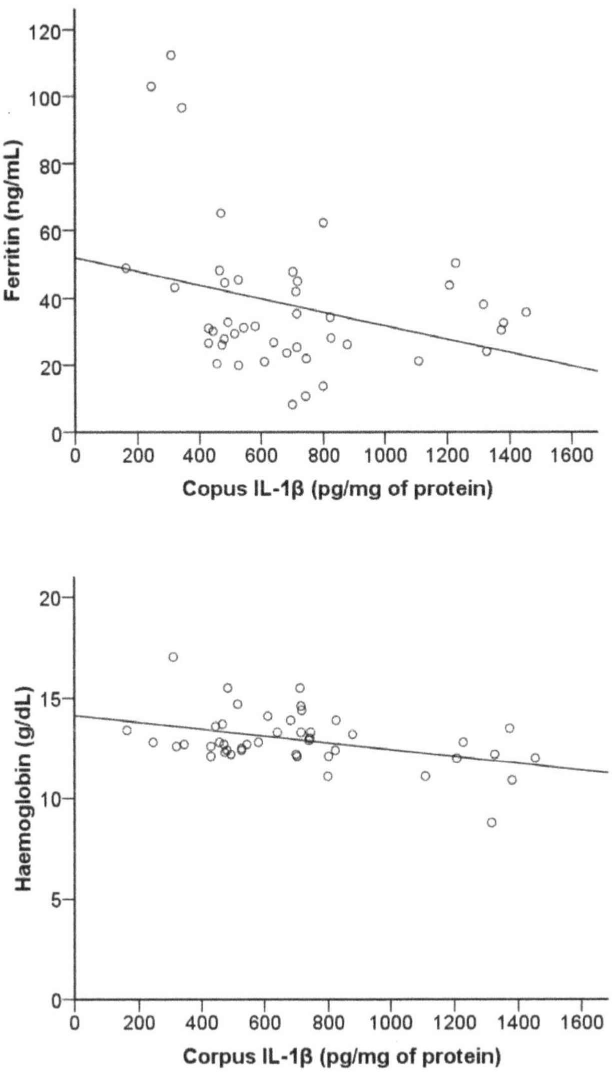

Figure 2. Correlations between corpus IL-1β concentrations and concentrations of ferritin and haemoglobin in *H. pylori*-positive children (n = 47). Statistical analysis by Pearson's correlation after log transformation in the case of IL-1β and ferritin.

624.7±183.1 pg/mg). In the *H. pylori*-positive group of children of 12 years of age or younger (16 non-carriers vs. 9 carriers), a significant negative association between *IL1RN* polymorphic genotype and haemoglobin (13.0±0.9 g/dL vs. 11.9±1.3 g/dL, p = 0.03) or haematocrit (39.5±2.2% vs. 36.0±4.2%, p = 0.01) was observed.

The mean gastric concentration of antral (p>0.12) and corpus IL-1β (p>0.15) and antral (p>0.32) and corpus TNF-α (p>0.28) did not differ between carriers and non-carriers of *IL1B* and *TNFA* polymorphic genotypes, independently of the *H. pylori*-status.

Discussion

ID is a very common micronutrient deficiency that affects individuals globally, but is a particular problem in developing countries. Children are considered to be at high-risk of ID that associates with deficits of immune, cognitive and motor functions [24,25], in addition to the possible development of anaemia.

Accumulating evidence from epidemiological studies and clinical trials implicates *H. pylori* infection in the aetiology of ID/IDA [22,26,27]. Notably, ID in *H. pylori* infected subjects is resistant to iron supplementation, but this resistance is reversible by *H. pylori* eradication [28,29]. However, the mechanism, or mechanisms, by which the infection might cause ID/IDA are still not determined. In the present study, we demonstrate that in *H. pylori*-infected children without common known causes of ID/IDA increased gastric IL-1β concentration is an independent predictor for low blood concentration of ferritin and haemoglobin.

Although it would be expected that in *H. pylori* infected children gastric IL-1β concentrations would be higher in the antrum, which is more inflamed than the corpus, a 2.5-fold increase in corpus IL-1β was observed. This could be explained either by increased corpus IL-1β production, or by a higher number of IL-1 receptors in the gastric corpus. In the former, as there was no corresponding increase in inflammation, IL-1β sources other than inflammatory cells have to be considered. However, taking in account that IL-1β inhibits gastric acid secretion by acting directly on parietal cells [14,17,30], the latter hypothesis seems more likely. Importantly, both murine gastric mucous and parietal cell lineages express the IL-1R1 receptor [31]. In contrast to IL-1β, the concentration of TNF-α was higher in the antrum than in the corpus, but TNF-α was not associated with blood iron parameters. However TNF-α concentrations were correlated with the scores of PMN cells in the corpus mucosa and inflammation has been considered a putative mechanism of disruption of the acid homeostasis.

Table 2. Histological comparison of antral and corpus gastric mucosa of *H. pylori (HP)*-positive (n = 47) and -negative (n = 78) children[a].

Inflammation	Absent n (%)	Mild n (%)	Moderate n (%)	Marked n (%)	P value
Antrum					
Chronic inflammation					
HP-positive	01 (2.2)	09 (19.5)	35 (76.1)	01 (2.2)	
HP-negative	34 (47.9)	37 (52.1)	0	0	<0.001
Active inflammation					
HP-positive	04 (8.7)	26 (56.5)	16 (34.8)	0	
HP-negative	66 (93.0)	5 (7.0)	0	0	<0.001
Corpus					
Chronic inflammation					
HP-positive	03 (6.8)	38 (86.4)	03 (6.8)	0	
HP-negative	42 (54.5)	35 (45.5)	0	0	<0.001
Active inflammation					
HP-positive	15 (34.1)	29 (65.9)	0	0	
HP-negative	74 (96.1)	03 (3.9)	0	0	<0.001

[a]One antral and 3 corpus gastric biopsy specimens from *HP*-positive and 7 antral and 1 corpus biopsy specimens from *HP*-negative children were deemed to be inadequate for histology assessment; n, number.
Neither atrophy, nor intestinal metaplasia was observed.

Table 3. *IL1B*-31, *IL1RN* and *TNFA*-307 genotypic frequencies in *H. pylori-positive* (n = 47) and *–negative* children (n = 78).

	All children n (%)	*H. pylori*-positive n (%)	*H. pylori*-negative n (%)
IL1B-31[a]			
T/T	37 (29.8)	16 (34.8)	21 (26.9)
T/C	63 (50.8)	20 (43.5)	42 (55.2)
C/C	24 (19.4)	10 (21.7)	14 (17.9)
IL1RN VNTR[b]			
1/1	82 (66.2)	30 (65.2)	52 (66.7)
1/2	35 (28.2)	15 (32.6)	20 (25.6)
2/2	07 (5.6)	01 (2.2)	06 (7.7)
TNFA-307			
G/G	87 (69.6)	32 (68.1)	55 (70.5)
G/A	38 (30.4)	15 (31.9)	23 (29.5)

[a]It was not possible to genotype 1 *H. pylori*-positive children for *IL1B*-31 and 1 for *IL1RN*.
[b]1 indicates all the long alleles and 2 the short allele. The loci did not deviate significantly from the expected Hardy-Weinberg distribution (P = 0.90 for *IL1B*-31, P = 0.26 for *IL1RN* and P = 0.08 for *TNFA*-307) and all segregated independently.

The negative correlation between gastric IL-1β and ID/IDA blood parameters observed in this study could be due to the powerful capability of IL-1β in inhibiting gastric acid secretion [14]. Gastric acid is essential for iron absorption by reducing the ferric iron to a more soluble and absorbable ferrous iron form [2,6]. The results of this study would support the argument that in the early phase of *H. pylori* infection, high gastric secretion of IL-1β that inhibits acid secretion impairs the absorption of iron. IL1β would also participate in the impairment of iron absorption by up-regulating hepcidin as demonstrated *in vivo* [31,32]. However, in a recent study, Schwarz *et al* [33] did not observe associations between the serum concentrations of hepcidin and *H. pylori* infection.

In chronic *H. pylori* infection in adulthood, gastric atrophy leading to hypochlorhydria is considered a mechanism of iron deficiency. Gastric corpus atrophic changes are more frequently observed in adult carriers of the *IL1* gene cluster polymorphisms [17]. In the present study, *IL1RN*, but not *IL1B* polymorphism, was associated with increased gastric IL-1β concentration in concordance with studies in our adult population [34]. The latter study demonstrated that polymorphism of *IL1RN*, but not *IL1B*, is associated with increased risk of atrophic gastric changes and gastric carcinoma in this region of Brazil. In the current study we demonstrate that in the group of the *H. pylori*-positive youngest children, the haemoglobin and haematocrit values are lower in carriers of *IL1RN* polymorphic alleles than in children with the wild genotype. The high production of IL-1β in the former group might account for a more severe hypochlorhydria in the acute phase of *H. pylori* infection that is mainly acquired in early childhood.

In conclusion, we provide additional and convincing evidence of a role of gastric IL-1β induced by *H. pylori* infection in decreasing iron absorption in children. Thus, *H. pylori* infected children with ID/IDA may benefit from *H. pylori* eradication therapy.

Author Contributions

Conceived and designed the experiments: DMMQ JEC. Performed the experiments: AMCR GAR FFM KNT SDC PFSB LPFC. Analyzed the data: DMMQJEC AMCR. Contributed reagents/materials/analysis tools: DMMQ JEC. Wrote the paper: DMMQ JEC AMCR.

References

1. WHO/UNICEF/UNU (2001) Iron deficiency anemia assessment, prevention, and control. Geneva: World Health Organization. Available: http://www.who.int/nutrition/publications/en/ida_assessment_prevention_control.pdf. Accessed 24 November 2012.
2. Zimmermann MB, Hurrell RF (2007) Nutritional iron deficiency. Lancet 370: 511–520.
3. Crompton DWT, Nesheim MC (2002) Nutritional impact of intestinal helminthiasis during the human life cycle. Annu Rev Nutr 22: 35–59.
4. Yip R, Limburg PJ, Ahlquist DA, Carpenter HA, ONeill A, et al. (1997) Pervasive occult gastrointestinal bleeding in an Alaska native population with prevalent iron deficiency. JAMA 277: 1135–1139.
5. Yokota S, Kono M, Mino E, Sato K, Takahashi M, et al. (2008) Enhanced Fe ion-uptake activity in *Helicobacter pylori* strains isolated from patients with iron-deficiency anemia. Clin Inf Dis 46: e31–33.
6. Annibale B, Capurso G, Lahner E, Passi S, Ricci R, et al. (2003) Concomitant alterations in intragastric pH and ascorbic acid concentrations in patients with *Helicobacter pylori* gastritis and associated iron deficiency anaemia. Gut 52: 496–501.
7. Windle HJ, Kelleher D, Crabtree JE (2007) Childhood *Helicobacter pylori* infection and growth impairment in developing countries: a vicious cycle? Pediatrics 119: E754–759.
8. Sobala GM, Crabtree JE, Dixon MF, Schorah CJ, Taylor JD, et al. (1991) Acute *Helicobacter pylori* infection: clinical features, local and systemic immune response, gastric mucosal histology, and gastric juice ascorbic acid concentrations. Gut 32: 1415–1418.
9. Harford WV, Barnett C, Lee E, Perez-Perez G, Blaser MJ, et al. (2000) Acute gastritis with hypochlorhydria: report of 35 cases with long term follow-up. Gut 47: 467–472.
10. Wilson KT, Crabtree JE (2007) Immunology of *Helicobacter pylori*: insights into the failure of the immune response and perspectives on vaccine studies. Gastroenterology 133: 288–308.

11. Fox JG, Otto G, Taylor NS, Rosenblad W, Murphy JC (1991) *Helicobacter mustelae*-induced gastritis and elevated gastric pH in the ferret (*Mustela putorius furo*). Infect Immun 59: 1875–1880.
12. Takashima M, Furuta T, Hanai H, Sugimura H, Kaneko E (2001) Effects of *Helicobacter pylori* infection on gastric acid secretion and serum gastrin levels in Mongolian gerbils. Gut 48: 765–773.
13. Correa P, Piazuelo MB (2008) Natural history of *Helicobacter pylori* infection. Dig Liver Dis 40: 490–496.
14. Beales IL, Calam J (1998) Interleukin 1 beta and tumour necrosis factor alpha inhibit acid secretion in cultured rabbit parietal cells by multiple pathways. Gut 42: 227–234.
15. Crabtree JE, Shallcross TM, Heatley RV, Wyatt JI (1991) Mucosal tumour necrosis factor alpha and interleukin-6 in patients with *Helicobacter pylori*-associated gastritis. Gut 32: 1473–1477.
16. Melo FF, Rocha AMC, Rocha GA, Pedroso SHSP, Batista SA (2012) A regulatory instead of an IL-17 T response predominates in *Helicobacter pylori*-associated gastritis in children. Microbes and Infection 14: 341–347.
17. El-Omar EM, Carrington M, Chow WH, McColl KE, Bream JH, et al. (2000) Interleukin-1 polymorphisms associated with increased risk of gastric cancer. Nature 404: 398–402.
18. Vannella L, Aloe Spirit MA, Gozza G, Tardellas L, Monarca B, et al. (2008) Benefit of concomitant gastrointestinal and gynaecological evaluation in premenopausal women with iron deficiency anaemia. Aliment Pharmacol Ther 28: 422–430.
19. Cardinali LC, Rocha GA, Rocha AM, Moura SB, Soares TF, et al. (2003) Evaluation of [^{13}C]urea-breath test and *Helicobacter pylori* stool antigen test for diagnosis of *H. pylori* infection in children from a developing country. J Clin Microbiol 41: 3334–3335.
20. Queiroz DMM, Guerra JB, Rocha GA, Rocha AMC, Santos A (2004) *IL1B* and *IL1RN* polymorphic genes and *Helicobacter pylori cagA* strains decrease the risk of reflux esophagitis. Gastroenterology 127: 73–79.
21. Dixon MF, Genta RM, Yardley JH, Correa P (1996) Classification and grading of gastritis. The updated Sydney System. Am J Surg Pathol 20: 1161–1181.
22. Mansfield JC, Holden H, Tarlow JK, Di Giovine FS, McDowell TL, et al. (1994) Novel genetic association between ulcerative colitis and the anti-inflammatory cytokine interleukin-1 receptor antagonist. Gastroenterology 106: 637–642.
23. Soares TF, Rocha GA, Rocha AM, Corrêa-Oliveira R, Martins-Filho AO, et al. (2005) Phenotypic study of peripheral blood lymphocytes and humoral immune response in *Helicobacter pylori* infection according to age. Scand J Immunol 62: 63–70.
24. Idiradinata P, Pollitt E (1993) Reversal of developmental delays in iron-deficient anaemic infants treated with iron. Lancet 341: 1–4.
25. Hurtado EK, Claussen AH, Scott KG (1999) Early childhood anemia and mild or moderate mental retardation. Am J Clin Nutr 69: 115–119.
26. Kurekci AE, Atay AA, Sarici SU, Yesilkaya E, Senses Z, et al. (2005) Is there a relationship between childhood *Helicobacter pylori* infection and iron deficiency anemia? J Trop Ped 51: 166–169.
27. Baggett H, Parkinson AJ, Muth PT, Gold BD, Gessner B (2006) Endemic iron deficiency associated with *Helicobacter pylori* infection among school-aged children in Alaska. Pediatrics 117: e396–404.
28. Choe YH, Lee JE, Kim SK (2000) Effect of *Helicobacter pylori* eradication on sideropenic refractory anaemia in adolescent girls with *Helicobacter pylori* infection. Acta Paediatr 89: 154–157.
29. Marignani M, Angeletti S, Bordi C, Malagnino F, Mancino C, et al. (1997) Reversal of long standing iron deficiency anaemia alter eradication of *Helicobacter pylori* infection. Scan J Gastroenterol 32: 617–622.
30. Waghray M, Zavros Y, Saqui-Salces M, El-Zaatari M, Alamelumangapuram CB (2010) Interleukin-1 promotes gastric atrophy through suppression of sonic hedgehog. Gastroenterology 138: 562–572.
31. Inamura J, Ikuta K, Jimbo J, Shindo M, Sato K, et al. (2005) Upregulation of hepcidin by interleukin-1β in human hepatoma cell lines. Hepatol Res 33: 198–205.
32. Lee P, Peng H, Gelbart T, Wang L, Beutler E (2005) Regulation of hepcidin transcription by interleukin-1 and interleukin 6. PNAS 102: 1906–1910.
33. Schwarz P, Kübler JAM, Strnad P, Katrin M, Barth TFE, et al. (2012) Hepcidin is localised in gastric parietal cells, regulates acid secretion and is induced by *Helicobacter pylori* infection. Gut 61: 193–201.
34. Rocha GA, Guerra JB, Rocha AM, Saraiva IE, Silva DA, et al. (2005) *IL1RN* polymorphic gene and *cagA*-positive status independently increase the risk of noncardia gastric carcinoma. Int J Cancer 115: 678–683.

22

The Role of Genetic Variants of Stromal Cell-Derived Factor 1 in Pediatric HIV-1 Infection and Disease Progression

Ketty Gianesin[1], Riccardo Freguja[1], Francesco Carmona[2], Marisa Zanchetta[2], Paola Del Bianco[2], Sandro Malacrida[3], Marco Montagna[2], Osvalda Rampon[4], Carlo Giaquinto[4], Anita De Rossi[1,2]*

1 Section of Oncology and Immunology, AIDS Reference Center, Department of Surgery, Oncology and Gastroenterology, University of Padova, Padova, Italy, **2** Istituto Oncologico Veneto – IRCCS, Padova, Italy, **3** Department of Neurosciences, University of Padova, Padova, Italy, **4** Department of Pediatrics, University of Padova, Padova, Italy

Abstract

Stromal cell-Derived Factor 1 (SDF1) is the natural ligand of CXCR4, the coreceptor of HIV-1 X4 viruses. This study investigated the role of the single nucleotide polymorphism (SNP) rs1801157 (NM_000609.5:c.*519G>A) of the *SDF1* gene in the natural history of mother-to-child transmission of HIV-1 and disease progression of HIV-1-infected children. The study was conducted in 428 children born to HIV-1-seropositive mothers, who had not undergone antiretroviral therapy (ART) during pregnancy, and in 120 HIV-1-infected children for whom the end-point was the onset of AIDS or the initiation of ART; 16 children developed early AIDS (<24 months of life), 13 from 24 to 84 months of age, and 14 had late AIDS (>84 months). The rs1801157 SNP was not associated with risk of perinatal infection in any genetic models tested. By contrast, this SNP influenced disease progression in a time-dependent manner. rs1801157 GA heterozygous children had a higher risk of late AIDS (HR = 6.3, 95%CI 1.9–20.7, p = 0.002) than children with the rs1801157 GG genotype. Children were studied for viral coreceptor usage at birth, after 84 months of age and/or at AIDS onset. While R5 viruses using CCR5 coreceptor were predominant at birth (94%) and at early AIDS (85%), viruses using CXCR4 coreceptor emerged during the course of infection and were detected in 49% of children older than 84 months and in 62% of late AIDS. The rs1801157 SNP did not influence the emergence of R5X4 viruses, but children with the rs1801157 GA genotype and R5X4 viruses were at significantly higher risk of late AIDS than children with rs1801157 GG genotype (OR = 8.0, 95% CI 1.2–52.2, p = 0.029). Our results indicate that the rs1801157 SNP does not influence perinatal infection, but impacts disease progression. This effect is time-dependent and linked to the coreceptor-usage of viral variants that undergo evolution during the course of HIV-1 infection.

Editor: Srinivas Mummidi, University of Texas Health Science Center/South Texas Veterans Health Care System, United States of America

Funding: The financial support for this research was received from the PENTA foundation. RF was supported by the PENTA Foundation. The funders had no role in study design, data collection and analysis, decision to publish, or preparation of the manuscript.

Competing Interests: The authors have declared that no competing interests exist.

* E-mail: anita.derossi@unipd.it

Introduction

The interaction of viral and host factors is believed to determine not only the risk for initial Human Immunodeficiency Virus type-1 (HIV-1) acquisition, but also the course of the infection. Increasing data support host genetic factors as important determinants of HIV-1 infection and pathogenesis.

The chemokine receptors CXCR4 and CCR5 have been identified as the major coreceptors for HIV-1 entry into target cells [1–4]. Mother-to-child transmission (MTCT) is the main source of pediatric HIV-1 infection. Viruses using CCR5 (R5 viruses) are the predominant viral variants transmitted from mother to child and detected in the newborn [5,6]. Evolution of HIV-1 coreceptor usage has been demonstrated during disease progression in adults as well as in children [7,8]. The evolution usually involved change from CCR5 usage to CXCR4 usage alone (X4 viruses) or in combination with CCR5 (R5X4 viruses). The switch from R5 phenotype to X4 or R5X4 phenotype, which occurred in approximately 50% of infected individuals [8,9], was associated with accelerated CD4 T cell decline and progression to AIDS [10,11].

Genetic polymorphisms of chemokine receptors and related ligands have been demonstrated to influence both HIV-1 transmission and disease progression [12]. The deletion of 32 bp (Δ32) in the *CCR5* gene impairs the expression of coreceptor on the cell membrane and Δ32 homozygosity confers resistance to infection by R5 viruses [13]. Heterozygotes express low levels of CCR5 receptors, slowing HIV-1 replication, spread and pathogenesis [14,15]. Furthermore, nucleotide variants in the *CCR5* promoter impact disease outcome; homozygosity for P1 haplotype is associated with rapid progression to AIDS in adults as well as in children [16,17].

The chemokine Stromal cell-Derived Factor 1 (SDF1) is the unique natural ligand of the CXCR4 receptor, and it may interfere with HIV-1 infection [18,19]. SDF1 exhibits genetic polymorphisms, including the single nucleotide polymorphism (SNP) rs1801157 (NM_000609.5:c.*519G>A, also known as SDF1 3′G>A). This SNP is located in the 3′ untranslated region of the gene that may serve as a target for cis-acting factors, thus influencing the chemokine's expression [20,21]. This SNP may thereby influence mRNA stability; *SDF1* mRNA containing the 3′A variant has a two-fold longer half-life compared to the 3′G variant [22]. Studies in adults have suggested that rs1801157 AA homozygosity was associated with increased plasma levels of SDF1 [23] and delayed progression to AIDS [24,25]. However, these findings were not confirmed by others [26,27]. Moreover, several studies suggested an association between the rs1801157 AA genotype and accelerated disease progression [28–30].

With regard to pediatric HIV-1 infection, there are very few data. One study in African population indicated that the mother's, but not the child's, rs1801157 GA genotype increases the risk of perinatal transmission of HIV-1, particularly during breastfeeding [31], but this association was not confirmed in breastfeeding mothers receiving zidovudine [32]. Few studies suggested that the rs1801157 AA genotype was associated with accelerated disease progression, but this variant occurred in a very small fraction of subjects [33,34]. Moreover, the protective effect of *CCR5*Δ32 heterozygosity appeared to be abrogated by the rs1801157 A allele [35]. None of these studies addressed the role of the rs1801157 genotype in relation to viral coreceptor usage at the onset of AIDS.

The aim of this study was to evaluate the role of *SDF1* rs1801157 polymorphism in the natural history of perinatal infection and disease progression of HIV-1-infected children, in relation to the coreceptor usage of the infecting viruses and time of AIDS onset.

Methods

Patients

The study population for the assessment of rs1801157 SNP in MTCT included 428 children (148 HIV-1-infected and 280 HIV-1-uninfected children), born to HIV-1-seropositive mothers between 1984 and 2002, whose virological analyses for diagnosis of HIV-1 infection were conducted at the AIDS Reference Center of Padova University. Inclusion criteria were the known HIV-1-seropositive status of the mother at delivery, and the absence of antiretroviral prophylaxis during pregnancy and/or at delivery. No child was breastfed. Diagnosis of HIV-1 infection was performed by virus isolation and polymerase chain reaction (PCR) [36,37]. The study population for the assessment of the rs1801157 SNP in disease progression involved 120 HIV-1-infected children followed from birth at the Pediatric Department of Padova University. Clinical and immunologic staging of the HIV-1-infected children was defined according to the classification system of the Centers for Disease Control and Prevention (CDC) [38].

The end-point of the study was the onset of severe clinical manifestations (stage C, CDC), or the initiation of antiretroviral therapy (ART). The median follow-up was 88 (interquartile range [IQR] 36-135) months. According to the natural history of pediatric HIV-1 infection [39–41], children were classified as early progressors if they developed severe symptoms of disease within two years, and late progressors if they developed severe symptoms of disease after seven years of age. The study was performed in accordance with the Helsinki Declaration and was approved by the Ethics Committee of the Istituto Oncologico Veneto, Prot. 2131, 2012/04 and Azienda Ospedaliera Padova, 30/01/2012. An informed verbal consent was obtained from the parents or the guardians of the children by a pediatrician and recorded on the clinical notes. According to the national law (General Authorization for the genetic data - Garante della Privacy 24 June 2011,G. U. no.159, 2011) the written consent was not required for this study. The Ethics Committees verified the requirements and approved this consent procedure.

SDF1 Genotyping

Genomic DNA was extracted from peripheral blood mononuclear cells (PBMC) with the QIAmp DNA Blood mini kit (Qiagen, Hilden, Germany), according to the manufacturer's instructions. Polymorphic sites in genomic DNA were analyzed by the TaqMan allelic discrimination assay. Primers for genotyping the rs1801157 SNP were F5′-CAAGCCTAGTGAAGGCTTCTCTC-3′ and R5′-TCAGGGTAGCCCTGCTGC-3′. The probes were as follows (allele-specific nucleotides are underlined): 5′-FAM-TGGGAGCC<u>G</u>GGTCTGCCTCT-BHQ1-3′ and 5′-HEX-ACATGGAGCC<u>A</u>GGTCTGCCTCTT-BHQ1–3′. PCR was performed in a thermal cycler (LightCycler 480, Roche Diagnostic, Mannheim, Germany) in a reaction volume of 20 µl containing 600 nM of each primer, 300 nM of probe for SNP G, 100 nM of probe for SNP A, 10 µl of 2x LightCycler 480 Probe Master (Roche Diagnostic) and 2 ng of sample DNA. The cycling conditions were 95°C for 10 min, followed by 45 cycles, each of 95°C for 10 sec, 62°C for 1 min and 72°C for 1 sec. Allele discrimination and genotype determination were based on the endpoint fluorescence measured by the LightCycler 480 detection system. Three positive controls, one for each of the possible genotypes, were included. Accuracy of genotyping was confirmed by direct sequencing of randomly selected samples, as previously described [42] using the same primers used in TaqMan assay.

CCR5 Genotyping

The P1/P1 haplotype on the promoter of the *CCR5* gene was determined by heteroduplex analysis, as described previously [17].

Viral Phenotype Analysis

Primary isolates were obtained by culturing PBMC from each subject with phytohemagglutinin (PHA)-stimulated PBMC from healthy donors, exactly as previously described [5]. Primary isolates were available from 53 children at birth, from 43 of 49 children older than 84 months of age, from 13 of 15 early AIDS and 13 of 14 late AIDS cases. Coreceptor usage of primary isolates was determined by viral infection in U87.CD4 cells that stably expressed CCR5 or CXCR4 coreceptors, as previously described [5]. On days 5 and 8, supernatants were collected and tested for p24 antigen using a commercially available assay (Vironostika® HIV Ag/Ab, Biomérieux SA, France). The laboratory strains HIV_{BAL} (R5-tropic) and HIV_{IIIB} (X4-tropic) were used as controls in all *in vitro* experiments.

V3 Genotyping

HIV-1 RNA was extracted from frozen plasma samples with the QIAmp RNA Viral Mini Kits (Qiagen), according to the manufacturer's instructions, and reverse transcribed by SuperScript III RT (Invitrogen, Milan, Italy) and random primers (Invitrogen). The cDNA obtained was used for nested PCR amplifications to sequence the *V3* region. The *V3* loop was amplified with the outer primer pair V3A (5′-TACAATGTACA-CATGGAATT-3′) and V3D (5′-ATTACAGTA-GAAAAATTCCCC-3′) and the inner primers V3B (5′-TGGCAGTCTAGCAGAAGAAG-3′) and V3C (5′-CTGGGTCCCCTCCTGAGG-3′). The first-round PCRs were performed with 5 ul of cDNA, in a 50 ul reaction mixture containing 5 ul of 10X PCR Buffer II (Applied Biosystems, Foster City, CA, USA), 700 nM of each of the outer primers, 200 nM of deoxyribonucleotide triphosphates, 1.6 mM of $MgCl_2$, and 1.5 U of AmpliTaq DNA polymerase (Applied Biosystems). Forty cycles were carried out in a thermal cycler (2720 thermal cycler, Applied Biosystem), each consisting of 30 sec at 94°C, 30 sec at 54°C, and 1 min at 72°C, followed by one cycle at 72°C for 7 min. Five microliters of the first-round PCR were amplified in a nested PCR with 100 uM of the inner primers; 40 cycles were run, each consisting of 30 sec at 94°C, 30 sec at 59°C, and 1 min at 72°C, followed by a final extension at 72°C for 7 min. All negative controls from the first round of amplification were included in the second amplification step. The amplified products were separated on a 2.5% agarose gel. Direct sequencing was performed as described previously [42], using the V3B and V3C primers. The sequence alignments were subsequently inspected manually. HIV-1 tropism was predicted from the *V3* genotype using position-specific scoring matrices $PSSM_{X4/R5}$ [43] (http://fortinbras.us/cgi-bin/fssm/fssm.pl). Standard sequencing with PSSM values below the predetermined cutoff of -6.96 were called R5, whereas those with scores greater than or equal to -6.96 were defined as R5X4 [43]. Where sequence ambiguity to the presence of nucleotide mixtures occurred, the permutation with the highest PSSM score was used to assign the score for a given replicate, to increase the sensitivity for detection of X4 variants [44]. For each HIV-1 RNA sample, the *V3* sequence with PSSM results were compared with the results of the viral phenotype assay. For discordant results, the test with the broadest prediction was considered.

Statistical Analyses

Genotype and allele frequencies, and Hardy-Weinberg equilibrium tests of the rs1801157 SNP were performed separately among cases and controls using the SNPStats program [45]. Estimation of the power of the study to detect association between SNP and HIV-1 infection was evaluated using the genetic power calculator available at http://pngu.mgh.harvard.edu/~purcell/gpc/for minimum detectable risk calculations using SNP effects under different study constrains. The minimum detectable effects with odds ratio (OR) was calculated at various allele frequencies of the SNP allele in a codominant model, based on an alpha of 0.05 and a prevalence 1/1.000 in the general population. With this sample size, we had 80% power to detect an OR of 4.3 if the risk allele frequency was 35%. Unconditional logistic regression analysis was performed with SNPStats to investigate the association between the SNP genotype and infection status. Because the mode of inheritance was unknown, to increase the power of the study four genetic models (codominant, dominant, recessive and overdominant) were considered and OR and 95% confidence intervals (CI) were calculated.

The probability of acquiring disease was calculated with the Kaplan-Meier method and the log-rank test was used to test for differences between genotype categories. Hazard ratios (HR) and their 95% CI based on the Cox proportional hazard model were estimated to test the association between genotypes, and risk of stage C. The assumption of proportional risk was evaluated using the Schoenfeld residuals test, which was significant for the rs1801157 ($p = 0.03$). To take into consideration this time-dependent effect, we added to the basic Cox proportional hazard model an interaction of the rs1801157 with a heaviside step function to get constant hazard ratios for different time intervals [46]. The function of risk was the following:

$h(t, SDF1) = h_0(t)\exp(\beta_1 \times SDF1 + \gamma_1 \times SDF1 \times g(t))$, where $g(t) = 0$ if $t \le t_0$ and $g(t) = 1$ if $t > t_0$, from which we obtain two different HR for the variable rs1801157: $HR(SDF1) = \exp(\beta_1)$ if $t \le t_0$, and $HR(SDF1) = \exp(\beta_1 + \gamma_1)$ if $t > t_0$. We chose visually the change point, t_0, as the integer year value were the two survivor curves appeared to diverge. OR and 95% CI were calculated to estimate association between the rs1801157 genotype and viral coreceptor usage. All tests were two-sided, and a p-value less than 0.05 was considered statistically significant. Statistical analyses were performed using Epi Info™ 3.5 and the SAS version 9.1.3 (SAS Institute, Cary, NC).

Results

Relationship between the rs1801157 SNP and Risk of Pediatric HIV-1 Infection

To analyze the impact of the rs1801157 SNP on HIV-1 perinatal infection, 148 HIV-1-infected and 280 exposed HIV-1-uninfected children were analyzed according to different genetic models. Genotype and allele frequencies for the rs1801157 were in Hardy-Weinberg equilibrium in both groups and were in agreement with frequencies reported in the NCBI database on the white population (data not shown). The rs1801157 AA genotype was very rare in both HIV-1-infected [3 (2.0%) of 148 children] and HIV-1-uninfected children [9(3.2%) of 280 children]. Forty-four (29.7%) of 148 HIV-1-infected and 97 (34.6%) of 280 HIV-1-uninfected children were heterozygous for the rs1801157 A allele. The SNP showed no significant association with the risk of HIV-1 infection in any genetic model considered (Table 1). Values of maternal viral load at delivery were available in a subgroup of 139 mothers (median $\log_{10}$ 3.74, range $\log_{10}$ 1.60-6.32, HIV-1 RNA copies/ml of plasma). After adjustment for maternal viral load, the rs1801157 SNP was found to not be significantly associated with the risk of HIV-1 infection.

Relationship between the rs1801157 SNP and Disease Progression

The relationship between the rs1801157 SNP and disease progression was studied in 120 HIV-1-infected children followed from birth. The end-point of the study was the onset of severe clinical manifestations (stage C, CDC) or the initiation of ART. Nine children were excluded from the study because of initiation of early ART within three months of age. Of the 111 children, seventy-seven children (69.4%) had the rs1801157 GG genotype and among them 24 (31.2%) developed AIDS. Thirty-two children (28.8%) had the rs1801157 GA genotype and 18 (56.3%) progressed to AIDS. Overall, the rs1801157 GA genotype tended to be associated with a worse prognosis and a rapid disease progression, with both Kaplan-Meier ($p = 0.051$) (Figure 1) and Cox analyses (HR = 1.83, 95% CI 0.99-3.41; $p = 0.055$) (Table 2). Children with the rs1801157 GA genotype had a median time to stage C of 114 (92;-) months *versus* children with the rs1801157 GG genotype who had a median time to stage C of 199 (140;-) months. Only 2 children had the rs1801157 AA genotype; one developed AIDS at 5 months and the other one entered ART at 135 months. These cases were excluded from the analysis, because there was not sufficient statistical power to evaluate the effect of rs1801157 AA homozygosity.

Interestingly, the effect of the rs1801157 SNP seemed to be time-dependent, with survival curves beginning to diverge at approximately 90 months of age, suggesting a change in the proportionality of risk (Figure 1). To better investigate this aspect, we divided the time periods into distinct intervals and fitted the proportional hazard models in each interval [46]. To determine the boundaries of the time intervals, we selected periods according to the natural history of pediatric HIV-1 infection [39–41] and the divergence of survival curves. Among children with the GG or GA genotype, 15 developed AIDS within the first 24 months of life (early AIDS), 13 developed AIDS between 24 and 84 months of

Table 1. Frequencies of the rs1801157 genotype and risk of pediatric HIV-1 infection.

Genetic model	rs1801157 genotype	Uninfected children, N. (%)	Infected children, N. (%)	OR (95% CI)	p-value
Codominant	GG	174 (62.1%)	101 (68.2%)	1.00	0.410
	GA	97 (34.6%)	44 (29.7%)	0.78 (0.51–1.20)	
	AA	9 (3.2%)	3 (2.0%)	0.57 (0.15–2.17)	
Dominant	GG	174 (62.1%)	101 (68.2%)	1.00	0.210
	GA + AA	106 (37.9%)	47 (31.7%)	0.76 (0.50–1.16)	
Recessive	GG + GA	271 (96.8%)	145 (98.0%)	1.00	0.470
	AA	9 (3.2%)	3 (2.0%)	0.62 (0.17–2.34)	
Overdominant	GG + AA	183 (65.4%)	104 (70.3%)	1.00	0.300
	GA	97 (34.6%)	44 (29.7%)	0.80 (0.52–1.23)	

age, and 14 developed AIDS after 84 months of age (late AIDS). Cox analyses revealed that the influence of the rs1801157 SNP was not relevant before 84 months, while it became strongly significant after 84 months of age: the rs1801157 GA genotype was associated with a higher risk of late AIDS than the rs1801157 GG genotype (HR = 6.32, 95% CI 1.93–20.72, p = 0.002) (Table 2). The same evidence emerged when analysis was performed considering two time intervals, before and after 84 months of age (Table 2).

Five infants in our cohort were Δ32 heterozygous in the *CCR5* gene. After adjustment for *CCR5*Δ32, the rs1801157 GA genotype did not influence the onset of AIDS before 84 months (HR = 0.74, 95% CI 0.30–1.30, p = 0.506), but remained significantly associated with a higher risk of late AIDS onset (HR = 15.79, 95% CI 2.56–97.15, p = 0.003).

Analysis of Viral Coreceptor Usage

Considering the different impact of the rs1801157 SNP in relation to the time of infection and taking into account that coreceptor usage of infecting viruses may evolve during the course of infection, we analyzed the viral coreceptor usage in all children for whom primary isolates were obtained at birth, after 84 months of age and/or at AIDS onset. At birth, primary isolates were available from 53 children, 34 of 77 (44.2%) with the rs1801157 GG genotype and 19 of 32 (59.4%) with the rs1801157 GA genotype; 50 of 53 (94%) primary isolates had an R5 phenotype (Figure 2A) and R5 viral strains were also predominant in early AIDS (11 of 13 analyzed cases; 85%) (Figure 2B). Viruses using the CXCR4 coreceptor emerged during the course of infection; and were detectable in 21 out of 43 (49%) children analyzed after 84 months of age (Figure 2A) and in the majority of late AIDS (8 of 13 analyzed cases; 62%) (Figure 2B). Overall, R5X4 viruses tended to be associated with an increased risk of AIDS (HR = 2.00, 95% CI 0.90–4.40; p = 0.088), but early AIDS was significantly more associated with R5 viruses than late AIDS (Fisher test p = 0.041).

The rs1801157 SNP was not associated with emergence of CXCR4-usage viral strain; indeed, after 84 months of age, R5X4 viruses were found in 56% (9 of 16) and in 44% (12 of 27) of children with the rs1801157 GA and GG genotype, respectively (Fisher test p = 0.537).

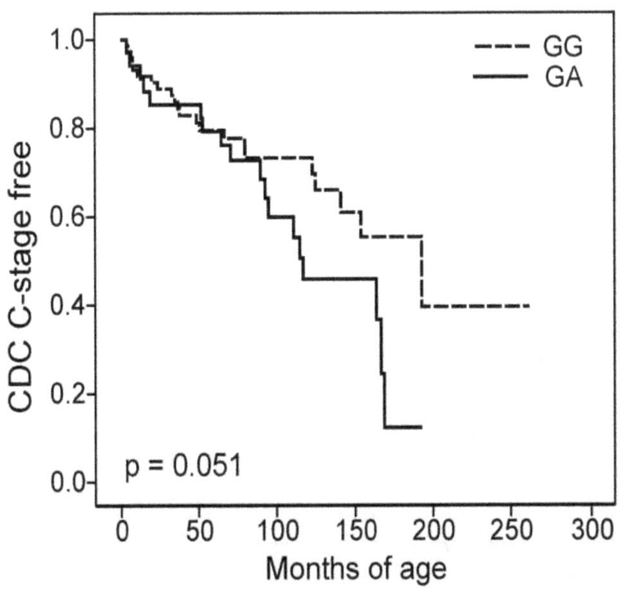

Figure 1. Kaplan-Meier curves showing the relationship between rs1801157 genotype and the onset of stage C CDC. The dashed line represents children with the GG genotype; the black line represents children with the GA genotype.

Table 2. rs1801157 genotypes and risk of disease progression according to different time period.

Time period age in months	rs1801157 genotype	AIDS/N.	HR (95% CI)	p-value
Overall	GG	24/77	1.00	0.055
	GA	18/32	1.83 (0.99–3.41)	
0-24 months	GG	10/77	1.00	0.768
	GA	5/32	1.18 (0.40–3.44)	
25-84months	GG	9/63	1.00	0.837
	GA	4/27	0.89 (0.27–2.87)	
>84 months	GG	5/31	1.00	0.002
	GA	9/18	6.32 (1.93–20.72)	
<84 months	GG	19/77	1.00	0.944
	GA	9/32	1.03 (0.47–2.28)	
>84 months	GG	5/31	1.00	0.002
	GA	9/18	6.32 (1.93–20.72)	

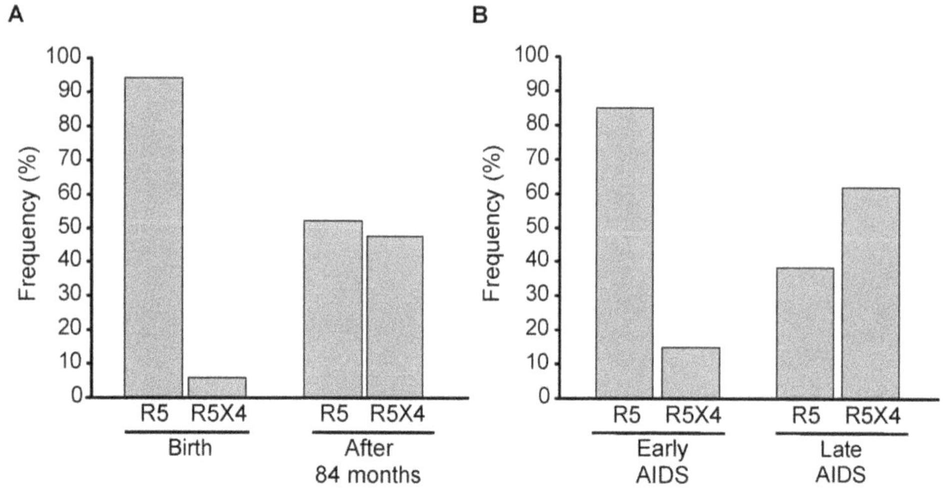

Figure 2. Viral coreceptor usage distribution in HIV-1-infected children. R5 and R5X4 viral strains in (A) HIV-1-infected children before and after 84 months of age; (B) at the onset of early AIDS (before 24 months of age) and late AIDS (after 84 months of age).

Association between the rs1801157 Genotype, *CCR5* Haplotype, Viral Coreceptor Usage and Disease Progression

Association analysis confirmed that the rs1801157 SNP was not related to early AIDS (p = 0.716), but strongly associated with late AIDS; children with rs1801157 GA genotype had a higher risk of late AIDS (OR = 5.20, 95% CI 1.38–19.67, p = 0.015) than children with the rs1801157 GG genotype (Table 3). This finding suggested an interaction between the rs1801157 SNP and viral coreceptor usage. This was supported by analysis of the *CCR5* promoter haplotype. In agreement with previous data [17], children carrying the P1/P1 haplotype showed a higher risk of developing early AIDS than children carrying other *CCR5* haplotypes (P1/P4, P2/P2, P2/P4, P4/P4). As opposed to that observed with the *SDF1* SNP, the effect of the P1/P1 *CCR5* haplotype was strongest in early AIDS (OR = 8.48, 95% CI 2.30–31.29; p = 0.001) when R5 viruses prevailed and lost after 84 months of age when R5X4 viral variants emerged in half of the studied children (Table 3).

Analysis of the association between the rs1801157 genotype, viral coreceptor usage and onset of late AIDS showed that children with the rs1801157 GA genotype and the R5X4 viral strain were at higher risk (OR = 8.00, 95% CI 1.23–52.25; p = 0.030) than children with the rs1801157 GG genotype and an R5 virus (Table 4). Of note, children with R5X4 variants and the rs1801157 GA genotype had a ten-fold higher risk of developing late AIDS (OR = 10.00, 95% CI 1.30–78.00; p = 0.028) than children with the rs1801157 GG genotype and a R5X4 virus, thus supporting the premise of a primarily protective role of the rs1801157 GG genotype against viruses using CXCR4 coreceptor.

Table 3. Association between the rs1801157 genotype, *CCR5* haplotype and early and late AIDS.

	Genotype	OR (95% CI)	p-value
Early AIDS			
SDF1	GG	1.00	0.716
rs1801157	GA	1.24 (0.39–3.97)	
CCR5	P1/P1	8.48 (2.30–31.29)	0.001
Haplotype	others*	1.00	
Late AIDS			
SDF1	GG	1.00	0.015
rs1801157	GA	5.20 (1.38–19.67)	
CCR5	P1/P1	0.78 (0.07–8.52)	0.837
Haplotype	others*	1.00	

*Others: CCR5 haplotypes P1/P4, P2/P2, P2/P4, P4/P4.

Discussion

Overall, these results demonstrated that rs1801157 polymorphism did not influence the susceptibility to perinatal HIV-1 infection, but strongly influenced in a time-dependent manner disease progression; children with the rs1801157 GA genotype had a 6–10 fold increased risk of developing late AIDS than children with the rs1801157 GG genotype.

To date, studies on the association between the rs1801157 genotype and HIV-1 susceptibility and disease progression have generated inconclusive results. These studies may have numerous confounding variables, such as differences in the characteristics of the study populations, the duration of follow-up, the definition of the study end-point, and the influence of antiretroviral therapy. Moreover, variation in coreceptor usage of infecting viruses and their evolution during the course of HIV-1 infection may contribute to generating different results. Our study, aimed at investigating the role of rs1801157 polymorphism in the natural history of perinatal HIV-1 infection and disease progression, was

Table 4. rs1801157 genotype and viral coreceptor usage in the onset of late AIDS.

Viral strain	rs1801157 genotype	AIDS/N.	OR (95% CI)	p-value
R5	GG	3/15	1.00	
R5	GA	2/7	1.60 (0.20–12.69)	0.657
R5X4	GG	2/12	0.80 (0.11–5.77)	0.825
R5X4	GA	6/9	8.00 (1.23–52.25)	0.030

conducted in a white population with no exposure to antiretroviral prophylaxis or therapeutic interventions. Furthermore, in a subset of the studied population viral coreceptor usage was defined.

In our study, the rs1801157 genotypes were similarly distributed among infants born HIV-1-infected and HIV-1-uninfected. In agreement with our results, a recent meta-analysis reported no significant association between the rs1801157 genotype and HIV-1 susceptibility in any genetic model [47]. Notably, most of the children in developed countries acquired infection around the time of delivery [37,48] and the transmitted viruses were predominantly of the R5 phenotype [49,50]. In agreement with this previous finding, 94% of studied children had an R5 virus at birth. Although a selection of transmitted variants cannot be excluded [51,52], this predominance of R5 isolates may explain the lack of a role of the rs1801157 SNP in perinatal HIV-1 infection.

SDF1 plays a strong role in disease progression. Notably, this role is time-dependent and selectively involves the onset of late AIDS. Conversely to adults, a fraction of perinatally HIV-1-infected children develop early AIDS within the first 24 months of age [53,54]. In this study, as well as in previous studies [5,17,55], most early AIDS were associated with an R5 virus. Polymorphisms in the *CCR5* promoter gene, such as the P1/P1 haplotype, may influence CCR5 expression and thus disease progression linked to R5 viruses [16]. This association may explain why genetic variants of the *CCR5*, but not the rs1801157 SNP, impact the risk of early AIDS.

In contrast, most of the late AIDS cases were associated with R5X4 viruses. While the role of P1/P1 was lost, the rs1801157 SNP acquired a strong influence, and its GA genotype was associated with a significantly higher risk of late AIDS than the GG genotype. It has been suggested that the rs1801157 A allele upregulates plasma chemokine levels [22,23]; upregulation of SDF1 levels in rs1801157 AA and GA patients may prevent the emergence of more pathogenic R5X4 strains, thus contributing to the slowing of disease progression [24]. Nonetheless, other studies did not correlate the rs1801157 A allele with chemokine production [27,56] and one study demonstrated that subjects with the rs1801157 A allele were also more likely to have detectable X4-tropic viruses [57]; the increased frequency of X4 viruses in subjects carrying the rs1801157 A allele may explain the observed adverse effect that this allele had on HIV-1 disease [28–30]. In our study we found no relationship between the rs1801157 genotype and emergence of CXCR4-usage viral strains. However, our study indicated that the impact of the rs1801157 SNP was linked to coreceptor usage of infecting viruses. In particular, while in children with the R5 virus, a GG or GA genotype did not influence the course of disease, in children with R5X4 viruses, those with the rs1801157 GA genotype had a 10-fold higher risk for developing late AIDS than those with the rs1801157 GG genotype.

These observations could have important implications for the clinical treatment of HIV-1-infected children. The discovery of CCR5 and CXCR4 as critical coreceptors for HIV-1 entry [1,2,4], coupled with the observation that patients heterozygous for *CCR5*Δ32 have a delayed disease progression [58], indicated that pharmacological blockade of the gp120-CCR5 interaction could be an effective strategy for inhibiting HIV-1 infection. Currently, entry inhibitors hold considerable potential for the treatment of HIV-1 infection, particularly in patients harbouring viruses resistant to traditional ART regimens with reverse transcriptase and protease inhibitors. Maraviroc, the first CCR5 inhibitor [59], is active against R5 viral strains [60]. Viruses using CXCR4 have become the dominant circulating strains in patients harboring R5X4 viruses prior to therapy [61]. The emergence of X4 strains as a result of CCR5 antagonist therapy, and the consequences on disease progression will need to be closely monitored. Data now available suggested that CCR5 antagonists might be more effective if utilized to treat patients at earlier stages of disease [62-65]. With this perspective, our study could be important in targeting therapy with CCR5 blockers in particular patients. Since our results suggest that the rs1801157 GA genotype is associated with a higher risk for developing AIDS, and that this effect is linked to the presence of viral strains using CXCR4, these patients may not be ideal candidates for a CCR5 inhibitor-based therapeutic regimens.

Acknowledgments

We thank Lisa Smith for editorial assistance.

Author Contributions

Conceived and designed the experiments: ADR CG. Performed the experiments: KG RF FC MZ. Analyzed the data: PDB SM KG RF MM CG ADR. Contributed reagents/materials/analysis tools: OR CG. Wrote the paper: KG ADR. Performed all the genotyping and sequencing analyses: KG RF. Performed the analyses of viral coreceptor usage: FC MZ. Performed the statistical analyses: PDB SM. Analyzed the data overall: KG RF MM CG ADR. Provided clinical samples and clinical data: OR CG.

References

1. Feng Y, Broder CC, Kennedy PE, Berger EA (1996) HIV-1 Entry Cofactor: Functional cDNA Cloning of a Seven-Transmembrane, G Protein-Coupled Receptor. Science 272: 872–877.
2. Deng H, Liu R, Ellmier W, Choe S, Unutmaz D, et al. (1996) Identification of a major co-receptor for primary isolates of HIV-1. Nature 381: 661–666.
3. Dragic T, Litwin V, Allaway GP, Martin SR, Huang Y, et al. (1996) HIV-1 entry into CD4+ cells is mediated by the chemokine receptor CC-CKR-5. Nature 381: 667–673.
4. Alkhatib G, Combadiere C, Broder CC, Feng Y, Kennedy PE, et al. (1996) CC CKR5: a RANTES, MIP-1alpha, MIP-1beta receptor as a fusion cofactor for macrophage-tropic HIV 1. Science 272: 1955–1958.
5. Ometto L, Zanchetta M, Mainardi M, De Salvo GL, Garcia-Rodriguez MC, et al. (2000) Co-receptor usage of HIV-1 primary isolates, viral burden, and CCR5 genotype in mother-to-child HIV-1 transmission. AIDS 14: 1721–1729.
6. Salvatori F, Scarlatti G (2001) HIV type 1 chemokine receptor usage in mother-to-child transmission. AIDS Res Hum Retroviruses 17: 925–935.
7. De Rossi A (2007) Virus-host interactions in paediatric HIV-1 infection. Curr Opin HIV AIDS 2: 399–404.
8. Coetzer M, Nedellec R, Salkowitz J, McLaughlin S, Liu Y, et al. (2008) Evolution of CCR5 Use before and during coreceptor switching. J Virol 82: 11758–11766.
9. Connor RI, Sheridan KE, Cerdani D, Choe S, Landau NR (1997) Change in Coreceptor Use Correlates with Disease Progression in HIV-1–Infected Individuals. J Exp Med 185: 621–628.
10. Berger EA, Murphy PM, Farber JM (1999) Chemokine receptors as HIV-1 coreceptors: roles in viral entry, tropism, and disease. Annu Rev Immunol 17: 657–700.
11. Raymond S, Delobel P, Mavigner M, Cazabat M, Encinas S, et al. (2010) CXCR4-using viruses in plasma and peripheral blood mononuclear cells during primary HIV-1 infection and impact on disease progression. AIDS 24: 2305–2312.
12. Arenzana-Seisdedos F and Parmentier M (2006) Genetics of resistance to HIV infection: Role of co-receptors and co-receptor ligands. Semin Immunol 18: 387–403.
13. Liu R, Paxton WA, Choe S, Ceradini D, Martin SR, et al. (1996) Homozygous defect in HIV-1 coreceptor accounts for resistance of some multiply-exposed individuals to HIV-1 infection. Cell 86: 367–377.
14. Wu L, Paxton WA, Kassam N, Ruffing N, Rottman JB, et al. (1997) CCR5 levels and expression, pattern correlate with infectability by macrophage-tropic HIV-1, in vitro. J Exp Med 185: 1681–1691.
15. Ometto L, Zanchetta M, Cabrelle A, Esposito G, Mainardi M, et al. (1999) Restriction of HIV type 1 infection in macrophages heterozygous for a deletion

in the CC-chemokine receptor 5 gene. AIDS Res Hum Retroviruses 15: 1441–1452.
16. Martin MP, Dean M, Smith MW, Winkler C, Gerrard B, et al. (1998) Genetic acceleration of AIDS progression by a promoter variant for CCR5. Science 282: 1907–1911.
17. Ometto L, Bertorelle R, Mainardi M, Zanchetta M, Tognazzo S, et al. (2001) Polymorphisms in the CCR5 promoter region influence disease progression in perinatally Human Immunodeficiency Virus Type 1- infected children. J Infect Dis 183: 814–818.
18. Bleul CC, Farzan M, Choe H, Parolin C, Clark-Lewis I, et al. (1996) The lymphocyte chemoattractant SDF-1 is a ligand for LESTR/fusin and blocks HIV-1 entry. Nature 382: 829–833.
19. Oberlin E, Amara A, Bachelerie F, Bessia C, Virelizier JL, et al. (1996) The CXC chemokine SDF-1 is the ligand for LESTR/fusin and prevents infection by T-cell-line-adapted HIV-1. Nature 382: 833–835.
20. Shirozu M, Nakano T, Inazawa J, Tashiro K, Tada H, et al. (1995) Structure and chromosomal localization of the human stromal cell-derived factor 1 (SDF1) gene. Genomics 28: 495–500.
21. Ross J (1996) Control of messenger RNA stability in higher eukaryotes. Trends Genet 12: 171–175.
22. Garcia-Moruja C, Rueda P, Torres C, Alcamí J, Luque F, et al. (2009) Molecular phenotype of CXCL12beta 3′UTR G801A polymorphism (rs1801157) associated to HIV-1 disease progression. Curr HIV Res 7: 384–389.
23. Tiensiwakul P (2004) Stromal cell-derived factor (SDF)1-3′A polymorphism may play a role in resistance to HIV-1 infection in seronegative high-risk Thais. Intervirology 47: 87–92.
24. Winkler C, Modi W, Smith MW, Nelson GW, Wu X, et al. (1998) Genetic restriction of AIDS pathogenesis by an SDF-1 chemokine gene variant. Science 279: 389–392.
25. Mahajan SD, Agosto-Mojica A, Aalinkeel R, Reynolds JL, Nair BB, et al. (2010) Role of chemokine and cytokine polymorphisms in the progression of HIV-1 disease. Biochem Biophys Res Commun 396: 348–352.
26. Ioannidis JP, Rosenberg PS, Goedert JJ, Ashton LJ, Benfield TL, et al. (2001) Effects of CCR5-Delta32, CCR2-64I, and SDF-1 3′A alleles on HIV-1 disease progression: An international meta-analysis of individual-patient data. Ann Intern Med 135: 782–795.
27. Soriano A, Martinez C, Garcia F, Plana M, Palou E, et al. (2002) Plasma Stromal-Derived Factor (SDF)-1 levels, SDF1-3′A genotype, and expression of CXCR4 on T lymphocytes: their impact on resistance to Human Immunodeficiency Virus Type 1 infection and its progression. J Infect Dis 186: 922–931.
28. Mummidi S, Ahuja SS, Gonzalez E, Anderson SA, Santiago EN, et al. (1998) Genealogy of the CCR5 locus and chemokine system gene variants associated with altered rates of HIV-1 disease progression. Nat Med 4: 786–793.
29. Van Rij RP, Broersen S, Goudsmit J, Coutinho RA, Schuitemaker H (1998) The role of a stromal cell-derived factor-1 chemokine gene variant in the clinical course of HIV-1 infection. AIDS 12: F85–F92.
30. Brambilla A, Villa C, Rizzardi G, Veglia F, Ghezzi S, et al. (2000) Shorter survival of SDF-1 3′A/3′A Homozygotes linked to CD4+ T cell decrease in advanced Human Immunodeficiency Virus Type 1 infection. J Infect Dis 182: 311–315.
31. John GC, Rousseau C, Dong T, Rowland-Jones S, Nduati R, et al. (2000) Maternal SDF1 3′A polymorphism is associated with increased perinatal human immunodeficiency virus type 1 transmission. J Virol 74: 5736–5739.
32. Katz DA, John-Stewart GC, Richardson BA, Majiwa M, Mabuka JM (2010) CCR5, RANTES and SDF-1 polymorphisms and mother-to-child HIV-1 transmission. Int J Immunogenet 37: 301–305.
33. Tresoldi E, Romiti ML, Boniotto M, Crovella S, Salvatori F, et al. (2002) Prognostic value of the Stromal-Derived Factor 1 3′A mutation in pediatric Human Immunodeficency Virus Type 1 infection. J Infect Dis 185: 696–700.
34. Singh KK, Barroga CF, Hughes MD, Chen J, Raskino C, et al. (2003) Genetic influence of CCR5, CCR2, and SDF1 variants on human immunodeficiency virus 1 (HIV-1)-related disease progression and neurological impairment, in children with symptomatic HIV-1 infection. J Infect Dis 188: 1461–1472.
35. Sei S, Boler AM, Nguyen GT, Stewart SK, Yang QE, et al. (2001) Protective effect of CCR5 delta 32 heterozygosity is restricted by SDF-1 genotype in children with HIV-1 infection. AIDS 15: 1343–1352.
36. De Rossi A, Ades AE, Mammano F, Ometto L, Giaquinto C, et al. (1991) Antigen detection, virus culture, polymerase chain reaction, and in vitro antibody production in the diagnosis of vertically transmitted HIV-1 infection. AIDS 5: 15–20.
37. De Rossi A, Ometto L, Mammano F, Zanotto C, Giaquinto C, et al. (1992) Vertical transmission of HIV-1: lack of detectable virus in peripheral blood cells of infected children at birth. AIDS 6: 1117–1120.
38. Centers for Disease Control and Prevention. Revised Classification System for Human Immunodeficiency Virus Infection in Children Less Than 13 Years of Age. MMWR 1994; 43 (RR-12) : 1–10.
39. Auger I, Thomas P, De Gruttola V, Morse D, Moore D, et al. (1988) Incubation periods for paediatric AIDS patients. Nature 336: 575–577.
40. The European Collaborative Study (1994) Natural history of vertically acquired human immunodeficiency virus-1 infection. Pediatrics 94: 815–819.
41. Pizzo PA, Wilfert CM (1995) Markers and determinants of disease progression in children with HIV infection. The Pediatric AIDS Siena Workshop II. J Acquir Immune Defic Syndr Hum Retrovirol 8: 30–44.
42. Ricci E, Malacrida S, Zanchetta M, Montagna M, Giaquinto C, et al. (2009) Role of β-defensin-1 polymorphisms in mother-child transmission of HIV-1. J Acquir Immune Defic Syndr 51: 13–19.
43. Jensen MA, Li FS, van't Wout AB, Nickle DC, Shriner D, et al. (2003) Improved coreceptor usage prediction and genotypic monitoring of R5-to-X4 transition by motif analysis of Human Immunodeficiency Virus type 1 env V3 loop sequences. J Virol 77: 13376–13388.
44. Low AJ, Dong W, Chan D, Sing T, Swanstrom R, et al. (2007) Current V3 genotyping algorithms are inadequate for predicting X4 co-receptor usage in clinical isolates. AIDS 21: F17–F24.
45. Solè X, Guinó E, Valls J, Iniesta R, Moreno V (2006) SNPStats: a web tool for the analysis of association studies. Bioinformatics 22: 1928–1929.
46. Kleinbaum DG, Klein M (1996) Survival Analysis: A Self-Learning Text. New York: Springer.
47. Liu S, Zhu H (2011) Association between polymorphism of SDF1 (CXCL12) gene and HIV-1 susceptibility: a meta-analysis. Curr HIV Res 9: 112–119.
48. Newell ML, Dunn DT, Peckham CS, Ades AE, Pardi G, et al. (European Collaborative Study) (1994). Caesarean section and risk of vertical transmission of HIV-1 infection. Lancet 343: 1464–1467.
49. Salvatori F, Masiero S, Giaquinto C, Wade CM, Brown AJ, et al. (1997) Evolution of human immunodeficiency virus type 1 in perinatally infected infants with rapid and slow progression to disease. J Virol 71: 4694–4706.
50. Cavarelli M, Karlsson I, Ripamonti C, Plebani A, Fenyo EM, et al. (2010) Flexible use of CCR5 in the absence of CXCR4 use explains the immune deficiency in HIV-1 infected children. AIDS 24: 2527–2533.
51. Casper C, Navér L, Clevestig P, Belfrage E, Leitner T, et al. (2002) Coreceptor change appears after immune deficiency is established in children infected with different HIV-1 subtypes. AIDS Res Hum Retroviruses 18: 343–352.
52. Clevestig P, Maljkovic I, Casper C, Carlenor E, Lindgren S, et al. (2005) The X4 phenotype of HIV type 1 evolves from R5 in two children of mothers, carrying X4, and is not linked to transmission. AIDS Res Hum Retroviruses 21: 371–378.
53. Italian Register for HIV Infection in Children (1994) Features of children perinatally infected with HIV-1 surviving longer than 5 years. Lancet 343: 191–195.
54. De Rossi A, Masiero S, Giaquinto C, Ruga E, Comar M, et al. (1996) Dynamics of viral replication in infants with vertically acquired human immunodeficiency virus type 1 infection. J Clin Invest 97: 323–330.
55. Cavarelli M, Karlsson I, Zanchetta M, Antonsson L, Plebani A, et al. (2008) HIV-1 with multiple CCR5/CXCR4 chimeric receptor use is predictive of immunological failure in infected children. PLoS One 3: e3292.
56. Petersen DC, Glashoff RH, Shrestha S, Bergeron J, Laten A, et al. (2005) Risk for HIV-1 infection associated with a common CXCL12 (SDF1) polymorphism and CXCR4 variation in an African population. J Acquir Immune Defic Syndr 40: 521–526.
57. Daar ES, Lynn HS, Donfield SM, Lail A, O'Brien SJ, et al. (2005) Stromal cell-derived factor-1 genotype, coreceptor tropism, and HIV type 1 disease progression. J Infect Dis 192: 1597–1605.
58. Dean M, Carrington M, Winkler C, Huttley GA, Smith MW, et al. (1996) Genetic restriction of HIV-1 infection and progression to AIDS by a deletion allele of the CKR5 structural gene. Science 273: 1856–1862.
59. Dorr P, Westby M, Dobbs S, Griffin P, Irvine B, et al. (2005) Maraviroc (UK-427,857), a potent, orally bioavailable, and selective small-molecule inhibitor of chemokine receptor CCR5 with broad-spectrum anti-human immunodeficiency virus type 1 activity. Antimicrob Agents Chemother 49: 4721–4732.
60. Westby M, Smith-Burchnell C, Mori J, Lewis M, Mosley M, et al. (2007) Reduced maximal inhibition in phenotypic susceptibility assays indicates that viral strains resistant to the CCR5 antagonist maraviroc utilize inhibitor-bound receptor for entry. J Virol 81: 2359–2371.
61. Westby M, Lewis M, Whitcomb J, Youle M, Pozniak AL, et al. (2006) Emergence of CXCR4-using human immunodeficiency virus type 1 (HIV-1) variants in a minority of HIV-1-infected patients following treatment with the CCR5 antagonist maraviroc is from a pretreatment CXCR4-using virus reservoir. J Virol 80: 4909–4920.
62. Koning FA, Koevoets C, van der Vorst TJ, Schuitemaker H (2005) Sensitivity of primary R5 HTV-1 to inhibition by RANTES correlates with sensitivity to small-molecule R5 inhibitors. Antivir Ther 10: 231–237.
63. Repits J, Oberg M, Esbjornsson J, Medstrand P, Karlsson A, et al. (2005) Selection of human immunodeficiency virus type 1 R5 variants with augmented replicative capacity and reduced sensitivity to entry inhibitors during severe immunodeficiency. J Gen Virol 86: 2859–2869.
64. Poveda E and Soriano V (2010) Optimizing management of treatment-naïve and treatment-experienced HIV+ patients: the role of maraviroc. HIV AIDS 2: 51–58.
65. Ruiz-Mateos E, González-Serna A, Genebat M, Machmach K, Vidal F, et al. (2011) Virological response after short-term CCR5 antagonist exposure in HIV-infected patients: frequency of subjects with virological response and associated factors. Antimicrob Agents Chemother 55: 4664–4669.

23

Comparative Analysis of rs12979860 SNP of the IFNL3 Gene in Children with Hepatitis C and Ethnic Matched Controls using 1000 Genomes Project Data

Giuseppe Indolfi[1]*, Giusi Mangone[2], Elisa Bartolini[1], Gabriella Nebbia[3], Pier Luigi Calvo[4], Maria Moriondo[2], Pier-Angelo Tovo[4], Maurizio de Martino[5], Chiara Azzari[2,5], Massimo Resti[1]

1 Paediatric and Liver Unit, Meyer Children's University Hospital of Florence, Florence, Italy, **2** Immunology Unit and Laboratory, Meyer Children's University Hospital of Florence, Florence, Italy, **3** U.O. Pediatria 2, Fondazione IRCCS Ca' Granda Ospedale Maggiore Policlinico, Milano, Italy, **4** Department of Pediatrics, Infectious Diseases Unit, University of Turin, Italy Regina Margherita Children's Hospital, Turin, Italy, **5** Department of Health Sciences, University of Florence, Florence, Italy

Abstract

The rs12979860 single nucleotide polymorphism located on chromosome 19q13.13 near the interferon L3 gene (formerly and commonly known as interleukin 28B gene) has been associated in adults with both spontaneous and treatment induced clearance of hepatitis C virus. Although the exact mechanism of these associations remains unclear, it suggests that variation in genes involved in the immune response against the virus favours viral clearance. Limited and preliminary data are available on this issue in children. The aim of the present study was to evaluate, in a representative cohort of children with perinatal infection, the potential association between rs12979860 single nucleotide polymorphism and the outcome of hepatitis C virus infection. Alleles and genotypes frequencies were evaluated in 30 children who spontaneously cleared the virus and in 147 children with persistent infection and were compared with a population sample of ethnically matched controls with unknown hepatitis C status obtained using the 1000 Genomes Project data. The C allele and the C/C genotype showed greater frequencies in the clearance group (76.7% and 56.7%, respectively) when compared with both children with viral persistence (C allele 56.5%, $p=0.004$; C/C genotype 32.7%, $p=0.02$) and with the ethnically matched individuals (C allele 59.7%, $p=0.02$; C/C genotype 34.7%, $p=0.03$). Children with the C/C genotype were 2 times more likely to clear hepatitis C virus relative to children with the C/T and T/T genotypes combined (odds ratio: 2.7; 90% confidence intervals: 1.3–5.8). The present study provides the evidence that the rs12979860 single nucleotide polymorphism influences the natural history of hepatitis C virus in children.

Editor: David R. Booth, University of Sydney, Australia

Funding: The authors have no support or funding to report.

Competing Interests: The authors have declared that no competing interests exist.

* E-mail: g.indolfi@meyer.it

Introduction

The rs12979860 single nucleotide polymorphism (SNP) on chromosome 19q13.13 near the *IFNL3* gene (formerly and commonly known as *IL28B*) has been associated in adults with both spontaneous and treatment induced clearance of hepatitis C virus (HCV) [1,2]. Three interferon (IFN)-λ genes, *IFNL1*, *IFNL2* (formerly *IL29* and *IL28A*, respectively) and *IFNL3* reside downstream of the rs12979860 SNP [3]. IFN-λ genes encode the type III IFNs. Type III IFNs (IFN-λs) like type I IFNs (IFN-α and IFN-β) induce antiviral activity and suppress HCV replication *in vitro* and *in vivo* through activation of the JAK-STAT pathway which leads to induction of several IFN stimulated genes which are responsible for antiviral activity [3]. Although the exact molecular phenotype of the genetic association between rs12979860 SNP of the *IFNL3* gene and clearance of HCV remains unclear, it is evident that variation in genes involved in the immune response against the virus favours viral clearance [3].

There is evidence that the frequency of the C allele of the rs12979860 SNP varies markedly across ethnic groups [1]. The C allele is less frequent among individuals of African ancestry relative to those of European ancestry and East Asians [1]. It is well known that that the probability of being cured by the combined treatment with pegylated IFN-α and ribavirin increases accordingly [4–6]. It has been estimated that approximately half of the difference in sustained virological response rates to combined treatment with pegylated IFN-α and ribavirin among these different ethnic groups can be accounted for by the difference in the frequency of the C allele [2].

Most of the studies published on the association between rs12979860 SNP of the *IFNL3* gene and spontaneous clearance of HCV have been performed in adults. Only two studies on small cohorts of children are available so far on the topic [7,8]. The natural history of hepatitis C in children is different when compared to adults [9,10]. Liver disease severity tends to be milder in children than in adults. This is thought to be the consequence of the different interplay between the virus and the immune system of the child and it is particularly true when the infection is acquired perinatally from the mother in the context of the high level of immune tolerance of the developing immune system of the newborn [11].

To confirm the potential effect of rs12979860 SNP of the *IFNL3* gene on the outcome of HCV infection in terms of spontaneous clearance and chronic infection in children, this variant was genotyped in an HCV cohort comprised of mono-ethnic children who spontaneously cleared the virus or had persistent infection. Allele and genotype frequencies in this cohort were compared with a population sample of ethnically matched controls with unknown hepatitis C status obtained using the 1000 Genomes Project data [12].

Materials and Methods

Study design

This is a cross-sectional study. All the children, born to an HCV-infected mother and older than 30 months evaluated between January 2011 to December 2012 during routine follow-up visits for perinatal HCV infection were recruited. Only children whose parents or guardians provided written informed consent were enrolled and genotyped for the SNP rs 12979860. Retrospective data to define the source and the outcome of the infection were collected at the time of the enrolment. All the children enrolled were negative for hepatitis B surface antigen and for antibodies against human immunodeficiency virus. The ethnic origin of the children enrolled was self-reported by the parents or guardians. The study received the approval of the ethical committee of the Meyer Children's University Hospital of Florence.

Definitions

Mother-to-child transmission of HCV was defined as transmission occurring during pregnancy or in the perinatal period from the HCV-infected mother to the foetus or to the child [13]. Maternal infection was confirmed basing on HCV antibodies testing in the last trimester before pregnancy or during pregnancy. Children were considered perinatally infected if HCV ribonucleic acid was detected in at least two serum samples at least three months apart during the first year of life, and/or when testing of antibodies against HCV was positive after 18 months of age [14]. Spontaneous clearance of HCV in children with perinatal infection is a well known phenomenon described in about 20% of the children with perinatal infection and occurring in the first 30 months of life [15]. Spontaneous clearance was therefore defined in children older than 30 months of age when polymerase chain reaction for HCV ribonucleic acid was negative and HCV antibodies were positive in at least three blood samples taken 6 months apart [9,15,16]. In the same age group positive polymerase chain reactions for HCV ribonucleic acid and HCV antibodies defined chronic hepatitis C [9,15]. Only children older than 30 months of age were recruited. Children with spontaneous clearance of HCV were routinely followed up to 18 years of age as part of the local research protocol.

Patients

One hundred and eighty six consecutive children were recruited. Nine of them (4.8%) were not enrolled as the parents did not provide the informed consent. Of the 177 children enrolled (95.2%), 30 consecutive children (16.9%) spontaneously cleared the virus and 133 (83.1%) were chronically infected.

Comparison with individuals studied in the 1000 Genomes Project

Allele and genotype frequencies for the rs12979860 SNP were examined for concordance with the individuals studied in the 1000 Genomes Project (http://www.1000genomes.org), October 2010 release [12].

Laboratory methods

Polymerase chain reaction for HCV was performed as previously described [15]. HCV antibodies were investigated by a third generation enzyme-linked immunosorbent assay (ELISA) (Ortho Diagnostic System Inc., Raritan, NJ) and confirmed by Western blot analysis (Innogenetics, Zwijndrecht, Belgium). *IFNL3* rs12979860 SNP genotyping was performed using Allelic Discrimination assays from Applied Biosystems following the instructions of the manufacturer. Genotyping was performed using Taqman custom-designed primers and probes as follows: forward primer GCCTGTCGTGTACTGAACCA, reverse primer GCGCGGAGTGCAATTCAAC, and probes TGGTTCGCGCCTTC (VIC) and CTGGTTCACGCCTTC (FAM) (Applied Biosystems). Before performing the PCR reactions DNA is added with Allelic Discrimination Assay Mix and TaqMan Universal PCR Master Mix to MicroAmp Optical 96-Well Reaction Plates (Applied Biosystems). Real-Time PCR reactions were performed using the 7500 Fast Real-Time PCR System. After preheating for 10 min. at 92°C, 40 cycles of 15 seconds at 95°C and one minute at 60°C followed. Data were analyzed using the ABI SDS software (Applied Biosystems).

Statistical analysis

Data were processed with the SPSSX statistical package (SPSS, Inc., Chicago, IL). Two tailed P values were used and a p value < 0.05 was defined as significant. Differences in frequencies were evaluated by chi^2 test or Fisher's exact probabilities. Odds ratio (OR) and 90% confidence intervals (CI) were calculated. Age was presented as median and interquartile range (IQR). Hardy-Weinberg Equilibrium (HWE) was tested. A deviation from HWE was defined with a criterion of p value <0.05.

Results

HCV infected children

Thirty children (16.9%) spontaneously cleared the virus and 133 (83.1%) were chronically infected. The characteristics of the children enrolled are summarized in table 1.

Data extracted from the 1000 Genomes Project database

Alleles and genotypes frequencies for the rs12979860 SNP were available in the 1000 Genomes Project database for 1,092 individuals. Rs12979860 alleles and genotypes frequencies according to the ethnic origin are summarized in table 2. The frequencies of the C and T alleles in each population sampled is described in figure 1. The highest frequencies of the C allele and of the C/C genotype were found in East Asians (92.5% and 85%, respectively). Among the 379 individuals of European ancestry, 98 (25.9%) were Italians. Italy was the nation where the present study was carried out. The frequency of the C allele and of the C/C genotype were significantly lower in the Italians when compared with the remaining Europeans (for the C allele: 59.7% and 71.2%, respectively, p = 0.003; for the C/C genotype: 34.7% and 51.2%, respectively, p = 0.005).

Comparison of the allele frequencies

In the HCV cohort, the frequency of the C allele was 76.7% among children who spontaneously cleared the virus *versus* 56.5% among children with chronic infection (p = 0.004; OR: 2.5; 90%CI: 1.4–4.6). The frequency of the C allele among children in the HCV cohort who spontaneously cleared the infection was

Table 1. Characteristics of the children enrolled in the hepatitis C virus cohort.

	Spontaneous clearance	Chronic infection
	30 (16.9%)	147 (83.1%)
Male/female	17/13	79/68
Age years, median (IQR)	12.7 (6.8)	11 (6.9)
Genotype		
1	9	89
2	0	17
3	5	25
4	0	15
multiple genotypes	2	1
not determined	14	0
C allele	46 (76.7%)*	166 (56.5%)*
T allele	14 (23.3%)	128 (43.5%)
C/C genotype	17 (56.7%)**	48 (32.7%)
C/T genotype	12 (40%)	70 (47.6%)
T/T genotype	1 (3.3%)***	29 (19.7%)

Note: IQR, interquartile range; * p = 0.004; OR 2.5; 90%CI 1.4–4.6; ** C/C genotype versus C/T and T/T combined p = 0.02; OR = 2.7; 90%CI 1.3–5.8; *** C/C genotype versus T/T p = 0.01; OR = 10.3; 90%CI 1.3–217.8

greater than that observed in the individuals of European ancestry but the difference did not reach the threshold of significance (75% *versus* 68.2%, p = 0.2). A significant difference was observed when the frequencies of C alleles of the children with spontaneous clearance and of Italians enrolled in the 1000 Genomes Project database were compared (76.7% *versus* 59.7%, p = 0.02; OR: 2.2; 90%CI: 1.2–4.1). The T-allele frequency was significantly greater in the chronically infected cohort compared with the European controls (43.5% *versus* 31.8%, p = 0.003).

Comparison of genotype frequencies

Genotypes were in Hardy-Weinberg equilibrium in the cohort of children with HCV infection (p = 0.63), in individuals of European ancestry and Italians selected from the 1000 Genomes Project database (table 2). Children with the C/C genotype were 2 times more likely to clear HCV relative to children with the C/T and T/T genotype combined (OR: 2.7; 90%CI: 1.3–5.8, p = 0.02). No difference was observed for clearance of HCV between the C/T and T/T genotypes and between the C/C and the C/T. Clearance was more common in children with the C/C genotype than in those with T/T (OR: 10.3; 90%CI: 1.3–217.8, p = 0.01). The C/C genotype was found in 56.7% of the children with spontaneous clearance of HCV and 47% in individuals of European ancestry (p = 0.7). The C/C genotype was more common in children with spontaneous clearance of HCV than in the Italians present in the 1000 Genomes Project database (56.7% versus 34.7%, p = 0.03; OR 2.5; 90%CI 1.1–5.4).

Table 2. Rs12979860 alleles and genotypes frequencies in the 1,092 individuals enrolled in the 1000 Genomes Project database.

Population	Alleles n (%)		Genotypes n (%)			HWE	
	C	T	C/C	C/T	T/T		n
EUROPEANS	**517 (68.2)**	**241 (31.8)**	**178 (47)**	**161 (42.5)**	**40 (10.5)**	**0.68**	**379**
Iberians (Spain)	22 (78.6)	6 (21.4)	9 (64.3)	4 (28.6)	1 (7.1)	0.57	14
Utah residents (U.S.A) with Northern and Western European ancestry	127 (74.7)	43 (25.3)	49 (57.6)	29 (34.2)	7 (8.2)	0.37	85
Finnish	133 (71.5)	53 (28.5)	47 (50.5)	39 (42)	7 (7.5)	0.77	93
British	118 (66.3)	60 (33.7)	39 (43.8)	40 (45)	10 (11.2)	0.95	89
Tuscans (Italy)	117 (59.7)*	79 (40.3)	34 (34.7)**	49 (50)	15 (15.3)	0.69	98
Europeans (without Tuscans)	400 (71.2)*	162 (28.8)	144 (51.2)**	112 (39.9)	25 (8.9%)	0.63	281
EAST ASIANS	**529 (92.5)**	**43 (7.5)**	**243 (85)**	**43 (15)**	**-**	**0.41**	**286**
Japanese (Tokyo)	159 (89.3)	19 (10.7)	70 (78.7)	19 (21.3)	-	0.26	89
Chinese (Beijing)	179 (92.3)	15 (7.7)	82 (84.5)	15 (15.5)	-	0.41	97
Chinese	191 (95.5)	9 (4.5)	91 (91)	9 (9)	-	0.63	100
AFRICANS	**195 (39.6)**	**297 (60.4)**	**38 (15.4)**	**119 (48.4)**	**89 (36.2)**	**0.86**	**246**
Kenyans	95 (49)	99 (51)	19 (19.6)	57 (58.8)	21 (21.6)	0.08	97
Nigerians	59 (33.5)	117 (66.5)	11 (12.5)	37 (42)	40 (45.5)	0.59	88
Afro-Americans	41 (33.6)	81 (66.4)	8 (13.1)	25 (41)	28 (45.9)	0.52	61
MIXED AMERICANS	**202 (55.8)**	**160 (44.2)**	**55 (30.4)**	**92 (50.8)**	**34 (18.8)**	**0.68**	**181**
Mexicans	69 (52.3)	63 (47.7)	17 (25.8)	35 (53)	14 (21.2)	0.61	66
Puertoricans	71 (64.5)	39 (35.5)	22 (40)	27 (49.1)	6 (10.9)	0.59	55
Colombians	62 (51.7)	58 (48.3)	16 (26.7)	30 (50)	14 (23.3)	0.99	60

Note: HWE, Hardy-Weinberg Equilibrium. * p = 0.003. ** p = 0.005.

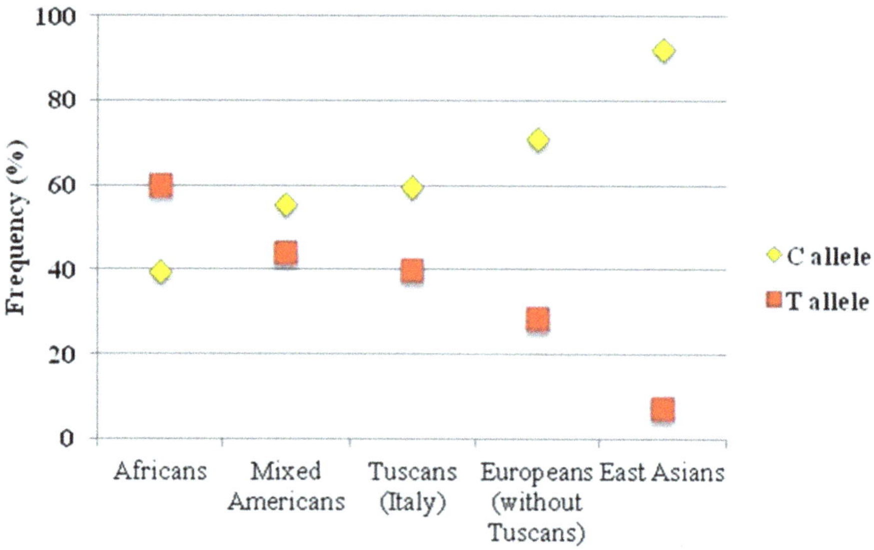

Figure 1. Frequency of rs12979860 C and T alleles in the diverse ethnic groups present in the 1000 Genomes Project database.

Discussion

The present study shows that the C allele and the C/C genotype of the rs12979860 SNP of the *IFNL3* gene are associated with spontaneous resolution of HCV infection in Italian children. The results of this study were obtained comparing the frequencies of the C and T allele and of the different genotypes of the rs12979860 SNP of the *IFNL3* gene between a cohort of children who spontaneously cleared or where chronically infected by HCV with ethnically matched controls. The rationale for this study was that, if the polymorphism influences natural clearance also in children, we would have obtained a frequency difference in these comparisons, since the children who naturally clear the virus will be excluded from the chronic infection cohort, thereby reducing the frequency of the allele that increases the likelihood of spontaneous clearance. The present results confirm the association demonstrated in adults [1]. Two preliminary paediatric studies were already published on the same topic [7,8] that enrolled a limited number of patients (n = 15 and n = 26, respectively) and used the classical approach of comparing the frequencies of the C/C genotypes in children with clearance and chronic infection. In the present study a significantly higher number of children was enrolled and the value of the results was enforced and validated by the comparisons of alleles and genotypes frequencies among children with chronic infection, spontaneous clearance and, differently by previous studies, with a cohort of ethnically matched controls.

One of the risks of the interpretation of genome wide association studies is to find spurious associations [17]. For this reason, the data extracted by the 1000 Genomes Project in this study were analyzed for consistency with the previous data published on the topic [1]. A higher frequency of the C allele was confirmed in East-Asians, followed by the Europeans and Africans-Americans [1]. The patterns of genetic variation across different populations are shaped by history, environment, and stochastic processes. It is noteworthy that, among the Europeans, a group of individuals from Italy (the country were the study was carried out) had significantly lower frequencies of the C allele and of the C/C genotype than the other Europeans. The European individuals therefore were not considered representative of the cohort of HCV infected children and Italians were selected as reference. The rationale for this choice was the observation that different studies have shown that, despite low average levels of genetic differentiation among Europeans, there is a close correspondence between genetic and geographic distances [17,18]. Two major axes of genetic variation have been observed within Europe, namely from North to South and from East to West and two representative populations have been identified, the CEU (Northwestern Europe) and the TSI populations (Tuscan Italians from Southern Europe). The pattern of variation of the rs12979860 SNP of the *IFNL3* gene observed among different European populations studied in the 1000 Genome Project is in line with the gradient of genetic variation described among Europeans following the North-Northwest/South-Southeast geographic axis [17]. When interpreting genome wide association studies the optimal solution is to select the geographically closer population as reference [17,18]. Spurious associations can arise if genetic structure is not properly accounted for and the results of the present article are the proof of it.

The present study contributes to the understanding of the mechanisms of clearance of HCV infection in children with perinatal infection. Spontaneous clearance of HCV in children perinatally infected has been associated so far with a transaminase flare in the first year of life and with HCV genotype 3 infection [15,19]. *IFNL3* is a human gene of the host system of innate antiviral defense. The outcome of HCV infection is dependent on the balance between innate immunity of the host and the multiple mechanisms to regulate and evade innate immunity evolved by HCV. Although early studies failed to find altered mRNA expression of *IFNL3* associated with different *IFNL3* genotypes, since the specificity of real-time PCR primers for *IFNL3* has increased (to differentiate between IFN-λ3 and the closely related IFN-λ2), it is now clear that SNPs of the *IFNL3* gene affect the expression of IFN-λ3 with the unfavourable allele resulting in less IFN-λ3 expression [20]. Furthermore, recently, a study showed that adults with the unfavourable *IFNL3* genotype have depressed innate immune function, particularly with respect to NK cells, suggesting that the decreased expression of *IFNL3* affects innate immunity and therefore clearance of HCV [21]. Quantitative and qualitative differences exist between adult and neonatal innate immune cells. Neonatal innate immune cells, for example, as compared with those of adults, have been described to produce lower levels of IFNs [22]. The activity of NK cells also differs between neonates and adults with many differences demonstrated in the pattern of cell-surface activating and inhibitory receptors [22]. Newborn and infant's immune responses are oriented towards immunological tolerance and neonatal innate immune defences are skewed towards protection against extracellular bacterial pathogens rather than intracellular bacterial pathogens and viruses [11]. Despite innate immunity in neonates and infants can be condidered physiologically depressed, it was of interest to evaluate if it still plays a role, in children as in adults, in spontaneous elimination of the virus. The results of the present study, confirming that the rs12979860 SNPs influences the natural history of hepatitis C virus in children, support that hypothesis.

SNPs of the *IFNL3* gene have been associated in adults with both spontaneous clearance of HCV infection and response to treatment with combined dual therapy with pegylated IFN and ribavirin. These results suggest that IFN-λ3 has a key role in determining both treatment-induced and spontaneous clearance of HCV. The association between rs12979860 SNP of the *IFNL3* gene and spontaneous clearance in children and the homology of this result with those obtained in adults, supports the hypothesis that *IFNL3* gene polymorphisms should be evaluated extensively as pretreatment predictor of virological response also in children.

In conclusion, the present result demonstrates that the frequencies of the C allele and the C/C genotype of the rs12979860 SNP of the *IFNL3* gene are higher in a cohort of children who spontaneously cleared HCV infection when compared to children with chronic hepatitis C and ethnically matched controls. The rs12979860 SNP of the *IFNL3* gene influences spontaneous resolution of HCV infection in Italian children.

Acknowledgments

We are grateful to the parents and to all the children enrolled in the present study. We are thankful to Dr Davide Mei for his precious scientific advice and technical assistance. This study has been carried out in the context of the "Progetto Giovani Ricercatori" of the Meyer Children's University Hospital.

Author Contributions

Conceived and designed the experiments: GI PLC GB PAT MdM CA MR. Performed the experiments: GM MM EB CA. Analyzed the data: GI GN PLC PAT EB CA MdM MR. Contributed reagents/materials/analysis tools: GM MM EB CA. Wrote the paper: GI MdM CA MR.

References

1. Thomas DL, Thio CL, Martin MP, Qi Y, Ge D, et al. (2009) Genetic variation in IL28B and spontaneous clearance of hepatitis C virus. Nature 461: 798–801.
2. Ge D, Fellay J, Thompson AJ, Simon JS, Shianna KV, et al. (2009). Genetic variation in IL28B predicts hepatitis C treatment-induced viral clearance. Nature 461: 399–401.
3. Urban T, Charlton MR, Goldstein DB (2012) Introduction to the genetics and biology of interleukin-28B. Hepatology 56: 361–366.
4. Yan KK, Guirgis M, Dinh T, George J, Dev A, et al. (2008) Treatment responses in Asians and Caucasians with chronic hepatitis C infection. World J Gastroenterol 14: 3416–3420.
5. Muir AJ, Bornstein JD, Killenberg PG; Atlantic Coast Hepatitis Treatment Group (2004) Peginterferon alfa-2b and ribavirin for the treatment of chronic hepatitis C in blacks and non-Hispanic whites. N Engl J Med 350: 2265–2271.
6. Liu CH, Liu CJ, Lin CL, Liang CC, Hsu SJ, et al. (2008) Pegylated interferon-alpha-2a plus ribavirin for treatment-naive Asian patients with hepatitis C virus genotype 1 infection: a multicenter, randomized controlled trial. Clin Infect Dis 47: 1260–1269.
7. Ruiz-Extremera A, Muñoz-Gámez JA, Salmerón-Ruiz MA, de Rueda PM, Quiles-Pérez R, et al. (2011) Genetic variation in interleukin 28B with respect to vertical transmission of hepatitis C virus and spontaneous clearance in HCV-infected children. Hepatology 53: 1830–1838.
8. Indolfi G, Sambrotta M, Moriondo M, Azzari C, Resti M (2011) Genetic variation in interleukin-28B locus is associated with spontaneous clearance of HCV in children with non-1 viral genotype infection. Hepatology 54: 1490–1491.
9. Bortolotti F, Verucchi G, Cammà C, Cabibbo G, Zancan L, et al. (2008) Long-term course of chronic hepatitis C in children: from viral clearance to end-stage liver disease. Gastroenterology 134: 1900–1907.
10. Afdhal NH (2004) The natural history of hepatitis C. Semin Liver Dis 24: 3–8.
11. Prendergast AJ, Klenerman P, Goulder PJ (2012) The impact of differential antiviral immunity in children and adults. Nat Rev Immunol 12: 636–648.
12. Genomes Project Consortium, Abecasis GR, Altshuler D, Auton A, Brooks LD, Durbin RM, et al. (2010) A map of human genome variation from population-scale sequencing. Nature 467: 1061–1073.
13. Indolfi G, Azzari C, Resti M (2013) Perinatal Transmission of Hepatitis C Virus. J Pediatr 163: 1549–1552.
14. Indolfi G, Resti M (2009) Perinatal transmission of hepatitis C virus infection. J Med Virol 81: 836–843.
15. Resti M, Jara P, Hierro L, Azzari C, Giacchino R, et al. (2003) Clinical features and progression of perinatally acquired hepatitis C virus infection. J Med Virol 70:373–377.
16. Indolfi G, Azzari C, Moriondo M, Lippi F, de Martino M, et al. (2006) Alanine transaminase levels in the year before pregnancy predict the risk of hepatitis C virus vertical transmission. J Med Virol 78: 911–914.
17. Novembre J, Johnson T, Bryc K, Kutalik Z, Boyko AR, et al. (2008) Genes mirror geography within Europe. Nature 456: 98–101.
18. Stathias V, Sotiris GR, Karagiannidis I, Bourikas G, Martinis G, et al. (2012) Exploring genomic structure differences and similarities between the Greek and European HapMap populations: implications for association studies. Ann Hum Genet 76: 472–483.
19. European Paediatric Hepatitis C Virus Network. (2005) Three broad modalities in the natural history of vertically acquired hepatitis C virus infection. Clin Infect Dis 41: 45–51.
20. Langhans B, Kupfer B, Braunschweiger I, Arndt S, Schulte W, et al. (2011) Interferon-lambda serum levels in hepatitis C. J Hepatol 54: 859–865.
21. Naggie S, Osinusi A, Katsounas A, Lempicki R, Herrmann E, et al. (2012) Dysregulation of innate immunity in hepatitis C virus genotype 1 IL28B-unfavorable genotype patients: impaired viral kinetics and therapeutic response. Hepatology 56: 444–454.
22. Kollmann TR, Crabtree J, Rein-Weston A, Blimkie D, Thommai F, et al. (2009) Neonatal innate TLR-mediated responses are distinct from those of adults. J Immunol 183: 7150–7160.

Serotypes and Patterns of Antibiotic Resistance in Strains Causing Invasive Pneumococcal Disease in Children Less than 5 Years of Age

Chunfeng Liu[1]*, Xiaoyu Xiong[1], Wei Xu[1], Jimei Sun[2], Lijie Wang[1], Jiujun Li[1]

1 Department of Pediatrics, Shengjing hospital of China Medical University, Shenyang, Liaoning, China, 2 Department of Bacteriology, Shengjing hospital of China Medical University, Shenyang, Liaoning, China

Abstract

Objective: The serotypes and patterns of antibiotic resistance of *Streptococcus pneumoniae (S. pneumoniae)* strains that cause invasive pneumococcal disease (IPD) in infants were analyzed to provide guidance for clinical disease prevention and treatment.

Methods: The clinical features of confirmed IPD were evaluated in 61 patients, less than 5 years of age, who were admitted to our hospital between January 2009 and December 2011. The serotypes and antibiotic resistance of strains of *S.pneumoniae* were determined using the capsular swelling method and the E-test.

Results: A total of 61 invasive strains were isolated. The serotype distribution of those isolates were 19A (41.0%), 14 (19.7%), 19F (11.5%), 23F (9.8%), 8 (4.9%), 9V (4.9%), 1 (3.3%), and 4, 6B, and 20 (each 1.6%). The percentage of *S. pneumoniae* strains resistant to erythromycin, clindamycin, and cotrimoxazole were 100%, 86.9%, and 100%, respectively. The percentage of *S. pneumoniae* strains resistant to penicillin, amoxicillin/clavulanic acid, cefuroxime, ceftriaxone, cefotaxime, cefepime, and meropenem were 42.6%, 18.0%, 82.0%, 18.0%, 13.1%, 13.1%, and 36.1%, respectively. The percentage of multidrug-resistant strains was 95.6%. Strains of all serotypes isolated in this study were highly resistant to erythromycin, cotrimoxazole, and clindamycin. Strains with serotype 19A had the highest rates of resistance.

Conclusions: Serotype 19A strains were most frequently isolated from children with IPD treated in our hospital. The strains causing IPD are highly resistant to antibiotics.

Editor: Willem van Schaik, University Medical Center Utrecht, The Netherlands

Funding: This is a sponsored study funded by Pfizer China. The authors declare that they have no financial interests that may influnce interpretation of the results and the others. The funders had no role in study design, data collection and analysis, decision to publish, or prepareation of the manuscript.

Competing Interests: This study has received funding from Pfizer China. The authors declare that they have no financial interests that may influence interpretation of the results and the others. This does not alter the authors' adherence to all the PLOS ONE policies on sharing data and materials.

* E-mail: zhliu258@hotmail.com

Introduction

Streptococcus pneumoniae (S. pneumoniae) is the predominant pathogen involved in bacterial infections and remains the leading cause of community-acquired respiratory infections in children. Pneumococcal disease is the leading cause of death worldwide among children less than 5 years of age [1–3] and endangers the health of Chinese children [4–7]. *S. pneumoniae* can result in bacteremia, meningitis, pericarditis, arthritis, and empyema; collectively these are referred to as invasive pneumococcal disease (IPD) [8] which can lead to severe illness, prolonged hospital stays, and death.

Currently, up to 13 serotypes are targeted in the available pneumococcal conjugate vaccines (PCVs). However, the formulations of these vaccines were initially designed to protect children against serotypes most commonly causing invasive disease in North America and may not reflect the serotype distribution across the world. Analysis of data from 6 ASEAN countries (defined as countries belonging to the Association of South East Asian Nations, ASEAN) showed that the most common disease causing serotypes of *S. pneumoniae* (in order of frequency) were 19F, 23F, 14, 6B, 1, 19A, and 3 [9]· Several studies showed the distribution of these serotypes to be diverse in various cities in China during different years [10,11]. In one study, conducted from 2006 to 2008 in 11 hospitals in China [12], 171 isolates of IPD-associated *S. pneumoniae*, taken from children under the age of 14 years, were analyzed for serotyping and antibiotic resistance. It is worthwhile to note that analysis of local serotype distribution showed that the non-7-valent pneumococcal conjugate vaccine (PCV-7) serotype 19A was very common (14.3%–50% of isolates) in some northern cities. On the other hand, serotype 19A was rarely found (0%–10.7% of isolates) in southern and eastern cities; a result similar to those found in Southeast Asian countries [9]. PCV-7 covered more strains found in southern and eastern cities (70.4% of isolates) than in northern cities (36.7% of isolates). The reasons for the difference in isolate serotype among the different regions are not very clear. In September 2008, PCV-7 became available in the private sector in China, however the vaccine was not widely used either in the south or in the north, so vaccination with PCV-7 in those areas cannot explain the serotype difference. In addition, antibiotic resistance rates, although variable, have been shown to be increasing over time in China [7,8,10–12]. This has resulted in tremendous difficulties in the treatment of *S. pneumoniae* infections.

Thus, it is important to determine the local serotypes and antibiotic resistance patterns of *S. pneumoniae* isolates, from children with IPD, in order to provide evidence and guidance for the use of vaccines and antibiotics. The current study examines the serotypes and patterns of antibiotic resistance in *S. pneumoniae* isolated from patients less than 5 years of age, who were hospitalized for IPD at Shengjing Hospital of China Medical University in Shenyang, a city in North China.

Methods

2.1 Patients

A total of 61 patients under 5 years of age, who were diagnosed with confirmed IPD between January 1, 2009 and December 31, 2011 in the Pediatrics Department, were studied. The diagnosis of IPD was based on cultures positive for *S. pneumoniae* that were taken from a normally sterile body site [13], such as blood, cerebrospinal fluid (CSF), or the pleural space. Forty-one strains were cultured from blood (60.3%), 20 from pleural effusion (29.4%), and 7 from the CSF (10.3%). The definition of pneumococcal meningitis was isolation of *S. pneumoniae* from the CSF or a clinical diagnosis of meningitis with pneumococcus isolated from another normally sterile site, such as blood. Among patients meeting these criteria, 7 had two isolates from different sites (7 isolates from blood, 4 isolates from pleural effusion, and 3 from CSF). In these 7 patients, only one isolate was included if both isolates expressed the same serotype.

This study was approved by the Medicine Ethics Committee of Shengjing Hospital affiliated with China Medical University (2011PS76K). Since this was a retrospective study, it was exempt from informed consent of the patients, parents, or guardians involved. Only *S. pneumoniae* strains preserved in the laboratory were used and no samples were taken directly from patients for this study; clinical data were collected in a manner that maintained patient privacy.

2.2 Isolation of bacterial strains

Blood samples were taken from children with IPD within 24 hours of admission. Cerebrospinal and pleural fluid samples were also taken from those children with clinical symptoms of sepsis, and/or meningitis or pleural effusion. *S. pneumoniae* isolates were analyzed and identified using standardized laboratory procedures, including colony morphology on blood agar, the optochin test, and the sodium deoxycholate solubility test. All of the isolates were confirmed as *S. pneumoniae* by testing for alpha hemolysis on blood agar, optochin susceptibility, and bile solubility (bioMérieux API system; France) and the Vitek 2 Compact system (bioMérieux) [14].

2.3 Serotyping of isolates

All isolates were serotyped by a capsule-quelling test using type-specific antisera (Statens Serum Institute, Copenhagen, Denmark). Typing was carried out by phase-contrast microscopy according to the published procedure [15].

2.4 Antimicrobial susceptibility testing

In vitro susceptibility tests were performed using Etest strips provided by the AB Biodisk Company (Solna, Sweden), and the minimum inhibitory concentrations (MICs) of 13 antimicrobial agents (penicillin, amoxicillin/clavulanic acid, cefotaxime, cefepime, ceftriaxone, cefuroxime, erythromycin, clindamycin, levofloxacin, cotrimoxazole, vancomycin, linezolid, and meropenem) were determined. Tests were performed following the recommended protocols of the United States Clinical and Laboratory Standard Institute (CLSI), and the 2008 amendments to the antibiotic susceptibility breakpoints for *S.pneumoniae* were adopted as criteria for determining drug resistance. The susceptibility medium was made using bioMérieux Mueller-Hinton agar. Multidrug-resistant *S. pneumoniae* isolates were defined as isolates that were resistant to 3 or more classes of antimicrobial agents.

2.5 Quality Control

The following strains were used for quality control: ATCC 49619 *S. pneumoniae*, ATCC 25923 *Staphylococcus aureus*, and *S. pneumoniae* standard strain 31001 serotype I (China Pharmaceutical and Biological Products).

2.6 Statistical Analysis

The data on antibiotic susceptibility and serotypes of the isolates were analyzed using SPSS version 17.0 (SPSS Inc., Chicago, IL) statistical software. The percentage of multidrug-resistant strains was calculated as the number of multidrug-resistant strains divided by total numbers of strains.

Results

3.1 Clinical data

The 61 patients with IPD included 37 boys and 24 girls. The age of the patients ranged from 3 months to less than 5 years. Patients less than 2 years of age accounted for 37 cases (60.7%). Thirty-seven patients received antibiotics before admission, including macrolides (erythromycin and azithromycin) and β-lactam antibiotics (penicillin, amoxicillin/clavulanic acid, cefuroxime, ceftriaxone, cefotaxime, cefoperazone, ticarcillin, cefpimizole, aztreonam, and cefepime). Of the 37 patients, 21 received β-lactam antibiotics alone, 8 received macrolides alone, and 8 received a combination of antibiotics (β-lactam and macrolides). Thirteen had been given antibiotics for less than 3 days (1–3 days) and 20 for more than 3 days (median 7 days, range 4–20 days). The mean hospital stay was 21 days, and the maximum stay was 113 days. There were 50 cases of pneumonia, which included 28 cases complicated by empyema. There were 11 cases of pneumococcal meningitis; 7 CSF samples and 4 blood samples were culture positive for *S. pneumoniae.* Five patients, all under 2 years of age, died. Four patients died from septic shock and one patient died from brain dysfunction. Twelve patients received mechanical ventilation for periods ranging from 1 to 39 days.

3.2 Serotyping

A total of 68 strains were isolated from 61 patients with IPD. Among those strains, 7 strains that were obtained from the same patients had the same serotype; therefore, 61 strains were serotyped. Ten serotypes were identified, including 19A (25, 41.0%), 14 (12, 19.7%), 19F (7, 11.5%), 23F (6, 9.8%), 8 (3, 4.9%), 9V (3, 4.9%), 1 (2, 3.3%), and 4, 6B and 20 (1 each, 1.6%). The 7-valent PCV covers 45.9% of the serotypes, the 10-valent PCV (PCV-10) covers 52.5% of the serotypes, and the 13-valent PCV (PCV-13) covers 91.8% of the serotypes. A total of 37 strains were isolated from patients less than 2 years of age, including 15 of 19A (18/37), 6 of 14 (6/37), 6 of 23F (6/37), 4 of 19F (4/37), 2 each of 9V and 8 (2/37), and 1 each of 4 and 6B (1/37). PCV-7 and PCV-10 cover 54.1% of these strains and PCV-13 covers 85.4% of these strains.

3.3 Antimicrobial susceptibility

The susceptibility results are shown in Table 1. The percentage of *S. pneumoniae* strains resistant to erythromycin, clindamycin, and cotrimoxazole were 100%, 86.9%, and 100%, respectively. The percentage of *S. pneumoniae* strains resistant to penicillin, amoxicillin/clavulanic acid, cefuroxime, ceftriaxone, cefotaxime, cefepime, and meropenem were 42.6%, 18.0%, 82.0%, 18.0%, 13.1%, 13.1%, and 36.1%, respectively. None of the strains were resistant to vancomycin, linezolid, or levofloxacin. The percentage of multidrug-resistant strains was 95.6%.

3.4 Correlation of serotype and drug resistance

As shown in Table 2, strains of all serotypes were highly resistant (with high MICs) to erythromycin, cotrimoxazole, and clindamycin, and no significant differences were detected between strains. Strains of some of the serotypes were also resistant to β-lactam antibiotics. Serotype 19A seemed to have a higher rate of resistance than other serotypes.

Discussion

S. pneumoniae is a highly virulent organism and is associated with a high rate of mortality [1–3,7]. Children, especially those below the age of 5, are particularly at risk from invasive infections. The data from our hospital [16] showed that approximately 74.4% of *S. pneumoniae* infections occurred in pediatric patients, and that pediatric patients accounted for 90% of invasive infections, with most occurring in patients less than 5 years of age.

Children under 2 years of age are known to be susceptible to IPD, and the mortality in these patients is high. In this study, patients less than 2 years of age accounted for 37 cases (60.7%) and 5 deaths, indicating that immature immunity among younger children may cause invasive infections to occur more easily. Consequently, special attention should be paid to young patients with *S. pneumoniae* infections. Compared with infections at other sites, pneumococcal meningitis is more severe and has a higher mortality rate, with a greater chance of adverse sequelae [17]. In this study, there were 3 deaths in patients with pneumococcal meningitis.

Based on the antigen profile of the polysaccharide capsule, *S. pneumoniae* can be divided into 46 serogroups, including more than 90 serotypes [18,19]. However, according to worldwide surveys, almost 90% of invasive infections are caused by about 16 *S. pneumoniae* serotypes, including 19F, 23F, 19A, 6B, 14, and 6A. Serotyping provides excellent guidance for choosing a specific PCV. Several studies, conducted in various cities in China during different years, demonstrated great diversity in the distribution of serotypes of *S. pneumoniae* [10–12]. These results indicate that the serotypes of the IPD-associated *S. pneumoniae* strains from different regions are varied. In our study, IPD serotyping revealed that 19A was most frequently isolated from children with IPD treated in our hospital, accounting for 41% of cases. It might be the most common IPD pathogen in infants in Shenyang and the surrounding areas, followed by 14 and 19F. The dominance of serotype 19A in Shenyang is similar to the recent trend seen in the Beijing area [5,12], possibly due to the close proximity of these 2 regions. The diversity of *S. pneumoniae* serotypes from different regions and differences in the serotypes that are covered by the various PCVs provide guidance for the selection of the appropriate vaccine in different regions. Our results indicated that PCV-7 would cover 45.9%, PCV-10 would cover 52.5%, and PCV-13 would cover 91.8% of the serotypes found in Shenyang. For vaccination and prevention, the major target population consists of children under the age of 2 years. PCV-7 and PCV-10 would cover 54.1% of this population and PCV-13 would cover 85.4% suggesting that PCV-13 should be the major target for future development and applications in the Shenyang areas. The spread of type 19A in western countries was found after the large-scale use of PCV-7, because 19A is not covered by PCV-7. However in North China, serotype 19A became prevalent in IPD before the introduction of PCV-7, and a similar phenomenon was observed in South Korea [20]. Our findings also indicated that serotype 19A was still one of the most common serotypes in Shenyang and was not related to the introduction of PCV-7, a vaccine not widely used in this area. The spread of highly resistant strains of serotype 19A reported in our study suggests that the widespread use of antimicrobials may provide the selective advantage necessary for resistant serotype expansion, similar to the situation in Korea [20].

Table 1. Antibiotic susceptibility of 61 invasive pneumococcal disease strains (minimum inhibitory concentration [MIC] method).

Antibiotics	% of isolates			MIC, mg/Ml		
	Susceptible	Intermediate	Resistant	50%	90%	Range
Penicillin	34.4	23.0	42.6	4	16	0.032–32
Amoxicillin/Clavulanic acid	50.8	31.1	18.1	3	8	0.025–32
Cefepime	39.3	47.5	13.2	4	17.6	0.064–32
Cefotaxime	57.4	29.5	13.1	1	4	0.016–16
Ceftriaxone	57.4	24.6	18.0	4	17.6	1–32
Cefuroxime	16.5	1.5	82.0	4	20.8	0.032–256
Erythromycin	0	0	100	>256	>256	2–>256
Trimoethoprim-sulfamethoxazole	0	0	100	32	1024	0.125–1024
Clindamycin	9.8	3.3	86.9	>256	>256	0.032–>256
Meropenem	14.8	49.2	36.0	0.5	1	0.008–2
Levofloxacin	100	0	0	1	1	0.25–2
Vancomycin	100	0	0	0.5	0.5	0.25–1
Linezolid	100	0	0	0.5	0.5	0.125–1

Table 2. Antibiotics resistance rates in different *Streptococcus pneumoniae* serotypes.

antibiotics	19A(25)		19F(7)		14(12)		23F(6)		Other serotypes(11)	
	No.	%	No.	%	No.	%	No.	%	No.	%
Penicillin	17	68.0	2	28.6	2	16.7	5	83.3	0	0
Amoxicillin/ Clavulanic acid	7	28.0	2	28.6	0	0	0	0	0	0
Cefepime	3	12.0	2	28.6	0	0	3	50	3	27.3
Cefotaxime	4	16.0	2	28.6	0	0	2	33.3	1	9.1
Ceftriaxone	3	12.0	4	57.1	1	8.3	1	16.7	1	9.1
Cefuroxime	24	96.0	6	85.7	11	91.7	5	83.3	2	18.2
Erythromycin	25	100	7	100	12	100	6	100	11	100
Trimoethoprim-sulfamethoxazole	25	100	7	100	6	50	5	83.3	8	72.7
Clindamycin	25	100	6	85.7	11	91.7	6	100	11	100
Meropenem	12	48.0	5	71.4	1	8.3	2	33.3	2	18.2
Levofloxacin	0	0	0	0	0	0	0	0	0	0
Vancomycin	0	0	0	0	0	0	0	0	0	0
Linezolid	0	0	0	0	0	0	0	0	0	0

Abbreviations: No., Number of isolates resistant to drug.

S. pneumoniae resistance to antibiotics is a growing problem and has become an important prognostic factor, since it is directly associated with persistent disease or disease mortality [21,22]. In this study, most of the 61 patients with IPD were treated for a period of time before being admitted to our hospital and were admitted because of exacerbation of disease. Our susceptibility analysis revealed that resistance to *S. pneumoniae* is a serious problem. The rate of multidrug resistance was 95.6%, and the rate of resistance to macrolides and clindamycin was as high as 100%. In addition, the rates of resistance and insensitivity to penicillins and cephalosporins showed an upward trend. This indicates that *S. pneumoniae* resistance to antibiotics plays a large role in the poor efficacy of antibiotics in both the inpatient and outpatient settings. Because most patients in our study had been treated before admission to the hospital, an unknown fraction of strains analyzed in the study could originate from IPDs that failed to respond to treatment. Thus, the strains tested could have been enriched for resistant isolates. Therefore, the high rates of antibiotic resistance among pneumococcal strains in our study may not completely represent resistance of pneumococcal strains circulating in the population of this region.

Studies have shown that *S. pneumoniae* strains resistant to penicillin and multidrug-resistant strains had significant correlations with specific serotypes [18–20]. Some of the multidrug-resistant serotypes may be disseminated worldwide. In this study, the rates of multidrug resistance of serotypes 19A, 19F, 14, 23F, 1, 4, and 6B were 100%. Generally, serotype 19A seemed to have a higher resistance rate than other serotypes, although no significant difference was found in most instances due to the low number of isolates in our study. Serotype 19A is not a serotype that is covered by the 7-valent vaccine, which should be of concern. Additional studies on the molecular mechanisms of resistance as well as on establishing the clonality of the resistant isolates are needed.

Studies in many countries have shown that use of PCV decreased the overall incidence of IPD among children [23–26]. The increase in cases of IPD among infants and toddlers and the increasing drug resistance of invasive *S. pneumoniae* also suggest the need for the implementation of vaccination in infants and young children. Because the non PCV-7 serotype is increasing in prevalence, broader serotype coverage such as PCV-13 might be optimal for future vaccination in Shenyang.

Acknowledgments

This study was completed under the joint efforts of the Departments of Pediatrics and Laboratory Medicine of Shengjing Hospital, China Medical University.

Author Contributions

Conceived and designed the experiments: CL. Performed the experiments: XX JS. Analyzed the data: CL XX LW. Contributed reagents/materials/ analysis tools: JS. Wrote the paper: CL JL WX.

References

1. WHO Publication (2012) Pneumococcal vaccines WHO position paper –2012–recommendations. Vaccine 30: 4717–4718.
2. UNICEF/WHO (2008) Pneumonia: The forgotten killer of children. Weekly Epidemiol Rec 83: 1–16.
3. Centers for Disease Control and Prevention (CDC) (2006) Vaccine preventable deaths and the global immunization vision and strategy, 2006–2015. MMWR Morb Mortal Wkly Rep 55: 511–515.
4. Liu SY, Dong L, Yang JH (2010) Clinical characteristics and antimicrobial resistance of invasive pneumococcal disease in children. Zhonghua er ke za zhi. Chinese journal of pediatrics 48: 95–99.
5. Xue L, Yao KH, Yu SJ, Liu ZJ, Qian J, et al. (2011) Molecular epidemiology of serotype 19A streptococcus pneumoniae isolated from children in Beijing, 1997–2006. Chin Med J 124: 1769–1774.
6. Yuan HY, Yu JX, Fu WL (2011) Antibiotics resistance of streptococcus pneumoniae in children lower respiratory infection. Zhonghua Yi Yuan Gan Ran Xue Za zhi. Chinese Journal of Nosocomiology 21: 2127–2128.
7. Yao KH, Yang YH (2008)Streptococcus pneumoniae diseases in Chinese children: Past, present and future. Vaccine 26: 4425–4433.
8. CDC (1997) Prevention Of pneumococcal disease: recommendations of the Advisory Committee on Immunization Practices (ACIP). MMWR Recomm Rep. 46: 1–24.

9. Jauneikaite E, Jefferies JM, Hibberd ML, Clarke SC (2012) Prevalence of Streptococcus pneumoniae serotypes causing invasive and non-invasive disease in South East Asia: a review. Vaccine 30: 3503–3514.
10. Liu Y, Wang H, Chen M, Sun Z, Zhao R, et al. (2008) Serotype distribution and antimicrobial resistance patterns of Streptococcus pneumoniae isolated from children in China younger than 5 years. Diagn Microbiol Infect Dis 61: 256–263.
11. Yao KH, Wang LB, Zhao GM, Zheng YJ, Deng L, et al. (2011) Pneumococcal serotype distribution and antimicrobial resistance in Chinese children hospitalized for pneumonia. Vaccine 29: 2296–2301.
12. Xue L, Yao K, Xie G, Zheng Y, Wang C, et al. (2010) Serotype distribution and antimicrobial resistance of streptococcus pneumoniae isolates that cause invasive disease among Chinese children. Clin Infect Dis 50: 741–744.
13. Centers for Disease Control and Prevention (1997) Case definitions for infectious conditions under public health surveillance. MMWR Recomm Rep 46: 1–55.
14. CLSI (2010) Performance Standards for Antimicrobial Susceptilibity Testing Sixteenth Informational Supplement. M100-S16. CLSI, 56–57.
15. Sorensen U (1993) Typing of pneumococci by using 12 pooled antisera. J Clin Microbiol 31: 2097–2100.
16. Sun J, Liu C, Wang Y, Zhou X, Zhang Z, et al. (2012) Changes in drug resistance and distribution of Streptococcus pneumonia infection from 2001 to 2011 in Shenyang area. Zhongguo Xiao Er Ji Jiu Yi Xue. Chin Pediatr Emerg Med 19: 368–371.
17. Nyasulu P, Cohen C, De Gouveia L, Feldman C, Klugman KP, et al. (2011) Increased Risk of Death in Human Immunodeficiency Virus-infected Children With Pneumococcal Meningitis in South Africa, 2003–2005. Pediatr Infect Dis J 30: 1075–1080.
18. Gareia-Suarez Mdel M, Villaverde R, CaldeviUa AF, Méndez FJ, Vázquez F (2006) Serotype distribution and antimicrobial resistance of invasive and non-invasive pneumococceal isolates in Asturias, Spain. Jpn J Infect Dis 59: 299–305.
19. Denham BC, Clarke SC (2005) Serotype incidence and antibiotic susceptibility of Streptococcus pneumoniae causing invasive disease in Scotland 1999–2002. J Med Microbiol 54: 327–331.
20. Choi EH, Kim SH, Eun BW, Kin SJ, Kim NH, et al. (2008) Streptococcus pneumoniae serotype 19A in children, South Korea. Emerg Infect Dis 14: 275–281.
21. McGee L, McDougal L, Zhou J, Spratt BG, Tenover FC, et al. (2001) Nomenclature of major antimicrobial-resistant clones of Streptococcus pneumoniae defined by the pneumococcal molecular epidemiology network. J Clin Microbiol 39: 2565–2571.
22. Lonks JR, Garau J, Gomez L, Xercavins M, Ochoa de Echagüen A, et al. (2002) Failure of Macrolide Antibiotic Treatment in Patients with Bacteremia Due to Erythromycin-Resistant Streptococcus pneumoniae. Clinical Infectious Diseases 35: 556–564.
23. Centers for Disease Control and Prevention (CDC) (2005) Direct and indirect effects of routine vaccination of children with 7-Valent pneumococcal conjugate vaccine on incidence of invasive pneumococcal disease-United States, 1998–2003. MMWR Morb Mortal Wkly Rep 54: 893–897.
24. Roche P, Krause V, Cook H, Barralet J, Coleman D, et al. (2007) Invasive pneumococcal disease in Australia, 2005. Commun Dis Intell, 31: 86–100.
25. Centers for Disease Control and Prevention (CDC). (2008) Progress in introduction of pneumococcal conjugate vaccine – worldwide, 2000–2008. MMWR Morb Mortal Wkly Rep 57: 1148–1151.
26. Weil-Olivier C, van der Linden M, de Schutter I, Dagan R, Mantovani L (2012) Prevention of pneumococcal diseases in the post-seven valent vaccine era: A European perspective. BMC Infect Dis. 7: 207.

25

The Predictive Value of the NICE "Red Traffic Lights" in Acutely Ill Children

Evelien Kerkhof[1], Monica Lakhanpaul[2], Samiran Ray[3], Jan Y. Verbakel[4], Ann Van den Bruel[5], Matthew Thompson[5], Marjolein Y. Berger[6], Henriette A. Moll[1], Rianne Oostenbrink[1]*, for the European Research Network on recognising serious InfEctions (ERNIE) members¶

1 Erasmus MC-Sophia Children's Hospital, Department of General Pediatrics, Rotterdam, The Netherlands, **2** Department of General and Adolescent Pediatrics, University College London, Institute of Child Health, London, United Kingdom, **3** Pediatric Intensive Care Unit, Great Ormond Street Hospital, London, United Kingdom, **4** Department of General Practice, Katholieke Universiteit Leuven, Leuven, Belgium, **5** Department of Primary Care Health Sciences, University of Oxford, Radcliffe Observatory Quarter, Oxford, United Kingdom, **6** Department of General Practice, University Groningen, University Medical Centre Groningen, Groningen, The Netherlands

Abstract

Objective: Early recognition and treatment of febrile children with serious infections (SI) improves prognosis, however, early detection can be difficult. We aimed to validate the predictive rule-in value of the National Institute for Health and Clinical Excellence (NICE) most severe alarming signs or symptoms to identify SI in children.

Design, Setting and Participants: The 16 most severe ("red") features of the NICE traffic light system were validated in seven different primary care and emergency department settings, including 6,260 children presenting with acute illness.

Main Outcome Measures: We focussed on the individual predictive value of single red features for SI and their combinations. Results were presented as positive likelihood ratios, sensitivities and specificities. We categorised "general" and "disease-specific" red features. Changes in pre-test probability versus post-test probability for SI were visualised in Fagan nomograms.

Results: Almost all red features had rule-in value for SI, but only four individual red features substantially raised the probability of SI in more than one dataset: "does not wake/stay awake", "reduced skin turgor", "non-blanching rash", and "focal neurological signs". The presence of $\geq$3 red features improved prediction of SI but still lacked strong rule-in value as likelihood ratios were below 5.

Conclusions: The rule-in value of the most severe alarming signs or symptoms of the NICE traffic light system for identifying children with SI was limited, even when multiple red features were present. Our study highlights the importance of assessing the predictive value of alarming signs in clinical guidelines prior to widespread implementation in routine practice.

Editor: Soren Gantt, University of British Columbia, Canada

Funding: EK is supported by ZonMW, a Dutch organisation for health research and development; RO is supported by an unrestricted grant of the Europe Container Terminals B.V and by a fellowship award of European Society of Pediatric Infectious Diseases. The funders had no role in study design, data collection and analysis, decision to publish, or preparation of the manuscript.

Competing Interests: ML was the clinical director leading the NICE fever guideline; we believe this improved the clinical contents of the study. RO is supported by an unrestricted grant of the Europe Container Terminals B.V, which does not alter our adherence to PLOS ONE policies on sharing data and materials.

* E-mail: r.oostenbrink@erasmusmc.nl

¶ Authors who wrote the paper on behalf of the (ERNIE) is provided in the Acknowledgments.

Introduction

Fever is one of the most common symptoms among children presenting to ambulatory care.[1–3] The majority of children presenting with an acute illness to ambulatory care will have self-limiting viral infections, with only a small proportion having a serious infection (SI).[1,4–6] Early recognition and treatment of children with SI are related to better prognosis,[7,8] however identification of SI at first presentation can be difficult.

The National Institute for Health and Clinical Excellence (NICE) 2013 guideline for the management of children with feverish illness provides comprehensive guidance on the assessment, investigation and management of children presenting at different settings, including primary care and pediatric specialty settings.[6,9] One of the key elements of the guideline is a "traffic light" system for the diagnostic assessment of children under five years of age presenting with a feverish illness. This evidence and consensus-based system includes clinical features identified from existing scoring systems for acutely ill children,[10–13] and disease-specific signs and symptoms. Children with the most alarming (or "red") features are considered at higher risk of SI, for whom subsequent management includes invasive investigations, treatment, and hospital admission.

As one of the few evidence-based guidelines for children with fever [14,15] and the only for both primary and secondary care, the NICE febrile child guideline has been implemented in many settings in not only the United Kingdom but also in other countries. Recently, two studies reported low specificities for the approach that any abnormal amber or red feature would indicate possible SI.[16,17] This could be due to the inclusion of amber features, whose association with SI may be weaker.

In this study we aimed to determine the predictive ("rule-in") value of the red features of the NICE traffic light system, both for the individual red features as their combinations for identifying children with SI in various acute pediatric settings in Europe.

Methods

Identification of datasets

We used data on seven independent cohorts [4,18–23] collected by collaborators of the European Research Network on recognising serious InfEctions (ERNIE) group.[24] Data were prospectively collected at first contact using standardised (site-specific) documentation of patient characteristics, except for Monteny et al [19] where data was collected using structured clinical proformas separate from the consultation. All datasets were cohort studies of children in various age ranges (0–16 years), presenting to ambulatory care settings (i.e. general or family practice, pediatric outpatient clinic, pediatric assessment unit or emergency department) with an acute illness or infection.

Two datasets based on primary care settings were considered as low prevalence settings of SI (<5%) and five datasets based on emergency care settings as high prevalence settings (>5%).[25] More details on the original cohorts have been published elsewhere ([4,18–23]).

Ethical approval

This research conforms to the Helsinki Declaration and to local legislation. The original study authors have all agreed to share their data, and had obtained ethical approval from their local research ethics committees for the initial data collection, prior to this study.

Processing of included datasets

Key characteristics of each dataset are shown in table 1. We selected children under the age of five years with an acute illness based on general symptoms [4,21,22] or specifically on the presence of fever [18–20,23], as this is the target group of the NICE guideline (table 1).

The NICE traffic light system includes 16 red features, which are categorised into 5 main domains: Colour (1 red feature), Activity (4 red features), Respiratory (3 red features), Hydration (1 red feature), and Other (7 red features).[6,9] When study variables were not entirely identical to the red features in the NICE febrile child guideline, we identified proxies where possible. Identification and handling of variables has been described earlier [17], a full list of all approximations is described in table S1. When a red feature was not recorded in the dataset and no suitable proxy was identified, this item was excluded from that specific dataset. Table S2 outlines the unrecorded and missing data from each dataset separately.

Missing values were not imputed because the necessary missing-at-random assumption was likely to be incorrect. We considered red features that were "not documented" in individual patient records as "absent", given that the red feature or its proxy was recorded in that particular dataset.[17]

The translation, recoding and data-checking were performed by two authors (EK, JV) and the results of each step were discussed with all primary study authors.[17]

Outcome measures

Serious infections (SI) were defined as sepsis (including bacteremia), meningitis, pneumonia, osteomyelitis, cellulitis, and complicated urinary tract infections. [25] Serious infections (SI) were not only based on clinical diagnosis, but reference standard test criteria were used to determine final diagnoses of SI. Detailed description on these reference standard test criteria are available in the original study papers.[4,18–23] Assessment of the diagnoses to ensure comparability of outcomes was discussed with the lead investigator of each study as described earlier.[17]

Statistical analysis

The individual red features were analysed in every dataset separately. Additionally, results were categorised as "general" red features (items 1–7 and 9–10) and "disease-specific" red features (items 8 and 11–16).

We assessed the rule-in value for SI for each red feature separately by calculating positive likelihood ratios (LR+). Red features were considered to have rule-in value if they raised the probability of illness with a positive likelihood ratio of more than 5.0.[25] The univariable association between each individual red feature and the presence of SI was tested by Chi-square analysis. Likelihood ratios, sensitivity and specificity were measured for the presence of ≥1 RTL, ≥2 RTLs and ≥3 RTLs. The sensitivity and specificity for "general" and "disease-specific" red features were plotted in receiver operating characteristic (ROC) space.

The incremental diagnostic value for up to more than four red features compared to one red feature was evaluated by logistic regression analyses with forward selection (Wald test, p-value <0.05).

We visualised the change in pre-test probability versus post-test probability for SI in a Fagan nomogram.[26]

No overall pooled likelihood ratios were calculated because of the substantial clinical heterogeneity between datasets (differences in setting, inclusion criteria, immunisation schedules and definition of serious infection).[17] All analyses were done with SPSS software (version 20.0, SPSS Inc, Chicago).

Results

Included datasets

We selected 6,260 children under five years of age of seven pre-existing datasets (n = 6,260/10,812, 58%) for diagnostic studies in children with an acute illness (table 1). Children were included based on fever,[19,20,23] acute illness,[4,18] acute infection,[21] and referral for meningeal signs.[22] Children with various severities of co-morbidity were excluded in five studies,[4,19–23], one study excluded children if the acute episode was caused by an exacerbation of a chronic condition[4] and one study excluded children who required immediate resuscitation [18] (table 1). All studies included sepsis, meningitis, pneumonia and complicated urinary tract infections in their outcome definition. Osteomyelitis and cellulitis were explicitly mentioned in five and three datasets, respectively.

The median age of the selected children ranged from 0.8 years to 1.9 years. The prevalence of SI ranged from 1.2% to 4.1% in two datasets from general practice [4,19] and from 9.3% to 40.2% in five datasets from emergency departments and a pediatric assessment unit [18,20–23].

Red traffic lights included in the datasets

Data on all red features included in domains "Colour" and "Hydration" were available in all datasets. The red features "no response to social cues", and "weak, high-pitched or continuous

Table 1. Characteristics of datasets with children <5 years of age suspected of acute illness*.

Dataset	Setting	Country	Inclusion Criteria	Exclusion Criteria	n/ original study population (%)	Prevalence Serious Infection % (CI)	Median Age (IQR)
1. Bleeker et al. 2007[23]	ED	NL	Children aged 1–36 months with fever (T>38) at emergency department, no clear focus identified after evaluation GP or history by pediatrician	Chronic disease, Immunodeficiency	595/595 (100)	23.0 (19.6–26.4)	0.8 (0.3–1.4)
2. Brent et al. 2011[18]	ED	UK	All children presenting with a medical problem to the pediatric emergency-care unit whatever their age	Children who required immediate resuscitation. Comorbidity and chronic illness	494/2777 (18)	9.3 (6.7–11.9)	1.5 (0.9–2.7)
3. Oostenbrink et al. 2004[22]	ED	NL	Children aged 1 month-16 years, meningeal signs at GP, pediatrician or self-referred with neck pain	Comorbidity, ventriculoperitoneal drain	423/593 (71)	40.2 (35.5–44.9)	1.1 (0.5–2.7)
4. Roukema et al. 2008[20]	ED	NL	Children aged 1 month-16 years with fever (T>38) at emergency department, without meningeal irritation	Chronic disease, Immunodeficiency	1459/1750 (83)	11.7 (10.1–13.4)	1.4 (0.7–2.6)
5. Thompson et al. 2009[21]	PAU	UK	Children aged 3 months-16 years with suspected acute infection	Children with diseases liable to cause repeated serious bacterial infection, and infections resulting from penetrating trauma	434/700 (62)	37.1 (32.5-41.7)	1.6 (0.9–2.7)
6. Monteny et al. 2008[19]	GP	NL	Children aged 3 months-6 years, contacting a GP cooperative after hours with fever as the presenting symptom	Language barriers, no repeated inclusion within the last two weeks	487/506 (96)	4.1 (2.3-5.9)	1.7 (0.9–3.0)
7. Van den Bruel et al. 2007[4]	GP/AP/ ED	BE	Non-referred children ≤16 years with acute illness for max 5 days	Traumatic or neurological illness, intoxication, psychiatric or behavioural problems without somatic cause or an exacerbation of a chronic condition. No repeated inclusion of same infant within 5 days. Exclusion of physicians if the assumption of consecutive inclusion was probably violated	2368/3891 (60)	1.2 (0.8–1.6)	1.9 (0.9–3.2)

*Using temperature >38.0°C or general symptoms of acute illness.

GP = General Practice; AP = Ambulatory Pediatric Care; ED = Emergency Department; PAU = Pediatric Assessment Unit; BE = Belgium; NL = the Netherlands; UK = United Kingdom; CI = Confidence Interval IQR= interquartile range.

cry" of domain "Activity" were not recorded in two [20,23], and one dataset [18], respectively. Other red features in this domain were available in all datasets. Red features related to the "Respiratory" domain were not recorded in four ("grunting") [4,21–23], one ("tachypnoea") [22], and two ("chest indrawing") [22,23], datasets respectively. "Disease-specific" red features (items 8 and 11–16) were recorded less frequently in all datasets but in particular in low prevalence settings (range missing values 0–50%), see table S2).

Performance of individual red traffic lights

Table 2 shows positive and negative likelihood ratios of the 16 individual red features for each dataset separately. All red features with high rule-in value (LR+ >5) are highlighted in bold.

Four of all 16 red features did not achieve high rule-in value (LR+ <5) including two red features which were not available in the datasets or were not reaching significance ($p<0.05$) when present.

The one red feature which provided high rule-in value in two datasets from both low and higher prevalence settings, was "does not wake or if roused does not stay awake" (LR+5.9 (95% CI 3.5–10.0) and LR+7.8, 95% CI 4.4–13.6, respectively). The red features "reduced skin turgor", "non-blanching rash", and "focal neurological signs" showed high rule-in value in two high prevalence settings each (range LR+5.0-9.7)[18,20,22]. The red features "pale/mottled/ashen/blue", "appears ill to a healthcare professional", "weak, high-pitched or continuous cry", "tachypnoea", "moderate or severe chest indrawing", and "age 0–3 months & temperature ≥38°C" showed high rule-in value in one low prevalence setting (range LR+5.9-83.6)[4]. High rule-in value for the red features "grunting" and "bulging fontanelle", was observed in one high prevalence dataset (range LR+7.8–11.3).[20] In two high prevalence settings for none of the red features high rule-in value was observed.[21,23]

Performance of multiple red traffic lights

The association between SI and the number of positive red features with the performance measures of positive likelihood ratios, sensitivity and specificity is shown in table 3. We measured the maximum predictive value of multiple red features by logistic regression analysis and the slope of the ROC-curve. We noted a significant increase of rule-in value with the number of positive red features in most datasets (range LR+2.1 – 10.0 when ≥3 red features), with the exception of Monteny et al.[19] (p-value <0.05). This was also observed in the increased values of specificity when more red features were present. The presence of 4 or more red features did not contribute to discriminative value compared to up to 3 red features. The proportion of children having ≥3 red features ranged from 2% to 50% and did not differ between low and high prevalence settings. "General" red features were almost entirely responsible for the total ROC-area (table 3). We did not test disease-specific red features on disease-specific outcome measures due to the small numbers of these events. In figure 1 we visualised the change in pre-test to post-test probability for SI when three or more (general or disease-specific) red features were present in a Fagan nomogram.[27] For example, the 9% pre-test probability of having a SI for a child in the Brent et al dataset increases to 28% (95% CI 17–42%) post-test probability when having three or more red features, but decreases only to 7% (95% CI 6–9%) if less than three red features were present.

Discussion

Main findings

This is the first study on broadly validating the diagnostic performance of the individual red features and their combinations of the NICE febrile child guideline in acutely ill children in various settings in Europe. Although we observed rule-in value for almost all individual red features in at least one dataset, only four red features raised the probability of SI with a positive likelihood ratio of more than 5.0 in more than one setting: "does not wake or if roused does not stay awake", "reduced skin turgor", "non-blanching rash", and "focal neurological signs". Children with more than one red feature had an increased risk of SI, however, more than three red features did not further increase disease probability.

Comparison with other studies

To our knowledge there are three previous studies that estimated the predictive value of any amber or red feature for the detection of SI, but they did not evaluate the individual features of the NICE traffic light system separately. De et al.[16] found that the NICE traffic light system failed to identify a substantial proportion of children with serious bacterial infections. Combining the amber and red feature categories resulted in a sensitivity of 85.8% and specificity of 28.5% for the detection of any serious bacterial infections. Within the original data of Thompson et al. the diagnostic value of vital signs and the NICE traffic light system for identifying children with SI was assessed in a pediatric assessment unit.[21] They stated that the presence of one or more amber and red features was 85% sensitive, but only 29% specific in identifying serious or intermediate infections.[21] However, this original study was performed in children up to 16 years of age in contrast to this present study limited to children up to 5 years of age. Finally, a previous study assessing the diagnostic value of any abnormal amber or red feature (not considering combinations) of the NICE traffic light system to rule-out SI, had sensitivity of 97–100% in low and intermediate prevalence settings and 87–99% in high prevalence settings.[17] The results of all three validation studies suggest possible clinical value for ruling-out SI using both amber and red features, but at the expense of a large group of children testing false positive. However, up to 15% of children with a serious infection will be missed. Alternatively, the presence of any amber or red feature does not allow ruling-in SI considering the very low specificity. In low prevalence settings, alarming signs are preferably highly sensitive to correctly rule-out SI in order to limit incorrect referral.[24] In high prevalence settings specificity is more important because a high rate of false positive children could result in high admission rates and unnecessary investigations.[24] Unfortunately there was too much heterogeneity in our datasets to stratify according to prevalence.

Clinical and research implications

With decreasing incidence of SI, clinicians may increasingly rely on alarming symptoms described in (inter)national clinical guidelines. Broad validation could support the wider adoption of the NICE guideline in various settings in Europe and other high-income countries. Although the traffic light system of the NICE febrile child guideline is mostly based on systematic literature reviews and consensus, only four red features achieved high rule-in value in more than one dataset and none of them across all settings. Moreover, in at least as many datasets these four red features did not achieved high rule-in value and therefore hampers strong conclusions.

Table 2. Likelihood ratios individual red traffic lights.

Dataset	LR (CI)	prevalence	COLOUR: Pale/ mottled/ ashen/ blue	ACTIVITY: No response to social cues	ACTIVITY: Ill appearance	ACTIVITY: Does not (stay) wake	ACTIVITY: Weak/ high/ continuous cry	RESPIRATORY: Grunting	RESPIRATORY: Tachypnoea	RESPIRATORY: Chest indrawings	HYDRATION: Reduced skin turgor	OTHER: Age <3 m & temp ≥38°C	OTHER: Non-blanching rash	OTHER: Bulging fontanelle	OTHER: Neck stiffness	OTHER: Status epilepticus	OTHER: Focal neurologic signs	OTHER: Focal seizures
			positive likelihood ratio (LR+) and negative likelihood ratio (LR-)															
Bleeker et al.[23]	LR +	High	2.3 (1.5–3.4)*	-	1.4 (1.2–1.7)*	2.6 (1.0–6.9)*	1.1 (0.9–1.3)	-	3.0 (1.9–4.6)*	-	1.9 (1.3–2.8)*	1.5 (1.1–2.1)*	-	1.8 (0.7–4.4)	-	-	-	-
(n = 595)	LR -		0.9 (0.8–0.9)	-	0.7 (0.6–0.9)	1.0 (0.9–1.0)	0.9 (0.8–1.1)		0.8 (0.8–0.9)		0.9 (0.8–1.0)	0.9 (0.8–1.0)	-	1.0 (0.9–1.0)	-	-	-	-
Brent et al.[18]	LR +	High	2.6 (1.8–3.8)*	1.6 (0.4–7.0)	2.7 (2.0–3.6)*	1.4 (0.2–11.1)	-	**7.8 (2.2–28.0)***	2.9 (1.7–4.9)*	4.9 (2.2–10.8)*	**9.7(0.6–153.1)***	1.9 (0.6–6.5)	**	**	**	**	**	**
(n = 494)	LR -		0.7 (0.5–0.9)	1.0 (0.9–1.0)	0.5 (0.4–0.7)	1.0 (1.0–1.0)	-	0.9 (0.8–1.0)	0.8 (0.6–0.9)	0.9 (0.7–1.0)	1.0 (0.9–1.0)	1.0 (0.9–1.0)	**	**	**	**	**	**
Oostenbrink et al. [22]	LR +	High	1.9 (1.0–3.5)*	1.9 (1.4–2.5)*	3.0 (0.8–11.7)	**7.8 (4.4–13.6)***	1.1 (0.7–1.8)	-	-	-	**7.4 (1.7–33.5)***	1.6 (0.9–2.9)	**7.2 (3.3–15.9)***	2.7 (1.6–4.4)*	1.8 (1.6–2.0)*	-	**7.4 (2.6–21.4)***	**
(n = 423)	LR -		0.9 (0.9–1.0)	0.8 (0.7–0.9)	1.0 (0.9–1.0)	0.6 (0.6–0.7)	1.0 (0.9–1.1)	-	-	-	0.9 (0.9–1.0)	0.9 (0.9–1.0)	0.8 (0.8–0.9)	0.8 (0.8–0.9)	0.2 (0.1–0.3)	-	0.9 (0.8–0.9)	**
Roukema et al. [20]	LR +	High	1.5 (0.2–12.8)	-	2.7 (1.6–4.5)*	2.8 (1.2–6.5)*	2.9 (1.4–6.3)*	2.9 (1.6–5.3)*	2.6 (1.4–4.7)*	1.2 (0.7–2.1)	1.9 (0.2–16.8)	1.8 (1.0–3.3)*	**7.5 (1.5–37.0)***	**11.3(1.9–67.1)***	4.8 (1.9–12.2)*	**	**5.0 (2.5–10.2)***	1.5 (0.2–12.8)
(n = 1459)	LR -		1.0 (1.0–1.0)	-	0.9 (0.9–1.0)	1.0 (1.0–1.0)	1.0 (0.9–1.0)	0.9 (0.9–1.0)	1.0 (0.9–1.0)	1.0 (0.9–1.0)	1.0 (1.0–1.0)	1.0 (0.9–1.0)	1.0 (1.0–1.0)	1.0 (1.0–1.0)	1.0 (1.0–1.0)	**	0.9 (0.9–1.0)	1.0 (1.0–1.0)
Thompson et al.[21]	LR +	High	1.3 (1.0–1.6)	2.4 (0.9–6.2)	**	1.5 (0.9–2.5)	1.5 (1.1–2.1)*	-	4.7 (1.5–14.4)*	1.5 (1.0–2.3)	2.0 (0.8–4.9)	**	1.7 (0.9–3.4)	-	**	-	-	-
(n = 434)	LR -		0.9 (0.8–1.0)	1.0 (0.9–1.0)	**	0.9 (0.9–1.0)	0.9 (0.8–1.0)	-	0.9 (0.9–1.0)	0.9 (0.8–1.0)	1.0 (0.9–1.0)	**	1.0 (0.9–1.0)	-	**	-	-	-
Monteny et al.[19]	LR +	Low	1.7 (1.1–2.5)*	1.4 (0.9–2.1)	1.7 (0.6–4.9)	1.8 (1.0–3.2)	0.8 (0.5–1.4)	1.5 (1.2–1.8)*	**	**	0.8 (0.1–5.4)	**	0.4 (0.1–2.8)	**	1.8 (1.1–2.9)*	-	-	-
(n = 487)	LR -		0.7 (0.4–1.1)	0.7 (0.5–1.2)	0.9 (0.8–1.1)	0.8 (0.5–1.1)	1.2 (0.8–1.7)	0.4 (0.1–1.0)	**	**	1.0 (0.9–1.1)	**	1.1 (1.0–1.2)	**	0.7 (0.4–1.1)	-	-	-
Van den Bruel et al.[4]	LR +	Low	**83.6 (12.2–572.4)***	3.2 (1.9–5.3)*	**6.6 (4.5–10.0)***	**5.9 (3.5–10.0)***	**7.0 (4.1–11.8)***	-	**7.3 (4.1–12.9)***	**8.0 (4.9–13.1)***	2.2 (0.3–15.5)	**9.3 (2.3–38.1)***	**	-	**	-	-	-
(n = 2368)	LR -		0.9 (0.8–1.0)	0.7 (0.5–1.0)	0.5 (0.4–0.8)	0.7 (0.5–0.9)	0.7 (0.5–0.9)	-	0.7 (0.6–0.9)	0.6 (0.5–0.9)	1.0 (0.9–1.1)	0.9 (0.8–1.0)	**	-	**	-	-	-

'General' red traffic lights: Pale/ mottled/ ashen/ blue; No response to social cues; Ill appearance; Does not (stay) wake; Weak/ high/ continuous cry; Grunting; Tachypnoea; Reduced skin turgor; Age <3 m & temp ≥38°C.
'Disease specific' red traffic lights: Chest indrawings; Non-blanching rash; Bulging fontanelle; Neck stiffness; Status epilepticus; Focal neurologic signs; Focal seizures.
CI: confidence interval.
*P-value <0.05 (Chi-square analysis).
**Red traffic light not positive in non SI- and/or SI population.
-Not recorded.

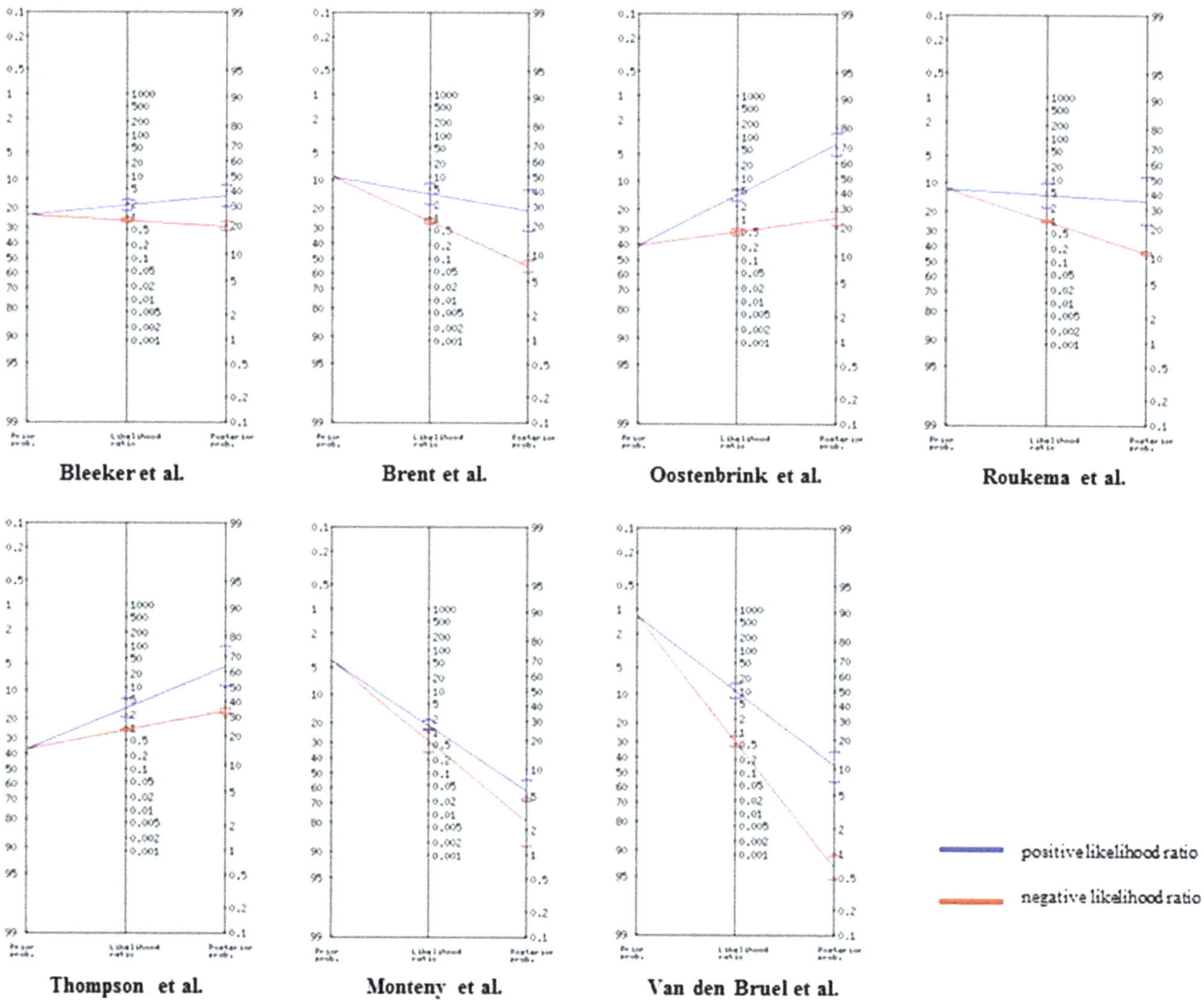

Figure 1. Calculation of post-test pobability for serious infections if ≥3 red traffic lights present using Fagan nomogram.

The rule-in value of several other red features was not confirmed in multiple settings either, questioning their inclusion in this setting-independent traffic light system.

Our observations of varying rule-in values of red features in the 7 databases did not support the development of one prediction model including the most important red features. However, we consistently observed an association between 3 or more red features and SI but combinations of red features will never be able to definitely rule-in a SI without uncertainty. This could be due to dilution of their accuracy by the inclusion of aspecific red features or because of the interaction between different red features.

The relatively lower recording of "disease-specific" features hampered our analyses, in particular in low prevalence settings. This may in part have been caused by the fact that it is more difficult to identify proxies for such features, in contrast to more general features.

The main findings in our study corresponds with the limited performance of the Yale Observation Scale, on which the NICE traffic light system is partly based.[17,25] In the revised 2013 guideline[9] two red features were deleted of the previous 2007 protocol[6] or transferred to amber features: "Age 3–6m & temperature ≥39°C" and "bile-stained vomiting". This is supported by our findings that we did not find rule-in value for the former but only had one dataset available for the latter which showed high rule-in value though. Next, as disease specific red features are strongly related to specific but rare diseases, their positive documentation rate is already expected to be low. Although these disease specific red features may be relevant for one specific outcome, it is difficult to evaluate these in the general population of fever with a broad differential diagnosis. However, achieving complete certainty with clinical features is not the goal here. Rather, red features should lift the probability of SI over a certain decision threshold: either to refer, request additional testing or start empiric treatment. As we do not know at what specific risk thresholds we (intuitively) undertake action, clinical interpretation of post-test probabilities as expressed in Fagan nomograms (figure 1) remains difficult. As diagnosis assessment is a dynamic process and may be influenced by evolution of symptoms in time, repeated assessment of deviating red features in those with only one or two features in particular, may improve the evaluation of SI.

Finally, the NICE traffic light system could also be improved by taking more recent evidence into account, such as on peripheral circulation, parental concern [25] or urine analysis [16].

Table 3. Likelihood ratios and ROC-areas of combinations of multiple red traffic lights.

		BLEEKER et al.[23]	BRENT et al.[18]	OOSTENBRINK et al.[22]	ROUKEMA et al.[20]	THOMPSON et al.[21]	MONTENY et al.[19]	VAN DEN BRUEL et al.[4]
		N_{total}=595 SI=137;23.0%	**N_{total}=494 SI=46;9.3%**	**N_{total}=423 SI=170;40.2%**	**N_{total}=1,459 SI=171;11.7%**	**N_{total}=434 SI=161;37.1%**	**N_{total}=487 SI=20;4.1%**	**N_{total}=2,368 SI=28;1.2%**
Number red features	LR +/- (CI)							
≥1 RTL	Likelihood ratio +	1.18 (1.10–1.27)*	1.94 (1.57–2.39)*	1.39 (1.27–1.51)*	1.75 (1.39–2.20)*	1.28 (1.12–1.46)*	1.08 (1.05–1.12)	3.33 (2.76–4.02)*
	Likelihood ratio -	0.41 (0.24–0.70)	0.42 (0.26–0.69)	0.13 (0.06–0.28)	0.81 (0.72–0.91)	0.59 (0.43–0.80)	-	0.24 (0.12–0.53)
≥2 RTLs	Likelihood ratio +	1.49 (1.25–1.79)*	3.70 (2.68–5.12)*	2.36 (1.94–2.87)*	3.40 (2.24–5.16)*	1.75 (1.31–2.33)*	1.25 (1.07–1.46)	6.38 (4.82–8.44)*
	Likelihood ratio -	0.68 (0.55–0.84)	0.49 (0.35–0.69)	0.35 (0.26–0.46)	0.88 (0.82–0.94)	0.78 (0.67–0.89)	0.36 (0.10–1.35)	0.36 (0.21–0.62)
≥3 RTLs	Likelihood ratio +	2.10 (1.50–2.93)*	3.90 (2.15–7.08)	4.65 (3.29–6.58)*	4.14 (2.02–8.50)	2.97 (1.66–5.31)*	1.44 (1.07–1.95)	10.0 (6.43–15.45)*
	Likelihood ratio -	0.81 (0.72–0.91)	0.79 (0.67–0.94)	0.47 (0.39–0.57)	0.95 (0.91–1.00)	0.88 (0.81–0.95)	0.58 (0.30–1.15)	0.56 (0.40–0.79)
	Sens/Spec (CI)							
≥1 RTL	Sensitivity	0.91 (0.84-0.94)	0.74 (0.60-0.84)	0.96 (0.92-0.98)	0.36 (0.29-0.43)	0.76 (0.69-0.82)	1.00 (0.84-1.00)	0.82 (0.64-0.92)
	Specificity	0.23 (0.20-0.27)	0.62 (0.57-0.66)	0.31 (0.25-0.37)	0.80 (0.77-0.82)	0.40 (0.35-0.46)	0.07 (0.05-0.10)	0.75 (0.74-0.77)
≥2 RTLs	Sensitivity	0.58 (0.50-0.66)	0.59 (0.44-0.72)	0.76 (0.70-0.82)	0.16 (0.12-0.23)	0.40 (0.33-0.48)	0.90 (0.70-0.97)	0.68 (0.49-0.82)
	Specificity	0.61 (0.56-0.65)	0.84 (0.81-0.87)	0.68 (0.62-0.73)	0.95 (0.94-0.96)	0.77 (0.72-0.82)	0.28 (0.24-0.32)	0.89 (0.88-0.91)
≥3 RTLs	Sensitivity	0.31 (0.24-0.39)	0.26 (0.16-0.40)	0.59 (0.51-0.66)	0.06 (0.03-0.11)	0.17 (0.12-0.24)	0.70 (0.48-0.85)	0.46 (0.30-0.64)
	Specificity	0.85 (0.82-0.88)	0.93 (0.91-0.95)	0.87 (0.83-0.91)	0.98 (0.98-0.99)	0.94 (0.91-0.96)	0.51 (0.47-0.56)	0.95 (0.94-0.96)
	ROC-area (CI)							
All red features		0.64 (0.59–0.70)	0.73 (0.65–0.82)	0.79 (0.74–0.84)	0.59 (0.54–0.63)	0.63 (0.57–0.68)	0.65 (0.53–0.77)	0.84 (0.75–0.93)
General#		0.64 (0.59–0.70)	0.73 (0.65–0.81)	0.69 (0.64–0.75)	0.59 (0.54–0.64)	0.60 (0.55–0.66)	0.65 (0.54–0.76)	0.82 (0.72–0.91)
Disease spec.^		0.51 (0.46–0.57)	0.56 (0.47–0.66)	0.77 (0.72–0.81)	0.53 (0.48–0.58)	0.56 (0.50–0.62)	0.56 (0.43–0.69)	0.69 (0.57–0.81)

*P-value <0.05 (added value of e.g. ≥3 RTLs above ≥2 RTLs, by logistic regression analysis).
LR: likelihood ratio (positive and negative).
Sens: sensitiviteit; Spec: specificiteit; CI: confidence interval.
#1. Colour: pale / mottled/ ashen/ blue; 2. No response to social cues; 3. Ill appearance; 4. Does not (stay) awake; 5. Weak/ high pitched/ continuous cry; 6. Grunting; 7. Tachypnoea; 9. Reduced skin turgor; 10. Age <3 m & temp ≥38°C;
^8. Chest indrawing 11. Non-blanching rash; 12. Bulging fontanelle; 13. Neck stiffness; 14. Status epilepticus; 15. Focal neurologic symptoms; 16. Focal seizures.

Strengths and limitations

We assessed the NICE red traffic lights in 6,260 children from seven existing datasets with various pediatric populations and settings including two low prevalence primary care settings, which are usually underrepresented in diagnostic studies in this area.[24] In addition, we validated the red features separately to identify their individual predictive value.

Despite the large amount of data, not all red features had been recorded in all datasets, necessitating the use of proxy variables.[17] Furthermore, differences in population characteristics (table 1), such as age distribution or prevalence of specific diagnoses within the group of SI, prevented the calculation of overall diagnostic performance measures.

Furthermore, by assuming missing red features as not present and more complete documentation of red features in ill children, we may have overestimated our likelihood ratios by increasing the contrast between children with and without SI.

However, the variability in variables and case-mix reflects clinical practice and therefore will strengthen generalizability of our results.

Conclusion

Our results support rule-in value of several individual red features from the NICE febrile child guideline in specific settings, although not consistent. However most features had little rule-in value across multiple settings. The NICE red traffic lights, even when three or more features are present, seem to have limited value for ruling-in serious infections. Our results underline the importance to widely validate the predictive value of individual and combinations of multiple red features in clinical guidelines, prior to widespread dissemination and adoption.

Acknowledgments

The authors wrote the paper on behalf of the European Research Network on Recognising Serious Infection (ERNIE). The principal investigators are: Marjolein Berger, Frank Buntinx, Bert Aertgeerts, Monica Lakhanpaul, David Mant, Henriette Moll, Rianne Oostenbrink, Richard Stevens, Matthew Thompson, Ann Van den Bruel and Jan Verbakel. We gratefully acknowledge the members of the ERNIE group for the collaboration and their advice on the message of the manuscript. We want to thank the emergency-personnel of all ambulatory care settings for their participation and careful collection of the required data. We acknowledge the researchers Sacha Bleeker, Andrew Brent, Samiran Ray, Jolt Roukema, Matthew Thompson, Miriam Monteny and Ann Van den Bruel for the data acquisition and contribution of the original studies.

Disclaimer: for this study we selected children with an acute illness from seven cohorts collected by the collaboration of the European Research Network on recognising serious InfEctions(ERNIE) group.[4,18,19,20–23]

Author Contributions

Conceived and designed the experiments: EK ML SR HAM RO. Performed the experiments: EK ML SR JV AVDB MT MYB HAM RO. Analyzed the data: EK RO. Contributed reagents/materials/analysis tools: ML JV AVDB MT MYB HAM RO. Wrote the paper: EK RO. Reviewed and revised the manuscript: EK ML SR JV AVDB MT MYB HAM RO. Translation, synopsis and recoding of the datasets: EK SR JV. Participated in recoding and data checking and in discussion about each step of the results: ML SR JV AVDB MT MYB HAM RO.

References

1. Armon K, MacFaul R, Hemingway P, Werneke U, Stephenson T (2004) The impact of presenting problem based guidelines for children with medical problems in an accident and emergency department. Arch Dis Child 89: 159–164.
2. Bruijnzeels MA, Foets M, van der Wouden JC, van den Heuvel WJ, Prins A (1998) Everyday symptoms in childhood: occurrence and general practitioner consultation rates. Br J Gen Pract 48: 880–884.
3. Moll van Charante EP, van Steenwijk-Opdam PC, Bindels PJ (2007) Out-of-hours demand for GP care and emergency services: patients' choices and referrals by general practitioners and ambulance services. BMC Fam Pract 8: 46.
4. Van den Bruel A, Aertgeerts B, Bruyninckx R, Aerts M, Buntinx F (2007) Signs and symptoms for diagnosis of serious infections in children: a prospective study in primary care. Br J Gen Pract 57: 538–546.
5. Craig JC, Williams GJ, Jones M, Codarini M, Macaskill P, et al. (2010) The accuracy of clinical symptoms and signs for the diagnosis of serious bacterial infection in young febrile children: prospective cohort study of 15 781 febrile illnesses. BMJ 340: c1594.
6. National Institute for Health and Clinical Excellence (2007) Feverish illness in children - Assessment and initial management in children younger than 5 years. London: National Institute for Health and Clinical Excellence.
7. Inwald DP, Tasker RC, Peters MJ, Nadel S, Paediatric Intensive Care Society Study G (2009) Emergency management of children with severe sepsis in the United Kingdom: the results of the Paediatric Intensive Care Society sepsis audit. Arch Dis Child 94: 348–353.
8. Kumar A (2009) Optimizing antimicrobial therapy in sepsis and septic shock.Crit Care Clin 25: 733–751, viii.
9. Chen SM, Chang HM, Hung TW, Chao YH, Tsai JD, et al. (2013) Diagnostic performance of procalcitonin for hospitalised children with acute pyelonephritis presenting to the paediatric emergency department. Emerg Med J 30: 406–410.
10. McCarthy PL, Sharpe MR, Spiesel SZ, Dolan TF, Forsyth BW, et al. (1982) Observation scales to identify serious illness in febrile children. Pediatrics 70: 802–809.
11. Teach SJ, Fleisher GR (1995) Efficacy of an observation scale in detecting bacteremia in febrile children three to thirty-six months of age, treated as outpatients. Occult Bacteremia Study Group. J Pediatr 126: 877–881.
12. McCarthy PL, Lembo RM, Baron MA, Fink HD, Cicchetti DV (1985) Predictive value of abnormal physical examination findings in ill-appearing and well-appearing febrile children. Pediatrics 76: 167–171.
13. Baker MD, Avner JR, Bell LM (1990) Failure of infant observation scales in detecting serious illness in febrile, 4- to 8-week-old infants. Pediatrics 85: 1040–1043.
14. Berger MY, Boomsma LJ, Albeda FW, Dijkstra RH, Graafmans TA, et al. (2008) Guideline Children with fever [NHG-standaard Kinderen met koorts]. Dutch College of General Practitioners [Nederlands Huisartsen Genootschap].
15. Chiappini E, Principi N, Longhi R, Tovo PA, Becherucci P, et al. (2009) Management of fever in children: summary of the Italian Pediatric Society guidelines. Clin Ther 31: 1826–1843.
16. De S, Williams GJ, Hayen A, Macaskill P, McCaskill M, et al. (2013) Accuracy of the "traffic light" clinical decision rule for serious bacterial infections in young children with fever: a retrospective cohort study. BMJ 346: f866.
17. Verbakel JY, Van den Bruel A, Thompson M, Stevens R, Aertgeerts B, et al. (2013) How well do clinical prediction rules perform in identifying serious infections in acutely ill children across an international network of ambulatory care datasets? BMC Med 11: 10.
18. Brent AJ, Lakhanpaul M, Thompson M, Collier J, Ray S, et al. (2011) Risk score to stratify children with suspected serious bacterial infection: Observational cohort study. Arch Dis Child 96: 361–367.
19. Monteny M, Berger MY, van der Wouden JC, Broekman BJ, Koes BW (2008) Triage of febrile children at a GP cooperative: determinants of a consultation. Br J Gen Pract 58: 242–247.
20. Roukema J, Steyerberg EW, van der Lei J, Moll HA (2008) Randomized trial of a clinical decision support system: impact on the management of children with fever without apparent source. J Am Med Inform Assoc 15: 107–113.
21. Thompson M, Coad N, Harnden A, Mayon-White R, Perera R, et al. (2009) How well do vital signs identify children with serious infections in paediatric emergency care? Arch Dis Child 94: 888–893.
22. Oostenbrink R, Moons KG, Derksen-Lubsen AG, Grobbee DE, Moll HA (2004) A diagnostic decision rule for management of children with meningeal signs. Eur J Epidemiol 19: 109–116.
23. Bleeker SE, Derksen-Lubsen G, Grobbee DE, Donders AR, Moons KG, et al. (2007) Validating and updating a prediction rule for serious bacterial infection in patients with fever without source. Acta Paediatr 96: 100–104.
24. Oostenbrink R, Thompson M, Steyerberg EW, ERNIE members (2012) Barriers to translating diagnostic research in febrile children to clinical practice: a systematic review. Arch Dis Child 97: 667–672.

26

Respiratory Viruses in Hospitalized Children with Influenza-Like Illness during the H1n1 2009 Pandemic in Sweden

Samuel Rhedin[1*❡], Johan Hamrin[2,3*❡], Pontus Naucler[4,5], Rutger Bennet[2,3], Maria Rotzén-Östlund[6], Anna Färnert[1,5] , Margareta Eriksson[2,3]

1 Department of Medicine Solna - Infectious Diseases Unit, Karolinska University Hospital, Stockholm, Sweden, **2** Department for Women and Child Health, Karolinska University Hospital, Stockholm, Sweden, **3** Astrid Lindgren Children's Hospital, Stockholm, Sweden, **4** Department of Microbiology, Tumor and Cell Biology, Karolinska Institutet, Stockholm, Sweden, **5** Department of Infectious Diseases, Karolinska University Hospital, Stockholm, Sweden, **6** Department of Clinical Microbiology, Karolinska University Hospital, Stockholm, Sweden

Abstract

Background: The swine-origin influenza A(H1N1)pdm09 pandemic of 2009 had a slower spread in Europe than expected. The human rhinovirus (HRV) has been suggested to have delayed the pandemic through viral interference. The importance of co-infections over time during the pandemic and in terms of severity of the disease needs to be assessed.

Objective: The aim of this study was to investigate respiratory viruses and specifically the presence of co-infections with influenza A(H1N1)pdm09 (H1N1) in hospitalized children during the H1N1 pandemic. A secondary aim was to investigate if co-infections were associated with severity of disease.

Methods: A retrospective study was performed on 502 children with influenza-like illness admitted to inpatient care at a pediatric hospital in Stockholm, Sweden during the 6 months spanning the H1N1 pandemic in 2009. Respiratory samples were analyzed for a panel of 16 viruses by real-time polymerase chain reaction.

Results: One or more viruses were detected in 61.6% of the samples. Of these, 85.4% were single infections and 14.6% co-infections (2–4 viruses). The number of co-infections increased throughout the study period. H1N1 was found in 83 (16.5%) children and of these 12 (14.5%) were co-infections. HRV and H1N1 circulated to a large extent at the same time and 6.0% of the H1N1-positive children were also positive for HRV. There was no correlation between co-infections and severity of disease in children with H1N1.

Conclusions: Viral co-infections were relatively common in H1N1 infected hospitalized children and need to be considered when estimating morbidity attributed to H1N1. Population-based longitudinal studies with repeated sampling are needed to improve the understanding of the importance of co-infections and viral interference.

Editor: Benjamin J. Cowling, University of Hong Kong, Hong Kong

Funding: No financial support for the study was received.

Competing Interests: The authors have declared that no competing interests exist.

* E-mail: samuel.rhedin@ki.se (SR); johan.hamrin@karolinska.se (JH)

❡ These authors contributed equally to this work.

¶ These authors also contributed equally to this work.

Introduction

Influenza pandemics have struck human societies throughout history, sometimes with devastating outcome [1]. In March 2009, the novel swine-origin influenza A(H1N1)pdm09 (referred throughout as H1N1) was reported in Mexico causing great fear in countries worldwide [2,3]. The spread in Europe was however slower than expected [4]. In Sweden, the first sporadic cases were diagnosed in May 2009 and not until October, after a smaller peak in July and August, the reported cases increased to peak in November 2009 [5]. Sweden was one of the countries that adopted countrywide vaccination against H1N1 reaching a coverage of approximately 60% of the population, with the first doses distributed in the middle of October 2009, and vaccination may have contributed to the rapid decline in reported cases in December [6].

The delayed spread of H1N1 in Sweden during the early autumn of 2009 has been suggested to be due to viral interference with human rhinovirus (HRV) [7]. Also in Norway and France, high PCR detection ratio of HRV in early autumn before the spread of H1N1 was reported [8,9], but the hypothesis of viral interference between H1N1 and HRV has been contradicted in studies from Italy and USA [10,11]. Viral interference refers to that infections with one virus affect the spread of other viruses reflecting either an epidemiological or a biological interaction, which in turn could be due to a cellular or immunological mechanism [7,12,13]. Although the H1N1 pandemic has been extensively investigated there are limited studies that have assessed viral co-infections over time and their importance in severity of disease during the pandemic.

We investigated viral real-time polymerase chain reaction (PCR) data of respiratory samples and clinical records in hospitalized children with influenza-like illness (ILI) in Stockholm, Sweden during the H1N1 pandemic in 2009. The aim of this study was to investigate respiratory viruses and specifically the presence of co-infections with influenza A(H1N1)pdm09 (H1N1) in hospitalized children during the H1N1 pandemic. A secondary aim was to investigate if co-infections were associated with severity of disease.

Materials and Methods

Study Design

The study was a retrospective study of children 0–17 years with suspected influenza admitted to inpatient care at Astrid Lindgren Children's Hospital at Karolinska University Hospital in Solna, a tertiary university hospital in Stockholm, Sweden between July 1 and December 30 2009, the period of the H1N1 pandemic in Stockholm. The catchment area covered 221 585 children 0–17 years [14]. The policy of the hospital during the H1N1 pandemic was to collect respiratory samples for viral PCR analyses from every child who was admitted to inpatient care with clinical suspicion of influenza i.e. ILI, including children with unspecific symptoms, such as abdominal pains, vomiting, diarrhea, seizures and apnea (in infants).

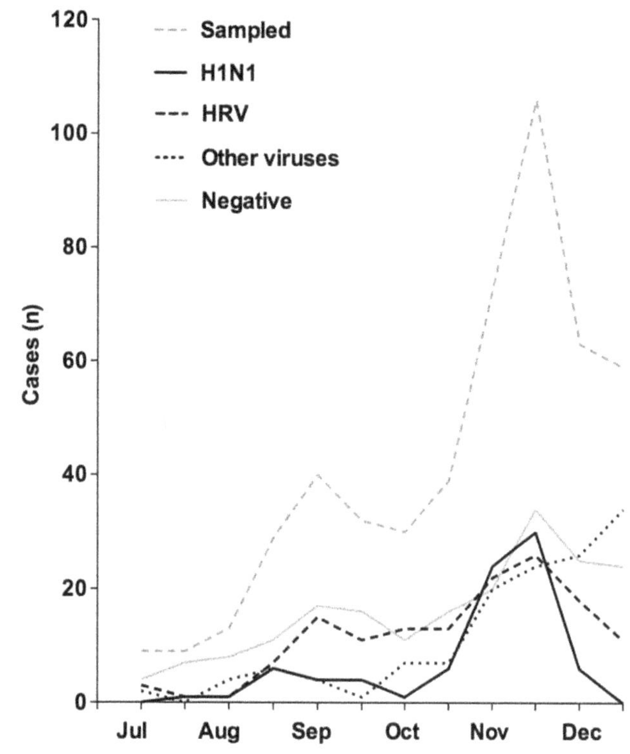

Figure 1. Prevalence over time. Total number of detected viruses among children with influenza-like illness at Astrid Lindgren Children's Hospital, Karolinska University Hospital, Stockholm during the influenza A(H1N1)pdm09 pandemic. Included is also the number of PCR-negative children (neg, n = 193) as well as total number of sampled children (n = 502).

Children admitted to inpatient care in which a respiratory sample was analyzed by viral PCR during the study period were identified at the accredited (ISO 15189:2007) Microbiological Laboratory at Karolinska University Hospital. The children were excluded if the respiratory samples had initially been tested solely for H1N1 and respiratory syncytial virus (RSV) and the material was insufficient for analysis of additional viruses or if the respiratory samples were taken without clinical suspicion of influenza i.e. surveillance testing when children were moved to the pediatric intensive care unit or elective bronchoscopy. If a child was sampled more than once, only the first sample was included in the analyses.

Demographic and clinical data were collected from the medical records. Data on vaccination were available for the children with H1N1 but were not systematically collected for all admitted children. Children were categorized according to underlying condition: 1) previously healthy, 2) asthma including children with multiple episodes of obstructive bronchitis, 3) neuromuscular disease, 4) immunosuppression, 5) preterm birth, congenital heart disease and chronic respiratory disease, and 6) other underlying conditions such as renal, metabolic and gastrointestinal diseases. Clinical manifestations during admission were further classified as: 1) uncomplicated (admitted for observation, slight dehydration), 2) respiratory problems such as wheezing, tracheitis, croup and obstructive apnea, 3) suspected bacterial infections such as pneumonia, empyema, bacterial tonsillitis and otitis media, 4) seizures (both febrile and afebrile), 5) other manifestations (gastroenteritis, ileus, metabolic acidosis, myocarditis, renal failure, encephalitis, viral meningitis and myositis). Moreover, admission to the pediatric intensive care unit (PICU) and duration of hospitalization were recorded.

Ethics Statement

The study was part of a large retrospective review of clinical data covering 20 years of influenza epidemics in Stockholm approved by the Regional Ethics Review Board in Stockholm (dnr2009/1878-31/1). The guardians consented verbally to the collection of microbiology samples and were informed about the results at the time of the child's admission according to routine clinical practice. Written consents from the guardian's were not collected due to the nature of the study.

Sampling and Microbiological Analyses

Respiratory samples were collected either at the emergency unit or at the pediatric inpatient ward. The majority of samples were obtained from nasopharyngeal aspirates (n = 427) or nasopharyngeal swabs (n = 60) and a few were obtained from tracheal secretion (n = 11), oropharyngeal secretion (n = 2) or bronchoalveolar lavage (n = 2). The samples were extracted with MagAttract Virus Mini M48 kit (Qiagen) in a BioRobot M48 instrument and analyzed by an in-house real-time PCR with a virus panel including the following 16 viruses: influenza A seasonal (FluA) as well as influenza A(H1N1)pdm09 (H1N1), influenza B (FluB), human adenovirus (HAdV), human rhinovirus (HRV), parainfluenzavirus 1–3 (PIV1-3), human bocavirus (HBoV), human metapneumovirus (HMPV), respiratory syncytial virus (RSV), human enterovirus (HEV) and coronavirus serotypes 229E, HKU1, NL63 and OC43 (HCoV) as previously described [15]. The PCR was mainly based on separate single PCRs, however duplex PCR was used for PIV1 and PIV3 and for PIV2 and HCoV-229E. The assay was limited at distinguishing HRV-RNA from HEV-RNA due to cross-reactivity [15]. Detection of both

Table 1. Viral co-detection among PCR-positive samples.

Detected virus, n (%)	H1N1	HAdV	HBoV	HCoV	HEV	HMPV	HRV	RSV	PIV1	PIV2	PIV3
Positive samples[a]	83 (16.5)	29 (5.8)	29 (5.8)	17 (3.4)	13 (2.6)	2 (0.4)	141 (28.1)	12 (2.4)	22 (4.4)	9 (1.8)	2 (0.4)
Single infections	71 (85.5)	18 (62.1)	11 (37.9)	6 (35.3)	12 (92.3)	1 (50.0)	111 (78.7)	11 (91.7)	15 (68.2)	8 (88.9)	1 (50.0)
Co-infections[b]	12 (14.5)	11 (37.9)	18 (62.1)	11 (64.7)	1 (7.7)	1 (50.0)	30 (21.3)	1 (8.3)	7 (31.8)	1 (11.1)	1 (50.0)
H1N1	–	3 (10.3)	4 (13.8)	1 (5.9)		1 (50.0)	5 (3.5)		1 (4.5)		
HAdV	3 (3.6)	–		1 (5.9)			8 (5.7)		1 (4.5)		
HBoV	4 (4.8)		–	3 (17.6)	1 (7.7)	1 (50.0)	9 (6.4)		1 (4.5)	1 (11.1)	
HCoV	1 (1.2)	1 (3.4)	3 (10.3)	–			6 (4.3)		1 (4.5)		1 (50.0)
HEV			1 (3.4)		–						
HMPV	1 (1.2)		1 (3.4)			–	1 (0.7)				
HRV	5 (6.0)	8 (27.6)	9 (31.0)	6 (35.3)		1 (50.0)	–	1 (8.3)	3 (13.6)	1 (11.1)	
RSV							1 (0.7)	–			
PIV1	1 (1.2)	1 (3.4)	1 (3.4)	1 (5.9)			3 (2.1)		–		
PIV2			1 (3.4)				1 (0.7)			–	
PIV3				1 (5.9)							–

[a]Number in brackets representing percentage of total children (n = 502).
[b]Triple and quadruple infections counted as multiple double infections.

HEV and HRV was determined as only HRV positive if the cycle threshold value (Ct-value) for HRV was at least 5 cycles lower than for HEV. If HEV and HRV were found at equally high reactivity (ΔCt-values <5), the infection was clinically determined as HRV when the predominant symptoms were respiratory tract infection and as only HEV when the predominant symptoms were fever and malaise with clinical suspicion of encephalitis or if HEV was also detected in stool or cerebrospinal fluid. If only a smaller virus panel including H1N1, FluA, FluB and RSV was initially performed, the analyses were complemented for the other viruses. Respiratory samples as well as extracted DNA were stored at −70°C.

Data Analysis

Data were analyzed in STATA version 12.0 and R version 1.40. Continuous data were analyzed using the Mann-Whitney U-test and categorical variables using Fisher exact test or chi-square test as appropriate. In order to address temporal variations and age co-infections were studied for every half-month and stratification for age (<1 year, 1 to 6 years and >6 years of age) was performed.

Results

Viral Findings in 502 Respiratory Samples from Children with ILI

During the study period 559 respiratory samples were analyzed for respiratory viruses. Twenty-three samples tested solely for H1N1 and RSV were excluded due to insufficient material for analysis of additional viruses, 14 samples were taken as surveillance samples without clinical suspicion of influenza and 20 samples were excluded from children with repeated sampling. In total, 502 unique children were included in the analyses, representing a large majority of the 599 admissions with a discharge diagnosis of infection or respiratory disease (ICD-10 diagnosis of A, B or J) during this period. The PCR panel was positive for at least one virus in 309 of the 502 episodes (61.6%). Out of the 16 viruses analyzed, all were detected during the study period except FluA, FluB and HCoV-NL63. HRV was the most frequent pathogen overall (45.6% of the PCR-positive samples, 28.1% of all samples, n = 141) followed by H1N1 (26.9% of the PCR-positive samples, 16.5% of all samples, n = 83) (Table 1). The most frequently detected virus at a specific time point was H1N1 at the peak of the pandemic in November 2009 (Fig. 1). When studying the number of PCR detections over time of HRV and H1N1, the viruses followed a similar pattern coinciding in time with the highest peak in November, also when most children were sampled (Fig. 1).

Analysis of H1N1/HRV Co-infections and Viral Dynamics

A single virus was detected in 264 samples (85.4% of the PCR-positive samples), two viruses in 41 samples (13.3%), three viruses in 3 (0.9%) and four concurrent viruses in one (0.3%) sample. HEV, RSV, PIV2, H1N1 and HRV were mainly found as single infections (in 92.3%, 91.7%, 88.9%, 85.5% and 78.7% respectively) whereas HBoV and HCoV were more rarely detected alone (in 37.9% and 35.3% of the samples respectively) (Table 1).

The number of co-infections increased through the study period with a significantly higher proportion of co-infections in October-December compared to July-September (p = 0.0008) (Fig. 2a). Co-infections in the H1N1-positive children were exclusively detected in October-December (Fig. 2b). Of the 83 H1N1-positive children 12 (14.5%) were co-infected with another virus of which 5 (6.0%) were positive for HRV, these co-infections all occurred in November, the peak of detection for both viruses (Fig. 2b). When H1N1-negative children where compared to H1N1-positive children, HAdV, HCoV, HEV, HRV, PIV1 and RSV where significantly more often detected in H1N1-negative children (Table 2).

Viral Findings and Age

Children positive for H1N1 were older (median age 3.3 years) than children positive for HCoV (median age 2.0, p = 0.02), HEV (median age 1.3, p<0.01), HRV (median age 1.5 years, p<0.001), and RSV (median age 0.4, p<0.0001), respectively (Table S1). In

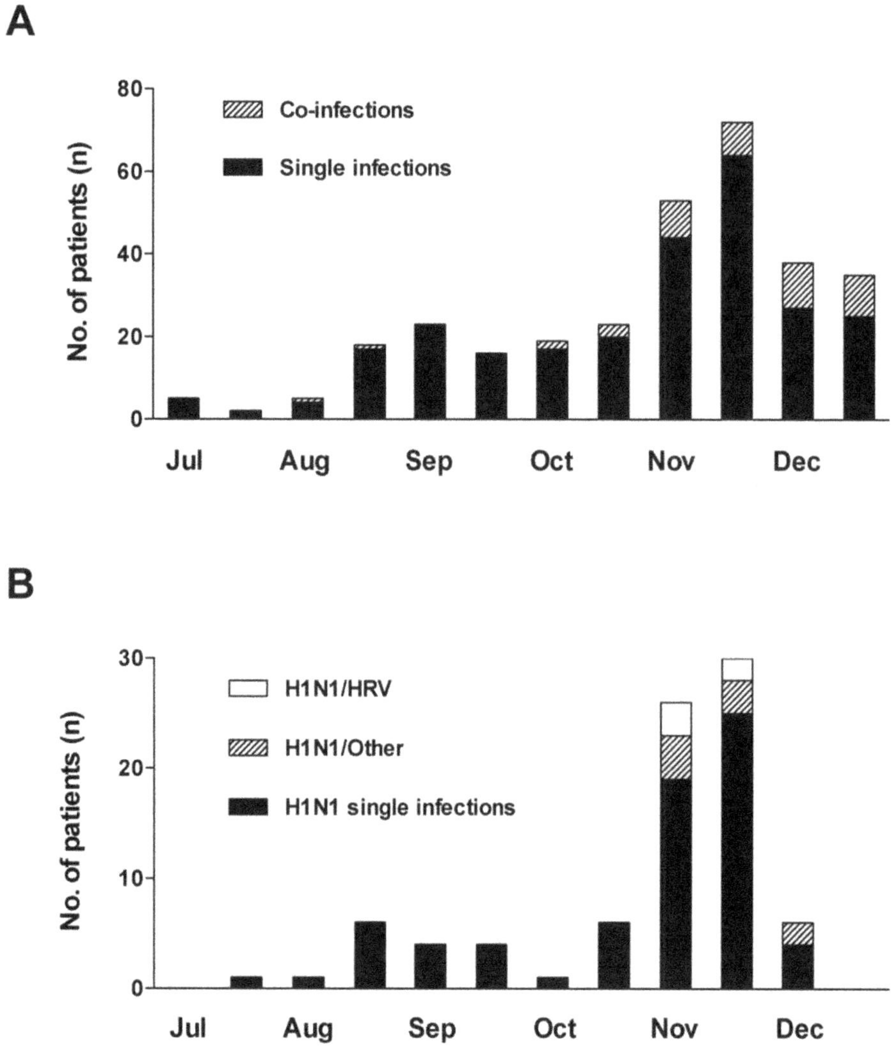

Figure 2. Co-infections over time. Number of children with co-infections over time in (a) all children and (b) H1N1-positive children. H1N1-positive co-infected children divided into co-infection with HRV (H1N1/HRV) and co-infection with other viruses (H1N1/other).

an age-stratified analysis, children between 1–6 years (i.e. the usual age of daycare attendance in Sweden) had a significantly higher proportion of co-infections compared to the rest of the children ($p = 0.02$), however there was no significant age difference when analyses where restricted to the H1N1-positive children ($p = 0.34$) (Fig. 3).

Host Factors and Severity of Disease in Relation to Viral Findings

Among the 502 children included in the study 51.4% were reported as previously healthy. The most common underlying condition was asthma or obstructivity (17.9%), followed by neurological disorders (10.9%). Children with asthma or obstructivity had a higher proportion of HRV and HBoV compared to non-asthmatic children ($p<0.0001$ and $p = 0.003$ respectively). Among the 83 children with H1N1 infections, 13 (15.7%) had been vaccinated, however, all within less than two weeks prior to admission. Host factors (age, sex and underlying conditions) as well as severity of disease were not found to be associated with co-infections in children with H1N1, except for a tendency of increased frequency of suspected bacterial infections in H1N1-coinfected children ($p = 0.07$) (Table 3).

Children with H1N1 were treated more often (10.8%) at the pediatric intensive care unit (PICU) than children with other viruses (3.3%) or negative PCR (2.6%) ($p = 0.01$ and $p = 0.004$ respectively). The most common PCR finding in the 21 children admitted to PICU during the study period was H1N1 (42.9%), followed by HRV (28.6%). Co-infections were seen in two of the children (9.5%), 14 were single infections (66.7%) and five children were PCR-negative (23.9%). Moreover, nine (42.9%) of the PICU treated children were reported as previously healthy and the most common underlying condition was neurological disorders (23.8%). Six of the children (four with terminal cancer and two with cerebral palsy) died during admission; two with H1N1, one PIV1, one HRV and two with negative PCR.

Discussion

Among 502 hospitalized children with ILI in Stockholm during the H1N1 pandemic in 2009, 61.6% had a respiratory virus detected by PCR and 16.5% were infected with H1N1. We assessed the impact of co-infections among these children over

Table 2. Distribution of virus in H1N1-positive and H1N1-negative samples.

Detected virus	Total n	H1N1-negative n (%)	H1N1-positive n (%)	p-value
HAdV	29	26 (11.5)	3 (3.6)	**0.046**
HBoV	29	25 (11.1)	4 (4.8)	0.12
HCoV	17	16 (7.1)	1 (1.2)	**0.049**
HEV	13	13 (5.8)	0 (0.0)	**0.023**
HMPV	2	1 (0.4)	1 (1.2)	0.47
HRV	141	136 (60.2)	5 (6.0)	**<0.0001**
RSV	12	12 (5.3)	0 (0.0)	**0.041**
PIV1	22	21 (9.3)	1 (1.2)	**0.012**
PIV2	9	9 (4.0)	0 (0.0)	0.12
PIV3	2	2 (0.9)	0 (0.0)	1.00
Co-infections		33 (14.6)	12 (14.5)	0.26
Single infections		193 (85.4)	71 (85.5)	
No. of positive samples		226	83	
Total no. of samples		419	83	

time and in relation to severity of disease. Although the retrospective study design has limitations with clinical data not being systematically collected, the strength of the study was the uniquely high sampling coverage with extended viral PCR-analyses in admitted children, as a result of the hospital policy during the H1N1 pandemic. The study thus provides a rather complete assessment of the viral panorama in hospitalized children with ILI in Northern Stockholm during this six-month period. Interestingly, among the positive samples only 26.9% were positive for H1N1, suggesting that several other respiratory viruses caused ILI.

Co-infections with two or more viruses were detected in 14.6% of the positive samples, and 14.5% of the H1N1 infected children were positive for an additional virus. Some viruses were more often found in combination with another virus e.g. HBoV and HCoV, while H1N1, HEV, HRV, PIV2 and RSV were mostly detected as single respiratory viral infections. Furthermore, when H1N1-negative children where compared to H1N1-positive children, HAdV, HCoV, HEV, HRV, RSV and PIV1 where more often detected in H1N1-negative children which suggest an association of these viruses with ILI. Although attempts have been made to attribute diseases to individual viruses by quantitative assessments of the PCR results (CT-values) [16] the single time point measurements cannot distinguish which virus that causes the disease. Our results indicate that the causal role of other respiratory viral infections needs to be considered when estimating morbidity attributed to H1N1.

Co-infections might be a result of acquiring two viruses concurrently. Nonetheless, detection of two viruses might rather be a result of a combination of a newly acquired virus together with an asymptomatic infection or shedding from a recent symptomatic infection. HRV is commonly detected in asymptomatic individuals and viral shedding is known to occur for several weeks after an infection [16–18], and can be prolonged in asthmatic children [19]. Co-infections were here mainly detected in children 1–6 years of age, indeed the age group attending daycare in Sweden and known to be at high risk of respiratory

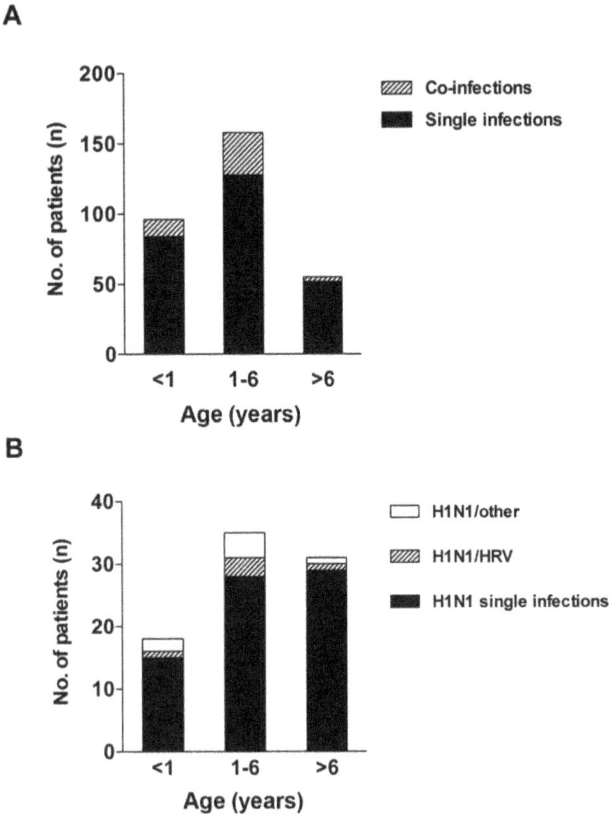

Figure 3. Co-infections and age. Comparison of number of co-infections according to age between children under 1 year (<1), children 1–6 years (1–6) and children over six years (>6) in (a) all children and (b) H1N1-positive children. H1N1-positive co-infected children divided into co-infection with HRV (H1N1/HRV) and co-infection with other viruses (H1N1/other).

viral infections. The increasing frequency of co-infections during the study period might also represent accumulation of persistent viral shedding during the autumn.

The children infected with H1N1 were older than children infected with HCoV, HEV, HRV and RSV. H1N1-positive children where also more often treated in the PICU compared to children with other viral infections indicating the pathogenicity of H1N1 in this population. Detection of additional viruses in H1N1-positive children were, as opposed to previous findings [11,20], not associated with the severity of disease. One explanation could be the low rate of RSV infections in our material since the study period included only the beginning of the RSV season and hence none of the H1N1-positive children were co-infected with RSV. In South America the two epidemics of H1N1 and RSV coincided with a reported high morbidity and a high frequency of severe disease [20]. Unfortunately, bacterial cultures where not systematically performed during the study period. This might bias our results as it has been reported that both influenza and HRV are associated with increased risk for bacterial infections, such as *Streptococcus pneumoniae* [21,22].

The importance of viral interference for the spread of respiratory disease needs further understanding, as does the role of co-infections in terms of severity of disease. Although a few epidemiological studies have assessed the role of viral interference during the H1N1 pandemic and pointed out HRV as a potential protective factor for H1N1 infection, the results and conclusions drawn have been diverging [7–11,23]. As opposed to previous

Table 3. Severity of disease and underlying conditions in children admitted with influenza-like illness.

	H1N1 single infection (n = 71) median/n (%)	H1N1 coinfection (n = 12) median/n (%)	p-value
Age	3.5	2.7	0.25
Male sex	41 (57.7)	8 (66.7)	0.75
UNDERLYING DISEASE			
Healthy	40 (56.3)	6 (50.0)	0.68
Asthma	11 (15.5)	0 (0.0)	0.35
Neuromuscular disease	6 (8.5)	3 (25.0)	0.12
Immunosuppression	5 (7.0)	1 (8.3)	1.00
Prematurity/VOC/chronic respiratory disease	4 (5.6)	2 (16.7)	0.21
Other[a]	5 (7.0)	0 (0.0)	1.00
SEVERITY OF DISEASE			
Uncomplicated	34 (47.9)	3 (25.0)	0.21
Respiratory problems	14 (19.7)	3 (25.0)	0.70
Bacterial infections	8 (11.3)	4 (33.3)	0.07
Seizures	4 (5.6)	1 (8.3)	0.55
Other[b]	9 (12.7)	1 (8.3)	1.00
Intensive care	7 (9.9)	2 (16.7)	0.61
Days admitted (range)	2 (1–23)	3 (1–12)	0.45
Deaths	2 (2.8)	0 (0.0)	1.00

[a]Renal, metabolic and gastrointestinal diseases.
[b]Including gastroenteritis, ileus, metabolic acidosis, myocarditis, renal failure, encephalitis, viral meningitis and myositis.

reports of low prevalence of H1N1 (or even reduction of H1N1) when HRV was prevalent [7–9], our data indicated co-circulation of the two viruses and 6.0% of the children with H1N1 were also positive for HRV. Our observation is in line with a recent report from Beijing [24].

The high detection of HRV during the study period might reflect seasonality of HRV disease, but could also be an effect of increased sampling due to the fear of influenza A(H1N1)pdm09 during the pandemic. Indeed, the frequency of HRV-detection seems to closely follow the sampling frequency in children at our hospital throughout the year (unpublished data).

The viruses detected in these hospitalized children are likely to only partly reflect the spread of different viruses in the catchment area during the study period. Our data can therefore not be used to address whether viral interference prevented the spread of H1N1 in Stockholm. It might be tempting to use hospital data to calculate the observed number of co-infections in relation to expected numbers based on the assumption that infections with different viruses occur independently of each other within the total number of hospital specimens [9,23,25,26]. However, these estimates do not take into account the incidence in the catchment population nor the hospitalization rate of the children infected by the respective viruses.

Interestingly, in a recent intervention study, children vaccinated with inactivated trivalent influenza vaccine carried a higher risk of future infections with respiratory picornaviruses compared to children who received placebo [27], suggesting possible interactions between influenza and other viruses. Sweden adopted countrywide vaccination against H1N1 reaching a coverage of approximately 60% of the population, with the first doses distributed in the middle of October 2009 [6] which might have affected the distribution of respiratory viruses in the studied population.

Our data indicate that in addition to H1N1, ILI during the pandemic was associated with a large number of other respiratory viruses. Viral co-infections in children with H1N1 were not associated with severity of disease; moreover the findings of additional viruses in H1N1-positive children need to be taken into account when attributing morbidity to H1N1. To further investigate interaction of respiratory viruses, population-based prospective studies with longitudinal sampling would be highly informative. Moreover the biological mechanism in viral interference needs to be better understood.

Acknowledgments

We would like to acknowledge the staff at Astrid Lindgren Children's Hospital in Stockholm and at the Karolinska Microbiological Laboratory. Further we would like to thank Benjamin Cowling, James Nokes, Kristina Broliden and Lars Öhrmalm for valuable points of view on the manuscript.

Author Contributions

Conceived and designed the experiments: SR JH RB MRÖ AF ME. Analyzed the data: SR JH. Contributed reagents/materials/analysis tools: SR PN RB MRÖ ME AF. Wrote the paper: SR JH PN AF.

References

1. Guan Y, Vijaykrishna D, Bahl J, Zhu H, Wang J, et al. (2010) The emergence of pandemic influenza viruses. Protein Cell 1: 9–13.
2. Dawood FS, Jain S, Finelli L, Shaw MW, Lindstrom, etal. (2011) Emergence of a Novel Swine-Origin Influenza A (H1N1) Virus in Humans. N Eng J Med 360: 2605–2615.
3. Itoh Y, Shinya K, Kiso M, Watanabe T, Sakoda Y, et al. (2009) In vitro and in vivo characterization of new swine-origin H1N1 influenza viruses. Nature 460: 1021–1025.
4. Falagas ME, Cholevas NV, Kapaskelis AM, Vouloumanou EK, Michalopoulos A, et al. (2010) Epidemiological aspects of 2009 H1N1 influenza: the accumulating experience from the Northern Hemisphere. Eur J Microbiol Infect Dis 29: 1327–1347.
5. Swedish Institute for Communicable Disease Control (2010) Influensarapport vecka 1 (4/1–10/1). [article in swedish] http://smi.se/publikationer/veckorapporter/influensarapporter/sasongen20092010/influensarapport-vecka1-2010/. [cited 7 june 2012].
6. Ortqvist A, Berggren I, Insulander M, de Jong B, Svenungsson B (2011) Effectiveness of an adjuvanted monovalent vaccine against the 2009 pandemic strain of influenza A(H1N1)v, in Stockholm County, Sweden. Clin Infect Dis 52: 1203–1211.
7. Linde A, Rotzen-Ostlund M, Zweygberg-Wirgart B, Rubinova S, Brytting M (2009) Does viral interference affect the spread of influenza? Euro Surveill 40:pii = 19354.
8. Ånestad G, Nordbø SA (2011) Virus interference. Did rhinoviruses activity hamper the progress of the 2009 influenza A (H1N1) pandemic in Norway? Med Hypotheses 77: 1132–1134.
9. Casalegno JS, Ottmann M, Duchamp MB, Escuret V, Billaud G, et al. (2010) Rhinoviruses delayed the circulation of the pandemic influenza A (H1N1) 2009 virus in France. Clin Microbiol Infect 16: 326–329.
10. Nisii C, Meschi S, Selleri M., Bordi L, Castilletti C, et al. (2010) Frequency of detection of upper respiratory tract viruses in patients tested for pandemic H1N1/09 viral infection. J Clin Microbiol 48: 3383–3385.
11. Esper FP, Spahlinger T, Zhou L (2011) Rate and influence of respiratory co-infection on pandemic (H1N1) influenza disease. J Infect 63: 260–266.
12. DaPalma T, Doonan BP, Trager NM, Kasman LM (2010) A systematic approach to virus-virus interactions. Virus Res 149: 1–9.
13. Wagner RR (1960) Viral interference, some considerations of basic mechanisms and their potential relationship to host resistance relationship to host resistance. Bacteriol Rev 24: 151–166.
14. Statistics Sweden (2009) Population by municipality, marital status, age and sex. http://www.scb.se/[cited 7 june 2012].
15. Tiveljung-Lindell A, Rotzén-Ostlund M, Gupta S, Ullstrand R, Grillner L, et al. (2009) Development and Implementation of a Molecular Diagnostic Platform for Daily Rapid Detection of 15 Respiratory Viruses. J Med Virol 175: 167–175.
16. Jansen RR, Wieringa J, Koekkoek SM, Visser CE, Pajkrt D, et al. (2011) Frequent Detection of Respiratory Viruses without Symptoms: Toward Defining Clinically Relevant Cutoff Values. J Clin Microbiol 49: 2631–2636.
17. van der Zalm MM, van Ewijk BE, Wilbrink B, Uiterwaal CS, Wolfs TF, et al. (2009) Respiratory pathogens in children with and without respiratory symptoms. J Pediatr 154: 396–400.
18. Wright PF, Deatly AM, Karron RA, Belshe RB, Shi JR, et al. (2007) Comparison of results of detection of rhinovirus by PCR and viral culture in human nasal wash specimens from subjects with and without clinical symptoms of respiratory illness. J Clin Microbiol 45: 2126–2129.
19. Kling S, Donninger H, Williams Z, Vermeulen J, Weinberg E, et al. (2005) Persistence of rhinovirus RNA after asthma exacerbation in children. Clin Exp Allergy 35: 672–678.
20. Libster R, Bugna J, Coviello S, Hijano DR, Dunaiewsky M, et al. (2010) Pediatric hospitalizations associated with 2009 pandemic influenza A (H1N1) in Argentina. N Eng J Med 362: 45–55.
21. McCullers J a, McAuley JL, Browall S, Iverson AR, Boyd KL, et al. (2010) Influenza enhances susceptibility to natural acquisition of and disease due to Streptococcus pneumoniae in ferrets. J Infect Dis 202: 1287–1295.
22. Wang JH, Kwon HJ, Jang YJ (2009) Rhinovirus enhances various bacterial adhesions to nasal epithelial cells simultaneously. Laryngoscope 119: 1406–1411.
23. Greer RM, McErlean P, Arden KE, Faux CE, Nitsche A, et al. (2009) Do rhinoviruses reduce the probability of viral co-detection during acute respiratory tract infections? J Clin Microbiol 45: 10–15.
24. Yang Y, Wang Z, Ren L, Wang W, Vernet G, et al. (2012) Influenza A/H1N1 2009 Pandemic and Respiratory Virus Infections, Beijing, 2009–2010. PloS One 7:e45807.
25. Tanner H, Boxall E, Osman H (2012) Respiratory viral infections during the 2009–2010 winter season in Central England, UK: incidence and patterns of multiple virus co-infections. Eur J Clin Microbiol 31: 3001–3006.
26. Brunstein JD, Cline CL, McKinney S, Thomas E (2008) Evidence from multiplex molecular assays for complex multipathogen interactions in acute respiratory infections. J Clin Microbiol 46: 97–102.
27. Cowling BJ, Fang VJ, Nishiura H, Chan KH, Ng S, et al. (2012) Increased risk of noninfluenza respiratory virus infections associated with receipt of inactivated influenza vaccine. Clin Infect Dis 54: 1778–83.

Spectrum and Inoculum Size Effect of a Rapid Antigen Detection Test for Group A Streptococcus in Children with Pharyngitis

Jérémie F. Cohen[1,2]*, Martin Chalumeau[1,2], Corinne Levy[3], Philippe Bidet[4], Franck Thollot[5], Alain Wollner[3], Edouard Bingen[4], Robert Cohen[3,6]

1 Unité de Recherche Epidémiologique en Santé Périnatale et Santé des Femmes et des Enfants (U953), Inserm, Paris, France, **2** Service de Pédiatrie Générale, Hôpital Necker-Enfants-Malades, AP-HP et Université Paris-Descartes, Paris, France, **3** Association Clinique et Thérapeutique du Val-de-Marne (ACTIV), Saint-Maur-des-Fossés, France, **4** Service de Microbiologie, Hôpital Robert Debré, AP-HP et Université Paris-Diderot, Paris, France, **5** Association Française de Pédiatrie Ambulatoire (AFPA), Essey-lès-Nancy, France, **6** Service de Microbiologie, Centre Hospitalier Intercommunal de Créteil, Créteil, France

Abstract

Background: The stability of the accuracy of a diagnostic test is critical to whether clinicians can rely on its result. We aimed to assess whether the performance of a rapid antigen detection test (RADT) for group A streptococcus (GAS) is affected by the clinical spectrum and/or bacterial inoculum size.

Methods: Throat swabs were collected from 785 children with pharyngitis in an office-based, prospective, multicenter study (2009–2010). We analysed the effect of clinical spectrum (i.e., the McIsaac score and its components) and inoculum size (light or heavy GAS growth) on the accuracy (sensitivity, specificity, likelihood ratios and predictive values) of a RADT, with laboratory throat culture as the reference test. We also evaluated the accuracy of a McIsaac-score–based decision rule.

Results: GAS prevalence was 36% (95CI: 33%–40%). The inoculum was heavy for 85% of cases (81%–89%). We found a significant spectrum effect on sensitivity, specificity, likelihood ratios and positive predictive value ($p<0.05$) but not negative predictive value, which was stable at about 92%. RADT sensitivity was greater for children with heavy than light inoculum (95% vs. 40%, $p<0.001$). After stratification by inoculum size, the spectrum effect on RADT sensitivity was significant only in patients with light inoculum, on univariate and multivariate analysis. The McIsaac-score–based decision rule had 99% (97%–100%) sensitivity and 52% (48%–57%) specificity.

Conclusions: Variations in RADT sensitivity only occur in patients with light inocula. Because the spectrum effect does not affect the negative predictive value of the test, clinicians who want to rule out GAS can rely on negative RADT results regardless of clinical features if they accept that about 10% of children with negative RADT results will have a positive throat culture. However, such a policy is more acceptable in populations with very low incidence of complications of GAS infection.

Editor: Bernard Beall, Centers for Disease Control & Prevention, United States of America

Funding: This study was funded by Dectrapharm, manufacturer of the RADT (Rapid Antigen Detection Test). JFC is a masters student supported by educational grants from Agence Régionale de Santé d'Ile-de-France and Laboratoires Guigoz - Société Française de Pédiatrie - Groupe de Pédiatrie Générale - Groupe de Recherches Epidémiologiques en Pédiatrie. This work was supported by a research grant from the Assistance Publique-Hôpitaux de Paris (PHRC Régional 2012, AOR 12089). The funders had no role in study design, data collection and analysis, decision to publish, or preparation of the manuscript.

Competing Interests: This study was funded by Dectrapharm, manufacturer of the RADT (Rapid Antigen Detection Test). Dectrapharm had no role in the design and conduct of the study, the collection, analysis, and interpretation of the data, or the review or approval of the manuscript. There are no patents, products in development or marketed products to declare. This does not alter the authors' adherence to all the PLoS ONE policies on sharing data and materials.

* E-mail: jeremie.cohen@inserm.fr

Introduction

Group A streptococcus (GAS) is found in 20% to 40% of cases of childhood pharyngitis; the remaining cases are considered viral [1]. Clinical examination cannot distinguish accurately between viral and GAS pharyngitis [2], and a diagnostic test based on a throat swab is recommended in most countries [3]. Throat culture on a blood agar plate in a microbiology laboratory for 48 hours is the reference test for diagnosis of GAS pharyngitis [4–7]. Rapid antigen detection tests (RADTs) have been proposed as an alternative to throat culture. Compared to laboratory culture, RADTs have high specificity (≈95%) and results are immediate. Their main drawbacks are low sensitivity (≈85%, range 65.6% to 98.9%) [8,9] and variations in sensitivity by clinical spectrum of the disease (spectrum effect, or spectrum bias) [10–12]. The major issue for the spectrum effect is the generalisability of test performance. First, the overall population estimate might not be generalisable to patient subpopulations; second, the diagnostic accuracy that was observed in one study might not be applicable to other patients. Three studies have shown a significant spectrum effect on RADT sensitivity, but these studies had methodological limitations suggesting selection, indication, partial verification, and measurement biases [13–15]. No studies investigated the effect of clinical spectrum on sensitivity, specificity, likelihood ratios and predictive values of RADTs at the same time [13–15]. As well, RADT sensitivity is affected by inoculum size [16–18] – the amount of GAS colonies identified on throat culture and considered a proxy of the bacterial load on the swab. In vitro, the threshold of positivity of RADTs is between 10^5 and 10^7 colony-forming units per ml [19]. To date, several studies evaluated the effects of clinical spectrum and inoculum size on RADT sensitivity, but these effects were studied only separately, and no study has analysed the potential relation of clinical spectrum and inoculum size.

Because of the need to reduce antibiotics consumption, clinical decision rules were developed to help clinicians determine which patients should undergo testing and/or treatment with antibiotics. A decision rule based on the McIsaac score was recently proposed for adults and children [20–22], but this McIsaac-score–strategy was insufficiently validated in children [21–23]. In one validation study by McIsaac *et al.*, the reader cannot evaluate the risk of selection bias because the distribution of scores in children was not reported [21]. Another validation study did not include children with low-risk scores (score ≤1) [22]. A third study aimed to validate the McIsaac score in children, but the rule was modified for application in low-resource settings and no longer integrated the use of a throat culture or RADT [23].

We aimed to determine whether the diagnostic accuracy of a RADT for GAS pharyngitis is affected by the clinical spectrum effect and/or bacterial inoculum size and to validate a McIsaac-score–based decision rule.

Methods

Study Design

This is a secondary analysis of data from an office-based, multicenter, prospective study that took place in France between October 2009 and June 2011 (unpublished data). The aims of the princeps study were to evaluate the frequency of GAS carriage in healthy children and to compare the performance of a RADT between children with pharyngitis and healthy children, with throat culture in a microbiology laboratory as the reference test (intermediate results presented at the 28th Annual Meeting of The European Society for Paediatric Infectious Diseases, Nice, France, 2010; abstract A-229-0021-00920). This ancillary analysis was restricted to patients with pharyngitis from the first year of inclusion. The STARD statement was followed for reporting the results of the study [24].

Patients

Eligible patients were 3 to 15 years old who were evaluated by their paediatrician between October 2009 and May 2010, who had a diagnosis of pharyngitis and did not receive antibiotics for 7 days before inclusion. Pharyngitis was defined by inflammation of the pharynx and/or tonsils. In total, 17 French paediatricians who are part of a research and teaching network (ACTIV) participated in the study [25].

Throat Swabs

Throat samples were obtained by use of a double-swab collection–transportation system (Venturi Transystem Amies agar, COPAN Diagnostics, Corona, CA, USA). The RADT (StreptAtest, Dectrapharm, France), a GAS-specific immuno-chromatographic strip assay, was performed immediately with swab #1 collected in the paediatrician's office. Swab #2 was held at ambient temperature and sent within 72 hr to the Robert Debré Hospital laboratory by an express messenger service. On receipt, the swab was rolled over one-quarter of a trypticase soy agar plate with 5% sheep blood, and the inoculum was further distributed on the plate by streaking with a sterile wire loop. The plates were incubated anaerobically at 37°C and read after 18 to 24 hr. Negative cultures were reexamined after an additional 24 hr of incubation (48 hr total). ß-haemolytic colonies were further investigated by latex agglutination (Prolex, Pro-Lab Diagnostics, Richmond Hill, ON, Canada). With GAS positivity, inoculum size was estimated as follows: 1+, <10 colonies; 2+, 11–50 colonies; and 3+, >50 colonies per plate. Data for patients with 1+ and 2+ cultures were combined to produce a dichotomized variable (light or heavy GAS growth). Microbiologists were blinded to individual clinical data and RADT results.

Clinical Data

We collected clinical data needed to calculate the McIsaac score for each patient. The McIsaac score predicts GAS pharyngitis and ranges from 0 to 5 [20–22]. McIsaac criteria include age 3 to 15 years, history of fever, tonsillar swelling or exudate, tender anterior cervical adenopathy, and absence of cough. As for other studies [13,26], the adenopathy criterion was modified to include any anterior cervical adenopathy ≥1 cm and/or presence of tenderness because tender lymph nodes can be difficult to assess in children. As for other authors [13–15], extreme McIsaac scores were combined (scores 1 and 2, and 4 and 5), and for analysis of clinical components of the score, age was re-coded into 2 categories of equal range (3–8 years; 9–14 years).

Sample Size

In the original study, sample size was estimated so that the 95% confidence interval (95CI) for RADT sensitivity would be a +/−5% estimation. Assuming sensitivity to vary between 75% and 95% and a GAS prevalence of 35%, a sample of 714 children with pharyngitis was needed. No other sample size calculation was performed for this secondary analysis.

Ethics

The study protocol was approved by the Institutional Review Board Comité de Protection des Personnes Ile-de-France XI (n°09016) and the French administrative authorities (CNIL, n°1354254; Afssaps, n°2009-A00086-51). Parent and patient approval for participation was obtained before inclusion. Data were double entered into 4D software version 6.4 (4D) and the database was fully anonymized.

Statistical Analysis

Hospital laboratory throat culture was considered the reference test. First, we described patient demographic features and overall prevalence of groups A, C and G β-haemolytic streptococci. Patients with group C or G β-haemolytic streptococci were considered GAS-negative in the analysis. Then, GAS prevalence by McIsaac score and each McIsaac criterion were described. Second, we used chi-square tests to investigate the clinical spectrum effect on RADT diagnostic accuracy (sensitivity, specificity, likelihood ratios and predictive values) by McIsaac score and each McIsaac criterion. Third, chi-square tests were used to compare the distribution of GAS inoculum size by office-to-laboratory delay (≤48 vs. >48 hr) and to study the effect of inoculum size (light or heavy GAS growth) on RADT sensitivity. Fourth, the distribution of heavy inocula by McIsaac score was explored by a chi-square test for trend, and the association of clinical signs and inoculum size was evaluated by comparing the frequency of heavy inoculum according to each clinical criterion by chi-square tests. Fifth, a binomial model with an identity link was used to evaluate the combination of clinical spectrum effect and inoculum size on RADT sensitivity [27]. Differences in RADT sensitivity were estimated by restricting the analysis to patients with a positive throat culture and using the result of the RADT as the outcome in the model. RADT sensitivity was investigated by univariate modeling according to each McIsaac criterion and then, multivariate modeling by all McIsaac criteria and inoculum size. Potential interaction between inoculum size and each McIsaac criterion was assessed by use of a Wald test. For multivariate modeling, variables were added one by one following the crescent univariate statistical significance order until non-convergence of the model. Significant interactions were managed by introducing corresponding interaction terms in the multivariate model and, in case of non-convergence, by stratification on inoculum size. Sixth, the accuracy of the following McIsaac-score–based decision rule was studied in terms of sensitivity and specificity: (a) scores <2, no further testing or antibiotic; (b) scores 2–3, culture all, antibiotics only with positive culture; (c) scores ≥4, treat empirically with antibiotics [22]. Statistical analysis involved use of Stata/SE 12 (StataCorp, College Station, TX, USA).

Results

Population Characteristics, GAS Prevalence

In total, 807 children met the inclusion criteria; 1 patient with unreadable RADT results, 2 with lost throat swabs and 19 with missing data for McIsaac score calculation were secondarily excluded. Therefore, analysis involved 785 children (351 girls [44.7%]), with mean (SD) age 6.1 (2.5) years. Overall, GAS prevalence was 36.3% (95CI, 32.9%–39.8%). In all, 4 (<1%) Group C and 7 (<1%) Group G β-haemolytic streptococci were identified on BAP. The mean age of secondarily excluded children was 5.9 (3.0) years and GAS was found in throat cultures for 4/20 (20.0% [7.9%–39.2%]).

GAS prevalence increased with increasing McIsaac score (p<0.001) (Tables 1 and 2), from 24.3% to 41.2% for children with ≤2 and ≥4 McIsaac score, respectively. Some clinical criteria were also associated with GAS: age <9 years, absence of cough, and presence of fever (Table 2).

Table 1. Distribution of the McIsaac scores and corresponding frequencies of positive results of rapid antigen detection test (RADT), group A streptococcus (GAS) and heavy GAS inocula (N =785).

	n (%)			
McIsaac score[a]	Total	RADT -positive	GAS -positive[b]	Heavy inoculum[c]
1	12 (1)	2/12 (17)	3/12 (25)	2/3 (67)
2	103 (13)	21/103 (20)	25/103 (24)	20/25 (80)
3	262 (33)	82/262 (31)	89/262 (34)	73/89 (82)
4	286 (36)	115/286 (40)	114/286 (40)	100/114 (88)
5	122 (16)	54/122 (44)	54/122 (44)	48/54 (89)

[a]All scores were ≥1 because all included patients were 3 to 15 years old.
[b]Laboratory throat culture positive for GAS.
[c]p =0.09, χ^2 test for trend for the frequency of heavy inoculum by McIsaac score.

Spectrum Effect

Overall, the sensitivity and specificity of the RADT was 86.7% (82.2%–90.4%) and 94.6% (92.2%–96.4%), respectively; positive and negative likelihood ratios 16.1 (11.1–23.2) and 0.14 (0.10–0.19), respectively; and positive and negative predictive values 90.1% (86.0%–93.4%) and 92.6% (89.9%–94.7%), respectively.

We found significant variations in RADT sensitivity and specificity by McIsaac score (Table 2). Sensitivity increased from 75% (55.1%–89.3%) to 84.3% (75.0%–91.1%) and to 89.9% (84.3%–94.0%; p =0.02), and specificity decreased from 97.7% (91.9%–99.7%) to 96.0% (91.8%–98.4%) and to 92.5% (88.4%–95.5%; p =0.04) with McIsaac scores ≤2, 3 and ≥4, respectively (Table 2). RADT likelihood ratios and predictive values varied, but not significantly, by McIsaac score.

The RADT performance varied significantly by McIsaac criteria. For example, sensitivity was significantly lower in children ≥9 years old than in younger children (66.7% [47.2%–82.7%] vs. 89.0% [84.5%–92.6%], p<0.01). The negative predictive value varied, but not significantly, by McIsaac score or clinical criteria, ranging from 88.8% (80.8%–94.3%) for children without tonsillar swelling or exudate to 94.6% (90.0%–97.5%) for children without fever.

Effect of Inoculum Size on RADT Sensitivity

Among 285 GAS-positive throat cultures, 243 (85% [80.6%–89.2%]) showed heavy inoculum. The distribution of inoculum size did not differ by office-to-laboratory delay (≤48 vs. >48 hr, p =0.97). RADT sensitivity varied widely and significantly between patients with light and heavy inoculum (40.5% [25.6%–56.7%] vs. 94.7% [91.0%–97.1%], p<0.001). Light inoculum was found in 65.8% (50.0%–81.6%) of false-negative RADT cases versus 6.9% (3.7%–10.1%) of true-positive cases (p<0.001).

Frequency of heavy inocula increased with increasing McIsaac score, although not significantly (p =0.09, table 1). Heavy inoculum was significantly more frequent in children <9 years old than in older children (87.1% [82.9%–91.2%] vs. 70.0% [52.6%–87.4%], p<0.05).

Combined Effect of Clinical Spectrum and Inoculum Size

The results of univariate binomial modeling for RADT sensitivity were almost identical to those of stratified analysis (Tables 2 and 3): age ≥9 years and presence of cough were significantly associated with decreased RADT sensitivity (p<0.05). After stratification on inoculum size, wide and statistically significant variations in RADT sensitivity were found in patients with light inoculum (e.g., 37.4% variation in sensitivity by age, p<0.01), but not widely (<6%) nor significantly in patients with heavy inoculum. Interactions were found between inoculum size and age (p =0.03), anterior cervical adenopathy (p =0.01), and tonsillar swelling or exudate (p =0.07).

Because of these multiple interactions and because of no convergence in the multivariate model after introducing interaction terms, 2 multivariate models of RADT sensitivity were fit by stratifying on inoculum size (Table 3). Results of multivariate modeling were close to those of univariate modeling. Light inoculum was associated with wide and statistically significant adjusted variation in RADT sensitivity (e.g., from 23.6% to 40.9%), but heavy inoculum was not widely (≤6%) or significantly associated.

Table 2. Spectrum effect analysis: performance of rapid antigen detection test by clinical spectrum.

	n (%)	GAS (%)	p^a	Sensitivity (95CI)	p^a	Specificity (95CI)	p^a	PLR (95CI)	p^b	NLR (95CI)	p^b	PPV (95CI)	p^a	NPV (95CI)	p^a
McIsaac score															
≤2	115 (14)	24.3	<0.001[c]	75.0 (55.1–89.3)	0.02[c]	97.7 (91.9–99.7)	0.04[c]	32.6 (8.2–130.5)	0.23	0.26 (0.13–0.49)	0.09	91.3 (72.0–98.9)	0.61[c]	92.4 (84.9–96.9)	0.83[c]
3	262 (33)	34.0		84.3 (75.0–91.1)		96.0 (91.8–98.4)		20.8 (10.0–43.3)		0.16 (0.10–0.27)		91.5 (83.2–96.5)		92.2 (87.3–95.7)	
≥4	408 (51)	41.2		89.9 (84.3–94.0)		92.5 (88.4–95.5)		12.0 (7.7–18.7)		0.11 (0.07–0.17)		89.3 (83.7–93.6)		92.9 (88.9–95.8)	
Age (years)															
3–8	663 (84)	38.5	<0.01	89.0 (84.5–92.6)	<0.001	94.1 (91.4–96.2)	0.45	15.1 (10.2–22.4)	0.62	0.12 (0.08–0.17)	<0.001	90.4 (86.1–93.8)	0.48	93.2 (90.3–95.4)	0.26
9–14	122 (16)	24.6		66.7 (47.2–82.7)		96.7 (90.8–99.3)		20.4 (6.5–64.0)		0.34 (0.21–0.57)		87.0 (66.4–97.2)		89.9 (82.2–95.0)	
Lack of cough															
Yes	428 (55)	44.4	<0.001	90.0 (84.8–93.9)	0.02	94.1 (90.3–96.7)	0.65	15.3 (9.2–25.5)	0.89	0.11 (0.07–0.16)	0.02	92.4 (87.6–95.8)	0.07	92.2 (88.1–95.2)	0.76
No	357 (45)	26.6		80.0 (70.5–87.5)		95.0 (91.7–97.3)		16.1 (9.4–27.7)		0.21 (0.14–0.31)		85.4 (76.3–92.0)		92.9 (89.2–95.7)	
Anterior cervical adenopathy															
No	407 (52)	34.6	0.32	83.0 (75.7–88.8)	0.07	97.7 (95.2–99.2)	0.001	36.8 (16.6–81.4)	0.003	0.17 (0.12–0.25)	0.12	95.1 (89.7–98.2)	0.01	91.5 (87.7–94.5)	0.33
Yes	378 (48)	38.1		90.3 (84.2–94.6)		91.0 (86.6–94.4)		10.1 (6.7–15.2)		0.11 (0.06–0.18)		86.1 (79.5–91.2)		93.8 (89.9–96.6)	
Tonsillar swelling or exudates															
No	157 (20)	42.0	0.10	83.3 (72.1–91.4)	0.36	95.6 (89.1–98.8)	0.80	19.0 (7.2–49.7)	0.71	0.17 (0.10–0.30)	0.38	93.2 (83.5–98.1)	0.47	88.8 (80.8–94.3)	0.11
Yes	628 (80)	34.9		87.7 (82.6–91.7)		94.4 (91.7–96.4)		15.6 (10.5–23.3)		0.13 (0.09–0.19)		89.3 (84.4–93.1)		93.5 (90.6–95.6)	
Fever															
No	246 (31)	31.3	0.049	88.3 (79.0–94.5)	0.62	93.5 (88.7–96.7)	0.43	13.6 (7.6–24.2)	0.47	0.13 (0.07–0.23)	0.66	86.1 (76.5–92.8)	0.15	94.6 (90.0–97.5)	0.22
Yes	539 (69)	38.6		86.1 (80.6–90.5)		95.2 (92.3–97.2)		17.8 (11.0–28.8)		0.15 (0.10–0.21)		91.8 (87.0–95.2)		91.6 (88.1–94.3)	
Total	785	36.3		86.7 (82.2–90.4)		94.6 (92.2–96.4)		16.1 (11.1–23.2)		0.14 (0.10–0.19)		90.1 (86.0–93.4)		92.6 (89.9–94.7)	

Abbreviations: GAS, group A streptococcus; PLR, positive likelihood ratio; NLR, negative likelihood ratio; PPV, positive predictive value; NPV, negative predictive value.
[a]χ^2 test; [b] Mantel-Haenszel's χ^2 test; [c] χ^2 test for trend.

Table 3. Analysis of combined spectrum and inoculum size effect on sensitivity of rapid antigen detection test (RADT).

Variable	Univariate analysis[a] All inocula (n = 285)	p	Light inoculum (n = 42)	p	Heavy inoculum (n = 243)	p	p[b]	Multivariate analysis[a] Light inoculum[c] (n = 42)	p	Heavy inoculum[d] (n = 243)	p
Age (years)											
3–8	*ref*	0.01	*ref*	<0.01	*ref*	0.49	0.03	*ref*	<0.001	*ref*	0.36
9–14	−22.4 (−39.7; −5.1)		−37.4 (−64.1; −10.7)		−4.6 (−17.4; 8.3)			−40.9 (−57.9; −24.0)		−5.7 (−17.9; 6.4)	
Lack of cough											
Yes	*ref*	0.03	*ref*	0.09	*ref*	0.14	0.19	*ref*	<0.001	*ref*	0.08
No	−10.0 (−19.1; −9.0)		−25.0 (−53.6; 3.6)		−5.2 (−12.1; 1.7)			−23.6 (−23.7; −23.5)		−6.0 (−12.5; 0.6)	
Anterior cervical adenopathy											
No	*ref*	0.07	*ref*	0.01	*ref*	0.88	0.01	*ref*	0.01	*ref*	0.37
Yes	7.3 (−0.6; 15.2)		36.1 (7.7; 64.5)		−0.4 (−6.1; 5.2)			40.5 (16.7; 64.3)		2.0 (−2.3; 6.2)	
Tonsillar swelling or exudate											
No	*ref*	0.40	*ref*	0.12	*ref*	0.21	0.07	n/a[e]		*ref*	0.29
Yes	4.3 (−5.6; 14.3)		−25.0 (−56.2; 6.2)		5.4 (−3.1; 13.9)					4.0 (−3.4; 11.4)	
Fever											
No	*ref*	0.61	*ref*	0.27	*ref*	0.77	0.26	n/a[e]		*ref*	0.41
Yes	−2.3 (−10.8; 6.3)		−19.1 (−53.0; 14.8)		1.0 (−5.6; 7.6)					2.3 (−3.3; 8.0)	

Data RADT sensitivity difference (95% confidence interval) unless indicated.
Abbreviations: ref, reference; n/a, not applicable.
[a]Binomial modelling.
[b]Interaction test between clinical variables and inoculum size (Wald test).
[c]Model adjusted on age, lack of cough, anterior cervical adenopathy.
[d]Model adjusted on age, lack of cough, anterior cervical adenopathy, tonsillar swelling or exudate and fever.
[e]Not included in the model because of non-convergence.

Performance of the McIsaac-score–based Decision Rule

Among 785 children, 522 (66%) would have received antibiotics according to the decision rule. The rule had 98.9% (97.0%–99.8%) sensitivity and 52.0% (47.5%–56.5%) specificity.

Discussion

Accuracy of a diagnostic test can vary across patient subgroups within a population, a phenomenon referred to as spectrum effect (or spectrum bias) [10–12]. In assessing the relation of clinical spectrum and inoculum size with RADT performance for GAS pharyngitis, we confirm that the spectrum effect has an impact on RADT sensitivity and report for the first time that it also affects the specificity, likelihood ratios and positive predictive value of the test. However, the spectrum effect had no impact on the negative predictive value of the RADT, which remained stable at about 92%, regardless of McIsaac score or its components. Clinicians do not want to expose their patients to GAS suppurative and nonsuppurative complications by withholding antibiotic treatment and therefore need a diagnostic test with high, stable negative predictive value. In this population with a GAS prevalence of 36%, a patient with a negative RADT result had a probability of GAS-positive throat culture close to 8% regardless of clinical features.

This study confirms the important effect of inoculum size on RADT sensitivity, already described in other studies, and reports for the first time an association of clinical spectrum and inoculum size. Our data suggest that having more streptococci in the throat (greater inoculum size) might be associated with more intense symptoms (higher McIsaac score) ($p = 0.09$), although we might not have had enough statistical power to validate this hypothesis. However, because we were not able to differentiate GAS carriers from truly infected patients (i.e., by assessment of streptococcal antibody response) [16,28], we cannot conclude on whether these patients with low McIsaac scores and light inocula were more likely to be GAS carriers rather than truly infected patients.

We chose to investigate the McIsaac score in 3 categories rather than compare the accuracy of the RADT above and below a defined breakpoint [15] because this corresponds to the original aims of the score – to stratify patients into 3 levels of risk and to suggest a subsequent course of action (low-risk: no test, no antibiotics; intermediate risk: culture or RADT, antibiotics only for positive results; high-risk: empirical antibiotic treatment without testing) [20–22]. According to our results, the McIsaac score alone does not allow for ruling out or affirming the diagnosis of GAS pharyngitis because the reported GAS prevalence ranged from 25% (too-high level to rule out) to 44% (too-low level to affirm) in children with a score of 1 and 5, respectively. Moreover, the McIsaac-score–based decision rule had only 52.0% (47.5%–56.5%) specificity, which does not seem consistent with the current need to reduce antibiotic consumption to contain antimicrobial resistance.

One of the strengths of this study is its prospective, multicenter design, which limits the selection bias potentially present in other studies [13,14]. All included children underwent RADT and laboratory culture, which excluded the possible indication and verification biases of other studies [13,14]. The results of our study are close to those reported in the literature. GAS prevalence was 36.3% (32.9%–39.8%), which is close to that from a recent meta-analysis (37%, 32%–43%) [1]. The overall RADT sensitivity was 86.7% (82.2%–90.4%), which is close to that from another recent meta-analysis (85%, 84%–87%) [9]. A limitation is that we used a modified adenopathy criterion for the analyses. However, univariate and multivariate modeling results and the performance of the McIsaac-score-based decision rule were stable in a sensitivity analysis involving the original McIsaac adenopathy criterion instead of our modified criterion.

Another limitation to our study is that some throat swabs were plated >48 hr after collection. This delay had no significant effect on the distribution of GAS inocula, but prolonged or inadequate shipping conditions could have resulted in the loss of viability of GAS if the original swab had only small numbers of bacteria. Therefore, some swabs with light inocula could have been falsely read as negative on throat culture. Because RADTs are more likely to give negative results with light inocula, these swabs might have led to a systematic decrease in number of RADT false-negative results and systematic increase in number of RADT true-negative results, with over-estimation of the negative predictive value of the RADT as a result. We can assume that this bias occurred at random because shipping and all bacteriologic investigations were blinded to clinical data and RADT results – non-differential measurement bias. Such a bias usually leads to loss of power, and our results regarding the stability of the negative predictive value of the RADT should be considered with caution until they are confirmed with a larger sample of patients.

The American Academy of Pediatrics advises that "*Children with manifestations highly suggestive of viral infection [...] generally should not be tested for GAS infection*" [7]. Such guidelines cannot be formally validated because the criteria proposed to determine patients who should be tested are not integrated in an explicit decision rule and remain subject to personal interpretation. Because of GAS carriage and because GAS complications have become uncommon in North America and Western Europe [29], we advocate that the target sensitivity of diagnostic strategies for GAS pharyngitis should not be 100%. Moreover, discussions should not focus on sensitivity alone. We showed that the negative predictive value of a test can be stable across patient subgroups because variations in prevalence can be balanced by concomitant variations in sensitivity and specificity. Therefore, clinicians who want to rule out GAS can rely on negative RADT results regardless of clinical features if they accept that about 10% of children with negative RADT results will have a positive throat culture. However, these results should be considered with caution because they depend highly on the study population, the training of clinical and laboratory personnel and the microbiological devices and protocols used. Moreover, available data suggest that false-negative RADT results are as likely to occur in truly infected patients as in GAS carriers [16,28]. Therefore, such a policy would be more acceptable in populations with very low incidence of suppurative and non-suppurative complications of GAS infection [30]. The McIsaac-score–based decision rule is insufficiently accurate for children, and efforts are needed to develop more specific selective testing strategies for GAS pharyngitis in children.

Acknowledgments

We thank A. Liboz (Department of Microbiology, Robert Debré Hospital), M. Boucherat, MD (database design), F. de La Rocque, MD (study conception), I. Ramay, D. Menguy, S. Tortorelli and M. de Pereira (ACTIV), Pr A. Morabia, MD, PhD (spectrum effect analysis methodological support) and all the physician investigators who participated in the RADT GAS study: M. Benani, MD, F. Corrard, MD, P. Deberdt, MD, A. Elbez, MD, M. Goldrey, MD, J. Gosselin, MD, M. Koskas, MD, P. Martin, MD, A.S. Michot, MD, N. Panis, MD, D. Qutob, MD, C. Romain, MD, O. Romain, MD, C. Schlemmer, MD.

Author Contributions

Conceived and designed the experiments: RC EB AW FT MC. Performed the experiments: RC AW FT. Analyzed the data: JFC CL RC MC. Contributed reagents/materials/analysis tools: PB EB. Wrote the paper: JFC MC CL EB RC. Approved the final version of the manuscript: JFC MC CL PB FT AW EB RC.

References

1. Shaikh N, Leonard E, Martin JM (2010) Prevalence of streptococcal pharyngitis and streptococcal carriage in children: a meta-analysis. Pediatrics 126: e557–564.
2. Shaikh N, Swaminathan N, Hooper EG (2011) Accuracy and Precision of the Signs and Symptoms of Streptococcal Pharyngitis in Children: A Systematic Review. J Pediatr.
3. Matthys J, De Meyere M, van Driel ML, De Sutter A (2007) Differences among international pharyngitis guidelines: not just academic. Ann Fam Med 5: 436–443.
4. Bisno AL, Gerber MA, Gwaltney JM, Jr., Kaplan EL, Schwartz RH (2002) Practice guidelines for the diagnosis and management of group A streptococcal pharyngitis. Infectious Diseases Society of America. Clin Infect Dis 35: 113–125.
5. Gerber MA (2005) Diagnosis and treatment of pharyngitis in children. Pediatr Clin North Am 52: 729–747, vi.
6. Choby BA (2009) Diagnosis and treatment of streptococcal pharyngitis. Am Fam Physician 79: 383–390.
7. American Academy of Pediatrics (2009) Group A Streptococcal Infections. In: Pickering L, Baker C, Long S, McMillan J, editors. Red Book: 2009 Report of the Comittee on Infectious Disease. 28th ed. Elk Grove Village, IL: American Academy of Pediatrics. 616–628.
8. Gerber MA, Shulman ST (2004) Rapid diagnosis of pharyngitis caused by group A streptococci. Clin Microbiol Rev 17: 571–580.
9. Ruiz-Aragon J, Rodriguez Lopez R, Molina Linde JM (2010) Evaluation of rapid methods for detecting Streptococcus pyogenes. systematic review and meta-analysis. An Pediatr 72: 391–402.
10. Mulherin SA, Miller WC (2002) Spectrum bias or spectrum effect? Subgroup variation in diagnostic test evaluation. Ann Intern Med 137: 598–602.
11. Goehring C, Perrier A, Morabia A (2004) Spectrum bias: a quantitative and graphical analysis of the variability of medical diagnostic test performance. Stat Med 23: 125–135.
12. Elie C, Coste J (2008) A methodological framework to distinguish spectrum effects from spectrum biases and to assess diagnostic and screening test accuracy for patient populations: application to the Papanicolaou cervical cancer smear test. BMC Med Res Methodol 8: 7.
13. Hall MC, Kieke B, Gonzales R, Belongia EA (2004) Spectrum bias of a rapid antigen detection test for group A beta-hemolytic streptococcal pharyngitis in a pediatric population. Pediatrics 114: 182–186.
14. Edmonson MB, Farwell KR (2005) Relationship between the clinical likelihood of group a streptococcal pharyngitis and the sensitivity of a rapid antigen-detection test in a pediatric practice. Pediatrics 115: 280–285.
15. Tanz RR, Gerber MA, Kabat W, Rippe J, Seshadri R, et al. (2009) Performance of a rapid antigen-detection test and throat culture in community pediatric offices: implications for management of pharyngitis. Pediatrics 123: 437–444.
16. Gerber MA, Randolph MF, Chanatry J, Wright LL, DeMeo KK, et al. (1986) Antigen detection test for streptococcal pharyngitis: evaluation of sensitivity with respect to true infections. J Pediatr 108: 654–658.
17. Kuhn S, Davies HD, Katzko G, Jadavji T, Church DL (1999) Evaluation of the Strep A OIA assay versus culture methods: ability to detect different quantities of group A Streptococcus. Diagn Microbiol Infect Dis 34: 275–280.
18. Kurtz B, Kurtz M, Roe M, Todd J (2000) Importance of inoculum size and sampling effect in rapid antigen detection for diagnosis of Streptococcus pyogenes pharyngitis. J Clin Microbiol 38: 279–281.
19. Charlier-Bret N, Boucher B, Poyart C, Quesne G, Bingen E, et al. (2004) Rapid antigen detection tests for diagnosis of group A streptococcal pharyngitis: comparative evaluation of sensitivity and practicability of 16 in vitro diagnostics medical devices performed in July 2002 by the French health products safety agency (Afssaps) as part of its market control mission. Pathol Biol (Paris) 52: 438–443.
20. McIsaac WJ, White D, Tannenbaum D, Low DE (1998) A clinical score to reduce unnecessary antibiotic use in patients with sore throat. CMAJ 158: 75–83.

21. McIsaac WJ, Goel V, To T, Low DE (2000) The validity of a sore throat score in family practice. CMAJ 163: 811–815.
22. McIsaac WJ, Kellner JD, Aufricht P, Vanjaka A, Low DE (2004) Empirical validation of guidelines for the management of pharyngitis in children and adults. JAMA 291: 1587–1595.
23. Fischer Walker CL, Rimoin AW, Hamza HS, Steinhoff MC (2006) Comparison of clinical prediction rules for management of pharyngitis in settings with limited resources. J Pediatr 149: 64–71.
24. Bossuyt PM, Reitsma JB, Bruns DE, Gatsonis CA, Glasziou PP, et al. (2003) The STARD statement for reporting studies of diagnostic accuracy: explanation and elaboration. Ann Intern Med 138: W1–12.
25. Cohen R, Levy C, Ovetchkine P, Boucherat M, Weil-Olivier C, et al. (2004) Evaluation of streptococcal clinical scores, rapid antigen detection tests and cultures for childhood pharyngitis. Eur J Pediatr 163: 281–282.
26. Dimatteo LA, Lowenstein SR, Brimhall B, Reiquam W, Gonzales R (2001) The relationship between the clinical features of pharyngitis and the sensitivity of a rapid antigen test: evidence of spectrum bias. Ann Emerg Med 38: 648–652.
27. Wacholder S (1986) Binomial regression in GLIM: estimating risk ratios and risk differences. Am J Epidemiol 123: 174–184.
28. Johnson DR, Kurlan R, Leckman J, Kaplan EL (2010) The human immune response to streptococcal extracellular antigens: clinical, diagnostic, and potential pathogenetic implications. Clin Infect Dis 50: 481–490.
29. Carapetis JR, Steer AC, Mulholland EK, Weber M (2005) The global burden of group A streptococcal diseases. Lancet Infect Dis 5: 685–694.
30. Pelucchi C, Grigoryan L, Galeone C, Esposito S, Huovinen P, et al. (2012) Guideline for the management of acute sore throat. Clin Microbiol Infect 18 Suppl 1: 1–28.

28

Diagnostic Testing of Pediatric Fevers: Meta-Analysis of 13 National Surveys Assessing Influences of Malaria Endemicity and Source of Care on Test Uptake for Febrile Children under Five Years

Emily White Johansson[1]*, Peter W. Gething[2], Helena Hildenwall[3], Bonnie Mappin[2], Max Petzold[4], Stefan Swartling Peterson[1,3,5], Katarina Ekholm Selling[1]

1 International Maternal and Child Health, Department of Women's and Children's Health, Uppsala University, Uppsala, Sweden, 2 Spatial Ecology and Epidemiology Group, Department of Zoology, University of Oxford, Oxford, United Kingdom, 3 Global Health, Department of Public Health Sciences, Karolinska Institutet, Stockholm, Sweden, 4 Center for Applied Biostatistics, University of Gothenburg, Gothenburg, Sweden, 5 School of Public Health, College of Health Sciences, Makerere University, Kampala, Uganda

Abstract

Background: In 2010, the World Health Organization revised guidelines to recommend diagnosis of all suspected malaria cases prior to treatment. There has been no systematic assessment of malaria test uptake for pediatric fevers at the population level as countries start implementing guidelines. We examined test use for pediatric fevers in relation to malaria endemicity and treatment-seeking behavior in multiple sub-Saharan African countries in initial years of implementation.

Methods and Findings: We compiled data from national population-based surveys reporting fever prevalence, care-seeking and diagnostic use for children under five years in 13 sub-Saharan African countries in 2009–2011/12 (n = 105,791). Mixed-effects logistic regression models quantified the influence of source of care and malaria endemicity on test use after adjusting for socioeconomic covariates. Results were stratified by malaria endemicity categories: low ($PfPR_{2-10}<5\%$), moderate ($PfPR_{2-10}$ 5–40%), high ($PfPR_{2-10}>40\%$). Among febrile under-fives surveyed, 16.9% (95% CI: 11.8%–21.9%) were tested. Compared to hospitals, febrile children attending non-hospital sources (OR: 0.62, 95% CI: 0.56–0.69) and community health workers (OR: 0.31, 95% CI: 0.23–0.43) were less often tested. Febrile children in high-risk areas had reduced odds of testing compared to low-risk settings (OR: 0.51, 95% CI: 0.42–0.62). Febrile children in least poor households were more often tested than in poorest (OR: 1.63, 95% CI: 1.39–1.91), as were children with better-educated mothers compared to least educated (OR: 1.33, 95% CI: 1.16–1.54).

Conclusions: Diagnostic testing of pediatric fevers was low and inequitable at the outset of new guidelines. Greater testing is needed at lower or less formal sources where pediatric fevers are commonly managed, particularly to reach the poorest. Lower test uptake in high-risk settings merits further investigation given potential implications for diagnostic scale-up in these areas. Findings could inform continued implementation of new guidelines to improve access to and equity in point-of-care diagnostics use for pediatric fevers.

Editor: Joshua Yukich, Tulane University School of Public Health and Tropical Medicine, United States of America

Funding: Uppsala University provides salary support for SSP, KES and also funds EWJ. Karolinska Institutet provides salary support for SSP. HH receives funding from the Swedish Research Council for Health, Working Life and Welfare/the European Commission under a COFAS Marie Curie Post-Doctoral Fellowship. Salary support for MP is from University of Gothenburg. PWG is a Medical Research Council Career Development Fellow and receives funding from the Bill and Melinda Gates Foundation that also funds BM. The funders had no role in study design, data collection and analysis, decision to publish, or preparation of the manuscript.

Competing Interests: The authors have declared that no competing interests exist.

* E-mail: emily.johansson@kbh.uu.se

Introduction

For many years presumptive anti-malarial treatment for febrile children was promoted in malaria-endemic African countries due to lack of diagnostic tools, resulting in widespread malaria over-diagnosis [1], non-rational use of anti-malarial drugs [2], and poor quality treatment of other fever causes [3]. In 2010, however, the World Health Organization (WHO) revised guidelines to recommend diagnosis of all suspected malaria cases before starting treatment based on expert recommendations and increasing availability of malaria rapid diagnostic tests (mRDTs) [4]. Higher anti-malarial drug costs also drive the need for better precision in treatment [5].

The shift from presumptive treatment of febrile children to test-based case management has great potential to improve malaria surveillance, rational drug use and appropriate management of febrile illnesses [6]. By 2010, 37 African countries had a malaria

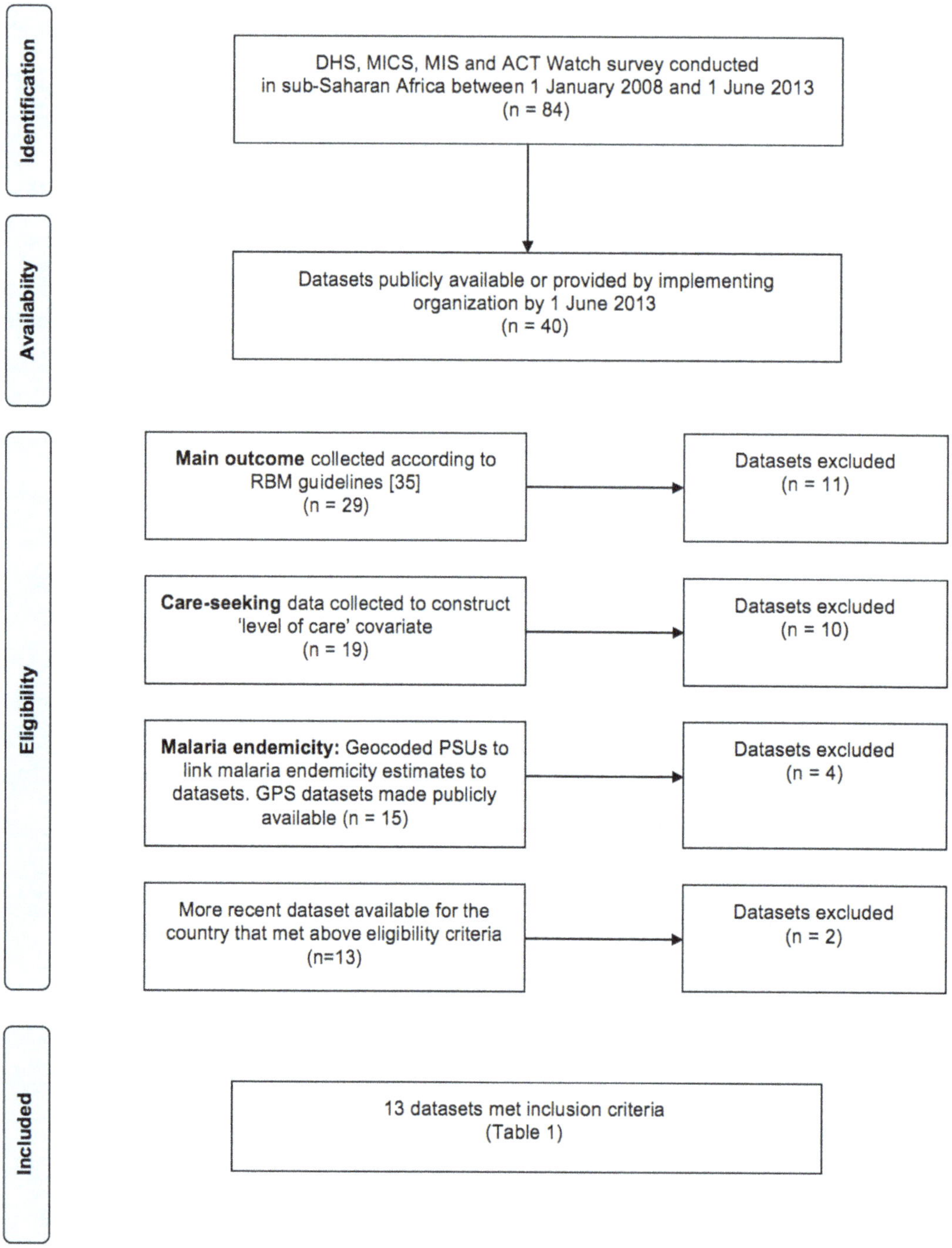

Figure 1. Flow chart of inclusion criteria for study.

diagnosis policy for all age groups and programs are now investing in wide-scale mRDT provision [7].

Despite this investment, evidence to date regarding malaria diagnostic test practices in sub-Saharan Africa is largely derived from adherence studies in limited health facility settings [8–22], or from qualitative interviews of health workers with limited external validity [23–27]. There has been no large-scale, systematic assessment of malaria test use at the population level as countries start scaling up diagnostics in line with revised international guidelines. There is also a limited understanding of factors associated with diagnostic test uptake for pediatric fevers, particularly in relation to patterns of malaria endemicity and treatment seeking behavior that may vary substantially within countries.

Malaria transmission intensity has long been known to influence the management of acute febrile illnesses in children, resulting in common malaria over-diagnosis in malaria-endemic settings [28]. Malaria endemicity has also been hypothesized to specifically affect malaria diagnostic testing practices [29] similar to how local disease epidemiology influences diagnostic use for pediatric infections in high-income countries [30]. Yet, there is currently limited understanding of this key relationship between local malaria epidemiology and the use of diagnostic tests to confirm malaria infection.

Similarly, it is likely that treatment-seeking behavior greatly influences whether a febrile child gets tested for malaria. Microscopy has historically been concentrated at hospitals and higher-level health facilities [31], and initial mRDT implementation has also targeted formal health system sources [6]. Yet, most pediatric febrile illnesses are managed at home or in community settings where diagnostic tests are near absent [32]. Recent research indicates that the largest contributor to reduced systems effectiveness of malaria case management in Zambia is where care was sought for the sick child [33]. Individual characteristics, notably maternal education, may also affect test use given their well-known role in the uptake of other child survival interventions [34]. Yet, there is no evidence about such factors, nor if these individual influences are conditioned by the child's residence or malaria risk.

In 2009, Roll Back Malaria (RBM) recommended asking a question on malaria diagnostic test use in national population-based surveys [35]. Since this time, comparable data have been collected in Demographic and Health Surveys (DHS) [36], Multiple Indicator Cluster Surveys (MICS) [37], Malaria Indicator Surveys (MIS) [38] and ACT Watch Household Surveys [39]. We analyzed these new data to assess extent and determinants of malaria diagnostic test use for pediatric fevers in multiple sub-Saharan African countries during initial years of implementing new guidelines. This paper represents an early assessment against which future progress in diagnostic scale-up may be measured.

Methods

Data Sources

National population-based cross-sectional surveys from DHS, MICS, MIS and ACT Watch conducted in sub-Saharan Africa since 2008 were systematically reviewed for inclusion in this study (Figure 1). 84 surveys were conducted in sub-Saharan African countries between 1 January 2008 and 1 June 2013; 40 datasets were publicly available by 1 June 2013 or were made available by the implementing organization. All datasets were included if they measured the outcome according to RBM guidelines [35], and main covariates as described below. 11 surveys did not collect the outcome measure, or data were collected using non-standard methods. 14 surveys did not collect information to measure main covariates (source of care or malaria endemicity). Two datasets were excluded because a more recent survey was available for the country.

13 DHS and MIS met inclusion criteria, which spanned the period 2009–2011/12 (Table 1). Survey methods are described elsewhere [36]. All surveys with one exception were conducted after national policies were changed to recommend parasitological diagnosis for all age groups prior to treatment, although countries were at different stages of operationalizing these policies at the time of survey fieldwork [40]. For this reason, country-level results are included as a supplement to this paper (Table S1).

Outcome and Explanatory Covariates

Malaria diagnostic test use is measured by asking caregivers of children under five with reported fever in the past two weeks if "At any time during the illness did (name) have blood taken from his/her finger or heel for testing?" This question does not differentiate between diagnostic tests, and is assumed to refer to either microscopy or mRDT.

There were two main covariates: source of care and malaria endemicity. Source of care is measured by asking caregivers of febrile children if they sought advice or treatment for the illness, and if so, from where care was sought. Multiple responses are allowed, and response categories are standardized across countries with some modifications to account for different health system structures. This covariate was categorized as: (1) hospital (2) non-hospital formal medical (3) community health worker (CHW) (4) pharmacy (5) other (6) no care sought. Hospital, CHW, and pharmacy include any such listed response. Non-hospital includes any formal health system source that is not a hospital or CHW, including health centers or posts, outreach or mobile clinics, and private doctors. Some countries include additional sources for this category, such as maternities or municipal clinics. Other includes shops, traditional practitioners, relatives, and non-specified sources. 'Hospital' and 'non-hospital' categories were further dichotomized into public or private sources to analyze test uptake across different managing authorities.

The questionnaire does not explicitly record where testing occurred, but plausibly happened where care was sought. If the child visited multiple sources (e.g. hospital and pharmacy), it was assumed testing occurred at the highest level attended and the covariate was coded using a hierarchical stepwise approach. We conducted a sensitivity analysis by comparing adjusted odds ratios with a covariate constructed by excluding febrile children visiting both hospital and non-hospital sources. In this approach, 732 febrile children visited multiple sources in 13 countries; 367 were excluded that visited both hospital and non-hospital sources. No significant difference was found between approaches (data not shown).

Malaria Atlas Project estimates of malaria endemicity were included in the model, which are described elsewhere [41]. Briefly, the geographical limits of malaria transmission were estimated using routine reporting data and biological models of transmission-limiting aridity and temperature conditions. Within these limits, parasite prevalence survey data were assembled, geolocated, and used within a Bayesian geostatistical model to interpolate a continuous space-time posterior prediction of age-standardized *Plasmodium falciparum* parasite rate in 2–10 year olds ($Pf\mathrm{PR}_{2-10}$) for every 5×5-km pixel for the year 2010. Malaria endemicity estimates were linked to survey datasets through geocoded PSUs. All individual observations were assigned their PSU-level malaria risk value, which was then categorized into one of five malaria endemicity classes: malaria free; unstable transmission; and low ($Pf\mathrm{PR}_{2-10}<5\%$), medium ($Pf\mathrm{PR}_{2-10}$ 5%–40%), and high ($Pf\mathrm{PR}_{2-10}>40\%$) stable endemic transmission.

Socioeconomic covariates associated with child survival intervention uptake were incorporated in the model. These included child's age and sex, maternal age and education, household wealth and density, and residence [42,43]. Child's age was categorized as 0–5, 6–11, 12–23, 24–35, 36–47, 48–59 months. Maternal age was categorized as 15–24, 25–29, 30–34, 35–39, 40–49 years. Maternal education was categorized as no education, primary and at least secondary education attendance. A household wealth index is pre-specified in datasets and described elsewhere [44]. Household density was categorized as 1–4, 5–8, 9–12 and 13 or more household members [45]. Residence was dichotomized as urban or rural.

Among 29,245 febrile children under five surveyed in 13 countries, 300 had missing values for the outcome, 312 for source of care, 752 for malaria endemicity, and one for maternal education. 36 had missing values for two or more variables. Listwise deletion was used to exclude observations with any missing value from the analysis.

Table 1. Survey information for 13 countries.

Country	Survey	Year	Fieldwork months	*n* PSUs	*n* Under-fives	Percent under-fives with fever (95% CI)[a]		*n* Febrile under-fives	Percent febrile under-fives tested (95% CI)[b]		Year of national policy change[c]
Angola	MIS	2011	January-May	240	7,782	34.1	(31.9–36.2)	2,652	25.9	(23.0–28.9)	2010
Burkina Faso	DHS	2010–2011	May-January	574	14,001	20.6	(19.5–21.7)	2,886	5.3	(4.3–6.3)	2009
Burundi	DHS	2010–2011	August-January	376	7,418	30.1	(28.6–31.7)	2,236	27.0	(24.4–29.6)	2007
Lesotho	DHS	2009–2010	October-January	400	3,348	17.2	(15.7–18.8)	577	10.0	(6.7–13.2)	–
Liberia	MIS	2011	September-December	150	2,876	49.2	(46.4–52.1)	1,416	33.3	(28.9–37.7)	2005
Madagascar	MIS	2011	April-May	268	6,377	14.7	(13.0–16.4)	938	6.2	(4.0–8.5)	2006
Malawi	DHS	2010	June-November	849	18,013	34.5	(33.0–36.0)	6,214	17.4	(15.8–19.1)	2011
Nigeria	MIS	2010	October-December	239	5,519	35.4	(32.3–38.6)	1,956	5.4	(4.1–6.8)	2006
Rwanda	DHS	2010–2011	September-March	492	8,605	15.8	(14.8–16.7)	1,355	21.0	(18.5–23.5)	2009
Senegal	DHS	2010–2011	October-April	391	10,893	22.6	(20.8–24.4)	2,463	9.7	(7.8–11.6)	2007
Tanzania	AIS/MIS	2011–2012	December-May	583	8,216	20.4	(18.8–22.0)	1,675	24.9	(21.2–28.7)	2009 (mainland); 2006 (Zanzibar)
Uganda	DHS	2011	June-December	404	7,535	40.4	(38.1–42.7)	3,042	25.9	(23.2–28.6)	1997
Zimbabwe	DHS	2010–2011	September-March	406	5,208	9.7	(8.8–10.7)	506	7.4	(4.9–9.8)	2008
Total					**105,791**	**26.5**	**(21.0–32.0)**	**27,916**	**16.9**	**(11.8–21.9)**	

DHS refers to Demographic and Health Survey. MIS refers to Malaria Indicator Survey. AIS refers to AIDS Indicator Survey. PSU refers to primary sampling unit.
[a]Children less than five years old reportedly having fever in the 2 weeks prior to the interview.
[b]Febrile children less than five years old reportedly receiving a finger or heel stick for testing.
[c][40] Refers to year national policy changed to recommend parasitological diagnosis in patients of all ages prior to treatment.

Data Analysis

Mixed-effects logistic regression models were used to quantify the influence of covariates on malaria test use in pooled and individual country datasets. PSUs were nested within country identifiers and normal distribution of the random effects was assumed. Covariates were included as categorical fixed effects nested within PSUs. Crude odds ratios of main covariates (malaria endemicity and source of care) were initially estimated for their effect on the outcome. Main covariates were then included simultaneously in one model and, subsequently, odds ratios were adjusted for the effect of all covariates, as listed above. We tested for an interaction between maternal education and malaria endemicity in the final model, and separately for an equivalent interaction between maternal education and residence. Results were stratified by malaria endemicity categories and separately by residence to examine effect differences across contexts. The level of statistical significance was set to 0.05. National point estimates were tabulated using sample weights pre-specified in datasets, and proportions for the pooled dataset were estimated using meta-analytical methods. Standard error estimation accounted for data clustering in survey designs. Stata 12 (STATA Corp, College Station, TX) was used for all analyses.

We also crudely estimated total pediatric fevers attending and tested at different sources of care in 2010 across studied countries to further contextualize findings in our discussion. This was done by applying proportions tested from our analysis to published estimates of total pediatric fevers updated to 2010 [46]. This crude analysis helps visualize the rough magnitude of tested and untested pediatric fevers at different sources of care in order to further inform discussion of results.

Results

105,791 children under five years old were surveyed in 13 countries (Table 1). 27,916 (26.5%, 95% CI: 21.0%–32.0%) had reported fever in the two weeks prior to the survey interview, and 4,990 (16.9%, 95% CI: 11.8%–21.9%) were tested.

Table 2 indicates that 35.3% (95% CI: 26.1%–44.6%) of febrile children attending hospitals were tested compared to 26.0% (95% CI: 18.2%–33.9%) visiting non-hospital formal medical sources, and 16.5% (95% CI: 10.6%–22.3%) visiting CHWs. 22.8% (95% CI: 14.5%–31.1%) of febrile children in low-risk areas were tested compared to 20.0% (95% CI: 13.6%–26.4%) in moderate stable transmission areas, and 16.3% (95% CI: 10.8%–21.7%) in high transmission settings. 11.1% (95% CI: 9.2%–13.1%) of febrile children in malaria-free areas were reportedly tested.

Main Covariates

Febrile children in high-risk areas were less often tested than those in low-risk areas (Table 3). Compared to low-risk areas, the odds of testing declined by 49% for febrile children in high-risk areas (OR: 0.51, 95% CI: 0.42–0.62), and by 54% (OR: 0.46, 95% CI: 0.34–0.63) in malaria-free areas. There was a non-significant difference in the odds of testing febrile children in moderate stable transmission areas when compared to low-risk areas (OR: 1.04, 95% CI: 0.86–1.25). Comparisons with unstable transmission areas are limited given few observations in these areas in our analysis.

Source of care was consistently and significantly associated with malaria test uptake after controlling for other covariates (Table 3). Compared to hospitals, the odds of testing febrile children decreased by 38% if attending non-hospital sources (OR: 0.62, 95% CI: 0.56–0.69), and by 69% (OR: 0.31, 95% CI: 0.23–0.43) if visiting CHWs. Nine countries had similar results (Figure 2 and Table S1). In Uganda, however, the odds of testing febrile children visiting non-hospital formal medical sources was 2.10 (95% CI: 1.67–2.64) times higher than if visiting hospitals. Figure 3 further illustrates the rough magnitude of tested and untested pediatric fevers at different sources of care in studied countries in 2010 to provide context to regression model results.

Crude analyses indicate a non-significant difference in test uptake among febrile children attending public (34.8%, 95% CI: 25.0%–44.5%) versus private (36.5%, 95% CI: 26.3%–46.8%) hospitals across studied countries ($p = 0.315$), and lower uptake at public (25.0%, 95% CI: 17.5%–32.5%) compared to private (30.8%, 95% CI: 16.5%–45.1%) non-hospital sources ($p = 0.022$).

Other Covariates

Residence was significantly associated with test use in the adjusted analysis (Table 3). Compared to urban areas, the odds of testing febrile children decreased by 29% in rural settings (OR: 0.71, 95% CI: 0.62–0.82). For febrile children in least poor households, the odds of testing was 1.63 (95% CI: 1.39–1.91) times higher than for those in poorest households after adjusting for other covariates. Febrile children of mothers that attended primary or at least secondary education had 1.32 (95% CI: 1.19–1.46) and 1.33 (95% CI: 1.16–1.54) times higher odds of getting tested, respectively, than those having mothers with no education. Febrile children over 12 months were more often tested than infants aged 0–11 months. Compared to older infants (6–11 months), the odds of younger infants (0–5 months) getting tested declined by 28% in the adjusted analysis (OR: 0.72, 95% CI: 0.59–0.87). Maternal age and child's sex were non-significant covariates.

Stratification by Malaria Endemicity

There was evidence of an interaction between categorical variables maternal education and malaria endemicity (p-values ranged from 0.009 to 0.467 for stable transmission categories) when incorporated into the final model. To further explore this result, the final model was stratified by low ($PfPR_{2-10}<5\%$), medium ($PfPR_{2-10}$ 5%–40%), and high ($PfPR_{2-10}>40\%$) stable malaria transmission categories. In high-risk settings, the odds of testing febrile children with mothers who attended primary or at least secondary education was 1.71 (95% CI: 1.44–2.02) and 2.23 (95% CI: 1.76–2.82) times higher, respectively, than if the mother had no education after controlling for other covariates (Figure 4). This effect was negligible in moderate- and low-risk areas. The stratified model by urban and rural residence indicated no significant difference in maternal education's effect on test use between contexts (data not shown).

Discussion

Overall, diagnostic testing of pediatric fevers was low and inequitable in studied countries at the outset of new guidelines. Test uptake was lowest at locations where pediatric fevers are more often managed, particularly for poorest children, and in areas with the highest risk of malaria infection. Our findings also demonstrate an important socioeconomic dimension to malaria testing.

We found seeking care from lower levels or less formal sources greatly reduced the likelihood of testing, as occurs with other facility-based interventions [47]. This is most plausibly explained by lower test availability at these locations, including their near absence among CHWs and pharmacies [48]. It is also possible that patients attending hospitals are systematically different from those

Table 2. Characteristics of febrile children less than five years old reportedly tested in 13 countries.

		n febrile under-fives[a]	Percent febrile under-fives tested (95% CI)[b]	
Total		*27,916*	*16.9*	*(11.8–21.9)*
Source of care[c]	Hospital	5,279	35.3	(26.1–44.6)
	Non-hospital formal medical	9,938	26.0	(18.2–33.9)
	Community health worker	381	16.5	(10.6–22.3)
	Pharmacy	1,742	6.2	(3.4–9.0)
	Other	1,769	6.9	(4.3–9.4)
	No care sought	8,618	3.3	(2.3–4.3)
Malaria endemicity[d]	No transmission	1,023	11.1	(9.2–13.1)
	Unstable transmission	7	42.9	(15.8–75.0)
	Low stable transmission	2,797	22.8	(14.5–31.1)
	Moderate stable transmission	12,211	20.0	(13.6–26.4)
	High stable transmission	11,287	16.3	(10.8–21.7)
Child's age (in months)	0–5	2,174	12.7	(8.3–17.0)
	6–11	4,094	17.1	(11.6–22.7)
	12–23	7,191	18.1	(12.5–23.8)
	24–35	6,006	17.8	(12.3–23.2)
	36–47	4,782	16.0	(11.3–20.7)
	48–59	4,021	15.9	(10.7–21.1)
Child's sex	Male	14,297	17.0	(12.0–22.0)
	Female	13,620	16.7	(11.7–21.8)
Maternal age (in years)	15–24	8,798	17.7	(12.7–22.8)
	25–29	7,725	16.8	(11.1–22.5)
	30–34	5,237	16.4	(11.2–21.5)
	35–39	3,829	16.3	(11.3–21.3)
	40–49	2,331	16.3	(11.5–21.2)
Maternal education	No education	9,989	14.0	(9.8–18.2)
	Primary attendance	13,883	17.4	(13.1–21.7)
	Secondary or higher attendance	4,047	27.0	(18.6–35.5)
Household wealth index	Poorest	6,107	12.4	(8.6–16.3)
	Second	5,797	12.8	(9.1–16.5)
	Middle	5,838	14.6	(10.1–19.1)
	Fourth	5,609	18.5	(12.6–24.5)
	Least poor	4,574	27.6	(18.0–37.3)
Number of household members	0–4	7,239	18.1	(12.8–23.4)
	5–8	14,156	17.0	(12.1–21.9)
	9–12	4,241	16.3	(10.9–21.6)
	13 or more	2,280	14.6	(10.1–19.1)
Residence	Urban	5,651	27.4	(17.8–37.1)
	Rural	22,264	14.6	(10.4–18.7)

[a]Children less than five years old reportedly having fever in the 2 weeks prior to the interview.
[b]Febrile children less than five years old reportedly receiving a finger or heel stick for testing.
[c]Non-hospital formal medical refers to any formal medical source that is not a hospital or CHW. Other refers to traditional practitioners, shops, relatives/friends, or other non-specified locations.
[d]No transmission refer to non-endemic areas. Unstable transmission refers to areas of very low but non-zero malaria transmission. Stable transmission categories refer to low ($PfPR_{2-10}<5\%$), moderate ($PfPR_{2-10}$ 5%–40%) and high ($PfPR_{2-10}>40\%$).

attending other sources in ways that influence testing (e.g. more severe illness).

Crude estimates of total pediatric fevers attending and tested at different sources of care further illustrates that diagnostic testing is not reaching sources of care bearing the disproportionate burden of fever cases. This is a particular challenge to improve equitable access to diagnostic testing in the future since these are the same sources where poor and marginalized families often seek care [32]. There is an urgent need to improve quantification of diagnostic

Table 3. Effect of source of care, malaria endemicity and socioeconomic covariates on test uptake.

		AOR[a]	95% CI	p-value
Source of care[b]	Hospital	1.00		
	Non-hospital formal medical	0.62	0.56–0.69	<0.001
	Community health worker	0.31	0.23–0.43	<0.001
	Pharmacy	0.06	0.05–0.09	<0.001
	Other	0.10	0.08–0.13	<0.001
	No care sought	0.05	0.04–0.06	<0.001
Malaria endemicity[c]	No transmission	0.46	0.34–0.63	<0.001
	Unstable transmission	1.32	0.11–15.50	0.823
	Low stable transmission	1.00		
	Moderate stable transmission	1.04	0.86–1.25	0.697
	High stable transmission	0.51	0.42–0.62	<0.001
Child's age (in months)	0–5	0.72	0.59–0.87	0.001
	6–11	1.00		
	12–23	1.24	1.09–1.41	0.001
	24–35	1.27	1.11–1.45	<0.001
	36–47	1.10	0.95–1.26	0.203
	48–59	1.18	1.02–1.37	0.030
Child's sex	Male	1.00		
	Female	0.98	0.91–1.06	0.676
Maternal age (in years)	15–24	1.00		
	25–29	1.01	0.91–1.12	0.891
	30–34	1.06	0.94–1.20	0.336
	35–39	1.06	0.92–1.21	0.425
	40–49	0.99	0.83–1.17	0.890
Maternal education	No education attendance	1.00		
	Primary attendance	1.32	1.19–1.46	<0.001
	Secondary or higher attendance	1.33	1.16–1.54	<0.001
Household wealth index	Poorest	1.00		
	Second	0.99	0.87–1.13	0.850
	Middle	1.03	0.90–1.18	0.670
	Fourth	1.21	1.06–1.40	0.006
	Least poor	1.63	1.39–1.91	<0.001
Number of household members	0–4	1.00		
	5–8	0.95	0.86–1.05	0.307
	9–12	0.87	0.76–0.99	0.036
	13 or more	0.66	0.54–0.80	<0.001
Residence	Urban	1.00		
	Rural	0.71	0.62–0.82	<0.001

CI refers to confidence interval. AOR refers to adjusted odds ratio. COR refers to crude odds ratio.

[a]Mixed-effects logistic regression model in pooled dataset of 13 surveys, adjusted for data clustering and above covariates.

[b]COR (source of care): non-hospital = 0.56 (95% CI: 0.51–0.62); community health worker = 0.30 (95% CI: 0.21–0.41); pharmacy = 0.06 (95% CI: 0.05–0.08); other = 0.09 (95% CI: 0.07–0.12); no care sought = 0.04 (95% CI: 0.04–0.05). Non-hospital formal medical refers to any formal medical source that is not a hospital or CHW. Other refers to traditional practitioners, shops, relatives/friends, or other non-specified locations.

[c]COR (malaria endemicity): no transmission = 0.51 (95% CI: 0.38–0.70); unstable transmission = 5.67 (95% CI: 0.44–73.6); moderate stable transmission = 1.35 (95% CI: 1.12–1.63); high stable transmission = 0.67 (95% CI: 0.55–0.81). No risk areas refer to non-endemic areas. Unstable malaria transmission refers to areas of very low but non-zero transmission. Stable transmission categories refer to low ($PfPR_{2-10}<5\%$), moderate ($PfPR_{2-10}$ 5%–40%) and high ($PfPR_{2-10}>40\%$).

need along these lines in order to inform mRDT forecasting and procurement as countries work toward universal test coverage.

Our results also indicate febrile children at the highest malaria risk are less often tested than those at lower risk. Some countries have prioritized mRDT to low-risk areas to increase diagnostic availability in these settings [49]. Reduced uptake in high-risk areas could also be due to entrenched presumptive treatment practices [50]. In locations where diagnostic tests commonly indicate malaria infection – or as malaria 'suspicion' rises – there may be less perceived value of testing over habitual presumptive

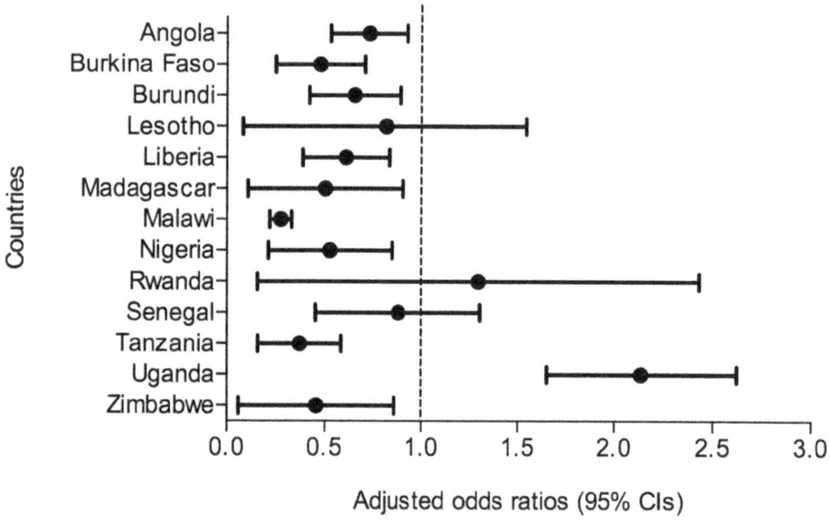

Figure 2. Forest plot of test uptake at non-hospital sources versus hospitals in each country. Figure legend: CI refers to confidence interval. Mixed-effects logistic regression models adjusted for data clustering and Table 3 covariates. AOR <1.0 indicates reduced odds of testing at non-hospital sources compared to hospitals.

treatment practices by caregivers and/or health workers. Similarly, less testing in malaria-free areas is likely due to lower malaria 'suspicion' in these settings. This finding merits further investigation given potential implications for mRDT scale-up in high-risk areas.

Different influences of maternal education on test use in low- and high-risk settings could further support this theory. Independent of other factors, our findings show febrile children of educated mothers in high-risk areas have twice the odds of getting tested than those with non-educated mothers, while this effect was negligible in low- and moderate-risk settings. Again, a perceived lesser value of testing in high-risk areas could exacerbate an 'early adopter' effect among better-educated mothers [51]. Poorly educated mothers, or those less open to new technologies or medical procedures, could be less inclined to change treatment habits in areas where testing commonly provides the same result as presumptive practices, particularly if time or cost is associated with testing. Health workers, too, could less often test children in high-risk settings without caregiver demand, which favors educated mothers. In low-risk areas where a malaria diagnosis is less clear, a wider range of caregivers and/or health workers may be more inclined toward testing, potentially coupled with higher test availability depending on country implementation strategies.

Results show infants are less often tested than older children, and younger infants (0–5 months) are less often tested than older ones (six to 11 months). This finding has not been previously reported to our knowledge. Mean age of malaria onset is about six months [52]. Health workers may therefore not suspect malaria in young infants and test less often. Alternatively, fever in infants is often a clinical 'red flag' given higher mortality rates in this age group. This could cause backsliding to habitual presumptive treatment practices. This result merits further investigation since malaria infection is still possible in young infants. In fact, testing could arguably be more informative for this group since diagnosis is less clear, and differential diagnosis of childhood illnesses with overlapping symptoms (e.g. malaria and pneumonia) is important [53].

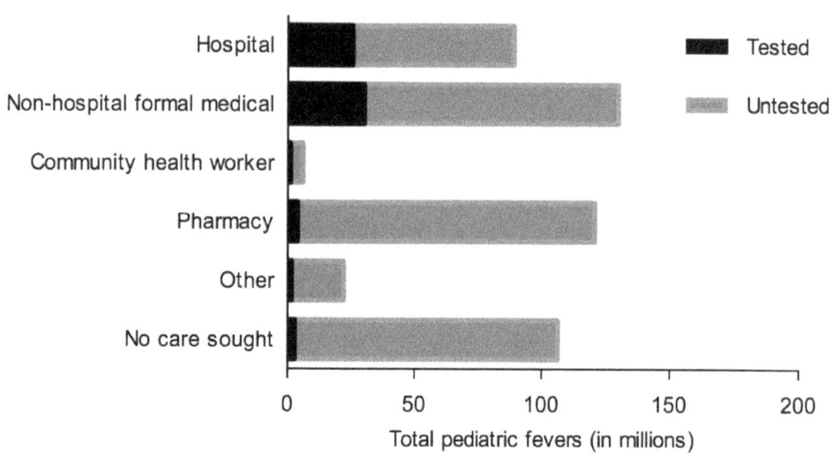

Figure 3. Estimated pediatric fevers attending and tested by source of care in 13 countries in 2010. Figure legend: All totals are given in '000 s.

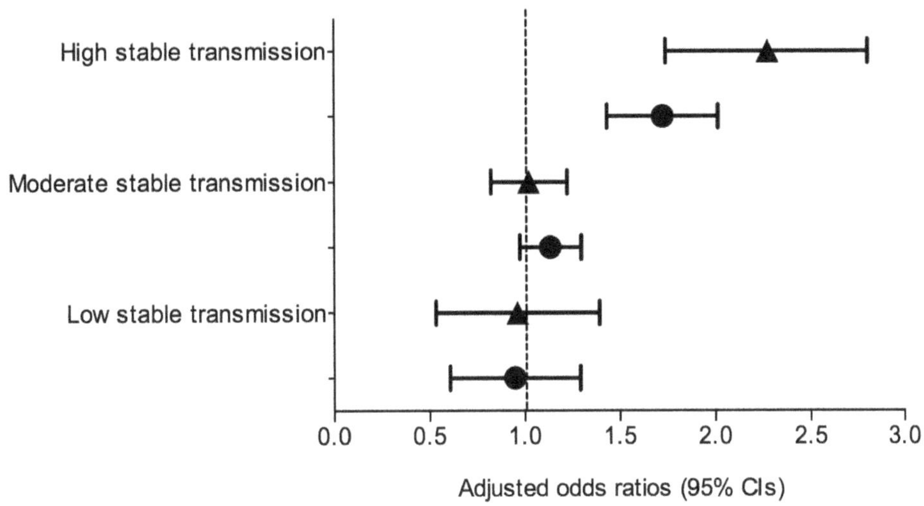

Figure 4. Effect of maternal education on test uptake in different malaria endemicities. Figure legend: ▲, Secondary or higher schooling versus no schooling; ●, Primary schooling versus no schooling. Mixed-effects logistic regression model in pooled dataset of 13 surveys, adjusted for data clustering and Table 3 covariates. Stable transmission categories refer to low (*Pf*PR_{2-10}<5%), moderate (*Pf*PR_{2-10} 5%–40%) and high (*Pf*PR_{2-10}> 40%).

Our study further demonstrates a socioeconomic dimension to malaria testing. Independent of other factors, febrile children in poorest households are less often tested, as are those with poorly educated mothers. Rural settings are associated with less testing, as are large households in the adjusted analysis. This is likely due to lower test availability where marginalized families often seek care. Integrated community case management is a promising approach to improve equitable access to testing and care [54]. Studies show that CHWs can appropriately use rapid diagnostic tests to manage pediatric fevers [55].

These results should be viewed in light of some data limitations. First, findings indicate differences in test uptake across population groups but do not explain reasons for observed practices. Second, surveys only measure whether blood was taken for testing, and as such, do not differentiate between microscopy and mRDT. Higher coverage at certain locations, such as hospitals, may be due to long-standing microscopy availability rather than targeted mRDT roll out. Moreover, testing practices could differ for microscopy and mRDT, particularly since mRDT requires less training and time to use effectively [56–58]. Data in this analysis may largely reflect testing by microscopy given our early assessment with countries at different stages of mRDT implementation. Future analyses based on more recent data, once available, could potentially provide a different result if a greater proportion of testing is conducted using mRDT rather than microscopy. Third, data indicate test use but not appropriate treatment based on test results. Fourth, surveys do not measure facility or clinician factors that may greatly influence uptake.

Finally, a recent validation study found caregiver recall of testing was not highly sensitive (61.9%) but had reasonable specificity (90.0%) when compared to direct facility observation of malaria diagnostic test receipt [59]. The authors found no significant differences in recall across examined caregiver characteristics. Other studies have shown poor caregiver recall of child morbidities or previous health events, particularly among poor, rural or less educated mothers [60,61]. Findings could overestimate differences in test uptake between these groups.

Conclusion

Based on 105,791 children under age five years surveyed in 13 countries in 2009–2011/12, our findings demonstrate low and inequitable testing of pediatric fevers as countries start to implement new guidelines. Malaria diagnostic testing has become increasingly important in the context of malaria control and elimination to improve surveillance, rational drug use and appropriate fever management [62]. Countries are now working toward universal test coverage of all suspected malaria cases in line with revised international guidelines. This paper represents an early assessment against which to measure future progress in diagnostic scale-up, and highlights inequities in testing that need to be addressed going forward. Research is urgently needed to better understand reasons for reduced testing among the youngest children and in high-risk settings, which could plausibly be due to a perceived lesser value of testing for these populations. This analysis should be repeated in the near-term as mRDT implementation matures, and additional data become available for the years 2012–2014. Similar analyses are also needed to examine testing practices for older children and adults. Current findings could inform continued mRDT implementation in order to improve access to and equity in point-of-care diagnostics use for pediatric fevers.

Author Contributions

Conceived and designed the experiments: EWJ KES SSP HH MP PWG. Performed the experiments: EWJ. Analyzed the data: EWJ MP KES SSP PWG BM HH. Contributed reagents/materials/analysis tools: EWJ KES MP SSP. Wrote the paper: EWJ. Analyzed and modeled populations at malaria risk: PWG BM. Estimated total pediatric fevers tested in 2010: PWG BM EWJ. Contributed to interpretation of findings: EWJ PWG SSP HH KES. Reviewed, revised and contributed writing to paper: EWJ PWG HH BM SSP MP KES.

References

1. Gwer C, Newton CJRC, Berkley JA (2007) Over-diagnosis and co-morbidity of severe malaria in African children: a guide for clinicians. Am J Trop Med Hyg 77: 6–13.
2. World Health Organization (2000) The use of anti-malarial drugs: report of a WHO informal consultation. Geneva: World Health Organization.
3. Källander K, Nsungwa-Sabiiti J, Peterson S (2004) Symptom overlap for malaria and pneumonia – policy implications for home management strategies. Acta Trop 90: 211–4.
4. World Health Organization (2010) Guidelines for the treatment of malaria. Geneva: World Health Organization.
5. Mosha JF, Conteh L, Tediosi F, Gesase S, Bruce J (2010) Cost implications of improving malaria diagnosis: findings from north-eastern Tanzania. PLoS One 5(1): e8707.
6. World Health Organization (2012) T3: Test. Treat. Track. Scaling up diagnostic testing, treatment and surveillance for malaria. Geneva: World Health Organization.
7. World Health Organization (2011) World malaria report 2011. Geneva: World Health Organization.
8. Bruxvoort K, Kalolella A, Nchimba H, Festo C, Taylor M, et al. (2013) Getting antimalarials on target: impact of national roll-out of malaria rapid diagnostic tests on health facility treatment in three regions of Tanzania. Trop Med Int Health 18: 1269–82.
9. Shakeley D, Elfving K, Aydin-Schmidt B, Msellem MI, Morris U, et al. (2013) The usefulness of rapid diagnostic tests in the new context of low malaria transmission in Zanzibar. PLoS One 8: e72912.
10. Mubi M, Kakoko D, Ngasala B, Premji Z, Peterson S, et al. (2013) Malaria diagnosis and treatment practices following introduction of rapid diagnostic tests in Kibaha District, Coast Region, Tanzania. Malar J 12: 293.
11. Bottieau E, Gillet P, De Weggheleire A, Scheirlinck A, Stokx J, et al. (2013) Treatment practices in patients with suspected malaria in Provincial Hospital of Tete, Mozambique. Trans R Soc Trop Med Hyg 107(3): 176–82.
12. Yukich JO, Bennett A, Albertini A, Incardona S, Moonga H, et al. (2012) Reductions in artemisinin-based combination therapy consumption after the nationwide scale up of routine malaria rapid diagnostic testing in Zambia. Am J Trop Med Hyg 87(3): 437–46.
13. Masanja IM, Selemani M, Amuri B, Kajungu D, Khatib R, et al. (2012) Increased use of malaria rapid diagnostic tests improves targeting of anti-malarial treatment in rural Tanzania: implications for nationwide rollout of malaria rapid diagnostic tests. Malar J 11: 221.
14. D'Acremont V, Kahama-Maro J, Swai N, Mtasiwa D, Genton B, et al. (2011) Reduction of anti-malarial consumption after rapid diagnostic tests implementation in Dar Es Salaam: a before-after and cluster randomized controlled study. Malar J 10: 107.
15. Bastiaens GJ, Schaftenaar E, Ndaro A, Keuter M, Bousema T, et al. (2011) Malaria diagnostic testing and treatment practices in three different Plasmodium falciparum transmission settings in Tanzania: before and after a government policy change. Malar J 10: 76.
16. Juma E, Zurovac D (2011) Changes in health workers' malaria diagnosis and treatment practices in Kenya. Malar J 10: 1.
17. Masanja MI, McMorrow M, Kahigwa E, Kachur SP, McElroy PD (2010) Health workers' use of malaria rapid diagnostic tests (RDTs) to guide clinical decision making in rural dispensaries, Tanzania. Am J Trop Med Hyg 83(6): 1238–41.
18. Kyabayinze DJ, Asiime C, Nakanjako D, Nabakooza J, Counihan H, et al. (2010) Use of RDTs to improve malaria diagnosis and fever case management at primary health care facilities in Uganda. Malar J 9: 200.
19. Skarbinski J, Ouma PO, Causer LM, Kariuki SK, Barnwell JW, et al. (2009) Effect of malaria rapid diagnostic tests on the management of uncomplicated malaria with artemethur-lumefantrine in Kenya: a cluster randomized trial. Am J Trop Med Hyg 80(6): 919–26.
20. Msellem MI, Mårtensson A, Rotllant G, Bhattarai A, Strömberg J, et al. (2009) Influence of rapid malaria diagnostic tests on treatment and health outcome in fever patients, Zanzibar: a crossover validation study. PLoS Med 6(4): e100070.
21. Zurovac D, Njogu J, Akhwale W, Hamer DH, Larson BA, et al. (2008) Effects of revised diagnostic recommendations on malaria treatment practices across age groups in Kenya. Trop Med Int Health 13(6): 784–7.
22. Hamer DH, Ndhlovu M, Zurovac D, Fox M, Yeboah-Antwi K, et al. (2007) Improved diagnostic testing and malaria treatment practices in Zambia. JAMA 297(20): 2227–31.
23. Ushasoro MD, Okoli CC, Uzochukwu BS (2013) Qualitative study of presumptive treatment of childhood malaria in third-tier tertiary hospitals in southeast Nigeria: a focus group and in-depth study. Malar J 12: 436.
24. Baltzell K, Elfving K, Shakely D, Ali AS, Msellem MI, et al. (2013) Febrile illness management in children under five years of age: a pilot study on primary health care workers' practices in Zanzibar. Malar J 12: 37.
25. Ezeoke OP, Ezumah NN, Chandler CC, Mangham-Jeffries LJ, Onwujekwe OE, et al. (2012) Exploring health providers' and community perceptions and experiences with malaria tests in South-East Nigeria: a critical step towards appropriate treatment. Malar J 11: 368.
26. Uzochukwu BS, Onwujekwe E, Ezuma NN, Exeoke OP, Ajuba MO, et al. (2011) Improving rational treatment of malaria: perceptions and influence of RDTs on prescribing behavior of health workers in southeast Nigeria. PloS One 6: e14627.
27. Chandler C, Jones C, Boniface G, Juma K, Reyburn H, et al. (2008) Guidelines and mindlines: why do clinical staff over-diagnose malaria in Tanzania? A qualitative study. Malar J 7: 53.
28. Reyburn H, Mbatia R, Drakeley C, Carneiro I, Mwakasungula E, et al. (2004) Overdiagnosis of malaria in patients with severe febrile illness in Tanzania: a prospective study. BMJ 329: 1212.
29. Graz B, Willcox M, Szeless T, Rougemont A (2011) "Test and treat" or presumptive treatment for malaria in high transmission situations? A reflection on the latest WHO guidelines. Malar J 10: 136.
30. Bisno AL, Gerber MA, Gwaltney JM, Kaplan EL, Schwartz RH (2002) Practice guidelines for the diagnosis and management of Group A Streptococcal Pharyngitis. Clin Inf D 35: 113–125.
31. Petti CA, Polage CR, Quinn TC, Ronald AR, Sande MA (2006) Laboratory medicine in Africa: a barrier to effective health care. Clin Infect Dis 42: 377–382.
32. Orem JM, Mugisha F, Okui AP, Musango L, Kirigia JM (2013) Health care seeking patterns and determinants of out-of-pocket expenditure for malaria for the children under-five in Uganda. Malar J 12: 175.
33. Littrell M, Miller JM, Ndhlovu M, Hamainza B, Hawela M, et al. (2013) Documenting malaria case management coverage in Zambia: a systems effectiveness approach. Malar J 12: 371.
34. Mosley WH, Chen L (1984) An analytic framework for the study of child survival in developing countries. Population and Development Review 10: 25–45.
35. Roll Back Malaria (2009) Guidelines for core population-based indicators. Calverton, Maryland: ICF Macro.
36. MEASURE DHS (2013) Demographic and health surveys. Available: http://www.measuredhs.com. Accessed 5 June 2013.
37. United Nations Children's Fund (2013) Childinfo: multiple indicator cluster surveys. Available: http://www.childinfo.org/mics.html. Accessed: 5 June 2013.
38. Roll Back Malaria (2013) Malaria indicator surveys. Available: http://www.malariasurveys.org. Accessed: 5 June 2013.
39. ACT Watch (2013) ACT Watch: Evidence for malaria medicine policy. Available: http://www.actwatch.info. Accessed 5 June 2013.
40. World Health Organization (2012) World malaria report 2012. Geneva: World Health Organization.
41. Hay SI, Smith DL, Snow RW (2008) Measuring malaria endemicity from intense to interrupted transmission. Lancet Infect Dis 8: 369–378.
42. Hwang J, Graves PM, Jima D, Reithinger R, Kachur SP, et al. (2010) Knowledge of malaria and its association with malaria-related behaviors – results from the malaria indicator survey, Ethiopia, 2007. PLoS ONE 5(7): e11692.
43. Watsierah CA, Jura WG, Raballah E, Kaseje D, Abong'o B, et al. (2011) Knowledge and behavior as determinants of anti-malarial drug use in a peri-urban population from malaria holoendemic region of western Kenya. Malar J 10: 99.
44. MEASURE DHS (2004) The DHS wealth index - DHS comparative reports. Calverton, Maryland: ICF Macro.
45. MEASURE DHS (1997) Demographic and socioeconomic characteristics of households - DHS comparative studies. Calverton, Maryland: ICF Macro.
46. Gething PW, Kirui VC, Alegana VA, Okiro EA, Noor AM, et al. (2010) Estimating the number of paediatric fevers associated with malaria infection presenting to Africa's public health sector in 2007. PLoS Med 7(7): e1000301.
47. Gabrysch S, Cousens S, Cox J, Campbell OMR (2011) The influence of distance and level of care on delivery place in rural Zambia: a study linked national data in a geographic information system. PLoS Med 8(1): e1000394.
48. Hamer DH, Marsh DR, Peterson S, Pagnoni F (2012) Integrated community case management: next steps in addressing the implementation research agenda. Am J Trop Med Hyg 87: 151–153.
49. Republic of Uganda (2009) Uganda national malaria strategic plan, 2011–2015. Kampala: Ministry of Health.
50. Mwanziva C, Shekalaghe S, Ndaro A, Mengerink B, Megiroo S, et al. (2008) Overuse of artemisinin-combination therapy in Mto wa Mbu (rivier of mosquitoes), an area misinterpreted as high endemic for malaria. Malar J 7: 232.
51. Pai NP, Vadnais C, Denkinger C, Engel N, Pai M (2012) Point-of-care testing for infectious diseases: diversity, complexity and barriers in low- and middle-income countries. PLoS Med 9(9): e1001306.
52. Achidi EW, Salimonu LS, Perlmann H, Perlmann P, Berzins K, et al. (1996) Lack of association between levels of transplacentally acquired Plasmodium falciparum-specific antibodies and age of onset of clinical malaria in infants in a malaria endemic area of Nigeria. Acta Trop 61: 315–326.

53. World Health Organization (1991) The overlap in the clinical presentation and treatment of malaria and pneumonia in children: report of a meeting. Geneva: World Health Organization.
54. Marsh DR, Hamer DH, Pagnoni F, Peterson S (2012) Evidence for the implementation, effects and impact of the integrated community case management strategy to treat childhood infection. Am J Trop Med Hyg 87: 2–5.
55. Mukanga DA, Tiono AB, Anyorigiya T, Källander K, Konate AT, et al. (2012) Integrated community case management of fevers in children under five using rapid diagnostic tests and respiratory rate counting: a multi-country cluster randomized trial. Am J Trop Med Hyg 87: 21–29.
56. Strom GE, Haanshuus CG, Fataki M, Langeland N, Blomberg B (2013) Challenges in diagnosing pediatric malaria in Dar Es Salaam, Tanzania. Malar J 12: 228.
57. Kahama-Maro J, D'Acremont V, Mtasiwa D, Genton B, Lengeler C (2011) Low quality of routine microscopy for malaria at different levels of the health system in Dar Es Salaam. Malar J 10: 332.
58. Harchut K, Standley C, Dobson A, Klaassen B, Rambaud-Althaus C, et al. (2013) Over-diagnosis of malaria by microscopy in the Kilombero Valley, Southern Tanzania: an evaluation of the utility and cost-effectiveness of rapid diagnostic tests. Malar J 12: 159.
59. Eisele TP, Silumbe K, Yukich J, Hamainza B, Keating J, et al. (2013) Accuracy of measuring diagnosis and treatment of childhood malaria from household surveys in Zambia. PLoS Med 10(5): e1001417.
60. Feiken DR, Audi A, Olack B, Bigogo GM, Polyak C, et al. (2010) Evaluation of the optimal recall period for disease symptoms in home-based morbidity surveillance in rural and urban Kenya. Int J Epidemiol 39(2): 450–8.
61. Hildenwall H, Lindkvist J, Tumwine JK, Bergqvist Y, Pariyo G, et al. (2008) Low validity of caretakers' reports on use of selected antimalarials and antibiotics in children with severe pneumonia at an urban hospital in Uganda. Trans Roy Soc Trop Med Hyg 103: 95–101.
62. Cotter C, Sturrock HJW, Hsiang MS, Liu J, Phillips AA, et al. (2013) The changing epidemiology of malaria elimination: new strategies for new challenges. Lancet 382: 900–911.

Permissions

All chapters in this book were first published in PLOS ONE, by The Public Library of Science; hereby published with permission under the Creative Commons Attribution License or equivalent. Every chapter published in this book has been scrutinized by our experts. Their significance has been extensively debated. The topics covered herein carry significant findings which will fuel the growth of the discipline. They may even be implemented as practical applications or may be referred to as a beginning point for another development.

The contributors of this book come from diverse backgrounds, making this book a truly international effort. This book will bring forth new frontiers with its revolutionizing research information and detailed analysis of the nascent developments around the world.

We would like to thank all the contributing authors for lending their expertise to make the book truly unique. They have played a crucial role in the development of this book. Without their invaluable contributions this book wouldn't have been possible. They have made vital efforts to compile up to date information on the varied aspects of this subject to make this book a valuable addition to the collection of many professionals and students.

This book was conceptualized with the vision of imparting up-to-date information and advanced data in this field. To ensure the same, a matchless editorial board was set up. Every individual on the board went through rigorous rounds of assessment to prove their worth. After which they invested a large part of their time researching and compiling the most relevant data for our readers.

The editorial board has been involved in producing this book since its inception. They have spent rigorous hours researching and exploring the diverse topics which have resulted in the successful publishing of this book. They have passed on their knowledge of decades through this book. To expedite this challenging task, the publisher supported the team at every step. A small team of assistant editors was also appointed to further simplify the editing procedure and attain best results for the readers.

Apart from the editorial board, the designing team has also invested a significant amount of their time in understanding the subject and creating the most relevant covers. They scrutinized every image to scout for the most suitable representation of the subject and create an appropriate cover for the book.

The publishing team has been an ardent support to the editorial, designing and production team. Their endless efforts to recruit the best for this project, has resulted in the accomplishment of this book. They are a veteran in the field of academics and their pool of knowledge is as vast as their experience in printing. Their expertise and guidance has proved useful at every step. Their uncompromising quality standards have made this book an exceptional effort. Their encouragement from time to time has been an inspiration for everyone.

The publisher and the editorial board hope that this book will prove to be a valuable piece of knowledge for researchers, students, practitioners and scholars across the globe.

List of Contributors

Eric D. McCollum
Baylor International Pediatric AIDS Initiative, Baylor College of Medicine, Lilongwe, Malawi

Geoffrey A. Preidis
Interdepartmental Program in Translational Biology and Molecular Medicine, Department of Pediatrics, Baylor College of Medicine, Houston, Texas, United States of America

Mark M. Kabue, Emmanuel B. M. Singogo and Peter N. Kazembe
Baylor Children's Foundation-Malawi, Baylor College of Medicine, Lilongwe, Malawi

Charles Mwansambo
Department of Pediatrics, Kamuzu Central Hospital, Lilongwe, Malawi

Mark W. Kline
Baylor International Pediatric AIDS Initiative, Baylor College of Medicine, Houston, Texas, United States of America

Sandrine Leroy
Centre for Statistics in Medicine, Oxford, United Kingdom
Epidemiology of Emerging Diseases Unit, Institut Pasteur, Paris, France
Inserm U953 Unit, Paris, France
Department of Pediatrics, Paris Descartes University, Necker Hospital, AP-HP, Paris, France

Franc¸ois Bouissou
Department of Pediatrics, Children's Hospital, Paul Sabathier University, CHU Purpan, Toulouse, France

Anna Fernandez-Lopez
Department of Pediatrics, Hospital Universitari Arnau de Vilanova, Lleida. Spain

Constantinos J. Stefanidis
Department of Nephrology "A. and P. Kyriakou" Childen's Hospital, Athens, Greece

Tim Ulinski
Department of Pediatric Nephrology, Trousseau Hospital and University Pierre et Marie Curie, Paris, France

Andrea L. Ciaranello
Division of Infectious Diseases, Massachusetts General Hospital, Boston, Massachusetts, United States of America

Rochelle P. Walensky
Division of Infectious Diseases, Massachusetts General Hospital, Boston, Massachusetts, United States of America
Division of General Medicine, Massachusetts General Hospital, Boston, Massachusetts, United States of America
Division of Infectious Disease, Brigham and Women's Hospital, Boston, Massachusetts, United States of America
Center for AIDS Research, Harvard Medical School, Boston, Massachusetts, United States of America

Kenneth A. Freedberg
Division of Infectious Diseases, Massachusetts General Hospital, Boston, Massachusetts, United States of America
Division of General Medicine, Massachusetts General Hospital, Boston, Massachusetts, United States of America
Center for AIDS Research, Harvard Medical School, Boston, Massachusetts, United States of America

Francois Dabis
INSERM U897 Africa Team, Institut de Santé Publique, d'Epidémiologie et de Développement (ISPED), Université Victor Segalen Bordeaux 2, Bordeaux, France

Freddy Perez
INSERM U897 Africa Team, Institut de Santé Publique, d'Epidémiologie et de Développement (ISPED), Université Victor Segalen Bordeaux 2, Bordeaux, France
Pan American Health Organization, HIV/AIDS Unit, Washington, D.C., United States of America

Matthews Maruva and Jo Keatinge
Elizabeth Glaser Pediatric AIDS Foundation: Zimbabwe Country Office, Harare, Zimbabwe

Jennifer Chu
Division of General Medicine, Massachusetts General Hospital, Boston, Massachusetts, United States of America

Barbara Engelsmann
Organization of Public Health Interventions and Development (OPHID) Trust, Harare, Zimbabwe

Angela Mushavi and Rumbidzai Mugwagwa
Ministry of Health and Child Welfare, Harare, Zimbabwe

Roberta Petrucci, Gregory Harper, Amin Ahmed Bawazir, Nabil Mohamed Abuamer and Luis Eduardo Cuevas
Liverpool School of Tropical Medicine, Liverpool, United Kingdom

Mohammed Ahmed Yassin
Liverpool School of Tropical Medicine, Liverpool, United Kingdom
Faculty of Medicine, University of Hawassa, Awassa, Ethiopia

Kefyalew Taye Garie and Zelalem Kebede
Faculty of Medicine, University of Hawassa, Awassa, Ethiopia

Isabel Arbide
Bushullo Major Health Centre, Awassa, Ethiopia

Melkamsew Aschalew and Yared Merid
Southern Region Health Bureau, Awassa, Ethiopia
Kemal Öztürk, Lia G. H. de Rond, Sabine C. de Greeff, Guy A. M. Berbers and Anne-Marie Buisman
Centre for Infectious Disease and Control (Clb), National Institute for Public Health and the Environment, Bilthoven, The Netherlands

Lotte H. Hendrikx
Centre for Infectious Disease and Control (Clb), National Institute for Public Health and the Environment, Bilthoven, The Netherlands
Research Centre Linnaeus institute, Spaarne Hospital Hoofddorp, Hoofddorp, The Netherlands

Elisabeth A. M. Sanders
Department of Pediatric Immunology and Infectious Diseases, University Medical Centre Utrecht, Utrecht, The Netherlands

Fangyou Yu and Xueqing Zhang
Department of Laboratory Medicine, The First Affiliated Hospital of Wenzhou Medical College, Wenzhou, China

Qiang Chen and Xiaojun Yu
Department of Laboratory Medicine, Jiangxi Provincial Children Hospital, Nanchang, China

Qiaoqiao Li, Lehe Yang and Liangxing Wang
Department of Respiratory Medicine, The First Affiliated Hospital of Wenzhou Medical College, Wenzhou, China

Baixing Ding, Cong Chen and Jingye Pan
Department of Intensive Care Unit, The First Affiliated Hospital of Wenzhou Medical College, Wenzhou, China

Zhiqiang Qin and Chris Parsons
Division of Infectious Diseases, Department of Medicine, Medical University of South Carolina, Charleston, South Carolina, United States of America

Jinwei Huang
Department of Laboratory Medicine, Lishui Center Hospital, Lishui, China

Yun Luo
Department of Microbiology, Zhejiang Provincial Center for Disease Control and Prevention, Hangzhou, China

Talley Andrews, David I. Buckley and Rick Deyo
Department of Family Medicine, Oregon Health and Science University, Portland, Oregon, United States of America

Matthew Thompson and Carl Heneghan
Department of Primary Care Health Sciences, University of Oxford, Oxford, United Kingdom

Niamh Redmond and Alastair D. Hay
Academic Unit of Primary Health Care, School of Social and Community Medicine, University of Bristol, Bristol, United Kingdom

Patricia J. Lucas
School for Policy Studies, University of Bristol, Bristol, United Kingdom

Peter S. Blair
School of Social and Community Medicine, St Michael's Hospital, University of Bristol, Bristol, United Kingdom

Nívea D. Amoêdo
Instituto de Bioquímica Médica, Universidade Federal do Rio de Janeiro, Rio de Janeiro, Brazil

Adriana O. Afonso
Departamento de Genética, Universidade Federal do Rio de Janeiro, Rio de Janeiro, Brazil
Centro de Ciências da Saúde, Universidade Católica de Petrópolis, Petrópolis, Brazil

Elizabeth S. Machado
Departamento de Genética, Universidade Federal do Rio de Janeiro, Rio de Janeiro, Brazil
Instituto de Puericultura e Pediatria Martagão Gesteira, Universidade Federal do Rio de Janeiro, Rio de Janeiro, Brazil

Marcelo A. Soares
Departamento de Genética, Universidade Federal do Rio de Janeiro, Rio de Janeiro, Brazil
Programa de Genética, Instituto Nacional de Câncer, Rio de Janeiro, Brazil

Sílvia M. Cunha
Hospital Municipal Jesus, Rio de Janeiro, Brazil

Ricardo H. Oliveira
Instituto de Puericultura e Pediatria Martagão Gesteira, Universidade Federal do Rio de Janeiro, Rio de Janeiro, Brazil

Emmanuel A. Temu
London School of Hygiene and Tropical Medicine, London, United Kingdom

Mike Coleman
Liverpool School of Tropical Medicine, Liverpool, United Kingdom

Ana Paula Abilio
National Institute of Health, Maputo, Mozambique

Immo Kleinschmidt
Tropical Epidemiology Group, London School of Hygiene and Tropical Medicine, London, United Kingdom

Marc Bonten
University Medical Center Utrecht, Utrecht, The Netherlands

Peter Klein Klouwenberg
University Medical Center Utrecht, Utrecht, The Netherlands
Kenya Medical Research Institute/Wellcome Trust Research Programme, Centre for Geographical Medicine Research - Coast, Kilifi, Kenya

Mahfudh Bashraheil, Ken Awuondo, James Berkley and Kevin Marsh
Kenya Medical Research Institute/Wellcome Trust Research Programme, Centre for Geographical Medicine Research - Coast, Kilifi, Kenya

Philip Sasi
Kenya Medical Research Institute/Wellcome Trust Research Programme, Centre for Geographical Medicine Research - Coast, Kilifi, Kenya
Muhimbili University, Dar es Salaam, Tanzania

Steffen Borrmann
Kenya Medical Research Institute/Wellcome Trust Research Programme, Centre for Geographical Medicine Research - Coast, Kilifi, Kenya
Department of Infectious Diseases, Heidelberg University School of Medicine, Heidelberg, Germany

Tim Lynch
Department of Pediatrics, Children's Hospital, University of Western Ontario, London, Ontario, Canada

Liza Bialy, Terry P. Klassen, Tamara Durec and Robin Leicht
Department of Pediatrics, University of Alberta, Edmonton, Alberta, Canada

James D. Kellner and David W. Johnson
Department of Pediatrics and Physiology and Pharmacology, University of Calgary and Alberta Children's Hospital, Calgary, Alberta, Canada

Martin H. Osmond
Clinical Research Unit, Children's Hospital of Eastern Ontario Research Institute, Ottawa, Ontario, Canada

Cynthia J. Snider, Stephen R. Cole, Pia D. M. MacDonald and Steven R. Meshnick
Department of Epidemiology, Gillings School of Global Public Health, University of North Carolina, Chapel Hill, North Carolina, United States of America

Kiprotich Chelimo and Peter Odada Sumba
Center for Global Health Research, Kenya Medical Research Institute, Kisumu, Kenya

Chandy C. John
Departments of Pediatrics and Medicine, University of Minnesota Medical School, Minneapolis, Minnesota, United States of America

Ann M. Moormann
Center for Global Health and Diseases, Case Western Reserve University, Cleveland, Ohio, United States of America
Departments of Pediatrics and Quantitative Health Services, University of Massachusetts Medical School, Worcester, Massachusetts, United States of America

Susan S. Chiu, Wilfred H. S. Wong and Eunice L. Y. Chan
Department of Paediatrics and Adolescent Medicine, The University of Hong Kong, Pokfulam, Hong Kong

Kwok-Hung Chan
Department of Microbiology, The University of Hong Kong, Pokfulam, Hong Kong

J. S. M. Peiris
Department of Microbiology, The University of Hong Kong, Pokfulam, Hong Kong
Hong Kong University Pasteur Research Centre, Pokfulam, Hong Kong

Sibhatu Biadgilign and Amare Deribew
Department of Epidemiology and Biostatistics, College of Public Health and Medical Science, Jimma University, Jimma, Ethiopia

Alemayehu Amberbir
Addis Ababa University, Addis Ababa, Ethiopia

Horacio Ruiseñor Escudero
Department of International Health, Bloomberg School of Public Health, Johns Hopkins University, Baltimore, Maryland, United States of America

Kebede Deribe
Department of General Public Health, College of Public Health and Medical Science, Jimma University, Jimma, Ethiopia

Renaud Becquet
Institut National de la Santéet de la Recherche Médicale (INSERM), Unité 897, Centre de Recherche "Epidé miologie et Biostatistique", Bordeaux, France
Institut de Santé Publique Epidé miologie Développement (ISPED), Université Victor Segalen Bordeaux 2, Bordeaux, France

Milly Marston
London School of Hygiene and Tropical Medicine, London, United Kingdom

Max Essex
Department of Immunology and Infectious Diseases, Harvard School of Public Health AIDS Initiative, Boston, Massachusetts, United States of America

Didier K. Ekouevi
PAC-CI program, ANRS site in Côte d'Ivoire, Abidjan, Côte d'Ivoire

Pablo Giusti, Stéphanie Boström and Marita Troye-Blomberg
Department of Immunology, Wenner-Gren Institute, Stockholm University, Stockholm, Sweden

Charles Arama
Department of Immunology, Wenner-Gren Institute, Stockholm University, Stockholm, Sweden
Malaria Research and Training Centre, Faculty of Medicine, Pharmacy and Dentistry, University of Bamako, Bamako, Mali

Stefania Varani
Department of Immunology, Wenner-Gren Institute, Stockholm University, Stockholm, Sweden
Department of Laboratory Medicine, Division of Clinical Microbiology, Karolinska University Hospital, Huddinge Sweden
Department of Haematology and Clinical Oncology, "L. and A. Seragnoli", University of Bologna, Bologna, Italy

Victor Dara, Boubacar Traore, Amagana Dolo and Ogobara Doumbo
Malaria Research and Training Centre, Faculty of Medicine, Pharmacy and Dentistry, University of Bamako, Bamako, Mali

Silvana Gomes Benzecry
Universidade do Estado do Amazonas, Manaus, Amazonas, Brazil

Márcia Almeida Araújo Alexandre
Universidade do Estado do Amazonas, Manaus, Amazonas, Brazil
Fundação de Medicina Tropical Dr. Heitor Vieira Dourado, Manaus, Amazonas, Brazil
Universidade Nilton Lins, Manaus, Amazonas, Brazil

Marcus Vinícius Guimarães Lacerda
Universidade do Estado do Amazonas, Manaus, Amazonas, Brazil
Fundação de Medicina Tropical Dr. Heitor Vieira Dourado, Manaus, Amazonas, Brazil
Universidade Nilton Lins, Manaus, Amazonas, Brazil
National Institute of Science and Technology for Innovation in Neglected Diseases, Rio de Janeiro, Brazil

André Machado Siqueira
Universidade do Estado do Amazonas, Manaus, Amazonas, Brazil
Fundação de Medicina Tropical Dr. Heitor Vieira Dourado, Manaus, Amazonas, Brazil
National Institute of Science and Technology for Innovation in Neglected Diseases, Rio de Janeiro, Brazil

Belisa Maria Lopes Magalhães and Sheila Vitor-Silva
Universidade do Estado do Amazonas, Manaus, Amazonas, Brazil
National Institute of Science and Technology for Innovation in Neglected Diseases, Rio de Janeiro, Brazil

Ellen Fátima Caetano Lança
Universidade do Estado do Amazonas, Manaus, Amazonas, Brazil
Universidade Federal do Amazonas, Manaus, Amazonas, Brazil

Connor O'Brien
Columbia University Medical Center, New York, New York, United States of America

Quique Bassat
Centre de Recerca en Salut Internacional de Barcelona (CRESIB)/Hospital Clı´nic, Universitat de Barcelona, Barcelona, Spain

Carol Portwine
Hematology/Oncology, McMaster Children's Hospital at Hamilton Health Sciences, Hamilton, Ontario, Canada

David Mitchell
Hematology/Oncology, Montreal Children's Hospital, Montreal, Québec, Canada

Donna Johnston
Hematology/Oncology, Children's Hospital of Eastern Ontario, Ottawa, Ontario, Canada

Rochelle Yanofsky
Hematology/Oncology, CancerCare Manitoba, Winnipeg, Manitoba, Canada

David Dix
Pediatric Hematology/Oncology, British Columbia Children's Hospital, Vancouver, British Columbia, Canada

Shayna Zelcer
Hematology/Oncology, London Health Sciences, London, Ontario, Canada

Elena Chiappini, Francesca Bonsignori, Sara Sollai and Luisa Galli and Maurizio de Martino
Anna Meyer University Hospital, Department of Science for Woman and Child Health, University of Florence, Florence, Italy

Chiara Della Bella, Amedeo Amedei, Elena Niccolai, Gianfranco Del Prete and Mario M. D'Elios
Department of Internal Medicine, University of Florence, Florence, Italy

Mahavir Singh
Lionex GmbH, Braunschweig, Germany

Sumita Pai, Sani Hussaini Aliyu and Johannis Andreas Karas
Clinical Microbiology & Public Health Laboratory, Health Protection Agency, Addenbrookes Hospital, Cambridge, United Kingdom

David Andrew Enoch
Peterborough & Stamford Hospitals NHS Foundation Trust, Peterborough City Hospital, Bretton Gate, Peterborough, United Kingdom
Dulciene Maria Magalhaes Queiroz andreia Maria Camargos Rocha, Fabricio Freire Melo, Gifone Aguiar Rocha and Kádima Nayara Teixeira
Laboratory of Research in Bacteriology, Faculdade de Medicina, Universidade Federal de Minas Gerais, Belo Horizonte, Brazil

Simone Diniz Carvalho and Paulo Fernando Souto Bittencourt
Endoscopy Service, University Hospital, Universidade Federal de Minas Gerais, Belo Horizonte, Brazil

Lucia Porto Fonseca Castro
Department of Pathology, Faculdade de Medicina, Universidade Federal de Minas Gerais, Belo Horizonte, Brazil

Jean E. Crabtree
Leeds Institute of Molecular Medicine, University of Leeds, Leeds, United Kingdom

Ketty Gianesin and Riccardo Freguja
Section of Oncology and Immunology, AIDS Reference Center, Department of Surgery, Oncology and Gastroenterology, University of Padova, Padova, Italy

Anita De Rossi
Section of Oncology and Immunology, AIDS Reference Center, Department of Surgery, Oncology and Gastroenterology, University of Padova, Padova, Italy
Istituto Oncologico Veneto- IRCCS, Padova, Italy

Francesco Carmona, Marisa Zanchetta, Paola Del Bianco and Marco Montagna
Istituto Oncologico Veneto- IRCCS, Padova, Italy

Sandro Malacrida
Department of Neurosciences, University of Padova, Padova, Italy

Osvalda Rampon and Carlo Giaquinto
Department of Pediatrics, University of Padova, Padova, Italy

Giuseppe Indolfi, Elisa Bartolini and Massimo Resti
Paediatric and Liver Unit, Meyer Children's University Hospital of Florence, Florence, Italy

Giusi Mangone and Maria Moriondo
Immunology Unit and Laboratory, Meyer Children's University Hospital of Florence, Florence, Italy

Chiara Azzari
Immunology Unit and Laboratory, Meyer Children's University Hospital of Florence, Florence, Italy
Department of Health Sciences, University of Florence, Florence, Italy

Gabriella Nebbia
U.O. Pediatria 2, Fondazione IRCCS Ca' Granda Ospedale Maggiore Policlinico, Milano, Italy

Pier Luigi Calvo and Pier-Angelo Tovo
Department of Pediatrics, Infectious Diseases Unit, University of Turin, Italy Regina Margherita Children's Hospital, Turin, Italy

Maurizio de Martino
Department of Health Sciences, University of Florence, Florence, Italy

Chunfeng Liu, Xiaoyu Xiong, Wei Xu, Lijie Wang and Jiujun Li
Department of Pediatrics, Shengjing hospital of China Medical University, Shenyang, Liaoning, China

Jimei Sun
Department of Bacteriology, Shengjing hospital of China Medical University, Shenyang, Liaoning, China

Evelien Kerkhof, Henriette A. Moll and Rianne Oostenbrink
Erasmus MC-Sophia Children's Hospital, Department of General Pediatrics, Rotterdam, The Netherlands

Monica Lakhanpaul
Department of General and Adolescent Pediatrics, University College London, Institute of Child Health, London, United Kingdom

Samiran Ray
Pediatric Intensive Care Unit, Great Ormond Street Hospital, London, United Kingdom

Jan Y. Verbakel
Department of General Practice, Katholieke Universiteit Leuven, Leuven, Belgium

Ann Van den Bruel and Matthew Thompson
Department of Primary Care Health Sciences, University of Oxford, Radcliffe Observatory Quarter, Oxford, United Kingdom

Marjolein Y. Berger
Department of General Practice, University Groningen, University Medical Centre Groningen, Groningen, The Netherlands

Samuel Rhedin
Department of Medicine Solna - Infectious Diseases Unit, Karolinska University Hospital, Stockholm, Sweden

Anna Färnert
Department of Medicine Solna - Infectious Diseases Unit, Karolinska University Hospital, Stockholm, Sweden
Department of Infectious Diseases, Karolinska University Hospital, Stockholm, Sweden

Johan Hamrin, Rutger Bennet and Margareta Eriksson
Department for Women and Child Health, Karolinska University Hospital, Stockholm, Sweden
Astrid Lindgren Children's Hospital, Stockholm, Sweden

Pontus Naucler
Department of Microbiology, Tumor and Cell Biology, Karolinska Institutet, Stockholm, Sweden
Department of Infectious Diseases, Karolinska University Hospital, Stockholm, Sweden

Maria Rotzén-Östlund
Department of Clinical Microbiology, Karolinska University Hospital, Stockholm, Sweden

Jérémie F. Cohen and Martin Chalumeau
Unitéde Recherche Epidé miologique en Santé Périnatale et Santédes Femmes et des Enfants (U953), Inserm, Paris, France
Service de Pédiatrie Générale, Hôpital Necker-Enfants-Malades, AP-HP et Université Paris-Descartes, Paris, France

Corinne Levy and Alain Wollner
Association Clinique et Thé rapeutique du Val-de-Marne (ACTIV), Saint-Maur-des-Fossés, France

Robert Cohen
Association Clinique et Thé rapeutique du Val-de-Marne (ACTIV), Saint-Maur-des-Fossés, France
Service de Microbiologie, Centre Hospitalier Intercommunal de Créteil, Créteil, France

Philippe Bidet and Edouard Bingen
Service de Microbiologie, Hôpital Robert Debré, AP-HP et Université Paris-Diderot, Paris, France

Franck Thollot
Association Franc¸aise de Pèdiatrie Ambulatoire (AFPA), Esseylès-Nancy, France

Emily White Johansson and Katarina Ekholm Selling
International Maternal and Child Health, Department of Women's and Children's Health, Uppsala University, Uppsala, Sweden

Stefan Swartling Peterson
International Maternal and Child Health, Department of Women's and Children's Health, Uppsala University, Uppsala, Sweden
Global Health, Department of Public Health Sciences, Karolinska Institutet, Stockholm, Sweden
School of Public Health, College of Health Sciences, Makerere University, Kampala, Uganda

Peter W. Gething and Bonnie Mappin
Spatial Ecology and Epidemiology Group, Department of Zoology, University of Oxford, Oxford, United Kingdom

Helena Hildenwall
Global Health, Department of Public Health Sciences, Karolinska Institutet, Stockholm, Sweden

Max Petzold
Center for Applied Biostatistics, University of Gothenburg, Gothenburg, Sweden

Index

www.ingramcontent.com/pod-product-compliance
Lightning Source LLC
LaVergne TN
LVHW060600210926
848485LV00005B/1346